Recent Progress in Osteoimmunology

Recent Progress in Osteoimmunology

Editor: Melonie Armstrong

AMERICAN
MEDICAL PUBLISHERS
www.americanmedicalpublishers.com

AMERICAN
MEDICAL PUBLISHERS
www.americanmedicalpublishers.com

Cataloging-in-Publication Data

Recent progress in osteoimmunology / edited by Melonie Armstrong.
p. cm.
Includes bibliographical references and index.
ISBN 979-8-88740-426-4
1. Immunology. 2. Musculoskeletal system--Immunology. 3. Bones--Immunology.
4. Musculoskeletal system--Diseases--Immunological aspects.
5. Bones--Diseases--Immunological aspects. I. Armstrong, Melonie.
QR181 .R43 2023
616.079--dc23

American Medical Publishers,
41 Flatbush Avenue,
1st Floor, New York,
NY 11217, USA

ISBN 979-8-88740-426-4 (Hardback)

Contents

Preface

The world is advancing at a fast pace like never before. Therefore, the need is to keep up with the latest developments. This book was an idea that came to fruition when the specialists in the area realized the need to coordinate together and document essential themes in the subject. That's when I was requested to be the editor. Editing this book has been an honour as it brings together diverse authors researching on different streams of the field. The book collates essential materials contributed by veterans in the area which can be utilized by students and researchers alike.

Osteoimmunology is the study of the correlation between bone and immune cells. It emphasizes the two sided communication that takes place among the immune cells and bones. The interactions taking place between the immune system and bone are critical in maintaining skeletal homeostasis. The bone marrow cavity is essential for the growth of the immune system. It also houses crucial stem cells for maintaining the immune system. Immune cells create cytokines, which have crucial effects on the modulation of bone homeostasis. There are a few critical cytokines, which are produced by the immune system, such as TNF-α, RANKL, IFNs, M-CSF and ILs. These affect the activity and differentiation of bone resorption and osteoclasts. This book is a valuable compilation of topics, ranging from the basic to the most complex advancements in the field of osteoimmunology. It will prove to be immensely beneficial to students and researchers in this field.

Each chapter is a sole-standing publication that reflects each author´s interpretation. Thus, the book displays a multi-facetted picture of our current understanding of application, resources and aspects of the field. I would like to thank the contributors of this book and my family for their endless support.

Editor

1

Effects of Vitamin E-Stabilized Ultra High Molecular Weight Polyethylene on Oxidative Stress Response and Osteoimmunological Response in Human Osteoblast

Luca Massaccesi[1], *Vincenza Ragone*[2], *Nadia Papini*[3], *Giancarlo Goi*[4], *Massimiliano Marco Corsi Romanelli*[1,5] *and Emanuela Galliera*[1,6*]

[1] Department of Biomedical Sciences for Health, Università degli Studi di Milano, Milan, Italy, [2] Research and Develpoment Department, Permedica S.p.A, Merate, Italy, [3] Department of Medical Biotechnology and Traslational Medicine, Università degli Studi di Milano, Milan, Italy, [4] Department of Biomedical, Surgical and Dental Sciences, Università degli Studi di Milano, Milan, Italy, [5] U.O.C SMEL-1 Patologia Clinica San Donato, IRCCS Policlinico San Donato, Milan, Italy, [6] IRCCS Istituto Ortopedico Galeazzi, Milan, Italy

***Correspondence:**
Emanuela Galliera
emanuela.galliera@unimi.it

High Crosslink process was introduced in the development of joint prosthetic devices, in order to decrease the wear rate of ultrahigh molecular weight polyethylene (UHMWPE), but it also triggers the formation of free radicals and oxidative stress, which affects the physiological bone remodeling, leading to osteolysis. Vitamin E stabilization of UHMWPE was proposed to provide oxidation resistance without affecting mechanical properties and fatigue strength. The aim of this study is to evaluate the antioxidant effect of vitamin E added to UHMWPE on oxidative stress induced osteolysis, focusing in particular on the oxidative stress response in correlation with the production of osteoimmunological markers, Sclerostin and DKK-1, and the RANKL/OPG ratio compared to conventional UHMWPE wear debris. Human osteoblastic cell line SaOS2 were incubated for 96 h with wear particles derived from crosslinked and not crosslinked Vitamin E-stabilized, UHMWPE without Vitamin E, and growth medium as control. Cellular response to oxidative stress, compared to not treat cells, was evaluated in terms of proteins O-GlcNAcylation, cellular levels of OGA, and OGT proteins by immunoblotting. O-GlcNAcylation and its positive regulator OGT levels are increased in the presence of Vitamin E blended UHMWPE, in particular with not crosslinked Vit E stabilized UHMWPE. Conversely, the negative regulator OGA increased in the presence of UHMWPE not blended with Vitamin E. Vitamin E-stabilized UHMWPE induced a decrease of RANKL/OPG ratio compared to UHMWPE without Vitamin E, and the same effect was observed for Sclerostin, while DKK-1 was not significantly affected. In conclusion, Vitamin E stabilization of UHMWPE increased osteoblast response to oxidative stress, inducing a cellular mechanism aimed at cell survival. Vitamin E antioxidant effect influences the secretion of osteoimmunological factors, shifting the bone turnover balance toward bone protection stimuli. This suggests that Vitamin E-Stabilization of UHMWPE could contribute to reduction of oxidation-induced osteolysis and the consequent loosening of the prosthetic devices, therefore improving the longevity of total joint replacements.

Keywords: vitamin E, high-molecular-weight polyethylene (HMWPE), oxidative stress, osteoblasts, proteins O-GlcNAcylation, osteoimmunological markers

INTRODUCTION

One of the main problems in total hip arthroplasty is osteolysis triggered by ultrahigh molecular weight polyethylene (UHMWPE) wear particles (1) and different strategies have been developed to improve the oxidation and wear resistance.

High crosslink process was developed in order to decrease the wear rate of UHMWPE (2), but it also triggers the formation of free radicals (3), leading to oxidative degradation of the material through a cascade reaction with oxygen (4). In order to reduce oxidation, Vitamin E was introduced in UHMWPE stabilization, to provide oxidation resistance without affecting mechanical and fatigue strength of the material (5, 6). Vitamin E in the most abundant and effective antioxidant in the body, able to react with free radicals in cell membrane and protect polyunsaturated fatty acids from degradation due to oxidation (7). Polyethylene has a lipid—like molecular structure and its oxidation follows a similar mechanism of oxidation of lipids *in vivo* (8).

The physiological intracellular redox state is maintained in equilibrium by the balance of antioxidants and reactive oxygen species (ROS)- producing enzyme. Oxidative stress occurs when the overproduction of ROS is not balanced by an adequate level of antioxidants (9). The redox state affects the physiological process of bone remodeling (9). Indeed, changes in the ROS/antioxidant balance are involved in the pathogenesis of bone loss. In particular, oxidative stress activates the differentiation of osteoclasts from their precursors, while inducing osteoblasts apoptosis, thus shifting the balance toward osteoclastogenesis and bone resorption (9). High levels of ROS reduce osteoblast differentiation and activity, therefore reducing mineralization and bone mass (10, 11). On the contrary, antioxidant may contribute to osteoblasts differentiation and activity, promoting bone formation (9, 11).

Moreover, oxidative stress promotes the inflammatory response and directly interferes with the osteoimmunological regulation of bone remodeling, based on the action of the RANKL/RANK/OPG system. The receptor activator of NF-κB (nuclear factor-κB) ligand (RANKL) is a key factor stimulating the differentiation and activation of osteoclasts, and therefore, is essential for bone remodeling. The binding of RANKL to its receptor RANK leads to osteoclasts differentiation, while the decoy receptor Osteoprotegerin (OPG) counteracts this effect by binding and blocking RANKL. ROS act as specific secondary messengers in signaling pathways involved in RANKL-induced osteoclast differentiation (12). The expression of RANKL and OPG is sensitive to oxidative status that reduces OPG expression and induces RANKL expression, thus shifting the balance toward bone loss. An excess of oxidative stress also induces apoptosis of osteocytes, resulting in the reduction OPG production and increase of Sclerostin and DKK-1, two inhibitors of the WNT pathway involved in the osteoimmunological regulation of bone remodeling (13, 14). The expression of WNT pathway inhibitors seems to be induced by inflammatory mediators and aging (15), both conditions characterized by an increase in oxidative stress.

In this context, knowing that oxidative stress plays an important role in bone remodeling disorders, it's extremely important to study the effect of antioxidant agent (Vitamin E) added to UHMWPE that may reduce oxidative stress, thus modulating the inflammatory process and the regulation of bone remodeling by osteoimmunological mediators, eventually protecting from periprosthetic bone loss. Several studies in the recent years evaluated the clinical advantages of Vitamin E added to UHMWPE (16–20), but there is little if no evidence focusing in particular on the protective role of Vitamin E from oxidative stress in correlation with inflammation and the consequent periprosthetic bone loss.

One of the main mechanisms of cellular oxidative stress response is the modification of intracellular proteins by monosaccharides of O-linked β-N- acetylglucosammine, known as O-GlcNAcylation (21). This is a post-translational modification of nuclear and cytoplasmic proteins, which consists in the attachment of a single N-acetylglucosamine (O-GlcNAc) to serine and threonine residues of a protein (22).Two enzymes regulate this process: O-GlcNAc transferase (OGT) that catalyzes the addition of O-GlcNAc to the hydroxyl group of serine or threonine residues of a protein, and O-GlcNAcase (OGA) that removes O-GlcNAc from proteins (23, 24). Levels of O-GlcNAc are induced in response to stress, in order to prevent apoptosis and promote cell survival mechanism, and are considered a target of mammalian stress response (25). The protein O-GlcNAcylation, OGA and OGT levels are therefore considered markers of cellular response to oxidative stress.

The aim of this study is to evaluate the antioxidant effect of vitamin E added to UHMWPE and the association with the main osteoimmunological biomarkers (RANKL/RANK/OPG), and WNT pathway inhibitors, in order to better understand how the antioxidant effect of Vitamin E can prevent periprosthetic inflammation and the consequent o and prosthetic loosening.

METHODS

UHMWPE Particles Generation

UHMWPE wear particles were generated as previously described in Galliera et al.(26) by four different UHMWPE articular inserts (raw material GUR 1020): Material (1) moderately cross-linked vitamin E-blended UHMWPE (60 kGy electron-beam irradiated) (vitamin E concentration 0.1 wt%), EtO sterilized (*Vital-XE®, Permedica S.p.A.*); Material (2) standard UHMWPE (without vitamin E and not cross-linked), EtO sterilized *(Permedica S.p.A);* Material (3) vitamin E-blended UHMWPE (vitamin E concentration 0.1 wt%) not cross-linked, EtO sterilized (*Vital-E®, Permedica S.p.A.*).

All UHMWPE wear particles were generated as described previously (26). Briefly, the articular inserts were rubbed for 10 days at 230 rpm against ceramic ball heads using a combined drilling and tapping machine (IM company, Italy), applying a load of 1,000 N. The resulting UHMWPE particles were released directly into a closed sterile recipient containing 500 mL of ultrapure water with 0.2% sodium azide (antibacterial additive).

Cell Culture and Treatment With Wear Particles

SAoS2 cells, a permanent line of human osteoblast-like cells, were obtained from a partner institute and grown in RPMI 1,640 (Invitrogen, Germany) with L-glutamine, 10% fetal bovine serum (FBS), 100 U/mL penicillin and 100 µg/mL streptomycin (GIBCO, USA). Cells were cultured in 5% CO_2 at 37°C in 12-well culture plates (Corning, USA).

Treatment with HUMWPE wear particles was performed as previously described (26). Briefly, after sterilization by UV irradiation overnight, the three types of wear particle (described above) diluted in growth media at a concentration of 1:1 or pure media (as control) were added to the cell culture. After 96 h of incubation, the supernatants of each well were collected and stocked at −20°C for ELISA assays, while cells were washed with PBS twice and then lysed for 15 min at 4°C in lysis buffer (25 mM Tris-HCl pH 7.4, 150 mM NaCl, 5 mM EDTA, 20 mM NaF, 1 mM Na3VO4, 0.5% v/v NP40, 10 mg/ml leupeptin, 10 mg/ml aprotinin, 1 mg/ml pepstatin A). Insoluble material was removed by centrifugation at 13,000 g for 10 min, supernatants were collected and assayed for protein concentration with Coomassie Protein Assay (Pierce). Then samples were analyzed by immunoblotting.

Evaluation of Oxidative Stress Parameters: Immunoblotting and Densitometry Analysis

Forty micrograms of cell proteins were separated by SDS electrophoresis under denaturating conditions using 6–10% polyacrylamide gels. SDS-PAGE gels were electrophoretically transferred on PVDF membrane in Tris-glicine buffer, using the Mini Transblot System (Bio-Rad Laboratories, Richmond, VA). O-GlcNAc levels were measured by anti-b-O-linked N-Acetylglucosamine (OGlcNAc) CTD 110.6, an antibody that specifically recognizes endogenous levels of O-GlcNAc, linked to both serine and threonine residues of proteins, 1:1000 dilution (Cell Signaling). Other primary antibodies were used as follows: anti-OGA 1:3000 dilution (Sigma-Aldrich), anti-OGT 1:500 dilution (Sigma–Aldrich), and anti-Histone H3 1:2000 dilution (Cell Signaling).

Each membrane was washed three times for 10 min and then incubated with the appropriate secondary antibody conjugated with horseradish peroxidase (Santa Cruz Biotechnology) for 1 h. For the immunological detection of proteins, MINI HD 9 System (Uvitec Limited, Cambridge UK) was used. Band density was quantified Quantity One Software (Bio-Rad Laboratories).

Evaluation of Oxidative Stress Parameters: ROS Generation Assay

ROS production was tested by OxiSelect™ *In vitro* ROS/RNS Assay kit [Green Fluorescence (Cell Biolabs)], according to manufacturer's protocol. Briefly, the OxiSelect™ *In vitro* ROS/RNS Assay Kit is an *in vitro* assay for measuring total ROS/RNS free radical activity. Unknown ROS or RNS samples or standards are added to the wells with a catalyst that helps accelerate the oxidative reaction. After a brief incubation, the prepared DCFH probe is added to all wells and the oxidation reaction is allowed to proceed. Samples are measured fluorometrically against a hydrogen peroxide or DCF standard. The assay is performed in a 96-well fluorescence plate format that can be read on a standard fluorescence plate reader. The free radical content in unknown samples is determined by comparison with the predetermined DCF or hydrogen peroxide standard curve.

Evaluation of Osteoimmunological Biomarkers: ELISA Assay

The osteoimmunological biomarkers were evaluated by ELISA assay in SaOS2 supernatant. In particular, RANKL was measured using an ELISA Duo Set assay (R&D System, Minneapolis, MN, USA), while DKK-1, OPG, and Sclerostin were measured by ELISA Quantikine colorimetric sandwich assays (R&D System, Minneapolis, MN, USA), according to the manufacturer's protocols.

RANKL: CV intra assay 8.01% and inter assay 6.2%; OPG: CV intra assay 7.3% and inter assay 6.9%; DKK-1: CV intra assay 2.7 % and inter assay 5.4 %, SOST: CV intra assay 2.1 %, and inter assay 8.2%.

Evaluation of Cell Vitality

Cell viability was assessed quantitatively using the resulting Alamar Blue® test, a non-toxic test for cells as it exploits the reducing power of living cells by measuring their metabolic activity quantitatively, which makes it possible to analyze, in different timing, the same proliferating cell population. This test was also used as an indirect index of cell proliferation. The assay exploits the mitochondrial activity of viable cells capable of maintaining an environment of reducing inside the cell. Resazurin, the active component of Alamar Blu, is a compound able to cross the membranes, and once it enters the cell, it gets reduced in Resorufin and its color turns from blue to red. The reduction was measured by a spectrophotometer at 560 and 600 nm (Glo Max, Promega). The results obtained by both the readings were analyzed following the indications provided by the assay protocol by calculating the percentage of cell viability as the difference in the reduction between the treated samples and the samples control (medium + Alamar Blue®).

Evaluation of Mineralization

The cells were seeded in 6-well plates at a density of 0.8 $\times 10^5$ cells/well and stabilized for 24 h. To induce osteoblast differentiation, Osteogenic medium (Promocell), containing 50 µg/ml L-ascorbic acid and 10 mM β-glycerophosphate, was added to culture for 11 days. The culture medium was changed every 3–4 days. Then, the cells were fixed in 10% formalin for 10 min and stained with the 40 mM Alizarin Red-S (pH 4.2; Sigma-Aldrich; Merck KGaA) for 15 min, all at RT. For quantification of Alizarin red S, 500 µl citrate solution containing 20% methanol and 10% acetic acid was added for 20 min at RT, and the absorbance of supernatants was measured at 570 nm using a GloMAx Fluorescence Reader (Promega). The plates were observed under the Leica Microscope DML B2/11888111 equipped with Leica camera DFC450 at ×100 magnification.

Statistical Analysis

Statistical analysis was performed with dedicated statistical software (GraphPad Prism 7); normality of distribution of the groups was verified by KS normality for all the parameters evaluated. Statistical analysis was performed with one-way ANOVA, considering $p < 0.05$ as significant and $p < 0.001$ as highly significant. Data are expressed as the mean ± standard deviation (SD).

RESULTS

Oxidative Stress Response

To investigate the effect of the of Vitamin E blended UHMWPE on O-GlcNAcylation process, we measured cellular O-GlcNAC levels by western blot using CTD110.6 antibody. As shown in **Figure 1,** Panel A, O-GlcNAcylation levels increased in the presence of Vitamin E blended UHMWPE (in particular with not crosslinked Vit E blended UHMWPE) while, conversely, they fall in the absence of Vitamin E.

Densitometric analysis showed a significative ($p < 0.005$) increase in O-GlcNAC levels in the presence of not-crosslinked Vit E blended HMWPE and a significative ($p < 0.005$) decrease in Vitamin E absence (**Figure 1B**).

In order to determine whether the observed variation in O-GlcNAC levels was caused by an alteration of the ratio between the two O-GlcNAc cycling enzymes, we examined protein expression of OGA and OGT by western blot analysis (**Figures 2A,B**). As shown in Panel A, a significant increase ($p < 0.01$) of OGT protein level was found in the presence of not-crosslinked Vitamin E blended UHMWPE, whereas a significant increase ($p < 0.05$) of OGA enzyme was observed in Vitamin E absence. The OGT/OGA expression ratio shows a behavior consistent with the observed O-GlcNAC levels (**Figure 2B**).

ROS production was evaluated during the treatment, at 24, 48, 72, and 96 h (**Figure 4C**).The results show that at early time points (24 h), there is a significative increase of ROS induced by M1 (crosslinked HUMWPE vitamin E added), while M3 (not crosslinked V, Vitamin E added UHMWPE) display a significative decrease compared to M2 (not crosslinked V, UHMWPE without Vitamin E). This effect attenuates at 48 h, resulting in an insignificant difference between M1 and M2, maintaining a low but weakly significant level in response to M3. At 72 h, there is a little and insignificant increase in ROS in response to M1 and M3, which then turns into comparable levels, with no significative difference between the three materials at 96 h.

Osteoimmunological Biomarkers

The secretion of osteoimmunological markers in the supernatant was measured after 96 h of incubation with material 1, 2, and 3, as described in the Method Session, and growth medium as control. The two main osteoimmunological pathways were evaluated: the RANK/RANKL/OPG, by measuring the secretion of RANKL and OPG from the osteoblast cell line SaOs2 pathway, and the Wnt pathway, by measuring the secretion of the two main Wnt inhibitors, Sclerostin (SOST), and DKK-1.

RANKL production (**Figure 3A**) displayed a insignificant increase in response to M1 material, compared to control, and it resulted comparable to control in response to M3 material. On the contrary, RANKL displayed a strong and significant increase in response to material M2. Conversely, OPG (**Figure 3B**) displayed a significant reduction in response to material M2, while it showed a significant increase in response to M1 and an even higher increase in response to material M3.

In order to evaluate the trend of bone remodeling regulators *in vitro*, the RANKL/OPG ratio was calculated (**Figure 3E**). In all the conditions, the RANKL/OPG ratio resulted largely <1.However, while in response to M1 and M3 the RANKL/OPG ratio was very low and comparable to control, in response to M2 the RANKL/OPG ratio displayed a very significant increase.

Sclerostin, a marker of bone resorption, displayed a significant increase in response to material M2, while it showed a significant decrease in response to material 1 and a little, even significant decrease in response to material M3 (**Figure 3C**). The secretion of the other Wnt inhibitor DKK-1 displayed no significant changes in response to material M1 compared to control (**Figure 3D**).

Cell Vitality and Mineralization After Exposure to M1, M2 and M3 Wear Debris

Cell were plated at the concentration of 10^3cells/mL, and 24 h after, when they resulted completely adherent, the incubation with wear particles started and lasted for 96 h, during the exponential growth phase. Doubling time of Saos cell is 37 h and they can be cultured in logaritimic growth for 7 days before splitting, when they reach the concentration of 3×10^5cells/mL.

Cells were equally plated for treatment with wear particles and control medium. The vitality and the growth rate of the Sa0S2 cell were evaluated by Alamar blue, and treated as well as not treated cells displayed exactly the same viability and growth rate, as shown in **Figure 4A**.

Mineralization assays were performed in the presence of material 1, 2, and 3, and only mineralization medium as control.

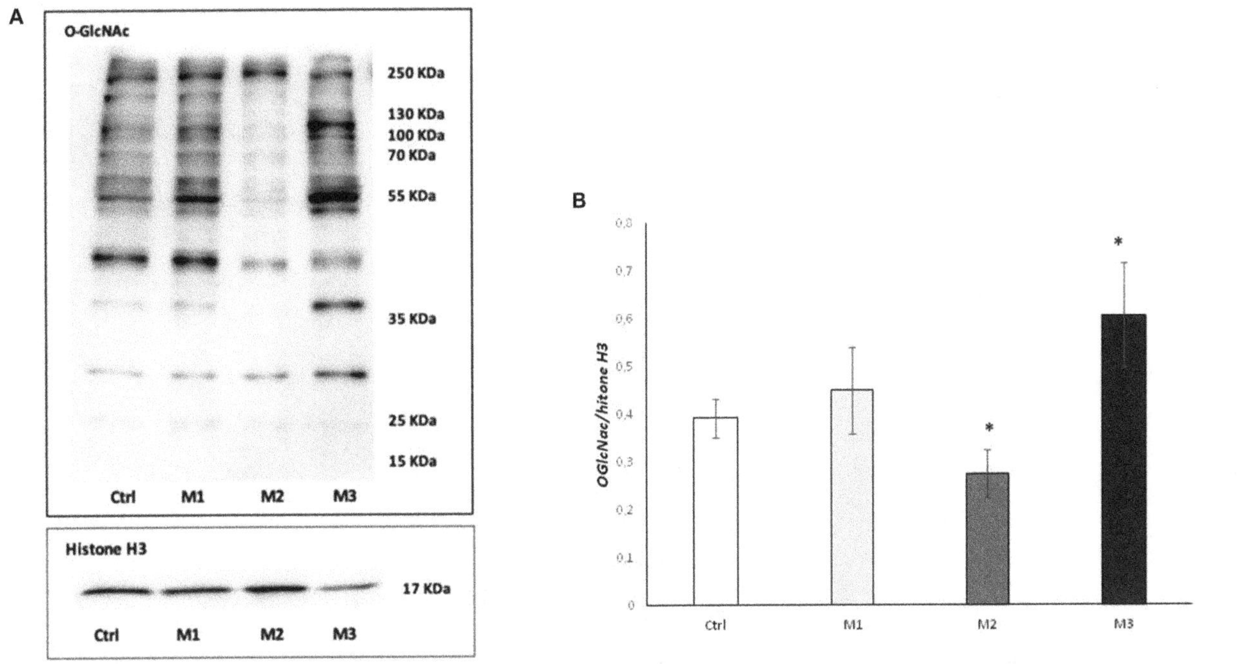

FIGURE 1 | Total O-GlcNAcylations after exposure to M1, M2, and M3 wear debris. **(A)** O-GlcNAcylations of cell proteins examined by western blotting. The western blot image is representative of three experiments. **(B)** Densitometric analysis of proteins expression was performed using Histone H3 as loading control. *$P < 0.05$ vs. Ctrl. Materials M1, M2, M3 are described in the Methods section, as follows: Material M1 a moderately cross-linked vitamin E-blended UHMWPE, EtO sterilized; Material M2 standard UHMWPE (without vitamin E and not cross-linked), EtO sterilized; Material M3 vitamin E-blended UHMWPE not cross-linked, EtO sterilized. Cnotrol (white bar) Material M1 (light gray bar), material M2 (medium gray bar), material M3 (dark gray bar).

As shown in **Figures 4B,D**. The three different kinds of material did not affect the mineralization of SaoS2.

DISCUSSION

Implant materials can release wear particles which may elicit adverse reactions in patients, such as local inflammatory response leading to tissue damage, which eventually results in loosening of the implant. In the case of ultra-high molecular weight polyethylene (UHMWPE), the inflammation is further boosted by the oxidation of the material, which has been recognized as a potential limiting factor for the longevity of total joint replacements (6). In order to reduce UHMWPE oxidation, chemical stabilization with Vitamin E was introduced over the past decade. Vitamin E, when added to UHMWPE, has been shown to suppress the oxidation cascade by reducing both alkyl and peroxy radicals (27). The antioxidant effect of Vitamin E has been extensively studied from the biochemical point of view (17, 28), but the comprehensive effect on cellular response to oxidative stress and the correlation with inflammatory response and bone resorption still needs to be fully elucidated. For this reason, this study aimed to evaluate the effects of Vitamin E addition to UHMWPE on both the aspects of inflammation leading to bone tissue damage: on the one hand the cellular response to oxidative stress and on the other hand the production of osteoimmunological mediators, that combine the regulation of inflammatory response to bone remodeling (23). In order to evaluate the effect of Vitamin E added, different variants of UHMWPE were evaluated. In the Vitamin E- UHMWPE production, the radiation cross linking process is required to reduce wear, but it also increases the oxidation of UHMWPE (24). For this reason, we evaluated two different types of Vitamin E-stabilized UHMWPE, one crosslinked, and one not crosslinked, compared to not crosslinked UHMWPE, without Vitamin E.

Cells and tissue respond to oxidative stress, environmental and injury by reprogramming gene expression, transcription, transduction, and post trasductional protein modification in order to stat pathways of repair and survival. In particular oxidative stress induces a dynamic O-GlcNAcylation (25, 29), promoting the glycosilation of some proteins and the deglycosilation of others, in order to prevent apoptosis and promote the cell survival mechanism (29). The dynamic O-GlcNAcylation is cycled by two enzymes, the O-GlcNAc transferase (OGT), which catalyzes the addition of O-GlcNAc residues, and the O-GlcNAcase (OGA), which removes O-GlcNAc residues. The level of O-GlcNAcylation, OGA, and OGT levels are therefore markers of cellular response to oxidative stress and were measured in the present study to evaluate the response of the osteoblastic cell line SaOs2 to wear debris from crosslinked Vitamin E—stabilized UHMWPE, not-crosslinked Vitamin E—stabilized UHMWPE and not-crosslinked UHMWPE without vitamin E, compared to not-treated cells. As shown in

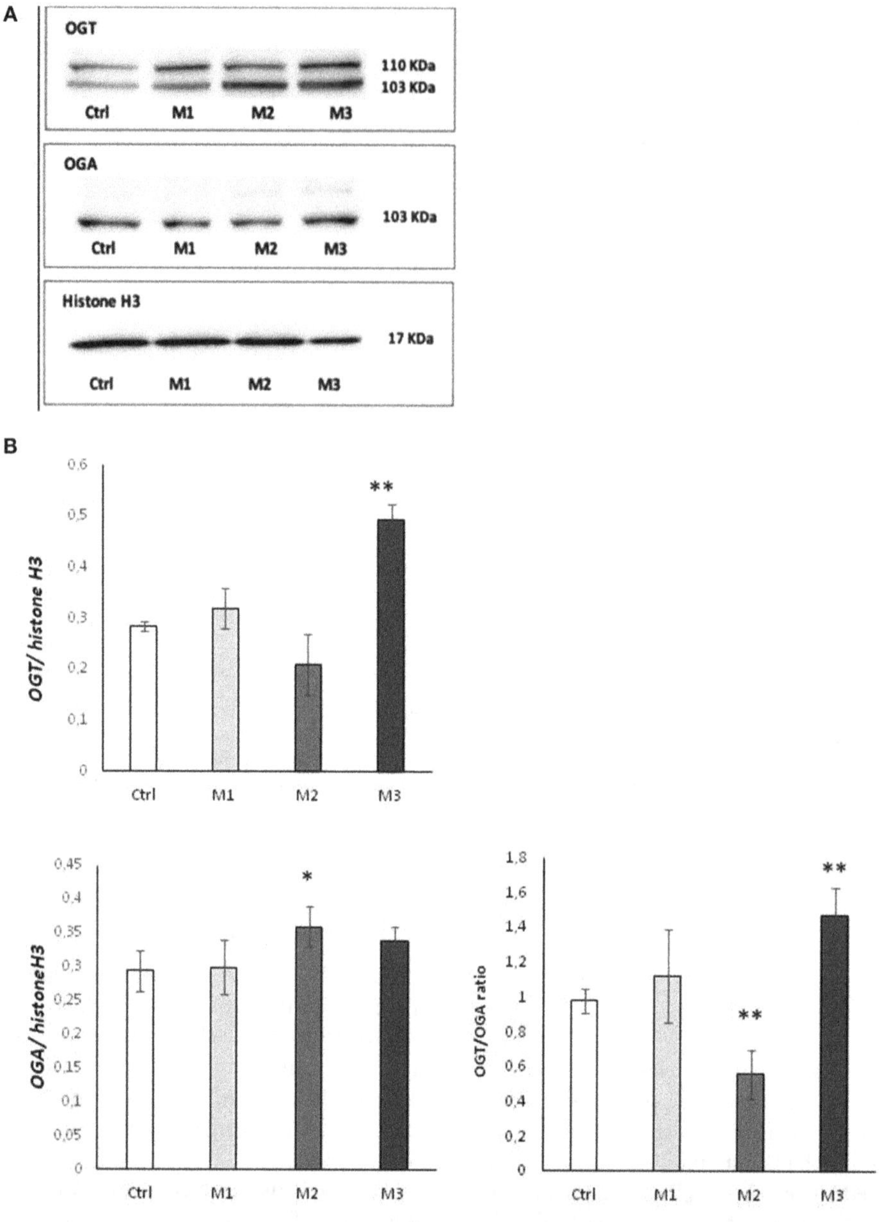

FIGURE 2 | OGA and OGT levels after exposure to M1, M2, and M3 wear debris. **(A)** Cellular levels of OGA and OGT proteins examined by western blotting. The western blot image is representative of three experiments. Densitometric analysis of proteins expression was performed using Histone H3 as loading control. **(B)** OGT/OGA expression ratio. $^*P < 0.05$ Vs. Ctrl; $^{**}P < 0.01$ Vs. Ctrl. Materials M1, M2, M3 are described in the Methods section, as follows: Material M1 a moderately cross-linked vitamin E-blended UHMWPE, EtO sterilized; Material M2 standard UHMWPE (without vitamin E and not cross-linked), EtO sterilized; Material M3 vitamin E-blended UHMWPE not cross-linked, EtO sterilized. Control (white bar) Material M1 (light gray bar), material M2 (medium gray bar), material M3 (dark gray bar).

Figure 1, O-GlcNAcylation is significantly reduced in response to notVitamin E-stabilized UHMWPE, while they are increased in response to Vitamin E—stabilized UHMWPE, compared to controls, with a significant increase in the case of not-crosslinked Vitamin E—stabilized UHMWPE (material 3), indicating that the presence of Vitamin E increase the ability of Saos2 Cells to respond to oxidative stress due to UHMWPE. This result is also confirmed by the specific evaluation of OGA and OGT: OGT production showed the same changes observed for O-GlcNAcylation, with a significant increase in response to not-crosslinked Vitamin E—stabilized UHMWPE, a little but not significant increase in response to crosslinked Vitamin E—stabilized UHMWPE and a decrease in response to not-crosslinked UHMWPE without Vitamin E. These results are in accordance with previous reports indicating that stress induced O-GlcNAcylation is coincident with increased protein expression of OGT of OGT (29–31). OGA exert the opposite role of OGT (21), and even though less is known about the regulation of OGA levels in stresses cells, recent studies reported that increased O-GlcNAcylation levels are associated with a decrease in OGA (29,

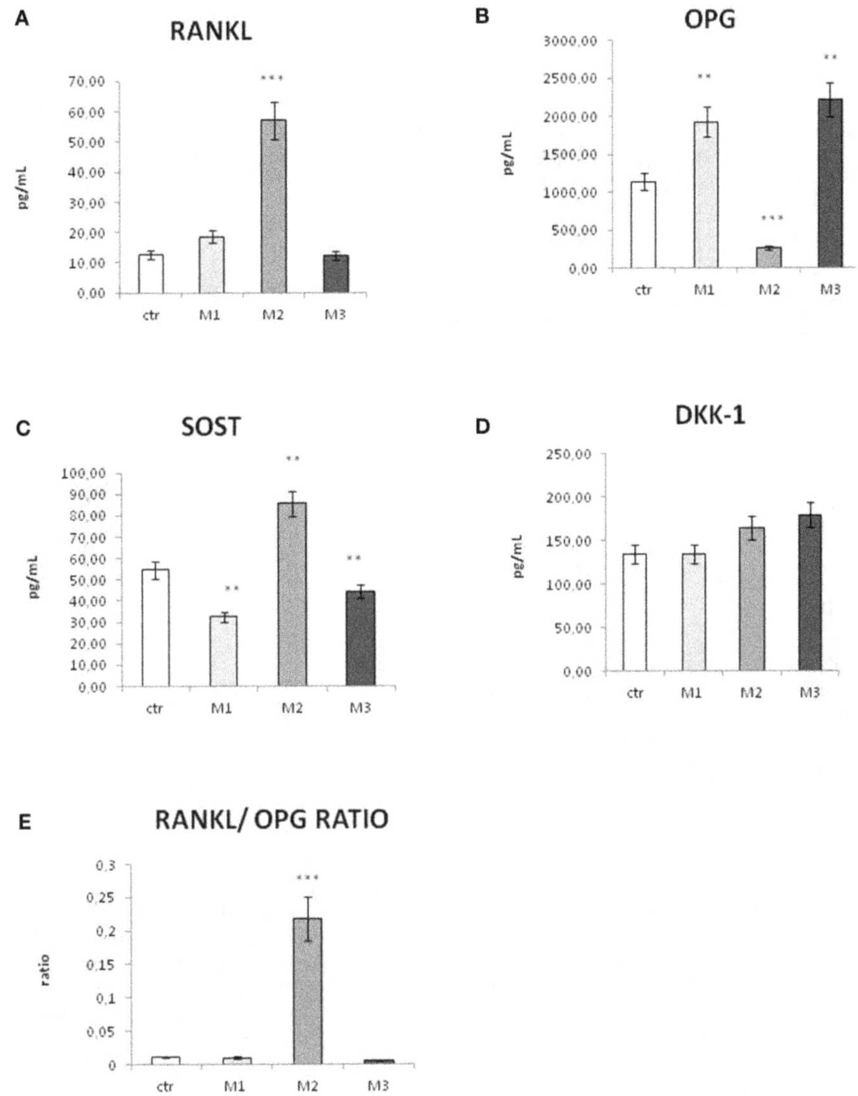

FIGURE 3 | Secretion of osteoimmunological biomarkers in the cell culture supernatant after exposure to M1, M2, and M3 wear debris. Concentrations (picograms per milliliter) of RANKL **(A)**, OPG **(B)**, Sclerostin (SOST, **C)**, and DKK-1 **(D)**, RANKL/OPG ratio **(E)** in the cell culture supernatant of control (white bar), material M1 (light gray bars), material M2 (medium gray bars), material M3 (dark gray bars). Materials M1, M2, M3 are described in the Methods section, as follows: Material M1 a moderately cross-linked vitamin E-blended UHMWPE, EtO sterilized; Material M2 standard UHMWPE (without vitamin E and not cross-linked), EtO sterilized; Material M3 vitamin E-blended UHMWPE not cross-linked, EtO sterilized. Control (white bar) Material M1 (light gray bar), material M2 (medium gray bar), material M3 (dark gray bar). *$p < 0.05$, statistically significant; **$p < 0.01$; ***$p < 0.005$.

31). Consistently with these evidences, we observed a significant increase of OGA in response to material 2 (UHMWPE without Vitamin E), in correspondence to a decrease of OGT, and no significant change in response to material 1 and 3 (UHMWPE with Vitamin E). The overall effect is more evident by evaluating OGT/OGA ratio, showing that UHMWPE without Vitamin E induced a very significant decrease in OGT/OGA ratio while not-crosslinked Vitamin E—stabilized UHMWPE induced a very significant increase in OGT/OGA ratio, shifting the balance toward increased cell survival. These results suggest that the addition of Vitamin E to UHMWPE increases the ability of SaOs2 cells to respond to oxidative stress induced by UHMWPE, while the absence of Vitamin E reduces the cell response to oxidative stress. Material 1 (crosslinked Vitamin E—stabilized UHMWPE) stimulated an increase in OGT/OGA ratio but in a minor extent of its not-crosslinked counterpart (material 3), indicating that the cross linking process contributes to generate oxidative stress and weakly reduces the beneficial effect of Vitamin E-stabilization. This is in accordance with the literature reporting that the cross linking process is a strong source of UHMWPE oxidation (6, 32, 33). Taken together, these results suggest that the Vitamin E-stabilization, in particular in absence of cross linking, stimulates cellular response to oxidative stress, in order to promote cell survival.

The results of ROS production are in line with recent literature evidences indicating that UHMWPE induce oxidative stress,

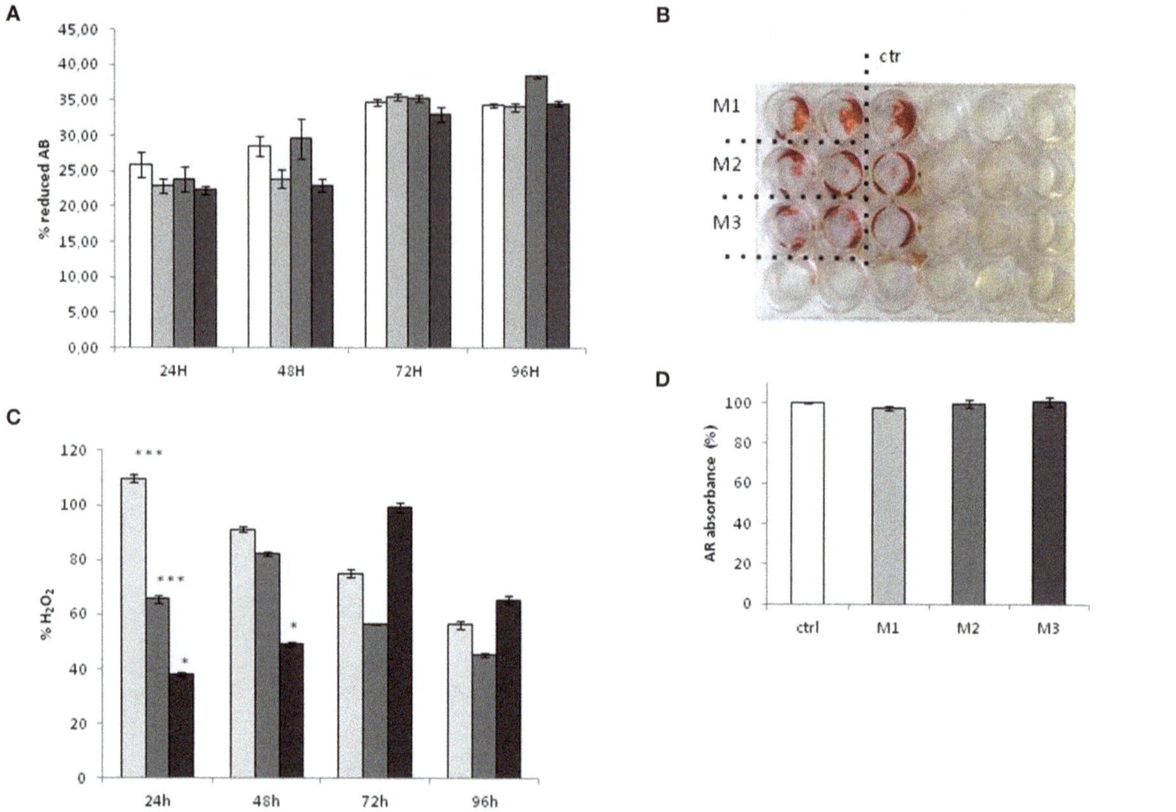

FIGURE 4 | Cell Vitality, mineralization, and ROS production after exposure to M1, M2, and M3 wear debris. **(A)** vitality and the growth rate of Sa0S2 cell evaluated by Alamar blue **(A,B)**. The vitality of the cells is expressed as percentage of reduced Alamar Blue (%AB), as indicated in Alamar Blue protocol. Mineralization Assay was evaluated by alizarin Red (AR) staining. The plates were observed under the Leica Microscope DML B2/11888111 equipped with Leica camera DFC450 at ×100 magnification **(B)**. For quantification of Alizarin red S, 500 μl citrate solution containing 20% methanol and 10% acetic acid was added for 20 min at RT, and the absorbance of supernatants was measured at 570 nm using an Fluorescence Reader (GloMAx). The mineralization is expressed as percentage of Alzarin Red staining (% ARS) of treated cells vs. untreated control **(D)**. **(C)** ROS production was tested by OxiSelect^{TM} *In vitro* ROS/RNS Assay kit. ROS production is expressed as percentage of H_2O_2 production vs. untreated control. Materials M1, M2, M3 are described in the Methods section, as follows: Material M1 a moderately cross-linked vitamin E-blended UHMWPE, EtO sterilized; Material M2 standard UHMWPE (without vitamin E and not cross-linked), EtO sterilized; Material M3 vitamin E-blended UHMWPE not cross-linked, EtO sterilized. Control (white bar) Material M1 (light gray bar), material M2 (medium gray bar), material M3 (dark gray bar). $^{*}p < 0.05$; $^{**}p < 0.01$, statistically very significant; $^{***}p < 0.005$.

even when modified (34) with Vitamin E. Indeed, Vitamin E exerts an antioxidant effect mainly *in vivo* as a scavenger of oxidant molecules, in particular lipid-soluble peroxyl radical, when they reach a high concentration, in order to prevent cell damage (35). On the other hand, is should be noted that low levels of oxidative stimuli, such as ROS generation (36), induce a cellular adaptive response to upregulate the defense capacity against subsequent oxidative stress (35, 37–39). Consistently, O-GlvNAcylation response proceeds as a two-step process. An initial ROS stimulus stimulates O-GlvNAcylation which, in turn, activates an intracellular signaling cascade leading to a long-term oxidative defense process. Indeed, a significative reduction in ROS generation is reported to be reduced by a sustained O-GlvNAcylation (40). In our results, the early and transient ROS production in response to M1 and M3 could be considered a priming factor that induces, at later time points, the O-GlvNAcylation as a mechanism of long-term antioxidant defense. Indeed, at a time point of 96 h, O-GlvNAcylation was observed in concordance with a decrease in ROS and a stabilization, with no significative difference between the three materials. These results indicate that Vitamin E added to WHMWPE does not have an immediate antioxidant effect (24 h) on the reduction ROS generation, but a more long term effect, stimulating, by an initial and transient ROS increase, the O-GlvNAcylation, which leads in turn to a antioxidant defense process.

These results are consistent with the final goal of Vitamin E adding to UHMWPE, to prevent the long-term effect of UHMWPE oxidation.

Oxidative stress is related to the inflammatory response, which in turn, affects bone turnover and remodeling by means of osteoimmunological mediators (9).

Vitamin E has also been shown to influence inflammatory cytokine production (17, 41). We recently showed the effect of Vitamin E—stabilized UHMWPE wear particles on osteoimmunological molecule's gene expression and secretion at early time points (26), so in this study, we aimed to analyze in parallel the effects of Vitamin E added to UHMWPE on oxidative stress response and osteoimmunological response. In particular, O-GlcNAcylation has been reported to affect the production of osteoimmunological factors (42). In our study, the osteoimmunological factors RANKL and its negative regulators confirmed our previous report, showing an increase in the bone-resorptive marker RANKL and a correspondent reduction of the osteo-protective marker OPG in response to UHMWPE without Vitamin E, while when vitamin E is added to stabilize UHMWPE, there is an strong reduction in RANKL, and an increase in OPG. In order to give a comprehensive result, we measured the RANKL/OPG ratio, which is considered a better parameter than the single RANKL and OPG values to evaluate the trend toward bone resorption or bone formation stimuli (43). A number of studies have shown that bone remodeling is dependent on the ratio of RANKL to OPG: if RANKL is higher bone resorption dominates, while when OPG is higher, the balance is shifted toward bone formation (44, 45). Thus, OPG acquired its name from its ability to protect bone from excessive resorption by counteracting the osteoclastic effects of RANKL (46, 47). Over the last decade, innovative, efficacious treatments for osteolysis have been developed specifically targeting the RANKL/OPG ratio, in order to reduce the incidence of related implant failures (43). In our study, RANKL/OPG ratio showed a trend toward an increase in this ratio when UHMWPE is not stabilized with Vitamin E, while the addition of Vitamin E restores the bone turnover stimuli to levels comparable to controls.

These results are also confirmed by the evaluation of two other main osteoimmunological factors, Sclerostin (SOST), and DKK-1, two inhibitors of the Wnt pathway involved in bone remodeling regulation. Wnt Signaling stimulates OPG expression, while the Wnt inhibitors Sclerostin and DKK-1 prevent this effect (13), thus promoting bone resorption. Our results confirmed an increase in Sclerostin expression in correspondence to a decrease in OPG expression, in response to material 2 (UHMWPE without Vitamin E), and a decrease of Sclerostin in correspondence to the treatment with Vitamin E-stabilized UHMWPE. In this case, no significant difference was observed among crosslinked and not-crosslinked Vitamin E-stabilized UHMWPE, suggesting that the cross linking process does not affect the expression of these osteoimmunological biomarkers. A different effect was observed for DKK-1 secretion, showing no significant decrease in response to material 1 and a little increase in response to material 3, while as expected it displayed an increase, even though not significant, in response to material 2. The exact mechanism of DKK-1 regulation of OPG production still needs to be elucidated, and these results suggest that it could be different from the Sclerostin mechanism. It is known that Sclerostin and DKK-1 can act separately and even alternatively in the regulation of bone turnover (48). We have already shown that Vitamin E-stabilized UHMWPE wear debris had different effects on Sclerostin and DKK-1 (26), and recent evidence indicated that these two Wnt inhibitors can be differently influenced by treatments (49) or pathological conditions (50). Consistently with these results, recent evidence showed that redox regulating mechanisms are able to affect cytokine and osteoimmunological factors produced by bone tissue and that the expression of RANKL, OPG and Sclerostin are redox regulated processes (51, 52). In particular, among Wnt pathway inhibitors, Sclerostin can be affected by oxidative stress, showing the same reduction in response to antioxidant as RANKL expression and RANKL/OPG ratio (52).

The limitation of this study is that the effect of Vitamin E stabilization was not tested on primary human osteoblasts, which could better reproduce the *in vivo* conditions, but on an immortalized human osteoblast cell line. Nevertheless, this choice was made in order to introduce as few variables as possible, since the effect of Vitamin E stabilization of UHMWPE on osteoblasts was unknown. Osteoblastic-like SaOS-2 cells are considered a valuable system for studying osteoblast functions and response to oxidative stress (10). Moreover, the choice for this immortalized cell line provides some advantages, such as a more stable and standardized growth condition than the primary cell culture.

In conclusion, taken together, these results suggest that the Vitamin E stabilization of UHMWPE produces two synergic effects on osteoblasts: on the one hand, it improves the ability of osteoblasts to respond to oxidative stress, inducing the cellular mechanism of defense, such as dynamic O-GlcNAcylation; on the other hand, the antioxidant effect influences the secretion on osteoimmunological factors, stimulating bone protective osteoimmunological factors such as OPG and reducing the RANKL/OPG ratio. This effect observed *in vitro*, could reflect *In vivo* through inducing a shift of the bone turnover balance toward bone protection. This suggests that the Vitamin E-Stabilization of UHMWPE could contribute to reduce oxidation- induced osteolysis (6, 32, 53) and the consequent loosening of the prosthetic device, therefore, improving the longevity of total joint replacements.

AUTHOR CONTRIBUTIONS

LM, EG, and VR contributed conception and design of the study. NP, LM, and GG performed the oxidative stress evaluation. MMCR and GG revised critically data interpretation. EG wrote the draft of the manuscript and performed osteoimmunological assays. All authors contributed to manuscript revision, read, and approved the submitted version.

FUNDING

This study was funded by a grant Ricerca Comissionata (#12973) of the University of Milan founded by Permedica.

REFERENCES

1. Oral E, Muratoglu OK. Vitamin E diffused, highly crosslinked UHMWPE: a review. *Int Orthop*. (2011) 35:215–23. doi: 10.1007/s00264-010-1161-y
2. Martell JM, Verner JJ, Incavo SJ. Clinical performance of a highly cross-linked polyethylene at two years in total hip arthroplasty: a randomized prospective trial. *J Arthroplasty*. (2003) 18 (7 Suppl. 1):55–9. doi: 10.1016/S0883-5403(03)00341-3
3. Esterbauer H, Gebicki J, Puhl H, Jurgens G. The role of lipid peroxidation and antioxidants in oxidative modification of LDL. *Free Radic Biol Med*. (1992) 13:341–90. doi: 10.1016/0891-5849(92)90181-F
4. Kashiwabara K, Nakajima T. Detection of human papillomavirus DNA in invasive cervical cancers by the polymerase chain reaction and its clinical significance. *Acta Pathol Jpn*. (1992) 42:876–83.
5. Oral E, Ghali BW, Muratoglu OK. The elimination of free radicals in irradiated UHMWPEs with and without vitamin E stabilization by annealing under pressure. *J Biomed Mater Res B Appl Biomater*. (2011) 97:167–74. doi: 10.1002/jbm.b.31799
6. Kurtz SM, Dumbleton J, Siskey RS, Wang A, Manley M. Trace concentrations of vitamin E protect radiation crosslinked UHMWPE from oxidative degradation. *J Biomed Mater Res A*. (2009) 90:549–63. doi: 10.1002/jbm.a.32122
7. Packer L, Suzuki YJ. Vitamin E and alpha-lipoate: role in antioxidant recycling and activation of the NF-kappa B transcription factor. *Mol Aspects Med*. (1993) 14:229–39.
8. Costa L, Luda MP, Trossarelli L, Brach del Prever EM, Crova M, Gallinaro P. Oxidation in orthopaedic UHMWPE sterilized by gamma-radiation and ethylene oxide. *Biomaterials*. (1998) 19:659–68. doi: 10.1016/S0142-9612(97)00160-9
9. Domazetovic V, Marcucci G, Iantomasi T, Brandi ML, Vincenzini MT. Oxidative stress in bone remodeling: role of antioxidants. *Clin Cases Miner Bone Metab*. (2017) 14:209–16. doi: 10.11138/ccmbm/2017.14.1.209
10. Romagnoli C, Marcucci G, Favilli F, Zonefrati R, Mavilia C, Galli G, et al. Role of GSH/GSSG redox couple in osteogenic activity and osteoclastogenic markers of human osteoblast-like SaOS-2 cells. *FEBS J*. (2013) 280:867–79. doi: 10.1111/febs.12075
11. Filaire E, Toumi H. Reactive oxygen species and exercise on bone metabolism: friend or enemy? *Joint Bone Spine*. (2012) 79:341–6. doi: 10.1016/j.jbspin.2012.03.007
12. Lee NK, Choi YG, Baik JY, Han SY, Jeong DW, Bae YS, et al. A crucial role for reactive oxygen species in RANKL-induced osteoclast differentiation. *Blood*. (2005) 106:852–9. doi: 10.1182/blood-2004-09-3662
13. Bellido T. Osteocyte-driven bone remodeling. *Calcif Tissue*. (2014) 94:25–34. doi: 10.1007/s00223-013-9774-y
14. Plotkin LI, Bellido T. Comment on osteocytes: masters orchestrators of bone. *Calcif Tissue Int*. (2014) 95:382–3. doi: 10.1007/s00223-014-9905-0
15. Rauner M, Sipos W, Pietschmann P. Age-dependent Wnt gene expression in bone and during the course of osteoblast differentiation. *Age*. (2008) 30:273–82. doi: 10.1007/s11357-008-9069-9
16. Shareghi B, Johanson PE, Karrholm J. Wear of vitamin E-infused highly cross-linked polyethylene at five years. *J Bone Joint Surg Am*. (2017) 99:1447–52. doi: 10.2106/JBJS.16.00691
17. Turner A, Okubo Y, Teramura S, Niwa Y, Ibaraki K, Kawasaki T, et al. The antioxidant and non-antioxidant contributions of vitamin E in vitamin E blended ultra-high molecular weight polyethylene for total knee replacement. *J Mech Behav Biomed Mater*. (2014) 31:21–30. doi: 10.1016/j.jmbbm.2012.12.006
18. Sillesen NH, Greene ME, Nebergall AK, Huddleston JI, Emerson R, Gebuhr P, et al. 3-year follow-up of a long-term registry-based multicentre study on vitamin E diffused polyethylene in total hip replacement. *Hip Int*. (2016) 26:97–103. doi: 10.5301/hipint.5000297
19. Salemyr M, Muren O, Ahl T, Boden H, Chammout G, Stark A, et al. Vitamin-E diffused highly cross-linked polyethylene liner compared to standard liners in total hip arthroplasty. A randomized, controlled trial. *Int Orthop*. (2015) 39:1499–505. doi: 10.1007/s00264-015-2680-3
20. Gigante A, Bottegoni C, Ragone V, Banci L. Effectiveness of vitamin-E-doped polyethylene in joint replacement: a literature review. *J Funct Biomater*. (2015) 6:889–900. doi: 10.3390/jfb6030889
21. Zachara N, Akimoto Y, Hart GW. Chapter 19. The O-GlcNAc modification. In: Varki A, Cummings RD, Esko JD, Freeze H, Hart G, Mart J, editors. *Essentials of Glycobiology*. 3rd ed. Cold Spring Harbor, NY: Cold Spring Harbor Laboratory Press (2015–2017). p. 239–51.
22. Comer FI, Hart GW. O-Glycosylation of nuclear and cytosolic proteins. Dynamic interplay between O-GlcNAc and O-phosphate. *J Biol Chem*. (2000) 275:29179–82. doi: 10.1074/jbc.R000010200
23. Jones D, Glimcher LH, Aliprantis AO. Osteoimmunology at the nexus of arthritis, osteoporosis, cancer, and infection. *J Clin Invest*. (2011) 121:2534–42. doi: 10.1172/JCI46262
24. Oral E, Neils A, Muratoglu OK. High vitamin E content, impact resistant UHMWPE blend without loss of wear resistance. *J Biomed Mater Res B Appl Biomater*. (2015) 103:790–7. doi: 10.1002/jbm.b.33256
25. Martinez MR, Dias TB, Natov PS, Zachara NE. Stress-induced O-GlcNAcylation: an adaptive process of injured cells. *Biochem Soc Trans*. (2017) 45:237–49. doi: 10.1042/BST20160153
26. Galliera E, Ragone V, Marazzi MG, Selmin F, Banci L, Corsi Romanelli MM. Vitamin E-stabilized UHMWPE: biological response on human osteoblasts to wear debris. *Clin Chim Acta*. (2018) 486:18–25. doi: 10.1016/j.cca.2018.07.012
27. Bracco P, Oral E. Vitamin E-stabilized UHMWPE for total joint implants: a review. *Clin Orthop Relat Res*. (2011) 469:2286–93. doi: 10.1007/s11999-010-1717-6
28. Bracco P, Bellare A, Bistolfi A, Affatato S. Ultra-high molecular weight polyethylene: influence of the chemical, physical and mechanical properties on the wear behavior. A Review. *Materials*. (2017) 10:791. doi: 10.3390/ma10070791
29. Zachara NE, O'Donnell N, Cheung WD, Mercer JJ, Marth JD, Hart GW. Dynamic O-GlcNAc modification of nucleocytoplasmic proteins in response to stress. A survival response of mammalian cells. *J Biol Chem*. (2004) 279:30133–42. doi: 10.1074/jbc.M403773200
30. Kazemi Z, Chang H, Haserodt S, McKen C, Zachara NE. O-linked beta-N-acetylglucosamine (O-GlcNAc) regulates stress-induced heat shock protein expression in a GSK-3beta-dependent manner. *J Biol Chem*. (2010) 285:39096–107. doi: 10.1074/jbc.M110.131102
31. Jensen RV, Zachara NE, Nielsen PH, Kimose HH, Kristiansen SB, Botker HE. Impact of O-GlcNAc on cardioprotection by remote ischaemic preconditioning in non-diabetic and diabetic patients. *Cardiovasc Res*. (2013) 97:369–78. doi: 10.1093/cvr/cvs337
32. Kurtz SM, Hozack WJ, Purtill JJ, Marcolongo M, Kraay MJ, Goldberg VM, et al. Otto Aufranc Award Paper: significance of *in vivo* degradation for polyethylene in total hip arthroplasty. *Clin Orthop Relat Res*. (2006) 453:47–57. doi: 10.1097/01.blo.0000246547.18187.0b
33. Reinitz SD, Currier BH, Levine RA, Collier JP, Van Citters DW. Oxidation and other property changes of a remelted highly crosslinked UHMWPE in retrieved tibial bearings. *J Biomed Mater Res B Appl Biomater*. (2017) 105:39–45. doi: 10.1002/jbm.b.33533
34. Gazzano E, Bracco P, Bistolfi A, Aldieri E, Ghigo D, Boffano M, et al. Ultra high molecular weight polyethylene is cytotoxic and causes oxidative stress, even when modified. *Int J Immunopathol Pharmacol*. (2011) 24(1 Suppl. 2):61–7. doi: 10.1177/03946320110241S212
35. Niki E. Role of vitamin E as a lipid-soluble peroxyl radical scavenger: *in vitro* and *in vivo* evidence. *Free Radic Biol Med*. (2014) 66:3–12. doi: 10.1016/j.freeradbiomed.2013.03.022
36. Reczek CR, Chandel NS. ROS-dependent signal transduction. *Curr Opin Cell Biol*. (2015) 33:8–13. doi: 10.1016/j.ceb.2014.09.010
37. Saito Y, Yoshida Y, Akazawa T, Takahashi K, Niki E. Cell death caused by selenium deficiency and protective effect of antioxidants. *J Biol Chem*. (2003) 278:39428–34. doi: 10.1074/jbc.M305542200
38. Girotti AW. Lipid hydroperoxide generation, turnover, and effector action in biological systems. *J Lipid Res*. (1998) 39:1529–42.
39. Chen ZH, Yoshida Y, Saito Y, Noguchi N, Niki E. Adaptive response induced by lipid peroxidation products in cell cultures. *FEBS Lett*. (2006) 580:479–83. doi: 10.1016/j.febslet.2005.12.045
40. Tan EP, McGreal SR, Graw S, Tessman R, Koppel SJ, Dhakal P, et al. Sustained O-GlcNAcylation reprograms mitochondrial function to regulate energy metabolism. *J Biol Chem*. (2017) 292:14940–62. doi: 10.1074/jbc.M117.797944
41. Chiba J, Rubash HE, Kim KJ, Iwaki Y. The characterization of cytokines in the interface tissue obtained from failed cementless total hip arthroplasty

with and without femoral osteolysis. *Clin Orthop Relat Res.* (1994) 8:304–12. doi: 10.1097/00003086-199403000-00043

42. Takeuchi T, Sugimoto A, Imazato N, Tamura M, Nakatani S, Kobata K, et al. Glucosamine suppresses osteoclast differentiation through the modulation of glycosylation including O-GlcNAcylation. *Biol Pharm Bull.* (2017) 40:352–6. doi: 10.1248/bpb.b16-00877
43. Kapasa ER, Giannoudis PV, Jia X, Hatton PV, Yang XB. The effect of RANKL/OPG balance on reducing implant complications. *J Funct Biomater.* (2017) 8:E42. doi: 10.3390/jfb8040042
44. Boyce BF, Xing L. The RANKL/RANK/OPG pathway. *Curr Osteoporos Rep.* (2007) 5:98–104. doi: 10.1007/s11914-007-0024-y
45. Boyce BF, Xing L. Biology of RANK, RANKL, and osteoprotegerin. *Arthritis Res Ther.* (2007) 9 (Suppl. 1):S1. doi: 10.1186/ar2165
46. Aubin JE, Bonnelye E. Osteoprotegerin and its ligand: a new paradigm for regulation of osteoclastogenesis and bone resorption. *Osteoporos Int.* (2000) 11:905–13. doi: 10.1007/s001980070028
47. Liu W, Zhang X. Receptor activator of nuclear factor-kappaB ligand (RANKL)/RANK/osteoprotegerin system in bone and other tissues (review). *Mol Med Rep.* (2015) 11:3212–8. doi: 10.3892/mmr.2015.3152
48. Witcher PC, Miner SE, Horan DJ, Bullock WA, Lim KE, Kang KS, et al. Sclerostin neutralization unleashes the osteoanabolic effects of Dkk1 inhibition. *JCI Insight.* (2018) 3:98673. doi: 10.1172/jci.insight.98673
49. Gatti D, Viapiana O, Fracassi E, Idolazzi L, Dartizio C, Povino MR, et al. Sclerostin and DKK1 in postmenopausal osteoporosis treated with denosumab. *J Bone Miner Res.* (2012) 27:2259–63. doi: 10.1002/jbmr.1681
50. Dovjak P, Dorfer S, Foger-Samwald U, Kudlacek S, Marculescu R, Pietschmann P. Serum levels of sclerostin and dickkopf-1: effects of age, gender and fracture status. *Gerontology.* (2014) 15:543–50. doi: 10.1159/000358303
51. Yu C, Huang D, Wang K, Lin B, Liu Y, Liu S, et al. Advanced oxidation protein products induce apoptosis, and upregulate sclerostin and RANKL expression, in osteocytic MLO-Y4 cells via JNK/p38 MAPK activation. *Mol Med Rep.* (2017) 15:543–50. doi: 10.3892/mmr.2016.6047
52. Fontani F, Marcucci G, Iantomasi T, Brandi ML, Vincenzini MT. Glutathione. N-acetylcysteine and lipoic acid down-regulate starvation-induced apoptosis, RANKL/OPG ratio and sclerostin in osteocytes: involvement of JNK and ERK1/2 signalling. *Calcif Tissue Int.* (2015) 96:335–46. doi: 10.1007/s00223-015-9961-0
53. Premnath V, Harris WH, Jasty M, Merrill EW. Gamma sterilization of UHMWPE articular implants: an analysis of the oxidation problem. *Ultra High Molecular Weight Poly Ethylene. Biomaterials.* (1996) 17:1741–53. doi: 10.1016/0142-9612(95)00349-5

2

S1P-S1PR1 Signaling: The "Sphinx" in Osteoimmunology

Lan Xiao [1,2†], *Yinghong Zhou* [1,2,3†], *Thor Friis* [1], *Kenneth Beagley* [1,2] *and Yin Xiao* [1,2,3*]

[1] *Institute of Health and Biomedical Innovation, Queensland University of Technology, Brisbane, QLD, Australia,* [2] *The Australia-China Centre for Tissue Engineering and Regenerative Medicine, Queensland University of Technology, Brisbane, QLD, Australia,* [3] *Key Laboratory of Oral Medicine, Guangzhou Institute of Oral Disease, Stomatology Hospital of Guangzhou Medical University, Guangzhou, China*

Correspondence:
Yin Xiao
yin.xiao@qut.edu.au

† These authors have contributed equally to this work

The fundamental interaction between the immune and skeletal systems, termed as osteoimmunology, has been demonstrated to play indispensable roles in the maintenance of balance between bone resorption and formation. The pleiotropic sphingolipid metabolite, sphingosine 1-phosphate (S1P), together with its cognate receptor, sphingosine-1-phosphate receptor-1 (S1PR1), are known as key players in osteoimmunology due to the regulation on both immune system and bone remodeling. The role of S1P-S1PR1 signaling in bone remodeling can be directly targeting both osteoclastogenesis and osteogenesis. Meanwhile, inflammatory cell function and polarization in both adaptive immune (T cell subsets) and innate immune cells (macrophages) are also regulated by this signaling axis, suggesting that S1P-S1PR1 signaling could aslo indirectly regulate bone remodeling *via* modulating the immune system. Therefore, it could be likely that S1P-S1PR1 signaling might take part in the maintenance of continuous bone turnover under physiological conditions, while lead to the pathogenesis of bone deformities during inflammation. In this review, we summarized the immunological regulation of S1P-S1PR1 signal axis during bone remodeling with an emphasis on how osteo-immune regulators are affected by inflammation, an issue with relevance to chronical bone disorders such as rheumatoid arthritis, spondyloarthritis and periodontitis.

Keywords: osteoimmunology, sphingosine 1-phosphate (S1P), sphingosine 1-phosphate receptor-1 (S1PR1), bone remodeling, immunomodulation

INTRODUCTION

Skeletal bone undergoes a life-long and continuous renovation termed "bone remodeling," a process that is necessary for bone homeostasis and consists of osteoclasts-driven bone resorption and osteoblasts-driven bone formation (1). Osteoclasts and osteoblasts—derived from immune progenitor cells and mesenchymal stem cells (MSCs), respectively—are linked *via* immune modulators and are the fundamental cell types of these two interconnected systems. Osteoimmunology, a term first coined at the beginning of this century (2), was identified over forty years ago (3), and describes the interaction between cells from the immune and skeletal systems. The realm of osteoimmunology has revealed a complex system of mutual regulation existing between immune cells and bone cells. This relationship sees the immune response greatly affecting osteoclast-osteoblast coupling, thus mediating the balance between bone resorption and formation, whereas, at another level, cells from the skeletal system have a profound effect on the differentiation and function of immune cells.

Sphingosine is one of the most important sphingolipid metabolites (4–6). It is named after the Sphinx, a mythical creature of Greek mythology famed for its mysterious features (7). Phosphorylation of sphingosine forms the pleiotropic and bioactive lipid sphingosine-1-phosphate (S1P) (8). S1P is produced by various cell types, which acts not only as an intracellular second messenger, but also an extracellular first messenger in both an autocrine and paracrine manner. It does this by binding with a class of G-protein-coupled receptors, known as sphingosine-1-phosphate receptors (S1PRs), of which there are currently five known subtypes, S1PR1 through to S1PR5 (9). Of these receptors, S1PR1 is expressed in most mammalian cell types and considered to be multifunctional in many biological processes. S1P-S1PR1 signaling has long been addressed as a key regulator of the immune response, due to its involvement in the chemotaxis, activation, differentiation, and function of immune cells (9–13). The elevated concentration of S1P, coupled with an up-regulation of S1PR1 expression locally within inflammatory tissues in many diseases, as well as the therapeutic effects of S1PR1 modulators, is an indication of the important role of S1P-S1PR1 signaling in inflammation (8, 13).

S1P-S1PR1 signaling is primarily thought to be a catalyst of inflammation and thereby inducing osteoclastogenesis; however, the fact that this pathway is also active during bone regeneration suggests an enigmatic and rather intriguing role in bone remodeling (14, 15). In this review, we will seek to highlight the interactions between the immune and skeletal systems, how these interactions affect bone remodeling, and what is known about the role of S1P-S1PR1 signaling in the emerging field of osteoimmunology.

THE FUNCTION OF S1P AND ITS RECEPTOR S1PR1

Sphingolipids are a key component of mammalian cell membranes and are metabolized in response to certain stimuli (4, 5). Sphingolipids are *de novo* biosynthesized from serine and palmitate in the endoplasmic reticulum (ER) (4, 5, 16, 17). The condensation of sphingolipids (*via* the action of serine palmitoyl transferase, SPT) forms 3-keto-dihydrosphingosine (16, 17), which is reduced to dihydrosphingosine, then subsequently acylated by (dihydro)-ceramide synthase (also known as Lass or CerS) to form dihydroceramide (18). The desaturation of dihydroceramide forms ceramides (19), the central player in sphingolipid metabolism (20), which could be deacylated by ceramidases (CERase) to produce sphingosines (21, 22). Sphingosine could be salvaged through reacylation, a process termed as "salvage pathway" which leading to ceramide regeneration; or it can be phosphorylated to form the multifunctional bioactive lipid S1P, which mediates a number of cellular processes, such as cell proliferation, survival, differentiation, migration, as well as cytokine and chemokine production (4, 5, 20, 23). S1P can be reversibly dephosphorylated to sphingosine by intracellular S1P phosphatases (SPPs) and extracellular lipid phosphate phosphatases, or irreversibly degraded by S1P lyase (SPL) (20, 24–27). In most mammalian cells, S1P levels are held in check by the actions of SPL and SPPs. SPL inhibition *via* both genetic and pharmacological tools results in tissue S1P accumulation *in vivo* (28). The exception is platelets, which lack SPL (29), and erythrocytes, which lack both SPL and SPPs (30). This absence explains why, under normal physiological conditions, circulating S1P levels are significantly higher (μM range) in peripheral blood than in solid tissues. S1P is also maintained at relatively high levels (>100 nM) in the lymphatic circulation, which is mainly due to the presence of lymphatic endothelial cells (31–33). Cells from the macrophage-monocyte lineage are also important producers of S1P (34).

The phosphorylation of sphingosine is performed by sphingosine kinases 1 and 2 (SPHK1 and SPHK2) (35). SPHK1 is mainly present in the cytoplasm which, after being activated by certain stimuli, is translocated to the cell membrane where it catalyzes sphingosine phosphoration (36). On the other hand, SPHK2 distributes not only in cell membrane, but also in organelles such as the ER, mitochondria, as well as in nucleus, which providing S1P for essential cellular processes, such as respiration, histone acetylation, and gene expression (37–39). For example, S1P is reported to regulate gene expression through modulating HDAC1 and HDAC2 activity (38, 40). Intracellular S1P also plays an essential part in tumor-necrosis factor-α (TNF-α) triggered NF-κB signaling *via* targeting TNF receptor-associated factor 2 (TRAF2), therefore participating the inflammatory, anti-apoptotic and immune processes (41). Once S1P is generated, it could be transported to activate its receptors, therefore functioning in a paracrine and/or autocrine manner (42, 43). This "inside-out relocation" of S1P is indispensable of special transports, as the polar head group in S1P makes it unable to move through the hydrophobic mammalian cell membranes (44). Transports such as the ATP-binding cassette (ABC) transporters family members have been demonstrated to facilitate S1P transporting in erythrocytes, platelets, and mammalian cells in an ATP-dependent manner (42, 45–49). Another transport, major facilitator superfamily transporter 2b (Mfsd2b) has also been found to play essential roles in exporting S1P in erythrocytes and platelets (50, 51). Especially, the transport spinster homolog 2 (SPNS2) is considered as a major regulator in S1P secretion in mammalian cells in a non-ATP dependent manner, which therefore playing essential roles in immune cell development and trafficking, as well as bone homeostasis (43, 52–57). Under inflammatory conditions, SPHK1 is abnormally activated to produce high levels of S1P, which is released into the local microenvironment. Inflammatory cytokines such as TNF-α, IL-1β, and interferon-γ (IFN-γ), have been shown to induce SPHK1 in an extracellular signal regulated kinase (ERK) signaling-dependent manner (38, 41, 58–60), and this partially explains the high S1P levels in the inflammatory tissues (61). Furthermore, inflammation is accompanied by vascular leakage, which may allow S1P to permeate from blood to tissues thereby raising the S1P concentrations within the inflammatory tissues (62).

The secreted S1P regulates pleiotropic biological functions by binding with its receptors (63). Upon activation, the S1P receptors couple with diverse heterotrimeric G-protein subunits (known as Gαi, Gαq/11, and Gα12/13), thereby directing different downstream signaling pathways (64). S1PR1 is the most widely expressed S1P receptor in most tissues, such as the lungs, brain, and especially immune organs (65–67). Following activation by S1P, S1PR1 interacts with Gαi, which then regulates the downstream signaling molecules (**Figure 1**), such as phospholipase C (PLC), phosphoinositide 3-kinase (PI3K), Ras guanosine triphosphatase (GTPase) and adenylyl cyclase (AC) (9, 68). These molecules subsequently activate their downstream signaling pathways (**Figure 1**), including Rac GTPase, mitogen-activated protein kinase (MAPK), Akt, and mammalian target of rapamycin (mTOR) (6, 9, 68, 69).

S1PR1 has a key role in the development of the vascular system and is highly expressed in differentiating endothelial cells (70). It is required to maintain the integrity of endothelial cell barrier and thus regulates vascular permeability responses, especially under inflammatory conditions (71). When SPHK1 is induced by inflammation, it enhances S1P production in endothelial cells, which then acts in a feed-forward manner to stimulate more S1PR1 expression, counteracting the increased permeability caused by pro-inflammatory mediators e.g., lipopolysaccharides (LPS), thereby preventing otherwise lethal cell-leakage in response to inflammation. The indispensable role of S1PR1 in vascular network stability has been further demonstrated by global *S1pr1* gene deletion, which results in defective vascular maturation and then embryonic lethality (70). Specific *S1pr1* deletion in endothelial cells results in deformities in the primary vascular plexus (angiogenic hypersprouting), limited blood flow, and vascular leakage (72–75). In epithelial cells, S1PR1 maintains cell barrier integrity and initiates the immune defense against the invading pathogens (76). S1PR1 is expressed in MSCs and regulates cell migration, proliferation, differentiation, and survival (77), whereas in osteoclast- and osteoblast-precursor cells S1PR1 expression is associated with their differentiation (78), further testament to its role in bone remodeling.

THE REGULATORY ROLES OF S1P-S1PR1 SIGNALING IN BONE REMODELING

Bone Remodeling and Osteoclast-Osteoblast Coupling

Osteoclasts and osteoblasts are the major players in the bone remodeling process. The hematopoietic stem cells (HSCs)-derived osteoclasts are considered as the major type of cells responsible for bone resorption (79). Osteoclastogenesis depends on receptor activator of nuclear factor-kappa B ligand (RANKL), a cytokine in the TNF family (80). RANKL activates its cognate receptor, receptor activator of nuclear factor-kappa B (RANK), initiating osteoclastogenic signals (**Figure S1**). The RANKL-RANK axis, together with the downstream NF-κB signaling pathway, is indispensable in osteoclastogenesis (81, 82). Another key factor in osteoclast formation is macrophage colony-stimulating factor (M-CSF), which is critical in regulating survival and proliferation of osteoclast precursors (83).

Osteoblasts are the major producer of RANKL and M-CSF (84), indicating that osteoclasts and osteoblasts are related "coupling" cells that link osteoclastogenesis to osteogenesis. Osteoblasts are derived from MSCs and are the main cell type responsible for bone formation (79). Factors such as alkaline phosphatase (ALP), runt-related transcription factor 2 (RUNX2), osteocalcin (OCN), and the Wnt/β-catenin and TGF-β signaling pathways, as well as the signal transducer and activator of transcription 3 (STAT3) signaling, are considered to be crucial in osteogenesis (85–89). Besides RANKL and M-CSF, osteoblasts also produce osteoprotegerin (OPG), which, conversely, acts as a decoy receptor of RANKL and thereby impeding osteoclastogenesis (90). Hence, osteoclasts and osteoblasts are interconnected by the RANKL/RANK/OPG axis, with the ratio of RANKL to OPG determining the balance between bone resorption and formation.

Bone remodeling is a strictly regulated process that must maintain bone formation at a rate equal to that of bone resorption (2). Skeletal pathologies arise when this balance is disrupted. The most common one of such disorders is when bone remodeling is skewed toward resorption—that is, when osteoclastogenesis is aberrantly stimulated so the rate of bone resorption exceeds bone formation, resulting in a net bone loss, as seen in inflammatory diseases, such as rheumatoid arthritis (RA) (91),periodontitis (92), and apical periodontitis (93).

The Roles of S1P-S1PR1 in Bone Remodeling

S1P has been found to induce both osteoclastogenesis and osteogenesis, a dual role that makes S1P-S1PR1 signaling more intriguing.

S1P-S1PR1 Signaling in Osteoclastogenesis

Together with its ligand S1P, S1PR1 directs chemotactic migration of osteoclast precursors *in vitro* and *in vivo*. S1P-S1PR1 signaling is thought to regulate osteoclast precursor trafficking to and from bone surface, where the precursor cells fuse and differentiate into osteoclasts, a process which dynamically regulates bone mineral homeostasis and osteoclastogenesis (78). S1PR1-dependent chemo-attraction is only activated when S1P concentration is comparably low. High concentrations of S1P activates the S1PR2 on the precursor cells and triggers an S1PR2-dependent chemo repulsion (94). This mechanism partially explains how these precursor cells are retained in bone marrow, where lower levels of S1P are found than in the peripheral blood. S1PR1 and S1PR2 act in a concerted manner to regulate osteoclast precursors egressing from bone marrow into circulation, depending on the relative concentrations of S1P. It is also found that the active form of vitamin D, 1,25-D, and its clinically used analog, eldecalcitol (ELD), effectively reduce bone resorption *via* inhibiting S1PR2 in circulating osteoclast precursors, as S1PR2-blockage directs the migration of osteoclast precursors from bone surface to blood. This study reveals the pharmacologic effect of vitamin D analog in therapy against osteoporosis (95), suggesting that the "S1PR1-S1PR2 concert" should be considered as a therapeutic target for diseases with bone loss. During RANKL-mediated osteoclast differentiation, the activity of SPHK1 is significantly enhanced and increases production of S1P by the precursor cells. Conversely, inhibition of SPHK1 leads to suppression of osteoclastogenesis (34).

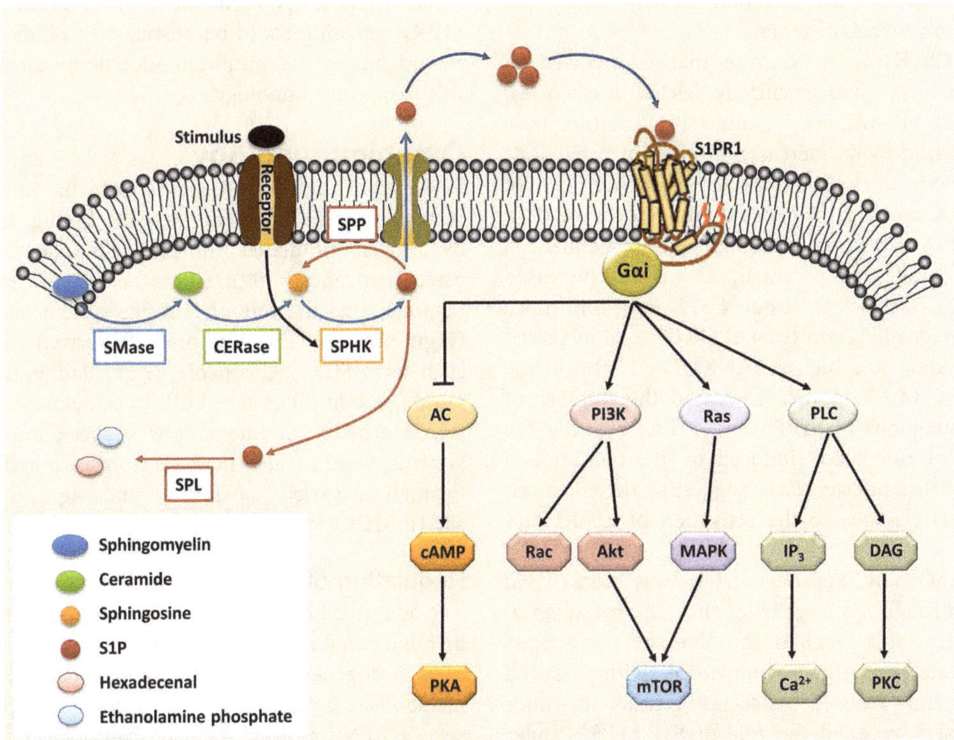

FIGURE 1 | The S1P-S1PR1 signaling. Sphingolipid (derived from cell membrane) is cleaved (by sphingomyelinases, SMase) to ceramide. Ceramide is then deacylated by ceramidases (CERase) to produce sphingosine. S1P is produced by phosphorylation of sphingosine, which is mediated by SPHKs (SPHK1 and SPHK2, which can be activated by certain stimulus). S1P can be reversibly degraded by S1P phosphatases (SPPs), or irreversibly degraded by S1P lyase (SPL). On the other hand, S1P can be transported outside the cells and acts in the autocrine or paracrine manners to activate its receptor S1PR1. The S1PR1 then activates its down-stream signal cascades and therefore regulates diverse cell activities. S1P, sphingosine-1-phosphate; S1PR1, sphingosine-1-phosphate receptor 1; PLC, phospholipase C; PI3K, phosphoinositide 3-kinase; AC, adenylyl cyclase; Ras, Ras GTPase; Rac, Rac GTPase; MAPK, mitogen-activated protein kinase; cAMP, cyclic adenosine monophosphate; mTOR, mammalian target of rapamycin; PKA, protein kinase A; PKC, protein kinase C; DAG, diacylglycerol; IP_3, Inositol trisphosphate.

S1P-S1PR1 Signaling in Osteogenesis

Although S1P is found to induce osteoclastogenesis, it also plays a positive role in osteogenesis. In the process of BMP-2-mediated osteoblast differentiation, S1P significantly induces ALP activity and the expressions of key bone formation markers, such as OCN and RUNX2. Enhanced BMP-2/SMAD signaling is the result of MEK (mitogen-activated protein kinase kinase) 1/2-ERK1/2 pathway activation (14). Another study indicates that S1P-S1PR1 signaling activation in osteoblasts mediates the activation of PI3K/Akt signaling and therefore inhibits glycogen synthase kinase-3β (GSK-3β), which leads to induced nuclear translocation of β-catenin, a key process in osteogenesis (96). S1P has also been found to induce RUNX2 expression in osteoblasts and thereby improve osteogenesis *in vitro* and *in vivo*, which is achieved through S1PR2-dependent activation of Smad1/5/8 signaling (97). Conditioned medium from osteoclasts can induce osteogenesis and is thought to be due to Wnt10b, BMP-6, and S1P secreted into the medium. And whereas S1P and BMP-6 can trigger the migration of pre-osteoblasts toward bone resorption sites, S1P can also induce osteogenic differentiation of the same cells by activating S1PR1, a finding that becomes apparent when S1PR1 is blocked (15). These properties of S1P-S1PR1 signaling to some degree explain how bone formation is initiated following bone resorption. Accordingly, hormone calcitonin (CT) has been found to block S1P secretion of osteoclast *via* SPNS2 inhibition, which consequently results in decreased bone formation *in vivo* in a S1PR3-dependent manner (55). In a more recent study, induced expression and activity of SPHK1 and SPHK2 have been observed during the *in vitro* osteoblast differentiation, accompanied with enhanced *Spns2* gene level, as well as increased S1P secretion. Blockage of SPHK1 or SPHK2 results in retarded osteogenic differentiation and mineralization, suggesting the indispensable role of S1P signaling in osteogenesis (54).

S1P-S1PR1 Signaling in Osteoclast-Osteoblast Coupling

Interestingly, intracellular S1P, which is produced during osteoclastogenesis, also inhibits this process, by suppressing p38-MAPK signaling, a key signaling pathway downstream of RANK (**Figure S1**). This is in contrast with extracellular S1P which has no effect on osteoclast differentiation, suggesting S1P can target cells other than osteoclasts, e.g., the coupling osteoblasts (34). S1P activates p38-MAPK and ERK signaling in osteoblasts, resulting in increased levels of cyclooxygenase-2 (COX2). COX2 induces the expression of prostaglandin E2 (PGE2), which prompts the production of RANKL by osteoblasts. RANKL binds to its receptor RANK on osteoclast precursors which promotes osteoclast differentiation and S1P secretion, thereby setting up a feed-forward loop for osteoclastogenesis.

Cathepsin K (CSTK) is an enzyme that is involved in bone degradation which, when specifically deleted in osteoclast lineage by targeted *in vivo* gene modification, results in a condition characterized by an increased number of osteoblasts and bone formation, as well as an increased number of dysfunctional osteoclasts and impaired bone resorption (98). The *in vitro* analysis of primary osteoblasts showed enhanced ALP activity and osteogenic potential, as well as increased RANKL/OPG ratio. Osteoclasts from *CSTK*-knockout mice presented with up-regulated expression of SPHK1 and increased S1P production leading to a higher RANKL/OPG ratio of the primary osteoblasts, which in turn increased the number of osteoclasts. The antagonist of S1PR1 and S1PR3 reduced the osteogenic ability of osteoblasts induced by the conditioned medium of *CSTK*-deficient osteoclasts, suggesting the enhanced *in vivo* osteogenesis was due to the activation of S1PR1 and S1PR3 (98).

In a more recent study, S1P degradation was blocked *via* SPL inhibition (through both genetic and pharmacological means) *in vivo*, and this resulted in increased bone mass and enhanced bone strength, accompanied with induced OPG expression and reduced osteoclastogenesis in mice (28). Further research revealed the role of S1P-S1PR2 under this phenomenon. In osteoblast, S1P-S1PR2 signaling played a significant role in bone remodeling, which not only promoting the osteogenic differentiation, but also inducing OPG production *via* p38–GSK3β-β-catenin and Wnt5A–LRP5 pathways, suggesting S1P-S1PR2 signaling should improve bone formation while limiting bone resorption. Accordingly, SPL inhibition ameliorated osteoporosis in OPG-deficient mice through inducing the activity and mineralization of osteoblast while reducing osteoclastogenesis. In addition, S1PR2-deficience resulted in osteopenia in mice, accompanied with reduced OPG expression and retarded differentiation of osteoblast (28). These results indicate that similar to S1PR1, S1P-S1PR2 signaling also acts as a coupling factor between osteoclast and osteoblast. However, S1PR2 activation leads to increased OPG production, which possibly neutralizing S1PR1-mediated RANKL expression and hence osteoclastogenesis. It is presumed that S1PR1-S1PR2 may act in a balanced way to maintain physiological bone remodeling, while this balance might be destroyed under pathological conditions such as inflammation, which needs further investigation. From these studies, it could be concluded that S1P acts as a coordinator between bone resorption and formation, which, in combination with its positive effects in both osteoclastogenesis and osteogenesis, suggesting a complicated role of this signaling in bone remodeling.

THE IMMUNOMODULATORY ROLE OF S1P-S1PR1 SIGNALING IN OSTEOIMMUNOLOGY

The balance of bone remodeling is maintained by the immune system, which, therefore, links the skeletal, and immune systems together. As a key regulator of the immune system, the S1P-S1PR1 signaling could be postulated to indirectly impact bone remodeling by the immunomodulation, indicating its enigmatic role in osteoimmunology.

Osteoimmunology

Evidence of the relationship between the immune and skeletal systems became apparent with the finding that IL-1, secreted by antigen-stimulated immune cells, plays a positive role in osteoclastogenesis (99). Since then, many more studies have demonstrated the role of immune system on bone remodeling (**Figure 2**) (100). Furthermore, cells derived from skeletal system, such as MSCs, are capable of regulating immune responses (101). Such findings gave birth to osteoimmunology, a field that is concerned with interactions between immune and skeletal systems, within which the cells from each system are correlated through a variety of factors and signaling pathways such as S1P-S1PR1.

Regulation of Bone Remodeling by Immune System

The adaptive immune cells—T-helper cells—play a critical role in bone remodeling by producing RANKL, the key factor in osteoclastogenesis, and also other factors that regulate bone metabolism. Cytokines derived from type 1 helper T (Th1) cells, such as IFNγ and granulocyte-macrophage colony-stimulating factor (GM-CSF), suppress osteoclastogenesis by interrupting the RANK signaling (**Figure 2**) (102–105). However, it is also reported that GM-CSF facilitates the fusion of pre-osteoclasts into multinucleated osteoclasts, suggesting a fundamental role of GM-CSF in the function of osteoclasts (106, 107). In addition, GM-CSF derived from breast tumor cells has been found as responsible for osteolytic bone metastasis *in vivo* (107). Other cytokines derived from type 2 helper T (Th2) cells, such as interleukin-4 (IL-4) and IL-10, also inhibit RANK signaling and osteoclast differentiation (108–110). IL-6, which is produced by Th2 cells and M1 macrophages, triggers osteoclastogenesis by promoting RANKL production, as well as stimulating IL-1 production, which amplifies the inflammatory response (111–113). IL-6 also induces the differentiation of type 17 helper T (Th17) cells, which secrete the pro-inflammatory cytokine IL-17 (114, 115), and in turn promote RANKL secretion and osteoclastogenesis (116, 117). The immune-suppressive regulatory T (Treg) cells (118), inhibit osteoclastogenesis in a direct cell-to-cell contact-dependent manner, by binding of cytotoxic T-lymphocyte-associated protein 4 (CTLA-4) on Treg cells with CD80 and CD86 on osteoclast precursors; Treg cells also reduce osteoclastogenesis by secreting IL-4 and IL-10 (119). Another Treg cell-derived factor, TGF-β, has pleiotropic effects on osteoclastogenesis. On one hand, TGF-β can induce osteoclast differentiation by promoting RANK expression and regulate activator protein 1 (AP-1) signaling (120, 121), a key downstream effector of RANK (**Figure S1**). However, in osteoclast-osteoblast co-cultures, TGF-β can also suppress RANKL expression in osteoblasts, effectively applying the brakes on osteoclastogenesis (120).

Cells from the innate immune system also contribute to the regulation of osteoclastogenesis. Macrophages, the

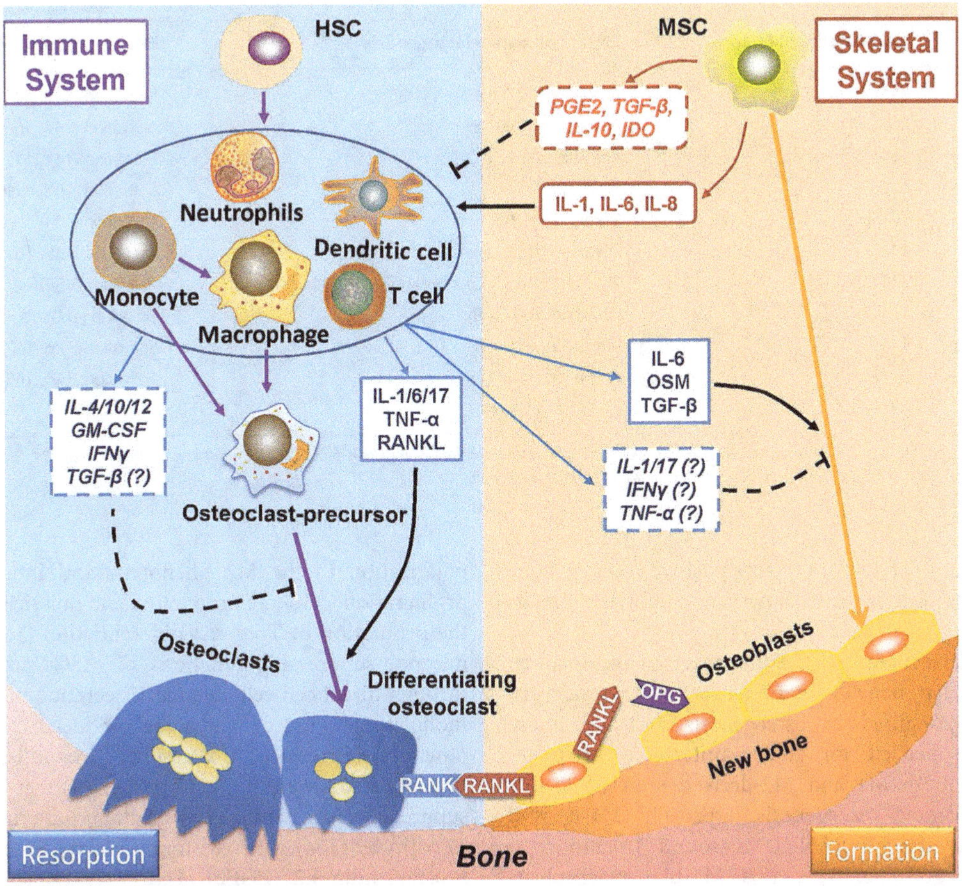

FIGURE 2 | Mutual regulations between the immune and skeletal systems. The two major players in bone remodeling—osteoclasts and osteoblasts are coupled through the RANKL-RANK-OPG axis: osteoblasts-derived RANKL combines with its ligand RANK in osteoclasts and plays an indispensable role in osteoclastogenesis; OPG (which is also derived from osteoblasts) reduces osteoclastogenesis by impairing the RANKL-RANK signaling. The immune system greatly takes part in osteoclastogenesis by producing RANKL; also, the immune-related factors either affect pre-osteoclasts, or interacts with osteoblasts to induce RANKL production to regulate osteoclastogenesis. The immune-derived regulators also affect the process of osteogenesis. On the other hand, the progenitor cells of the skeleton system—MSCs suppress immune response either by cell to cell intact or by secreting functional regulators; whereas under certain conditions, MSCs upon TLR4 stimulation secret factors which induce immune response. RANKL, receptor activator of nuclear factor factor-kappa B ligand; RANK, receptor activator of nuclear factor-kappa B; OPG, osteoprotegerin.

major components of innate immunity, constitute three sub-populations of cells: (1) non-activated M0 macrophages; (2) pro-inflammatory M1 macrophages, which are classically activated by LPS or Th1 cell cytokines such as IFNγ; and (3) M2 macrophages, which is alternatively activated by Th2 cell cytokines, such as IL-4 or IL-13, and are classified as anti-inflammatory macrophages (122–125). Macrophages are precursors of osteoclasts (126) and secrete factors that actively affect osteoclastogenesis. M1 macrophages express IL-1α and IL-1β which activates RANK signaling thereby inducing osteoclastogenesis, under both physiological and pathological conditions (127, 128). M1 macrophages also express TNF-α, which stimulates osteoclast differentiation by activating the NF-κB signaling (129, 130). Moreover, TNF-α promotes RANKL expression of osteoblasts to induce osteoclastogenesis (131, 132). On the contrary, M2 macrophages-derived IL-10 (133) is a negative regulator of osteoclastogenesis (110).

These immune-derived factors also participate in the regulation of osteogenic process. Originated from Treg cells and M2 macrophages, TGF-β has been identified as a crucial factor in osteoblast differentiation and mineralization (134). M2 macrophages also recruit MSCs (osteoblast precursors) by producing the transmembrane glycoprotein Osteoactivin (OA)/Glycoprotein non-metastatic melanoma protein B (GPNMB) (135). Interestingly, some pro-inflammatory factors, known as osteoclastogenic promoters, have also been found to induce osteogenesis. For instance, IL-6 can enhance ALP activity *in vivo via* STAT3 signaling, a further indication of the ability of IL-6 to affect osteogenesis (136–140). Originated from M1 macrophages, oncostatin M (OSM) facilitates osteogenesis by activating RUNX2 *via* STAT3 signaling pathway. Studies with OSM or OSM receptor (OSMR) deficient mice show reduced bone healing, evidence for its critical role in osteogenesis (141, 142). There are studies indicate that IL-1 (143, 144),

TABLE 1 | Effects of immune cells on bone remodeling.

Immune cells	Main functional factors	Effects on osteoclastogenesis	Effects on osteogenesis
M1 macrophages	IL-1	Activation (127, 128)	Activation (143, 144)/Inhibition (148, 149)
	TNF-α	Activation (129–132)	Activation (147, 150)/Inhibition (148, 149)
	OSM	Activation (151, 152)	Activation (141, 142)
M2 macrophages	IL-10	Inhibition (110)	Activation (153)/Inhibition (154, 155)
	TGF-β	Dural (120, 121)	Activation (134)
Th1 cells	IFNγ	Inhibition (105)	Activation (156, 157)/Inhibition (238)
	GM-CSF	Activation(106, 107)/Inhibition (102–104)	Activation (158)
Th2 cells	IL-4	Inhibition (108, 109)	Inhibition (159)
	IL-6	Activation (111–113)	Activation (136–140)
Th17 cells	IL-17	Activation (114, 115)	Activation (145, 146)/Inhibition (160)
Treg cells	CTLA-4	Inhibition (119)	–

CTLA-4, cytotoxic T-lymphocyte-associated protein 4; GM-CSF, granulocyte-macrophage colony-stimulating factor; IFNγ, interferon-γ; IL, interleukin; OSM, oncostatin M; TGF-β, transforming growth factor-β; Th, T helper; TNF-α: tumor necrosis factor α; Treg, regulatory T.

IL-17 (145, 146), and TNF-α (147) play positive roles in bone formation *in vitro* and *in vivo*, however, conflicting results exist (**Table 1**).

Accumulating evidences indicate that macrophages play an indispensable role in bone formation. The bone residential macrophages are required in osteogenesis and are, more importantly, also needed for the maintenance of bone-forming surfaces. Both M1 and M2-derived secreted factors are found to promote osteogenesis, especially M1-derived OSM (142). Interestingly, RANKL is found to induce a M1-like macrophage phenotype; this M1-like macrophage infiltration appears during the early stage of bone repair and is identified to facilitate osteogenesis (167). Furthermore, the conversion of M1 to M2 macrophages significantly improves mineralization of the co-cultured osteoblasts *in vitro* (168). This is consistent with the *in vivo* macrophage polarization during bone healing, that the infiltration of M1-like macrophages during the early inflammatory phase is indispensable for bone healing, while the M2-like macrophage infiltration becomes dominant in the later stage of bone repair (167). It can be presumed that the transient activation of M1 macrophages are essential for the early osteoblast activation, while M2 macrophages are indispensable for the later mineralization. Especially, cells from the macrophage—monocyte lineage are considered as important source of S1P (28), a crucial regulator in bone remodeling as discussed above, suggesting that macrophage-derived modulation on bone remodeling might also due to S1P-S1PR1 signaling, which needs further study in the future.

Immune-Regulation Mediated by Cells From Skeletal System

The skeletal system exerts a regulatory effect on the immune system *via* the actions of MSCs, which are capable of suppressing the differentiation and function of effector immune cells, such as Th1, Th17, and M1. MSCs can inhibit differentiation of M0 macrophages to dendritic cells (DCs) and suppress their maturation and function. MSCs also induce macrophage polarization to the M2 phenotype and interfere with T cell proliferation, cytokine production and polarization, in particular the promotion of Treg cell differentiation (101, 169–172). The immune-suppressing functions of MSCs are achieved either through direct cell-cell contact or secretion of soluble immune-modulators, some of which are produced constitutively while others are produced in response to inflammatory factors or activated immune cells (173). Direct cell-cell contact suppression is achieved through the programmed death 1 (PD-1) pathway (174), whereas immune suppressive factors include prostaglandin E2 (PGE2), TGF-β, IL-10, leukemia inhibitory factor (LIF), IL-1 receptor antagonist (IL-1RA) (173, 175). Of these factors, PGE2 is considered to be one of the most potent in MSCs' immunosuppressive arsenal, especially in term of macrophage polarization (101, 176). MSCs secrete PGE2 in response to pro-inflammatory factors, such as IFNγ or LPS (171, 177) and convert M1 macrophages to M2 phenotype (178). This process, which depends on PGE2, induces the production of immune suppressive cytokines (such as IL-10), while impeding the secretion of pro-inflammatory cytokines (such as TNF-α and IL-6), resulting in a microenvironment more suitable for tissue regeneration (171, 179). These effects of PGE2 directly affect the immune response and acts as a coupling factor between macrophages and MSCs/pre-osteoblasts in a way that facilitates osteogenesis (180).

However, when toll-like receptors (TLRs) are activated by LPS, IFN-α/γ, or TNF-α, MSCs can respond by producing pro-inflammatory cytokines (173) such as IL-1β and IL-6 and the chemokine IL-8, which attract the migration of neutrophils and augment the inflammatory response (181). It has emerged that similar to macrophages, human MSCs also polarizes into two distinct phenotypes: pro-inflammatory MSC1 and immunosuppressive MSC2 (182). TLR signaling plays an active role in this polarization, in which acute and low-level activation of TLR4 directs MSCs toward the MSC1 phenotype, whereas the TLR3 activation induces an MSC2 phenotype. The MSC1 phenotype can also be induced by IFNs or direct contact with certain pro-inflammatory cells. Polarized MSCs

TABLE 2 | Possible effects of S1P-derived immune-regulation on bone remodeling.

Cell type	Immune-regulation of S1P	Possible effects on bone remodeling	
		Osteoclasto-genesis	Osteogenesis
M1 macrophages	Differentiation↓ (161)	↓	↑
M2 macrophages	Differentiation↑ (161)	↓	↑
Th1 cells	Response↓ (162)	↓	↑
Th2 cells	Response↑ (163)	↓	↑
Th17 cells	Differentiation↑ (164, 165) Response↑ (164, 165)	↑	↑(?)
Treg cells	Differentiation↓ (165, 166)	↑	-

Th, T helper; Treg, regulatory T.

are thought to play roles similar to that of M1 and M2 macrophages in tissue repair (183), with MSC1s contributing to early stage inflammation and MSC2s contributing to late tissue regeneration. Of note, a recent study has found that macrophage-derived inflammatory factors could induce the RANKL production of bone marrow stromal cells through the SPHK1-S1PR1 axis (184), suggesting that S1P-S1PR1 signaling might participate in MSC polarization and therefore in turn regulate immune response.

Roles of S1P-S1PR1 in Osteoimmunology

When S1P binds with S1PR1, it forms a complex that governs a diverse range of immune cell activities, such as cell migration, proliferation, and differentiation (185). This immunomodulatory effect is thought to be pivotal for bone remodeling (**Figure 3**).

S1P-S1PR1 signaling plays a decisive role in regulating the traffic and egression of immune cells, such as HSCs, DCs, macrophages (monocytes), neutrophils, mast cells, T and B lymphocytes, natural killer T (NKT) cells (78, 186–193). Under both homeostatic and pathological conditions, S1P-S1PR1 signaling is required for mature thymocytes to egress from the thymus, as are T/B cells from secondary lymphoid tissues into blood or lymph (188, 194–196). S1PR1 deficiency results in blocked lymphocyte egression, a condition known as lymphopenia (196), suggesting a vital role for S1PR1 in the timely and appropriate distribution of immune cells, a process that aids homeostasis of the immune system. During inflammation, there is a spike of the local concentration of S1P, results in activated S1PR1 and the recruitment of immune cells—such as effector T cells—to the inflamed tissues and their *in situ* retention (61), which therefore promotes the inflammatory response—a process that induces bone resorption (100).

S1P-S1PR1 signaling is also an essential modulator of immune cell differentiation and function. S1P is required for the maturation and function of DCs, which further affects the activation and polarization of $CD4^{+}$T cells (197, 198). S1P regulates the function and especially the polarization of $CD4^{+}$T cell subsets. S1PR1 activation in $CD4^{+}$T cells impairs the production of IFNγ by Th1 cells, while enhance the production of Th2 cells-derived effector cytokine IL-4, thereby downregulating the Th1 cell response while upregulating that of Th2 cells (162, 163, 199, 200). On the other hand, S1P can induce the differentiation and activation of Th17 cells, as well as the production of IL-17 *in vitro* (**Table 2**)—both of which promote osteoclastogenesis (201). This is accompanied by reduced production of Th1 and Th2 cell-derived cytokines, a process that is considered to be S1PR1-dependent (164, 165). Furthermore, signaling through S1PR1 impedes the differentiation and function of Treg cells, the vital suppressor in immune response and osteoclast differentiation (118), by activating the downstream Akt-mTOR signaling pathway (166, 202), thereby exacerbating bone resorption (**Table 2**). More importantly, by enhancing RANKL production in $CD4^{+}$T cells S1P contributes to osteoclastogenesis (203).

However, in macrophage polarization, S1P-S1PR1 signaling tends to favor differentiation to an anti-inflammatory phenotype, inducing a conversion of the M1 to M2 subset (161). The S1P-derived induction of Th2 response and IL-4 secretion may indirectly affect this process. The shift from M1 toward the M2 subset (161) could be considered as reducing osteoclastogenesis, since the M1 macrophage-derived cytokines are recognized as inducers for osteoclast differentiation (**Table 1**). A similar shift may also take place in osteogenesis in which M1 macrophages, indispensable during the early stages of bone repair, shift toward the M2 phenotype that is required in the later stages of bone formation (142, 168). Therefore, in contrast to its immune-inductive role in $CD4^{+}$ T cell polarization, S1P-S1PR1 signaling has an immune-suppressive role in determining macrophage polarization, which complicates its role in bone remodeling (**Table 2**).

From these studies, a picture emerges of how S1P modulate osteoimmunology (**Figure 4**). Under physiological conditions, S1P secreted from osteoclasts during normal bone resorption may initiate bone formation. S1P prompts the migration and subsequent differentiation of MSCs to the resorption pits and also promotes the secretion of PGE2. The combined effect of S1P and PGE2 determines macrophage phenotype and creates a microenvironment suitable for bone regeneration. On the other hand, S1P and PGE2 induce the RANKL expression of osteoblasts. Osteoclast-precursors, which are also recruited by S1P, migrate to the resorption site where they are exposed to osteoblast-derived RANKL, which promotes their differentiation into mature osteoclasts, thus underpinning the continuous process of bone remodeling. Under pathological conditions, such as inflammation, the effects of S1P and PGE2 on macrophages are counteracted by inflammatory cytokines, which interfere with the conversion of M1 to M2 macrophages, resulting in a microenvironment that is unfavorable to osteogenesis. This is further exacerbated once the MSCs stop being immunosuppressive and exhibit a pro-inflammatory phenotype. T cells are also activated by S1P, which infiltrate in the site of resorption and secrete more RANKL into the local microenvironment. The high concentration of RANKL and inflammatory cytokines leads to a catabolic

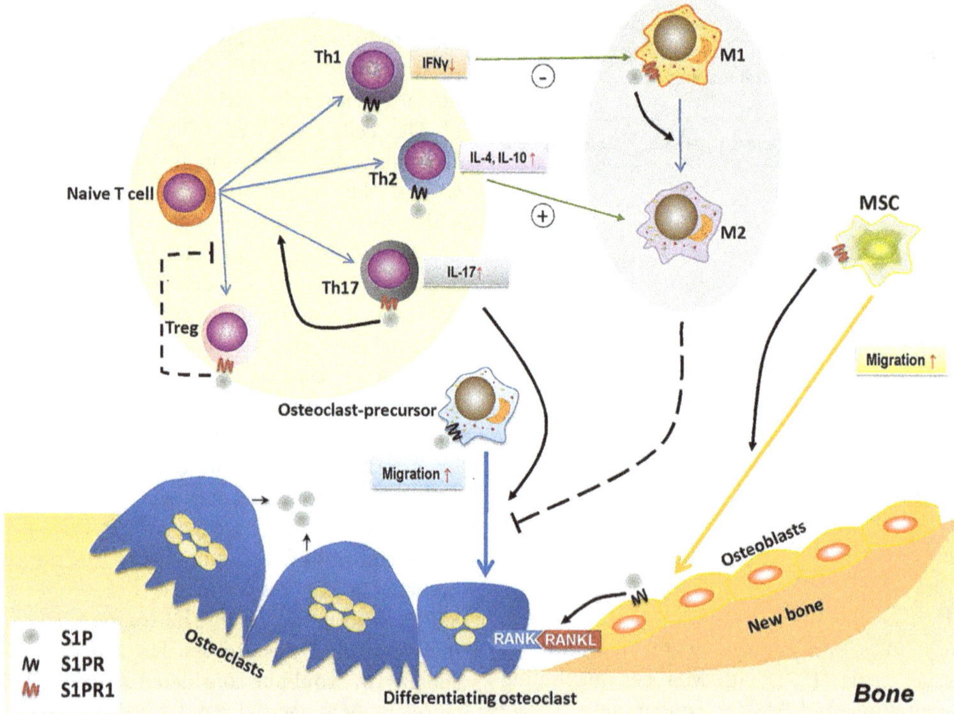

FIGURE 3 | The role of S1P-S1PR1 signaling in osteoimmunology. S1P-S1PR1 signaling is greatly involved in the interaction between immune system and bone remodeling. On one hand, S1PR1 directly affects osteoclastogenesis by inducing the migration of osteoclast-precursors. The direct effect of S1P on osteoclast-precursors results in reduced osteoclastogenesis; however, it induces RANKL production of osteoblasts and facilitating the RANKL-RANK mediated osteoclastogenesis. S1P also induces the migration of MSCs and osteogenesis by activating S1PR1. On the other hand, S1P-S1PR1 signaling participates in immune regulation, which affects the polarization and function of T-helper cells. S1P-S1PR1 signaling induces the differentiation and function of Th17 cells (known as inducing osteoclastogenesis) while impedes that of Treg cells (known as reducing osteoclastogenesis); therefore facilitating osteoclastogenesis. S1P also induces the function of Th2 cells while reduces that of Th1 cells, which affects the macrophage phenotype; also, S1P directly induces the transition of M1 to M2 phenotype by activating S1PR1. This conversion of pro-inflammatory M1 macrophages to tissue-engineering M2 macrophages therefore impedes osteoclastogenesis, which might also affect osteogenesis. S1P, sphingosine-1-phosphate; S1PR, sphingosine-1-phosphate receptor(s); S1PR1, sphingosine-1-phosphate receptor 1; MSC, mesenchymal stem cell; Th1/2/17, type 1/2/17 helper T cell; M1/M2, M1/M2 macrophage; Treg, regulatory T cell; IFNγ, interferon-γ; IL-4/10/17, interleukin-4/10/17.

imbalance that favors bone resorption. Of note, it is still unclear whether S1P signaling leads to "normal" or "abnormal" bone formation, as elevated S1P has also been found in diseases with unwanted excessive bone formation such as spondyloarthritis (54, 204).

Taken together, the weight of evidence all points to S1P-S1PR1 signaling having a pivotal role in osteoimmunology. At one level there is a direct link between S1P-S1PR1 and osteoclast-osteoblast coupling; however, there is also an indirect link that affects bone remodeling *via* S1P-S1PR1 regulation of immune response. Under certain pathological conditions, this finely tuned system is thrown into disequilibrium resulting in an overactive immune environment where bone resorption outstrips formation.

S1P-S1PR1 SIGNALING IN BONE DISEASES

Abnormally activated S1P-S1PR1 signaling has been observed in many diseases, such as RA, multiple sclerosis and cancer (205–207). The importance of S1P-S1PR1 signaling in osteoimmunology highlights the need to assess its roles in the pathogenesis of bone diseases. In addition, S1P regulation *via* SPL inhibition has been demonstrated to enhance bone mass and strength in a S1PR2-dependant manner *in vivo*, which also effectively ameliorating osteoporosis in S1PR2-deficient mice, suggesting S1P is a potential therapeutic target for bone diseases (28).

RA is an autoimmune disorder of the joints characterized by excessive osteoclastogenesis—the result of inflammatory immune response (206). Activated S1P-S1PR1 signaling is found in the synovial tissues of RA joints (206), which is considered to promote RANKL production of CD4$^+$T cells and synoviocytes in a COX-2-dependant manner (203). The joint and bone destruction is significantly alleviated in *Sphk1*-deficient mice: the reduced circulating S1P leads to limited COX-2 expression and Th17 differentiation, with a resulting inhibition of osteoclastogenesis in inflammatory joints (208). Fingolimod, also known as FTY720, is a sphingosine analog that acts as a modulator of S1P-S1PR1 signaling, which has been clinically used in treatment against multiple sclerosis

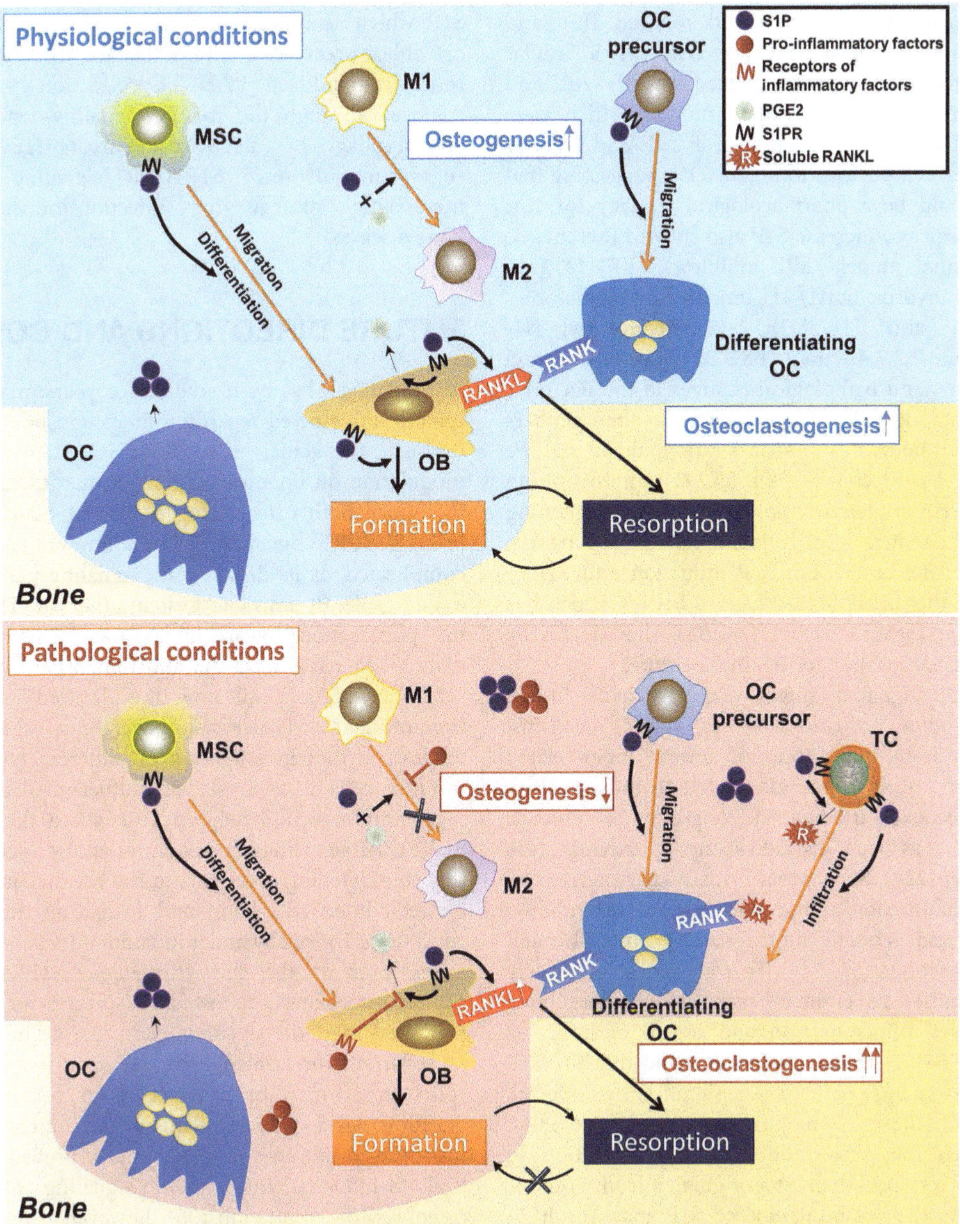

FIGURE 4 | Speculations on the regulatory roles of S1P on osteoimmunology under physiological and pathological conditions. In the physiological condition, osteoclast-derived S1P initiates bone formation by triggering MSCs migration to the resorption cite and by inducing osteoblasts differentiation. During the osteogenic process, S1P also induces the production of PGE2, which, together with S1P, leads the polarization of macrophages toward the M2 phenotype, thereby facilitating bone formation. S1P also induces RANKL production of osteoblasts, as well as the migration of osteoclast-precursors, initiating a new round of osteoclastogenesis. This makes the constant remodeling and bone metastasis. However, in the pathological condition (inflammation), the over-accumulated S1P results in infiltration of inflammatory cells (i.e., T-helper cells), which not only secret large amounts of pro-inflammatory cytokines, but also produce a lot of RANKL (in stimulation of S1P), which greatly induces osteoclastogenesis. On the other hand, the pro-inflammatory factors neutralize the immune-suppressive function of S1P and PGE2 on macrophages, result in failed conversion from M1 to M2 phenotype–an unsuitable circumstance for osteogenesis. This eventually makes to the imbalance between bone resorption and formation and thereby bone loss. S1P, sphingosine-1-phosphate; S1PR, sphingosine-1-phosphate receptor(s); MSC, mesenchymal stem cell; M1/M2, M1/M2 macrophage; OC, osteoclast; OB, osteoblast; TC, T cell; PGE2, prostaglandin E2.

(209). FTY720 is phosphorylated by SPHK2 (FTY720-P) *in vivo* to gain high affinity to S1PR1 (210, 211). Although both S1P and FTY720-P induce S1PR1 internalization (212, 213), the endocytosed S1PR1 following S1P binding is eventually recycled back to cell surface (212); while the endocytosed S1PR1 induced by FTY720-P is then irreversibly degraded (184, 213–217), resulting a pharmacologic deletion of S1PR1 from cell surface (218). FTY720 has been demonstrated to be effective in a mouse RA model, which inhibited the infiltration of effector CD4$^+$T cells and reduced IL-6 and TNF-α expression in synovial fibroblast cells (219). Similar results have been found in adjuvant-induced arthritis (AA) and collagen-induced arthritis (CIA) rodent models, which were achieved *via* modulating the migration of T cells and DCs, as well as regulating T cell polarization (220–222), suggesting that S1PR1-deletion could be a pharmacological strategy for RA. Interestingly, strategies to increase S1P also showed therapeutic effects in RA animal models. SPL inhibitors, (E)-1-(4-((1R, 2S,3R)-1,2,3,4-Tetrahydroxybutyl)-1H-imidazol-2-yl)ethanone Oxime (LX2931) and (1R,2S,3R)-1-(2-(Isoxazol-3-yl)-1H-imidazol-4-yl)butane-1,2,3,4-tetraol (LX2932) have been found to reduce symptoms and pathological changes in the RA mice model, which could dose-dependently decrease the numbers of circulating lymphocytes by sequestrating them in the thymus (223). In phase I clinical trial, LX2931 administration effectively decreased peripheral lymphocyte counts, suggesting it could potentially reduce local inflammation in RA patient (223). The similar effects between S1P induction and S1PR1 reduction indicate that other S1PRs such as S1PR2, which has demonstrated effects against S1PR1 (28, 94), should also be considered as therapeutic target for RA in the future.

Besides RA, S1P signaling might also participate in the pathogenesis of other arthritis such as spondyloarthritis. Spondyloarthritis (SpA) is a group of several inner-related disorders: psoriatic arthritis, arthritis related to inflammatory bowel disease, reactive arthritis, a subgroup of juvenile idiopathic arthritis, as well as ankylosing spondylitis (the prototypic subtype) (224). Spondyloarthritis is characterized by enthesopathy—inflammation at the cites (named as enthesis) where ligaments and tendons attach to the bone through fibrocartilage connections (54, 224). SpA at later stage usually results in abnormities at enthesis such as excessive bone formation, increased mineralization and fusion of bone, as well as ankyloses (54). A recent study has found that the S1P levels in serum from SpA patients are significantly induced, as compared with those from healthy donors (54, 204). S1P has also been found to induce the mineralization of primary chondrocytes and osteoblasts originated from enthesis (54). This suggests the accumulation of S1P may result in the excessive ossification in SpA, which still needs further verification (54).

S1P is also strongly associated with the pathogenesis of infection-related inflammatory bone loss, as seen in periodontitis and periapical lesions: an inflammatory condition caused by teeth-related bacterial infections that erodes alveolar bone. In a mouse periodontitis model, the ablation of SPHK1 can significantly attenuate alveolar bone loss and is accompanied by a reduction in the numbers of leukocytes and osteoclasts in the periodontal tissues (225). S1P-S1PR1 signaling is also linked to periapical lesions: an upregulation of S1PR1 positively correlates with RANKL and osteoclast expression and negatively with the number of Treg cells during the pathogenesis of periapical bone destruction (226). Further research into this phenomenon indicates that infection-induced M1 macrophages interact with osteoblast—precursors to enhance the production of S1P, which acts in an autocrine manner to activate S1PR1 on osteoblast-precursors. The activation of S1P-S1PR1 signaling results in induced RANKL production, which is partially achieved through the mTOR signaling-dependent inhibition of autophagy in osteoblast-precursors (184). These studies suggest modulation of S1P-S1PR1 signaling could be a novel therapeutic strategy for infection-induced inflammatory bone diseases.

FUTURE DIRECTIONS AND CONCLUSION

Although S1P has been studied for years, many questions still remain un-resolved regarding its role in bone remodeling. For instance, the actual outcome of S1P-S1PR1 signaling-derived modulation on bone remodeling is unknown, since it is found to induce both osteoclastogenesis and osteogenesis. The role of S1P-S1PR1 signaling in osteoimmunology is even more complicated, as its downstream signaling pathway, mTOR, has a dual role in immune system, that in Th cells it directs the polarization toward inflammatory phenotype, while in macrophages it directs the anti-inflammatory M2 polarization (125, 227–229). Until now the detailed cross-talk between immune and skeletal systems over bone regeneration remains unclear, further investigation on different types of infiltrating immune cells, as well as their mutual-regulations during bone regeneration, would help to understand the ultimate role of S1P-S1PR1 signaling in osteoimmunology. It could be presumed that this signaling takes part in the maintenance of the balance between bone resorption and formation under physiological conditions. Especially under inflammatory conditions, a question arises about whether the activated S1P-S1PR1 signaling would trigger osteogenesis in osteoblast-precursors, and it could be proposed that this signaling plays a role in the pathogenesis of inflammation-related bone sclerosis lesions, such as bone spurs in arthritis or sequestrum in osteomyelitis. Another question lies in the mechanism and outcome of S1P-S1PR1 mediated osteogenesis: it has been proved that S1P-S1PR1 leads to induced Wnt-β-catenin signaling pathway to improve osteoblast differentiation (96); however, if β-catenin induction continues, it would result in interrupted Notch signaling and therefore should interfere the terminal differentiation toward osteocytes, as it has been identified that Wnt and Notch pathways are mutually exclusive during osteogenesis; and the up-regulated Notch signaling plays indispensable roles in osteocyte differentiation, while Wnt signaling is more dominant during osteoblast differentiation (230). Also, S1P-S1PR1 activation will leads to the activation of mTOR signaling (166, 202). Although mTOR has been found to play decisive roles in the transition from pre-osteoblasts to osteoblasts (231–233), however, it acts as an inhibitor in the autophagy—an indispensable process in extracellular calcium deposition during mineralization (234–239). It could be presumed that S1P-S1PR1-Akt-mTOR signaling pathway should play positive roles during early stage osteoblast differentiation, however, the later stage osteocyte differentiation as well as mineralization might be affected; also, the quality of such mineralization might be abnormal or even pathological, as compared with the physiological ones.

In summary, S1P, a key coupling factor for osteoclasts and osteoblasts, plays a complex role in bone remodeling by targeting both osteoclastogenesis and osteogenesis. The immunomodulatory feature of S1P-S1PR1 signaling further indicates that favors the inflammatory cell phenotypes in the adaptive immune system (T cell subsets), while induces macrophage polarization toward the anti-inflammatory phenotype. This dual role in immune system indicates that S1P-S1PR1 signaling might take part in the maintenance of continuous bone turnover under physiological conditions, while lead to the pathogenesis of bone deformities during inflammation. Further investigation of the S1P-S1PR1 signaling pathway should help to get a better understanding about osteoimmunology and therefore benefit the clinical approach for inflammatory bone disorders.

AUTHOR CONTRIBUTIONS

All authors listed have made a substantial, direct and intellectual contribution to the work, and approved it for publication. LX involved in the concept and design of the article, wrote the manuscript. YZ involved in the conception and design of the article, reviewed the manuscript. TF assisted with manuscript preparation. KB reviewed the manuscript. YX involved in the conception and design of the article, and reviewed the manuscript.

FUNDING

This study was provided by the National Natural Science Foundation of China (NSFC, Grant No. 31771025), the National Natural Science Foundation of China (NSFC) Young Scientists Fund (Grant No. 81700969), the National Health and Medical Research Council (NHMRC) Early Career Fellowship (Grant No. 1105035).

ACKNOWLEDGMENTS

This study includes content from LX's thesis Dissecting the role of sphingosine 1-phosphate sphingosine 1-phosphate receptor 1 in inflammatory bone remodeling (240). This study has only appeared in this thesis, and the inclusion is in line with the policy of Queensland University of Technology.

SUPPLEMENTARY MATERIAL

Figure S1 | The RANKL-RANK axis mediated osteoclastogenic signals. RANK is activated when combining with its ligand RANKL. Activated RANK then triggers the down-stream osteoclastogenic signaling cascades. Activated TRAF6 induces the MAPK, IKK, and NF-κB signaling, which eventually result in activation of NFATc1 and osteoclastogenesis. RANKL: receptor activator of nuclear factor factor-kappa B ligand. RANK, receptor activator of nuclear factor-kappa B; TRAF6, tumor-necrosis factor (TNF) receptor-associated factor 6; IKK, inhibitor of nuclear factor kappa-B kinase; MAPK, mitogen-activated protein kinase; NF-κB, nuclear factor kappa B; AP-1, activator protein1; ERK, extracellular signal regulated kinase; JNK, c-Jun N-terminal kinase; NFATc1, nuclear factor of activated T-cells, cytoplasmic 1.

REFERENCES

1. Raggatt LJ, Partridge NC. Cellular and molecular mechanisms of bone remodeling. *J Biol Chem.* (2010) 285:25103–8. doi: 10.1074/jbc.R109.041087
2. Arron JR, Choi Y. Osteoimmunology: bone versus immune system. *Nature.* (2000) 408:535–6. doi: 10.1038/35046196
3. Horton JE, Raisz LG, Simmons HA, Oppenheim JJ, Mergenhagen SE. Bone resorbing activity in supernatant fluid from cultured human peripheral blood leukocytes. *Science.* (1972) 177:793–5. doi: 10.1126/science.177.4051.793
4. Gault CR, Obeid LM, Hannun YA. An overview of sphingolipid metabolism: from synthesis to breakdown. *Sphingolipids Signal Regulat Molecules.* (2010) 688:1–23. doi: 10.1007/978-1-4419-6741-1_1
5. Hannun YA, Obeid LM. Sphingolipids and their metabolism in physiology and disease. *Nat Rev Molecul Cell Biol.* (2018) 19:175–91. doi: 10.1038/nrm.2017.107
6. Takabe K, Paugh SW, Milstien S, Spiegel S. "Inside-out" signaling of sphingosine-1-phosphate: therapeutic targets. *Pharmacol Rev.* (2008) 60:181–95. doi: 10.1124/pr.107.07113
7. Thudichum JLW. *A Treatise on the Chemical Constitution of the Brain.* London: Archon Books (1962).
8. Maceyka M, Harikumar KB, Milstien S, Spiegel S. Sphingosine-1-phosphate signaling and its role in disease. *Trends Cell Biol.* (2012) 22:50–60. doi: 10.1016/j.tcb.2011.09.003
9. Kihara Y, Maceyka M, Spiegel S, Chun J. Lysophospholipid receptor nomenclature review: IUPHAR Review 8. *Br J Pharmacol.* (2014) 171:3575–94. doi: 10.1111/bph.12678
10. Yanagida K, Hla T. Vascular and immunobiology of the circulatory sphingosine 1-phosphate gradient. *Annu Rev Physiol.* (2017) 79:67–91. doi: 10.1146/annurev-physiol-021014-071635
11. Obinata H, Hla T. Sphingosine 1-phosphate and inflammation. *Int Immunol.* (2019) 2019:dxz037. doi: 10.1093/intimm/dxz037
12. Mendoza A, Fang V, Chen C, Serasinghe M, Verma A, Muller J, et al. Lymphatic endothelial S1P promotes mitochondrial function and survival in naive T cells. *Nature.* (2017) 546:158. doi: 10.1038/nature22352
13. Aoki M, Aoki H, Ramanathan R, Hait NC, Takabe K. Sphingosine-1-phosphate signaling in immune cells and inflammation: roles and therapeutic potential. *Mediat Inflamm.* (2016) 2016:8606878. doi: 10.1155/2016/8606878
14. Sato C, Iwasaki T, Kitano S, Tsunemi S, Sano H. Sphingosine 1-phosphate receptor activation enhances BMP-2-induced osteoblast differentiation. *Biochem Biophys Res Commun.* (2012) 423:200–5. doi: 10.1016/j.bbrc.2012.05.130
15. Pederson L, Ruan M, Westendorf JJ, Khosla S, Oursler MJ. Regulation of bone formation by osteoclasts involves Wnt/BMP signaling and the chemokine sphingosine-1-phosphate. *Proc Natl Acad Sci USA.* (2008) 105:20764–9. doi: 10.1073/pnas.0805133106
16. Hannun YA, Obeid LM. The ceramide-centric universe of lipid-mediated cell regulation: stress encounters of the lipid kind. *J Biol Chem.* (2002) 277:25847–50. doi: 10.1074/jbc.R200008200
17. Linn S, Kim H, Keane E, Andras L, Wang E, Merrill A. Regulation of *de novo* sphingolipid biosynthesis and the toxic consequences of its disruption. *Biochem Soc Trans.* (2001) 29(Pt 6):831–5. doi: 10.1042/0300-5127:0290831

18. Pewzner-Jung Y, Ben-Dor S, Futerman AH. When do Lasses (longevity assurance genes) become CerS (ceramide synthases)? Insights into the regulation of ceramide synthesis. *J Biol Chem.* (2006) 281:25001-5. doi: 10.1074/jbc.R600010200
19. Causeret C, Geeraert L, Van der Hoeven G, Mannaerts GP, Van Veldhoven PP. Further characterization of rat dihydroceramide desaturase: tissue distribution, subcellular localization, and substrate specificity. *Lipids.* (2000) 35:1117–25. doi: 10.1007/s11745-000-0627-6
20. Hannun YA, Obeid LM. Principles of bioactive lipid signalling: lessons from sphingolipids. *Nat Rev Molecul Cell Biol.* (2008) 9:139–50. doi: 10.1038/nrm2329
21. Xu R, Jin J, Hu W, Sun W, Bielawski J, Szulc Z, et al. Golgi alkaline ceramidase regulates cell proliferation and survival by controlling levels of sphingosine and S1P. *FASEB J.* (2006) 20:1813–25. doi: 10.1096/fj.05-5689com
22. Galadari S, Wu BX, Mao C, Roddy P, El Bawab S, Hannun YA. Identification of a novel amidase motif in neutral ceramidase. *Biochem J.* (2006) 393:687–95. doi: 10.1042/BJ20050682
23. Spiegel S, Milstien S. The outs and the ins of sphingosine-1-phosphate in immunity. *Nat Rev Immunol.* (2011) 11:403–15. doi: 10.1038/nri2974
24. Mechtcheriakova D, Wlachos A, Sobanov J, Kopp T, Reuschel R, Bornancin F, et al. Sphingosine 1-phosphate phosphatase 2 is induced during inflammatory responses. *Cell Signal.* (2007) 19:748–60. doi: 10.1016/j.cellsig.2006.09.004
25. Peest U, Sensken SC, Andréani P, Hänel P, Van Veldhoven PP, Gräler MH. S1P-lyase independent clearance of extracellular sphingosine 1-phosphate after dephosphorylation and cellular uptake. *J Cell Biochem.* (2008) 104:756–72. doi: 10.1002/jcb.21665
26. Johnson KR, Johnson KY, Becker KP, Bielawski J, Mao C, Obeid LM. Role of human sphingosine-1-phosphate phosphatase 1 in the regulation of intra- and extracellular sphingosine-1-phosphate levels and cell viability. *J Biol Chem.* (2003) 278:34541–7. doi: 10.1074/jbc.M301741200
27. Sigal YJ, Mcdermott MI, Morris AJ. Integral membrane lipid phosphatases/phosphotransferases: common structure and diverse functions. *Biochem J.* (2005) 387:281–93. doi: 10.1042/BJ20041771
28. Weske S, Vaidya M, Reese A, Lipinski KV, Keul P, Bayer JK, et al. Targeting sphingosine-1-phosphate lyase as an anabolic therapy for bone loss. *Nat Med.* (2018) 24:667–8. doi: 10.1038/s41591-018-0005-y
29. Ito K, Anada Y, Tani M, Ikeda M, Sano T, Kihara A, et al. Lack of sphingosine 1-phosphate-degrading enzymes in erythrocytes. *Biochem Biophys Res Commun.* (2007) 357:212–7. doi: 10.1016/j.bbrc.2007.03.123
30. Rosen H, Gonzalez-Cabrera PJ, Sanna MG, Brown S. Sphingosine 1-phosphate receptor signaling. *Annual Rev Biochem.* (2009) 78:743–68. doi: 10.1146/annurev.biochem.78.072407.103733
31. Pappu R, Schwab SR, Cornelissen I, Pereira JP, Regard JB, Xu Y, et al. Promotion of lymphocyte egress into blood and lymph by distinct sources of sphingosine-1-phosphate. *Science.* (2007) 316:295–8. doi: 10.1126/science.1139221
32. Schwab SR, Pereira JP, Matloubian M, Xu Y, Huang Y, Cyster JG. Lymphocyte sequestration through S1P lyase inhibition and disruption of S1P gradients. *Science.* (2005) 309:1735–9. doi: 10.1126/science.1113640
33. Venkataraman K, Lee YM, Michaud J, Thangada S, Ai Y, Bonkovsky HL, et al. Vascular endothelium as a contributor of plasma sphingosine 1-phosphate. *Circul Res.* (2008) 102:669–76. doi: 10.1161/CIRCRESAHA.107.165845
34. Ryu J, Kim HJ, Chang EJ, Huang H, Banno Y, Kim HH. Sphingosine 1-phosphate as a regulator of osteoclast differentiation and osteoclast–osteoblast coupling. *EMBO J.* (2006) 25:5840–51. doi: 10.1038/sj.emboj.7601430
35. Hait NC, Oskeritzian CA, Paugh SW, Milstien S, Spiegel S. Sphingosine kinases, sphingosine 1-phosphate, apoptosis and diseases. *Biochim Biophys Acta.* (2006) 1758:2016–26. doi: 10.1016/j.bbamem.2006.08.007
36. Pitson SM. Regulation of sphingosine kinase and sphingolipid signaling. *Trends Biochem Sci.* (2011) 36:97–107. doi: 10.1016/j.tibs.2010.08.001
37. Strub GM, Paillard M, Liang J, Gomez L, Allegood JC, Hait NC, et al. Sphingosine-1-phosphate produced by sphingosine kinase 2 in mitochondria interacts with prohibitin 2 to regulate complex IV assembly and respiration. *FASEB J.* (2011) 25:600–12. doi: 10.1096/fj.10-167502
38. Hait NC, Allegood J, Maceyka M, Strub GM, Harikumar KB, Singh SK, et al. Regulation of histone acetylation in the nucleus by sphingosine-1-phosphate. *Science.* (2009) 325:1254–7.
39. Selvam SP, De Palma RM, Oaks JJ, Oleinik N, Peterson YK, Stahelin RV, et al. Binding of the sphingolipid S1P to hTERT stabilizes telomerase at the nuclear periphery by allosterically mimicking protein phosphorylation. *Sci Signal.* (2015) 8:ARTN ra58. doi: 10.1126/scisignal.aaa4998
40. Riccio A. New endogenous regulators of class I histone deacetylases. *Sci Signal.* (2010) 3:ARTN pe1. doi: 10.1126/scisignal.3103pe1
41. Alvarez SE, Harikumar KB, Hait NC, Allegood J, Strub GM, Kim EY, et al. Sphingosine-1-phosphate is a missing cofactor for the E3 ubiquitin ligase TRAF2. *Nature.* (2010) 465:1084–8. doi: 10.1038/nature09128
42. Nishi T, Kobayashi N, Hisano Y, Kawahara A, Yamaguchi A. Molecular and physiological functions of sphingosine 1-phosphate transporters. *Bba-Mol Cell Biol L.* (2014) 1841:759–65. doi: 10.1016/j.bbalip.2013.07.012
43. Spiegel S, Maczis MA, Maceyka M, Milstien S. New insights into functions of the sphingosine-1-phosphate transporter SPNS2. *J Lipid Res.* (2019) 60:484–9. doi: 10.1194/jlr.S091959
44. Kim RH, Takabe K, Milstien S, Spiegel S. Export and functions of sphingosine-1-phosphate. *Bba-Mol Cell Biol L.* (2009) 1791:692–6. doi: 10.1016/j.bbalip.2009.02.011
45. Kobayashi N, Kobayashi N, Yamaguchi A, Nishi T. Characterization of the ATP-dependent Sphingosine 1-phosphate transporter in rat erythrocytes. *J Biol Chem.* (2009) 284:21192–200. doi: 10.1074/jbc.M109.006163
46. Kobayashi N, Nishi T, Hirata T, Kihara A, Sano T, Igarashi Y, et al. Sphingosine 1-phosphate is released from the cytosol of rat platelets in a carrier-mediated manner. *J Lipid Res.* (2006) 47:614–21. doi: 10.1194/jlr.M500468-JLR200
47. Nieuwenhuis B, Luth A, Jakobi M, Kleuser B. Involvement of the Abc-Transporter Abcc1 and the Sphingosine 1-Phosphate Receptor Subtype S1p3 in the cytoprotection of human fibroblasts by the glucocorticoid dexamethasone. *Naunyn Schmiedebergs Arch. Pharmacol.* (2010) 382:21. doi: 10.1007/s00109-009-0468-x
48. Takabe K, Kim RH, Allegood JC, Mitra P, Ramachandran S, Nagahashi M, et al. Estradiol induces export of sphingosine 1-phosphate from breast cancer cells via ABCC1 and ABCG2. *J Biol Chem.* (2010) 285:10477–86. doi: 10.1074/jbc.M109.064162
49. Tanfin Z, Serrano-Sanchez M, Leiber D. ATP-binding cassette ABCC1 is involved in the release of sphingosine 1-phosphate from rat uterine leiomyoma ELT3 cells and late pregnant rat myometrium. *Cell Signal.* (2011) 23:1997–2004. doi: 10.1016/j.cellsig.2011.07.010
50. Vu TM, Ishizu AN, Foo JC, Toh XR, Zhang FY, Whee DM, et al. Mfsd2b is essential for the sphingosine-1-phosphate export in erythrocytes and platelets. *Nature.* (2017) 550:524–8. doi: 10.1038/nature24053
51. Kobayashi N, Kawasaki-Nishi S, Otsuka M, Hisano Y, Yamaguchi A, Nishi T. MFSD2B is a sphingosine 1-phosphate transporter in erythroid cells. *Sci Rep.* (2018) 8:ARTN4969. doi: 10.1038/s41598-018-23300-x
52. Kawahara A, Nishi T, Hisano Y, Fukui H, Yamaguchi A, Mochizuki N. The Sphingolipid Transporter Spns2 Functions in Migration of Zebrafish Myocardial Precursors. *Science.* (2009) 323:524–7. doi: 10.1126/science.1167449
53. Hisano Y, Kobayashi N, Kawahara A, Yamaguchi A, Nishi T. The Sphingosine 1-phosphate transporter, SPNS2, functions as a transporter of the phosphorylated form of the immunomodulating agent FTY720. *J Biol Chem.* (2011) 286:1758–66. doi: 10.1074/jbc.M110.171116
54. Bougault C, El Jamal A, Briolay A, Mebarek S, Boutet MA, Garraud T, et al. Involvement of sphingosine kinase/sphingosine 1-phosphate metabolic pathway in spondyloarthritis. *Bone.* (2017) 103:150–8. doi: 10.1016/j.bone.2017.07.002
55. Keller J, Catala-Lehnen P, Huebner AK, Jeschke A, Heckt T, Lueth A, et al. Calcitonin controls bone formation by inhibiting the release of sphingosine 1-phosphate from osteoclasts. *Nat Commun.* (2014) 5:5215 doi: 10.1038/ncomms6215
56. Fukuhara S, Simmons S, Kawamura S, Inoue A, Orba Y, Tokudome T, et al. The sphingosine-1-phosphate transporter Spns2 expressed on endothelial cells regulates lymphocyte trafficking in mice. *J Clin Invest.* (2012) 122:1416–26. doi: 10.1172/JCI60746

57. Nijnik A, Clare S, Hale C, Chen J, Raisen C, Mottram L, et al. The role of sphingosine-1-phosphate transporter Spns2 in immune system function. *J Immunol.* (2012) 189:102–11. doi: 10.4049/jimmunol.1200282
58. Pettus BJ, Bielawski J, Porcelli AM, Reames DL, Johnson KR, Morrow J, et al. The sphingosine kinase 1/sphingosine-1-phosphate pathway mediates COX-2 induction and PGE2 production in response to TNF-α. *FASEB J.* (2003) 17:1411–21. doi: 10.1096/fj.02-1038com
59. Park ES, Choi S, Shin B, Yu J, Yu J, Hwang J M, et al. Tumor necrosis factor (TNF) receptor-associated factor (TRAF)-interacting protein (TRIP) negatively regulates the TRAF2 ubiquitin-dependent pathway by suppressing the TRAF2-sphingosine 1-phosphate (S1P) interaction. *J Biol Chem.* (2015) 290:9660–73. doi: 10.1074/jbc.M114.609685
60. Harikumar KB, Yester JW, Surace MJ, Oyeniran C, Price MM, Huang WC, et al. K63-linked polyubiquitination of transcription factor IRF1 is essential for IL-1-induced production of chemokines CXCL10 and CCL5. *Nat Immunol.* (2014) 15:231–8. doi: 10.1038/ni.2810
61. Ledgerwood LG, Lal G, Zhang N, Garin A, Esses SJ, Ginhoux F, et al. The sphingosine 1-phosphate receptor 1 causes tissue retention by inhibiting the entry of peripheral tissue T lymphocytes into afferent lymphatics. *Nat Immunol.* (2008) 9:42–53. doi: 10.1038/ni1534
62. Kono M, Proia RL. Imaging S1P1 activation *in vivo*. *Exp Cell Res.* (2015) 333:178–82. doi: 10.1016/j.yexcr.2014.11.023
63. Sanchez T, Hla T. Structural and functional characteristics of S1P receptors. *J Cell Biochem.* (2004) 92:913–22. doi: 10.1002/jcb.20127
64. Davis MD, Kehrl JH. The influence of sphingosine-1-phosphate receptor signaling on lymphocyte trafficking: how a bioactive lipid mediator grew up from an "immature" vascular maturation factor to a "mature" mediator of lymphocyte behavior and function. *Immunol Res.* (2009) 43:187–97. doi: 10.1007/s12026-008-8066-5
65. Cahalan SM, Gonzalez-Cabrera PJ, Sarkisyan G, Nguyen N, Schaeffer MT, Huang L, et al. Actions of a picomolar short-acting S1P1 agonist in S1P1-eGFP knock-in mice. *Nat Chem Biol.* (2011) 7:254–6. doi: 10.1038/nchembio.547
66. Chae SS, Proia RL, Hla T. Constitutive expression of the S1P 1 receptor in adult tissues. *Prostagland Other Lipid Med.* (2004) 73:141–50. doi: 10.1016/j.prostaglandins.2004.01.006
67. Kono M, Tucker AE, Tran J, Bergner JB, Turner EM, Proia RL. Sphingosine-1-phosphate receptor 1 reporter mice reveal receptor activation sites *in vivo*. *J Clin Invest.* (2014) 124:2076–86. doi: 10.1172/JCI71194
68. Cuvillier O. Sphingosine 1-phosphate receptors: from biology to physiopathology. *Med Sci.* (2012) 28:951–7. doi: 10.1051/medsci/20122811013
69. Nayak D, Huo Y, Kwang W, Pushparaj P, Kumar S, Ling EA, et al. Sphingosine kinase 1 regulates the expression of proinflammatory cytokines and nitric oxide in activated microglia. *Neuroscience.* (2010) 166:132–44. doi: 10.1016/j.neuroscience.2009.12.020
70. Liu Y, Wada R, Yamashita T, Mi Y, Deng CX, Hobson JP, et al. Edg-1, the G protein–coupled receptor for sphingosine-1-phosphate, is essential for vascular maturation. *J Clin Invest.* (2000) 106:951–61. doi: 10.1172/JCI10905
71. Camerer E, Regard JB, Cornelissen I, Srinivasan Y, Duong DN, Palmer D, et al. Sphingosine-1-phosphate in the plasma compartment regulates basal and inflammation-induced vascular leak in mice. *J Clin Invest.* (2009) 119:1871–9. doi: 10.1172/JCI38575
72. Shoham AB, Malkinson G, Krief S, Shwartz Y, Ely Y, Ferrara N, et al. S1P1 inhibits sprouting angiogenesis during vascular development. *Development.* (2012) 139:3859–69. doi: 10.1242/dev.078550
73. Gaengel K, Niaudet C, Hagikura K, Laviña B, Muhl L, Hofmann JJ, et al. The sphingosine-1-phosphate receptor S1PR1 restricts sprouting angiogenesis by regulating the interplay between VE-cadherin and VEGFR2. *Dev Cell.* (2012) 23:587–99. doi: 10.1016/j.devcel.2012.08.005
74. Jung B, Obinata H, Galvani S, Mendelson K, Ding BS, Skoura A, et al. Flow-regulated endothelial S1P receptor-1 signaling sustains vascular development. *Dev Cell.* (2012) 23:600–10. doi: 10.1016/j.devcel.2012.07.015
75. Mendelson K, Evans T, Hla T. Sphingosine 1-phosphate signalling. *Development.* (2014) 141:5–9. doi: 10.1242/dev.094805
76. Eskan MA, Rose BG, Benakanakere MR, Zeng Q, Fujioka D, Martin MH, et al. TLR4 and S1P receptors cooperate to enhance inflammatory cytokine production in human gingival epithelial cells. *Eur J Immunol.* (2008) 38:1138–47. doi: 10.1002/eji.200737898
77. Pitson SM, Pébay A. Regulation of stem cell pluripotency and neural differentiation by lysophospholipids. *Neurosignals.* (2009) 17:242–54. doi: 10.1159/000231891
78. Ishii M, Egen JG, Klauschen F, Meier-Schellersheim M, Saeki Y, Vacher J, et al. Sphingosine-1-phosphate mobilizes osteoclast precursors and regulates bone homeostasis. *Nature.* (2009) 458:524–8. doi: 10.1038/nature07713
79. Kini U, Nandeesh B. Physiology of bone formation, remodeling, and metabolism. In: Fogelman I, Gnanasegaran G, van der Wall H, editors. *Radionuclide and Hybrid Bone Imaging.* Berlin; Heidelberg: Springer (2012). p. 29–57. doi: 10.1007/978-3-642-02400-9_2
80. Lacey D, Timms E, Tan HL, Kelley M, Dunstan C, Burgess T, et al. Osteoprotegerin ligand is a cytokine that regulates osteoclast differentiation and activation. *Cell.* (1998) 93:165–76. doi: 10.1016/S0092-8674(00)81569-X
81. Theill LE, Boyle WJ, Penninger JM. RANK-L and RANK: T cells, bone loss, and mammalian evolution. *Annu Rev Immunol.* (2002) 20:795–823. doi: 10.1146/annurev.immunol.20.100301.064753
82. Kong YY, Yoshida H, Sarosi I, Tan HL, Timms E, Capparelli C, et al. OPGL is a key regulator of osteoclastogenesis, lymphocyte development and lymph-node organogenesis. *Nature.* (1999) 397:315–23. doi: 10.1038/16852
83. Yoshida H, Hayashi SI, Kunisada T, Ogawa M, Nishikawa S, Okamura H, et al. The murine mutation osteopetrosis is in the coding region of the macrophage colony stimulating factor gene. *Nature.* (1990) 345:442–4. doi: 10.1038/345442a0
84. Udagawa N, Takahashi N, Akatsu T, Tanaka H, Sasaki T, Nishihara T, et al. Origin of osteoclasts: mature monocytes and macrophages are capable of differentiating into osteoclasts under a suitable microenvironment prepared by bone marrow-derived stromal cells. *Proc Natl Acad Sci USA.* (1990) 87:7260–4. doi: 10.1073/pnas.87.18.7260
85. Komori T. Signaling networks in RUNX2-dependent bone development. *J Cell Biochem.* (2011) 112:750–5. doi: 10.1002/jcb.22994
86. Cai T, Sun D, Duan Y, Wen P, Dai C, Yang J, et al. WNT/β-catenin signaling promotes VSMCs to osteogenic transdifferentiation and calcification through directly modulating Runx2 gene expression. *Exp Cell Res.* (2016) 345:206–17. doi: 10.1016/j.yexcr.2016.06.007
87. Wu M, Chen G, Li YP. TGF-β and BMP signaling in osteoblast, skeletal development, and bone formation, homeostasis and disease. *Bone Res.* (2016) 4:16009. doi: 10.1038/boneres.2016.9
88. Potier E, Ferreira E, Andriamanalijaona R, Pujol JP, Oudina K, Logeart-Avramoglou D, et al. Hypoxia affects mesenchymal stromal cell osteogenic differentiation and angiogenic factor expression. *Bone.* (2007) 40:1078–87. doi: 10.1016/j.bone.2006.11.024
89. Yue R, Zhou BO, Shimada IS, Zhao Z, Morrison SJ. Leptin receptor promotes adipogenesis and reduces osteogenesis by regulating mesenchymal stromal cells in adult bone marrow. *Cell Stem Cell.* (2016) 18:782–96. doi: 10.1016/j.stem.2016.02.015
90. Simonet W, Lacey D, Dunstan C, Kelley M, Chang MS, Lüthy R, et al. Osteoprotegerin: a novel secreted protein involved in the regulation of bone density. *Cell.* (1997) 89:309–19. doi: 10.1016/S0092-8674(00)80209-3
91. Rodan GA, Martin TJ. Therapeutic approaches to bone diseases. *Science.* (2000) 289:1508–14. doi: 10.1126/science.289.5484.1508
92. Taubman MA, Valverde P, Han X, Kawai T. Immune response: the key to bone resorption in periodontal disease. *J Periodontol.* (2005) 76:2033–41. doi: 10.1902/jop.2005.76.11-S.2033
93. Wang CY, Stashenko P. Characterization of bone-resorbing activity in human periapical lesions. *J Endodont.* (1993) 19:107–11. doi: 10.1016/S0099-2399(06)80503-0
94. Ishii M, Kikuta J, Shimazu Y, Meier-Schellersheim M, Germain RN. Chemorepulsion by blood S1P regulates osteoclast precursor mobilization and bone remodeling *in vivo*. *J Exp Med.* (2010) 207:2793–8. doi: 10.1084/jem.20101474
95. Kikuta J, Kawamura S, Okiji F, Shirazaki M, Sakai S, Saito H, et al. Sphingosine-1-phosphate-mediated osteoclast precursor monocyte migration is a critical point of control in antibone-resorptive action

of active vitamin D. *Proc Natl Acad Sci USA.* (2013) 110:7009–13. doi: 10.1073/pnas.1218799110

96. Matsuzaki E, Hiratsuka S, Hamachi T, Takahashi-Yanaga F, Hashimoto Y, Higashi K, et al. Sphingosine-1-phosphate promotes the nuclear translocation of β-catenin and thereby induces osteoprotegerin gene expression in osteoblast-like cell lines. *Bone.* (2013) 55:315–24. doi: 10.1016/j.bone.2013.04.008
97. Higashi K, Matsuzaki E, Hashimoto Y, Takahashi-Yanaga F, Takano A, Anan H, et al. Sphingosine-1-phosphate/S1PR2-mediated signaling triggers Smad1/5/8 phosphorylation and thereby induces Runx2 expression in osteoblasts. *Bone.* (2016) 93:1–11. doi: 10.1016/j.bone.2016.09.003
98. Lotinun S, Kiviranta R, Matsubara T, Alzate JA, Neff L, Lüth A, et al. Osteoclast-specific cathepsin K deletion stimulates S1P-dependent bone formation. *J Clin Invest.* (2013) 123:666–81. doi: 10.1172/JCI64840
99. Dewhirst FE, Stashenko PP, Mole JE, Tsurumachi T. Purification and partial sequence of human osteoclast-activating factor: identity with interleukin 1 beta. *J Immunol.* (1985) 135:2562–8. Available online at: http://www.jimmunol.org/content/135/4/2562
100. Takayanagi H. Osteoimmunology: shared mechanisms and crosstalk between the immune and bone systems. *Nat Rev Immunol.* (2007) 7:292–304. doi: 10.1038/nri2062
101. Nauta AJ, Fibbe WE. Immunomodulatory properties of mesenchymal stromal cells. *Blood.* (2007) 110:3499–506. doi: 10.1182/blood-2007-02-069716
102. Kim MS, Day CJ, Morrison NA. MCP-1 is induced by RANKL, promotes osteoclast fusion and rescues GM-CSF suppression of osteoclast formation. *J Biol Chem.* (2005) 280:16163–9. doi: 10.1074/jbc.M412713200
103. Miyamoto T, Ohneda O, Arai F, Iwamoto K, Okada S, Takagi K, et al. Bifurcation of osteoclasts and dendritic cells from common progenitors. *Blood.* (2001) 98:2544–54. doi: 10.1182/blood.V98.8.2544
104. Lari R, Fleetwood AJ, Kitchener PD, Cook AD, Pavasovic D, Hertzog PJ, et al. Macrophage lineage phenotypes and osteoclastogenesis—Complexity in the control by GM-CSF and TGF-β. *Bone.* (2007) 40:323–36. doi: 10.1016/j.bone.2006.09.003
105. Takayanagi H, Ogasawara K, Hida S, Chiba T, Murata S, Sato K, et al. T-cell-mediated regulation of osteoclastogenesis by signalling cross-talk between RANKL and IFN-γ. *Nature.* (2000) 408:600–5. doi: 10.1038/35046102
106. Lee MS, Kim HS, Yeon JT, Choi SW, Chun CH, Kwak HB, et al. GM-CSF regulates fusion of mononuclear osteoclasts into bone-resorbing osteoclasts by activating the Ras/ERK pathway. *J Immunol.* (2009) 183:3390–9. doi: 10.4049/jimmunol.0804314
107. Park BK, Zhang H, Zeng Q, Dai J, Keller ET, Giordano T, et al. NF-κB in breast cancer cells promotes osteolytic bone metastasis by inducing osteoclastogenesis via GM-CSF. *Nat Med.* (2007) 13:62–9. doi: 10.1038/nm1519
108. Abu-Amer Y. IL-4 abrogates osteoclastogenesis through STAT6-dependent inhibition of NF-κB. *J Clin Invest.* (2001) 107:1375–85. doi: 10.1172/JCI10530
109. Moreno JL, Kaczmarek M, Keegan AD, Tondravi M. IL-4 suppresses osteoclast development and mature osteoclast function by a STAT6-dependent mechanism: irreversible inhibition of the differentiation program activated by RANKL. *Blood.* (2003) 102:1078–86. doi: 10.1182/blood-2002-11-3437
110. Park-Min KH, Ji JD, Antoniv T, Reid AC, Silver RB, Humphrey MB, et al. IL-10 suppresses calcium-mediated costimulation of receptor activator NF-κB signaling during human osteoclast differentiation by inhibiting TREM-2 expression. *J Immunol.* (2009) 183:2444–55. doi: 10.4049/jimmunol.0804165
111. Kudo O, Sabokbar A, Pocock A, Itonaga I, Fujikawa Y, Athanasou N. Interleukin-6 and interleukin-11 support human osteoclast formation by a RANKL-independent mechanism. *Bone.* (2003) 32:1–7. doi: 10.1016/S8756-3282(02)00915-8
112. Hashizume M, Hayakawa N, Mihara M. IL-6 trans-signalling directly induces RANKL on fibroblast-like synovial cells and is involved in RANKL induction by TNF-α and IL-17. *Rheumatology.* (2008) 47:1635–40. doi: 10.1093/rheumatology/ken363
113. Kurihara N, Bertolini D, Suda T, Akiyama Y, Roodman GD. IL-6 stimulates osteoclast-like multinucleated cell formation in long term human marrow cultures by inducing IL-1 release. *J Immunol.* (1990) 144:4226–30.
114. Korn T, Mitsdoerffer M, Croxford AL, Awasthi A, DardalhonVA, Galileos G, et al. IL-6 controls Th17 immunity in vivo by inhibiting the conversion of conventional T cells into Foxp3+ regulatory T cells. *Proc Natl Acad Sci USA.* (2008) 105:18460–5. doi: 10.1073/pnas.0809850105
115. Kimura A, Naka T, Kishimoto T. IL-6-dependent and-independent pathways in the development of interleukin 17-producing T helper cells. *Proc Natl Acad Sci USA.* (2007) 104:12099–104. doi: 10.1073/pnas.0705268104
116. Lubberts E, van den Bersselaar L, Oppers-Walgreen B, Schwarzenberger P, Coenen-de Roo CJ, Kolls JK, et al. IL-17 promotes bone erosion in murine collagen-induced arthritis through loss of the receptor activator of NF-κB ligand/osteoprotegerin balance. *J Immunol.* (2003) 170:2655–62. doi: 10.4049/jimmunol.170.5.2655
117. Van Den Berg WB, Miossec P. IL-17 as a future therapeutic target for rheumatoid arthritis. *Nat Rev Rheumatol.* (2009) 5:549–53. doi: 10.1038/nrrheum.2009.179
118. Sakaguchi S, Yamaguchi T, Nomura T, Ono M. Regulatory T cells and immune tolerance. *Cell.* (2008) 133:775–87. doi: 10.1016/j.cell.2008.05.009
119. Zaiss MM, Axmann R, Zwerina J, Polzer K, Gückel E, Skapenko A, et al. Treg cells suppress osteoclast formation: a new link between the immune system and bone. *Arthrit Rheumat.* (2007) 56:4104–12. doi: 10.1002/art.23138
120. Quinn JM, Itoh K, Udagawa N, Häusler K, Yasuda H, Shima N, et al. Transforming growth factor β affects osteoclast differentiation via direct and indirect actions. *J BoneMineral Res.* (2001) 16:1787–94. doi: 10.1359/jbmr.2001.16.10.1787
121. Galvin RJS, Gatlin CL, Horn JW, Fuson TR. TGF-β enhances osteoclast differentiation in hematopoietic cell cultures stimulated with RANKL and M-CSF. *Biochem Biophys Res Commun.* (1999) 265:233–9. doi: 10.1006/bbrc.1999.1632
122. Mills CD, Kincaid K, Alt JM, Heilman MJ, Hill A. M. M-1/M-2 macrophages and the Th1/Th2 paradigm. *J Immunol.* (2000) 164:6166–73. doi: 10.4049/jimmunol.164.12.6166
123. Horwood NJ. Macrophage polarization and bone formation: a review. *Clin Rev Allergy Immunol.* (2016) 51:79–86. doi: 10.1007/s12016-015-8519-2
124. Mantovani A, Sica A, Sozzani S, Allavena P, Vecchi A, Locati M. The chemokine system in diverse forms of macrophage activation and polarization. *Trends Immunol.* (2004) 25:677–86. doi: 10.1016/j.it.2004.09.015
125. Murray PJ, Allen JE, Biswas SK, Fisher EA, Gilroy DW, Goerdt S, et al. Macrophage activation and polarization: nomenclature and experimental guidelines. *Immunity.* (2014) 41:14–20. doi: 10.1016/j.immuni.2014.06.008
126. Takeshita S, Kaji K, Kudo A. Identification and characterization of the new osteoclast progenitor with macrophage phenotypes being able to differentiate into mature osteoclasts. *J Bone Mineral Res.* (2000) 15:1477–88. doi: 10.1359/jbmr.2000.15.8.1477
127. Wei S, Kitaura H, Zhou P, Ross FP, Teitelbaum SL. IL-1 mediates TNF-induced osteoclastogenesis. *J Clin Invest.* (2005) 115:282–90. doi: 10.1172/JCI200523394
128. Zwerina J, Redlich K, Polzer K, Joosten L, Krönke G, Distler J, et al. TNF-induced structural joint damage is mediated by IL-1. *Proc Natl Acad Sci USA.* (2007) 104:11742–7. doi: 10.1073/pnas.0610812104
129. Lam J, Takeshita S, Barker JE, Kanagawa O, Ross FP, Teitelbaum SL. TNF-α induces osteoclastogenesis by direct stimulation of macrophages exposed to permissive levels of RANK ligand. *J Clin Invest.* (2000) 106:1481–8. doi: 10.1172/JCI11176
130. Kobayashi K, Takahashi N, Jimi E, Udagawa N, Takami M, Kotake S, et al. Tumor necrosis factor α stimulates osteoclast differentiation by a mechanism independent of the ODF/RANKL–RANK interaction. *J Exp Med.* (2000) 191:275–86. doi: 10.1084/jem.191.2.275
131. Kitaura H, Sands MS, Aya K, Zhou P, Hirayama T, Uthgenannt B, et al. Marrow stromal cells and osteoclast precursors differentially contribute to TNF-α-induced osteoclastogenesis *in vivo*. *J Immunol.* (2004) 173:4838–46. doi: 10.4049/jimmunol.173.8.4838
132. Zou W, Hakim I, Tschoep K, Endres S, Bar-Shavit Z, Tumor necrosis factor-α mediates RANK ligand stimulation of osteoclast differentiation by an autocrine mechanism. *J Cell Biochem.* (2001) 83:70–83. doi: 10.1002/jcb.1202

133. Ho VW, Sly LM. Derivation and characterization of murine alternatively activated (M2) macrophages. *Methods Mol Biol.* (2009) 531:173–85. doi: 10.1007/978-1-59745-396-7_12

134. Bonewald L, Dallas S. Role of active and latent transforming growth factor β in bone formation. *J Cell Biochem.* (1994) 55:350–7. doi: 10.1002/jcb.240550312

135. Wu B, Sondag G, Malcuit C, Kim MH, Safadi FF. Macrophage-associated osteoactivin/GPNMB mediates mesenchymal stem cell survival, proliferation, and migration via a CD44-dependent mechanism. *J Cellul Biochem.* (2015) 117:1511–21. doi: 10.1002/jcb.25394

136. Cho TJ, Kim J, Chung C, Yoo W, Gerstenfeld L, Einhorn T, et al. Expression and role of interleukin-6 in distraction osteogenesis. *Calcified Tissue Int.* (2007) 80:192–200. doi: 10.1007/s00223-006-0240-y

137. Sammons J, Ahmed N, El-Sheemy M, Hassan H. The role of BMP-6, IL-6, and BMP-4 in mesenchymal stem cell-dependent bone development: effects on osteoblastic differentiation induced by parathyroid hormone and vitamin D3. *Stem Cells Dev.* (2004) 13:273–80. doi: 10.1089/154732804323099208

138. Blanchard F, Duplomb L, Baud'huin M, Brounais B. The dual role of IL-6-type cytokines on bone remodeling and bone tumors. *Cytokine Growth Factor Rev.* (2009) 20:19–28. doi: 10.1016/j.cytogfr.2008.11.004

139. Itoh S, Udagawa N, Takahashi N, Yoshitake F, Narita H, Ebisu S, et al. A critical role for interleukin-6 family-mediated Stat3 activation in osteoblast differentiation and bone formation. *Bone.* (2006) 39:505–12. doi: 10.1016/j.bone.2006.02.074

140. Bellido T, Borba VZ, Roberson P, Manolagas SC. Activation of the janus kinase/STAT (Signal Transducer and Activator of Transcription) signal transduction pathway by interleukin-6-type cytokines promotes osteoblast differentiation 1. *Endocrinology.* (1997) 138:3666–76. doi: 10.1210/en.138.9.3666

141. Song HY, Jeon ES, Kim JI, Jung JS, Kim JH. Oncostatin M promotes osteogenesis and suppresses adipogenic differentiation of human adipose tissue-derived mesenchymal stem cells. *J Cell Biochem.* (2007) 101:1238–51. doi: 10.1002/jcb.21245

142. Guihard P, Danger Y, Brounais B, David E, Brion R, Delecrin J, et al. Induction of osteogenesis in mesenchymal stem cells by activated monocytes/macrophages depends on oncostatin M signaling. *Stem Cells.* (2012) 30:762–72. doi: 10.1002/stem.1040

143. Sonomoto K, Yamaoka K, Oshita K, Fukuyo S, Zhang X, Nakano K, et al. Interleukin-1β induces differentiation of human mesenchymal stem cells into osteoblasts via the Wnt-5a/receptor tyrosine kinase–like orphan receptor 2 pathway. *Arthr Rheum.* (2012) 64:3355–63. doi: 10.1002/art.34555

144. Ma T, Miyanishi K, Trindade MC, Genovese M, Regula D, Smith RL, et al. Interleukin 1 receptor antagonist inhibits localized bone formation *in vivo*. *J Rheumatol.* (2003) 30:2547–52.

145. Huang H, Kim H, Chang E, Lee Z, Hwang S, Kim H, et al. IL-17 stimulates the proliferation and differentiation of human mesenchymal stem cells: implications for bone remodeling. *Cell Death Differen.* (2009) 16:1332–43. doi: 10.1038/cdd.2009.74

146. Ono T, Okamoto K, Nakashima T, Nitta T, Hori S, Iwakura Y, et al. IL-17-producing γδ T cells enhance bone regeneration. *Nat Commun.* (2016) 7:10928. doi: 10.1038/ncomms10928

147. Hess K, Ushmorov A, Fiedler J, Brenner RE, Wirth T. TNFα promotes osteogenic differentiation of human mesenchymal stem cells by triggering the NF-κB signaling pathway. *Bone.* (2009) 45:367–76. doi: 10.1016/j.bone.2009.04.252

148. Nanes MS. Tumor necrosis factor-α: molecular and cellular mechanisms in skeletal pathology. *Gene.* (2003) 321:1–15. doi: 10.1016/S0378-1119(03)00841-2

149. Perrien DS, Brown EC, Fletcher TW, Irby DJ, Aronson J, Gao GG, et al. Interleukin-1 and tumor necrosis factor antagonists attenuate ethanol-induced inhibition of bone formation in a rat model of distraction osteogenesis. *J Pharmacol Exp Therapeut.* (2002) 303:904–8. doi: 10.1124/jpet.102.039636

150. Ding J, Ghali O, Lencel P, Broux O, Chauveau C, Devedjian J, et al. TNF-α and IL-1β inhibit RUNX2 and collagen expression but increase alkaline phosphatase activity and mineralization in human mesenchymal stem cells. *Life Sci.* (2009) 84:499–504. doi: 10.1016/j.lfs.2009.01.013

151. Bozec A, Bakiri L, Hoebertz A, Eferl R, Schilling AF, Komnenovic V, et al. Osteoclast size is controlled by Fra-2 through LIF/LIF-receptor signalling and hypoxia. *Nature.* (2008) 454:221–5. doi: 10.1038/nature07019

152. Richards CD, Langdon C, Deschamps P, Pennica D, Shaughnessy SG. Stimulation of osteoclast differentiation in vitro by mouse oncostatin M, leukaemia inhibitory factor, cardiotrophin-1 and interleukin 6: synergy with dexamethasone. *Cytokine.* (2000) 12:613–21. doi: 10.1006/cyto.1999.0635

153. Dresner-Pollak R, Gelb N, Rachmilewitz D, Karmeli F, Weinreb M. Interleukin 10-deficient mice develop osteopenia, decreased bone formation, and mechanical fragility of long bones. *Gastroenterology.* (2004) 127:792–801. doi: 10.1053/j.gastro.2004.06.013

154. Van Vlasselaer P, Borremans B, Van Den Heuvel R, Van Gorp U, de Waal Malefyt R. Interleukin-10 inhibits the osteogenic activity of mouse bone marrow. *Blood.* (1993) 82:2361–70.

155. Van Vlasselaer P, Borremans B, Van Gorp U, Dasch J, De Waal-Malefyt R. Interleukin 10 inhibits transforming growth factor-beta (TGF-beta) synthesis required for osteogenic commitment of mouse bone marrow cells. *J Cell Biol.* (1994) 124:569–77. doi: 10.1083/jcb.124.4.569

156. Croes M, Öner FC, van Neerven D, Sabir E, Kruyt MC, Blokhuis TJ, et al. Proinflammatory T cells and IL-17 stimulate osteoblast differentiation. *Bone.* (2016) 84:262–70. doi: 10.1016/j.bone.2016.01.010

157. Duque G, Huang DC, Macoritto M, Rivas D, Yang XF, Ste-Marie LG, et al. Autocrine regulation of interferon γ in mesenchymal stem cells plays a role in early osteoblastogenesis. *Stem Cells.* (2009) 27:550–8. doi: 10.1634/stemcells.2008-0886

158. Postiglione L, Di Domenico G, Montagnani S, Di Spigna G, Salzano S, Castaldo C, et al. Granulocyte-macrophage colony-stimulating factor (GM-CSF) induces the osteoblastic differentiation of the human osteosarcoma cell line SaOS-2. *Calcified Tissue Int.* (2003) 72:85–97. doi: 10.1007/s00223-001-2088-5

159. Liu Y, Wang L, Kikuiri T, Akiyama K, Chen C, Xu X, et al. Mesenchymal stem cell-based tissue regeneration is governed by recipient T lymphocytes via IFN-γ and TNF-α. *Nat Med.* (2011) 17:1594–601.

160. Kim YG, Park JW, Lee JM, Suh JY, Lee JK, Chang BS, et al. IL-17 inhibits osteoblast differentiation and bone regeneration in rat. *Arch Oral Biol.* (2014) 59:897–905. doi: 10.1016/j.archoralbio.2014.05.009

161. Hughes JE, Srinivasan S, Lynch KR, Proia RL, Ferdek P, Hedrick CC. Sphingosine-1-phosphate induces an antiinflammatory phenotype in macrophages. *Circul Res.* (2008) 102:950–8. doi: 10.1161/CIRCRESAHA.107.170779

162. Dorsam G, Graeler MH, Seroogy C, Kong Y, Voice JK, Goetzl EJ. Transduction of multiple effects of sphingosine 1-phosphate (S1P) on T cell functions by the S1P1 G protein-coupled receptor. *J Immunol.* (2003) 171:3500–7. doi: 10.4049/jimmunol.171.7.3500

163. Wang W, Huang MC, Goetzl EJ. Type 1 sphingosine 1-phosphate G protein-coupled receptor (S1P1) mediation of enhanced IL-4 generation by CD4 T cells from S1P1 transgenic mice. *J Immunol.* (2007) 178:4885–90. doi: 10.4049/jimmunol.178.8.4885

164. Huang MC, Watson SR, Liao JJ, Goetzl EJ. Th17 augmentation in OTII TCR plus T cell-selective type 1 sphingosine 1-phosphate receptor double transgenic mice. *J Immunol.* (2007) 178:6806–13. doi: 10.4049/jimmunol.178.11.6806

165. Liao JJ, Huang MC, Goetzl EJ. Cutting edge: alternative signaling of Th17 cell development by sphingosine 1-phosphate. *J Immunol.* (2007) 178:5425–8. doi: 10.4049/jimmunol.178.9.5425

166. Liu G, Yang K, Burns S, Shrestha S, Chi H. The S1P1-mTOR axis directs the reciprocal differentiation of TH1 and Treg cells. *Nat Immunol.* (2010) 11:1047–56. doi: 10.1038/ni.1939

167. Huang R, Wang X, Zhou Y, Xiao Y. RANKL-induced M1 macrophages are involved in bone formation. *Bone Res.* (2017) 5:17019. doi: 10.1038/boneres.2017.19

168. Loi F, Córdova LA, Zhang R, Pajarinen J, Lin TH, Goodman SB, et al. The effects of immunomodulation by macrophage subsets on osteogenesis *in vitro*. *Stem Cell Res Ther.* (2016) 7:15. doi: 10.1186/s13287-016-0276-5

169. Aggarwal S, Pittenger MF. Human mesenchymal stem cells modulate allogeneic immune cell responses. *Blood.* (2005) 105:1815–22. doi: 10.1182/blood-2004-04-1559

170. Gur-Wahnon D, Borovsky Z, Beyth S, Liebergall M, Rachmilewitz J. Contact-dependent induction of regulatory antigen-presenting cells by human mesenchymal stem cells is mediated via STAT3 signaling. *Exp Hematol.* (2007) 35:426–33. doi: 10.1016/j.exphem.2006.11.001
171. Németh K, Leelahavanichkul A, Yuen PS, Mayer B, Parmelee A, Doi K, et al. Bone marrow stromal cells attenuate sepsis via prostaglandin E2–dependent reprogramming of host macrophages to increase their interleukin-10 production. *Nat Med.* (2009) 15:42–9. doi: 10.1038/nm.1905
172. Fibbe WE, Nauta AJ, Roelofs H. Modulation of immune responses by mesenchymal stem cells. *Annals N Y Acad Sci.* (2007) 1106:272–8. doi: 10.1196/annals.1392.025
173. Bunnell BA, Betancourt AM, Sullivan DE. New concepts on the immune modulation mediated by mesenchymal stem cells. *Stem Cell Res Ther.* (2010) 1:34. doi: 10.1186/scrt34
174. Augello A, Tasso R, Negrini SM, Amateis A, Indiveri F, Cancedda R, et al. Bone marrow mesenchymal progenitor cells inhibit lymphocyte proliferation by activation of the programmed death 1 pathway. *Eur J Immunol.* (2005) 35:1482–90. doi: 10.1002/eji.200425405
175. Auletta JJ, Deans RJ, Bartholomew AM. Emerging roles for multipotent, bone marrow–derived stromal cells in host defense. *Blood.* (2012) 119:1801–9. doi: 10.1182/blood-2011-10-384354
176. Bianco P, Robey PG, Simmons PJ. Mesenchymal stem cells: revisiting history, concepts, and assays. *Cell Stem Cell.* (2008) 2:313–9. doi: 10.1016/j.stem.2008.03.002
177. Chen K, Wang D, Du WT, Han ZB, Ren H, Chi Y, et al. Human umbilical cord mesenchymal stem cells hUC-MSCs exert immunosuppressive activities through a PGE 2-dependent mechanism. *Clin Immunol.* (2010) 135:448–58. doi: 10.1016/j.clim.2010.01.015
178. Maggini J, Mirkin G, Bognanni I, Holmberg J, Piazzón IM, Nepomnaschy I, et al. Mouse bone marrow-derived mesenchymal stromal cells turn activated macrophages into a regulatory-like profile. *PLoS ONE.* (2010) 5:e9252. doi: 10.1371/journal.pone.0009252
179. MacKenzie KF, Clark K, Naqvi S, McGuire VA, Nöehren G, Kristariyanto Y, et al. PGE2 induces macrophage IL-10 production and a regulatory-like phenotype via a protein kinase A–SIK–CRTC3 pathway. *J Immunol.* (2013) 190:565–77. doi: 10.4049/jimmunol.1202462
180. Chyun YS, Raisz LG. Stimulation of bone formation by prostaglandin E2. *Prostaglandins.* (1984) 27:97–103. doi: 10.1016/0090-6980(84)90223-5
181. Raicevic G, Rouas R, Najar M, Stordeur P, Boufker HI, Bron D, et al. Inflammation modifies the pattern and the function of Toll-like receptors expressed by human mesenchymal stromal cells. *Hum Immunol.* (2010) 71:235–44. doi: 10.1016/j.humimm.2009.12.005
182. Waterman RS, Tomchuck SL, Henkle SL, Betancourt AM. A new mesenchymal stem cell (MSC) paradigm: polarization into a pro-inflammatory MSC1 or an Immunosuppressive MSC2 phenotype. *PLoS ONE.* (2010) 5:e10088. doi: 10.1371/journal.pone.0010088
183. Verreck FA, de Boer T, Langenberg DM, van der Zanden L, Ottenhoff TH. Phenotypic and functional profiling of human proinflammatory type-1 and anti-inflammatory type-2 macrophages in response to microbial antigens and IFN-γ-and CD40L-mediated costimulation. *J Leukocyte Biol.* (2006) 79:285–93. doi: 10.1189/jlb.0105015
184. Xiao L, Zhou Y, Zhu L, Yang S, Huang R, Shi W, et al. SPHK1-S1PR1-RANKL axis regulates the interactions between macrophages and BMSCs in inflammatory bone loss. *J Bone Miner Res.* (2018) 3:1090–104. doi: 10.1002/jbmr.3396
185. Rivera J, Proia RL, Olivera A. The alliance of sphingosine-1-phosphate and its receptors in immunity. *Nat Rev Immunol.* (2008) 8:753–63. doi: 10.1038/nri2400
186. Wang F, Van Brocklyn JR, Hobson JP, Movafagh S, Zukowska-Grojec Z, Milstien S, et al. Sphingosine 1-phosphate stimulates cell migration through a Gi-coupled cell surface receptor potential involvement in angiogenesis. *J Biol Chem.* (1999) 274:35343–50. doi: 10.1074/jbc.274.50.35343
187. Schwab SR, Cyster JG. Finding a way out: lymphocyte egress from lymphoid organs. *Nat Immunol.* (2007) 8:1295–301. doi: 10.1038/ni1545
188. Zachariah MA, Cyster JG. Neural crest–derived pericytes promote egress of mature thymocytes at the corticomedullary junction. *Science.* (2010) 328:1129–35. doi: 10.1126/science.1188222
189. Cinamon G, Zachariah MA, Lam OM, Foss FW, Cyster JG. Follicular shuttling of marginal zone B cells facilitates antigen transport. *Nat Immunol.* (2008) 9:54–62. doi: 10.1038/ni1542
190. Jenne CN, Enders A, Rivera R, Watson SR, Bankovich AJ, Pereira JP, et al. T-bet–dependent S1P5 expression in NK cells promotes egress from lymph nodes and bone marrow. *J Exp Med.* (2009) 206:2469–81. doi: 10.1084/jem.20090525
191. Rathinasamy A, Czeloth N, Pabst O, Förster R, Bernhardt G. The origin and maturity of dendritic cells determine the pattern of sphingosine 1-phosphate receptors expressed and required for efficient migration. *J Immunol.* (2010) 185:4072–81. doi: 10.4049/jimmunol.1000568
192. König K, Diehl L, Rommerscheidt-Fuss U, Golletz C, Quast T, Kahl P, et al. Four-and-a-half LIM domain protein 2 is a novel regulator of sphingosine 1-phosphate receptor 1 in CCL19-induced dendritic cell migration. *J Immunol.* (2010) 185:1466–75. doi: 10.4049/jimmunol.0903449
193. Jolly PS, Bektas M, Olivera A, Gonzalez-Espinosa C, Proia RL, Rivera J, et al. Transactivation of sphingosine-1–phosphate receptors by FcεRI triggering is required for normal mast cell degranulation and chemotaxis. *J Exp Med.* (2004) 199:959–70. doi: 10.1084/jem.20030680
194. Zhang L, Orban M, Lorenz M, Barocke V, Braun D, Urtz N, et al. A novel role of sphingosine 1-phosphate receptor S1pr1 in mouse thrombopoiesis. *J Exp Med.* (2012) 209:2165–81. doi: 10.1084/jem.20121090
195. Allende ML, Tuymetova G, Lee BG, Bonifacino E, Wu YP, Proia RL. S1P1 receptor directs the release of immature B cells from bone marrow into blood. *J Exp\ Med.* (2010) 207:1113–24. doi: 10.1084/jem.20092210
196. Sinha RK, Park C, Hwang IY, Davis MD, Kehrl JH. B lymphocytes exit lymph nodes through cortical lymphatic sinusoids by a mechanism independent of sphingosine-1-phosphate-mediated chemotaxis. *Immunity.* (2009) 30:434–46. doi: 10.1016/j.immuni.2008.12.018
197. Czeloth N, Schippers A, Wagner N, Müller W, Küster B, Bernhardt G, et al. Sphingosine-1 phosphate signaling regulates positioning of dendritic cells within the spleen. *J Immunol.* (2007) 179:5855–63. doi: 10.4049/jimmunol.179.9.5855
198. Maeda Y, Matsuyuki H, Shimano K, Kataoka H, Sugahara K, Chiba K. Migration of CD4 T cells and dendritic cells toward sphingosine 1-phosphate (S1P) is mediated by different receptor subtypes: S1P regulates the functions of murine mature dendritic cells via S1P receptor type *J Immunol.* (2007) 178:3437–46. doi: 10.4049/jimmunol.178.6.3437
199. Gräler MH, Huang MC, Watson S, Goetzl EJ. Immunological effects of transgenic constitutive expression of the type 1 sphingosine 1-phosphate receptor by mouse lymphocytes. *J Immunol.* (2005) 174:1997–2003. doi: 10.4049/jimmunol.174.4.1997
200. Song J, Matsuda C, Kai Y, Nishida T, Nakajima K, Mizushima T, et al. A novel sphingosine 1-phosphate receptor agonist, 2-amino-2-propanediol hydrochloride (KRP-203), regulates chronic colitis in interleukin-10 gene-deficient mice. *J Pharmacol Exp Therapeut.* (2008) 324:276–83. doi: 10.1124/jpet.106.119172
201. Sato K, Suematsu A, Okamoto K, Yamaguchi A, Morishita Y, Kadono Y, et al. Th17 functions as an osteoclastogenic helper T cell subset that links T cell activation and bone destruction. *J Exp Med.* (2006) 203:2673–82. doi: 10.1084/jem.20061775
202. Liu G, Burns S, Huang G, Boyd K, Proia RL, Flavell RA, et al. The receptor S1P1 overrides regulatory T cell–mediated immune suppression through Akt-mTOR. *Nat Immunol.* (2009) 10:769–77. doi: 10.1038/ni.1743
203. Takeshita H, Kitano M, Iwasaki T, Kitano S, Tsunemi S, Sato C, et al. Sphingosine 1-phosphate (S1P)/S1P receptor 1 signaling regulates receptor activator of NF-κB ligand (RANKL) expression in rheumatoid arthritis. *Biochem Biophys Res Commun.* (2012) 419:154–9. doi: 10.1016/j.bbrc.2012.01.103
204. Barra G, Lepore A, Gagliardi M, Somma D, Matarazzo MR, Costabile F, et al. Sphingosine Kinases promote IL-17 expression in human T lymphocytes. *Sci Rep.* (2018) 8:13233. doi: 10.1038/s41598-018-31666-1
205. Choi JW, Gardell SE, Herr DR, Rivera R, Lee CW, Noguchi K, et al. FTY720 (fingolimod) efficacy in an animal model of multiple sclerosis requires astrocyte sphingosine 1-phosphate receptor 1 (S1P1) modulation. *Proc Natl Acad Sci USA.* (2011) 108:751–6. doi: 10.1073/pnas.1014154108
206. Kitano M, Hla T, Sekiguchi M, Kawahito Y, Yoshimura R, Miyazawa K, et al. Sphingosine 1-phosphate/sphingosine 1-phosphate receptor

1 signaling in rheumatoid synovium: Regulation of synovial proliferation and inflammatory gene expression. *Arthr Rheum.* (2006) 54:742–53. doi: 10.1002/art.21668
207. Ogretmen B. Sphingolipid metabolism in cancer signalling and therapy. *Nat Rev Cancer.* (2018) 18:33–50. doi: 10.1038/nrc.2017.96
208. Baker DA, Barth J, Chang R, Obeid LM, Gilkeson GS. Genetic sphingosine kinase 1 deficiency significantly decreases synovial inflammation and joint erosions in murine TNF-α-induced arthritis. *J Immunol.* (2010) 185:2570–9. doi: 10.4049/jimmunol.1000644
209. Kappos L, Antel J, Comi G, Montalban X, O'Connor P, Polman CH, et al. Oral fingolimod (FTY720) for relapsing multiple sclerosis. *N Engl J Med.* (2006) 355:1124–40. doi: 10.1056/NEJMoa052643
210. Sanchez T, Estrada-Hernandez T, Paik JH, Wu MT, Venkataraman K, Brinkmann V, et al. Phosphorylation and action of the immunomodulator FTY720 inhibits vascular endothelial cell growth factor-induced vascular permeability. *J Biol Chem.* (2003) 278:47281–90. doi: 10.1074/jbc.M306896200
211. Kharel Y, Lee S, Snyder AH, Sheasley-O'Neill SL, Morris MA, Setiady Y, et al. Sphingosine kinase 2 is required for modulation of lymphocyte traffic by FTY. *J Biol Chem.* (2005) 280:36865–72. doi: 10.1074/jbc.M506293200
212. Liu CH, Thangada S, Lee MJ, Van Brocklyn JR, Spiegel S, Hla T. Ligand-induced trafficking of the sphingosine-1-phosphate receptor EDG. *Molecul Biol Cell.* (1999) 10:1179–90. doi: 10.1091/mbc.10.4.1179
213. Gräler MH, Goetzl EJ. The immunosuppressant FTY720 down-regulates sphingosine 1-phosphate G-protein-coupled receptors. *FASEB J.* (2004) 18:551–3. doi: 10.1096/fj.03-0910fje
214. Jo E, Sanna MG, Gonzalez-Cabrera PJ, Thangada S, Tigyi G, Osborne DA, et al. S1P 1-selective in vivo-active agonists from high-throughput screening: off-the-shelf chemical probes of receptor interactions, signaling, and fate. *Chem Biol.* (2005) 12:703–15. doi: 10.1016/j.chembiol.2005.04.019
215. Oo ML, Thangada S, Wu MT, Liu CH, Macdonald TL, Lynch KR, et al. Immunosuppressive and anti-angiogenic sphingosine 1-phosphate receptor-1 agonists induce ubiquitinylation and proteasomal degradation of the receptor. *J Biol Chem/.* (2007) 282:9082–9. doi: 10.1074/jbc.M610318200
216. Oo ML, Chang SH, Thangada S, Wu MT, Rezaul K, Blaho V, et al. Engagement of S1P1-degradative mechanisms leads to vascular leak in mice. *J Clin Invest.* (2011) 121:2290–300. doi: 10.1172/JCI45403
217. Gonzalez-Cabrera PJ, Hla T, Rosen H. Mapping pathways downstream of sphingosine 1-phosphate subtype 1 by differential chemical perturbation and proteomics. *J Biol Chem.* (2007) 282:7254–64. doi: 10.1074/jbc.M610581200
218. Dyckman AJ. Modulators of Sphingosine-1-phosphate pathway biology: recent advances of sphingosine-1-phosphate Receptor 1 (S1P1) agonists and future perspectives. *J Med Chem.* (2017) 60:5267–89. doi: 10.1021/acs.jmedchem.6b01575
219. Tsunemi S, Iwasaki T, Kitano S, Imado T, Miyazawa K, Sano H. Effects of the novel immunosuppressant FTY720 in a murine rheumatoid arthritis model. *Clin Immunol.* (2010) 136:197–204. doi: 10.1016/j.clim.2010.03.428
220. Matsuura M, Imayoshi T, Okumoto T. Effect of FTY720, a novel immunosuppressant, on adjuvant- and collagen-induced arthritis in rats. *Int J Immunopharmacol.* (2000) 22:323–31. doi: 10.1016/S0192-0561(99)00088-0
221. Han YP, Li X, Zhou QY, Jie HY, Lao XB, Han JC, et al. FTY720 Abrogates collagen-induced arthritis by hindering dendritic cell migration to local lymph nodes. *J Immunol.* (2015) 195:4126–35. doi: 10.4049/jimmunol.1401842
222. Miller DC, Whittington KB, Brand DD, Hasty KA, Rosloniec EF. The CII-specific autoimmune T-cell response develops in the presence of FTY720 but is regulated by enhanced Treg cells that inhibit the development of autoimmune arthritis. *Arthrit Res Ther.* (2016) 18:ARTN8. doi: 10.1186/s13075-015-0909-6
223. Bagdanoff JT, Donoviel MS, Nouraldeen A, Carlsen M, Jessop TC, Tarver J, et al. Inhibition of Sphingosine 1-Phosphate Lyase for the treatment of rheumatoid arthritis: discovery of (E)-1-(4((1R,2S,3R)-1,2,3,4-Tetrahydroxybutyl)-1H-imidazol-2-yl)ethanone Oxime (LX2931) and (1R,2S,3R)-1-(2-(Isoxazol-3-yl)-1H-imidazol-4-yl)butane-1,2,3,4-tetraol (LX2932). *J Med Chem.* (2010) 53:8650–62. doi: 10.1021/jm101183p
224. Dougados M, Baeten D. Spondyloarthritis. *Lancet.* (2011) 377:2127–37. doi: 10.1016/S0140-6736(11)60071-8
225. Yu H, Sun C, Argraves K. Periodontal inflammation and alveolar bone loss induced by Aggregatibacter actinomycetemcomitans is attenuated in sphingosine kinase 1-deficient mice. *J Periodontal Res.* (2016) 51:38–49. doi: 10.1111/jre.12276
226. Xiao L, Zhu L, Yang S, Lei D, Xiao Y, Peng B. Different correlation of sphingosine-1-phosphate receptor 1 with receptor activator of nuclear factor Kappa B ligand and regulatory T cells in rat periapical lesions. *J Endodont.* (2015) 41:479–86. doi: 10.1016/j.joen.2014.10.010
227. Byles V, Covarrubias AJ, Ben-Sahra I, Lamming DW, Sabatini DM, Manning, BD, et al. The TSC-mTOR pathway regulates macrophage polarization. *Nat Commun.* (2013) 4:2834. doi: 10.1038/ncomms3834
228. Gulen MF, Kang Z, Bulek K, Youzhong W, Kim TW, Chen Y, et al. The receptor SIGIRR suppresses Th17 cell proliferation via inhibition of the interleukin-1 receptor pathway and mTOR kinase activation. *Immunity.* (2010) 32:54–66. doi: 10.1016/j.immuni.2009.12.003
229. Zhu L, Yang T, Li L, Sun L, Hou Y, Hu X, et al. TSC1 controls macrophage polarization to prevent inflammatory disease. *Nat Commun.* (2014) 5:4696. doi: 10.1038/ncomms5696
230. Shao J, Zhou Y, Xiao Y. The regulatory roles of Notch in osteocyte differentiation via the crosstalk with canonical Wnt pathways during the transition of osteoblasts to osteocytes. *Bone.* (2018) 108:165–78. doi: 10.1016/j.bone.2018.01.010
231. Chen J, Long F. mTORC1 signaling promotes osteoblast differentiation from preosteoblasts. *PLoS ONE.* (2015) 10:e0130627. doi: 10.1371/journal.pone.0130627
232. Fitter S, Matthews MP, Martin SK, Xie J, Ooi SS, Walkley CR, et al. mTORC1 plays an important role in skeletal development by controlling preosteoblast differentiation. *Mol Cell Biol.* (2017) 37:e00668–16. doi: 10.1128/MCB.00668-16
233. Chen J, Long F. mTOR signaling in skeletal development and disease. *Bone Res.* (2018) 6:1. doi: 10.1038/s41413-017-0004-5
234. Nollet M, Santucci-Darmanin S, Breuil V, Al-Sahlanee R, Cros C, Topi M, et al. Autophagy in osteoblasts is involved in mineralization and bone homeostasis. *Autophagy.* (2014) 10:1965–77. doi: 10.4161/auto.36182
235. Ravikumar B, Vacher C, Berger Z, Davies JE, Luo S, Oroz LG, et al. Inhibition of mTOR induces autophagy and reduces toxicity of polyglutamine expansions in fly and mouse models of Huntington disease. *Nat Genet.* (2004) 36:585–95. doi: 10.1038/ng1362
236. Ching JK, Weihl CC. Rapamycin-induced autophagy aggravates pathology and weakness in a mouse model of VCP-associated myopathy. *Autophagy.* (2013) 9:799–800. doi: 10.4161/auto.23958
237. Kim J, Kundu M, Viollet B, Guan KL. AMPK and mTOR regulate autophagy through direct phosphorylation of Ulk. *Nat Cell Biol.* (2011) 13:132–41. doi: 10.1038/ncb2152
238. Noda T, Ohsumi Y. Tor, a phosphatidylinositol kinase homologue, controls autophagy in yeast. *J Biol Chem.* (1998) 273:3963–6. doi: 10.1074/jbc.273.7.3963
239. Schmelzle T, Hall MN. TOR, a central controller of cell growth. *Cell.* (2000) 103:253–62. doi: 10.1016/S0092-8674(00)00117-3
240. Xiao L. *Dissecting the Role of Sphingosine 1-Phosphate-Sphingosine 1-Phosphate Receptor 1 in Inflammatory Bone Remodelling.* Brisbane: Queensland University of Technology (2017).

3

The Role of Mast Cells in Bone Metabolism and Bone Disorders

*Deniz Ragipoglu[1], Anne Dudeck[2], Melanie Haffner-Luntzer[1], Martin Voss[2], Jochen Kroner[1], Anita Ignatius[1] and Verena Fischer[1]**

[1] Trauma Research Center Ulm, Institute of Orthopedic Research and Biomechanics, Ulm University Medical Center, Ulm, Germany, [2] Medical Faculty, Institute for Molecular and Clinical Immunology, Otto-von-Guericke University Magdeburg, Magdeburg, Germany

***Correspondence:**
Verena Fischer
verena.fischer@uni-ulm.de

Mast cells (MCs) are important sensor and effector cells of the immune system that are involved in many physiological and pathological conditions. Increasing evidence suggests that they also play an important role in bone metabolism and bone disorders. MCs are located in the bone marrow and secrete a wide spectrum of mediators, which can be rapidly released upon activation of mature MCs following their differentiation in mucosal or connective tissues. Many of these mediators can exert osteocatabolic effects by promoting osteoclast formation [e.g., histamine, tumor necrosis factor (TNF), interleukin-6 (IL-6)] and/or by inhibiting osteoblast activity (e.g., IL-1, TNF). By contrast, MCs could potentially act in an osteoprotective manner by stimulating osteoblasts (e.g., transforming growth factor-β) or reducing osteoclastogenesis (e.g., IL-12, interferon-γ). Experimental studies investigating MC functions in physiological bone turnover using MC-deficient mouse lines give contradictory results, reporting delayed or increased bone turnover or no influence depending on the mouse model used. By contrast, the involvement of MCs in various pathological conditions affecting bone is evident. MCs may contribute to the pathogenesis of primary and secondary osteoporosis as well as inflammatory disorders, including rheumatoid arthritis and osteoarthritis, because increased numbers of MCs were found in patients suffering from these diseases. The clinical observations could be largely confirmed in experimental studies using MC-deficient mouse models, which also provide mechanistic insights. MCs also regulate bone healing after fracture by influencing the inflammatory response toward the fracture, vascularization, bone formation, and callus remodeling by osteoclasts. This review summarizes the current view and understanding of the role of MCs on bone in both physiological and pathological conditions.

Keywords: mast cells, inflammation, bone disorders, osteoporosis, fracture healing

INTRODUCTION

Mast cells (MCs) are tissue-resident immune cells and are best known for promoting allergic reactions (1). However, research over recent decades has revealed important functions of MCs in numerous physiological conditions, including the regulation of angiogenesis and tissue homeostasis, but also in pathological conditions, such as gastrointestinal and cardiovascular diseases. MCs are distributed throughout several tissues, including the skeletal system (2). They are suitable candidates to be involved in bone metabolism and bone disorders, because MCs store and de novo synthesize many mediators, including cytokines and enzymes (3), which have been shown to regulate bone homeostasis and to be involved in the pathogenesis of several skeletal diseases (4). Indeed, increased numbers of MCs have been found in patients with reduced bone mass observed in mastocytosis or postmenopausal osteoporosis (5, 6). Furthermore, it has been shown that the synovial fluids of patients suffering from rheumatoid arthritis (RA) or osteoarthritis (OA) contain increased MC numbers and elevated concentrations of certain MC mediators including tryptase or histamine (7, 8). Importantly, numerous experimental studies using MC-deficient mouse models confirmed the involvement of MCs in the pathologies of osteoporosis and arthritis (9, 10). Interestingly, several groups using MC-deficient mouse models discovered that MCs also play an important role in the process of bone fracture healing and might be involved in the regulation of osteoclastogenesis (10, 11). However, further research needs to elucidate the molecular mechanisms of MC actions in these various physiological and pathological conditions.

The scope of this review is to provide an overview of the physiological role of MCs in bone homeostasis based on the current state of knowledge. Moreover, the role of MCs in bone disorders will be discussed, focusing on osteoporosis and bone fracture healing, including both current clinical and experimental data. The involvement of MCs in RA and OA will be discussed only briefly, because there are several comprehensive reviews from other authors, which summarize the important function of MCs in these bone disorders (12–14).

MAST CELLS AND THEIR PHYSIOLOGICAL ROLES

MCs are tissue-resident hematopoietic cells and are identified by their large number of secretory granules, which contain a broad variety of preformed mediators, including biogenic amines (e.g., histamine), heparin, cytokines [e.g., tumor necrosis factor (TNF), interleukin-6 (IL-6)], enzymes (e.g., chymases, tryptases), and various growth factors [e.g., vascular endothelial growth factor (VEGF), fibroblast growth factor (FGF)] (3). Unlike most other hematopoietic cells, mature MCs are not found in the circulation under physiological conditions. They are released from the bone marrow as MC progenitors (MCps). MCps are characterized by their expression of CD34, as are other early hematopoietic cells, and by MC-related surface markers, including CD117 (c-Kit), also known as stem cell factor (SCF) receptor (15). c-Kit is highly expressed on hematopoietic stem cells and its activity is crucial for hematopoiesis. Interestingly, only MCs retain c-Kit expression throughout their lifetime, whereas it is lost in other hematopoietic lineages during differentiation. SCF/c-Kit signaling is essential for MC growth, differentiation, and survival. Late MCps also express the high-affinity immunoglobulin E (IgE) receptor (FcεRI), as do mature MCs, however, MCps are less or non-granulated in contrast to mature MCs, which have many metachromatic granules (15–17). Committed MCps enter the target tissues and complete their maturation based on the local microenvironment (18). That is why their types and amounts of mediators can vary during MC maturation depending on the respective tissue (19). While MCs are located in almost all tissues, high numbers are found in tissues facing the external environment, including the skin, lungs, and intestines, where pathogen exposure is most likely. Thereby, MCs serve as immunological sentinels in the first line of defense. Their long lifespan of up to several months as well as their perivascular, perilymphatic, and perineuronal locations potentiate MCs to respond rapidly to pathogens. Moreover, they can also react to humoral and neuronal stimuli as well as tissue damage (e.g., physical injury inducing damage-associated molecular patterns) or environmental insults (20, 21).

Mature MCs are mainly divided into two subsets in both humans and rodents, which differ in their anatomical distribution and the types of proteases produced (22). In humans, so-called MC_T express only tryptases and are located predominantly in the lungs and small intestinal mucosa, whereas MC_{TC} produce both tryptases and chymases as well as carboxypeptidase A3 (Cpa3). MC_{TC} predominate in the skin and the submucosa of the small intestine (23). In rodents, MCs are classified into connective tissue MCs (CTMCs) and mucosal MCs (MMCs). In terms of tissue localization and protease content, CTMCs are thought to resemble human MC_{TC}, whereas MMCs closely correspond to human MC_T. CTMCs are particularly located in the skin, peritoneal cavity, and submucosa of the intestine, while MMCs occupy the mucosal epithelium of the lungs and the gastrointestinal tract (24). Both MC subtypes are mainly identified via their protease content. While MMCs predominantly express the chymases MC protease-1 (Mcpt-1) and Mcpt-2, CTMCs express the chymases Mcpt-4 and Mcpt-5 as well as the tryptases Mcpt-6 and Mcpt-7, and additionally Cpa3. Furthermore, both subclasses react differently in response to stimulation and inhibition by drugs and interactions with T cells. MMCs expand remarkably during T cell-dependent immune responses, whereas CTMCs do not require T cells for expansion (22–24).

MCs can be activated by numerous factors, including immunoglobulins, cytokines, neuropeptides, complement proteins, and pathogen-associated molecular patterns (e.g., by

---

Abbreviations: CIA, Collagen-Induced Arthritis; Cpa3, Carboxypeptidase A3; CTMCs, Connective Tissue Mast Cells; CXCL, Chemokine (C-X-C Motif) Ligand; DT, Diphtheria Toxin; DTR, Diphtheria Toxin Receptor; ER, Estrogen Receptor; f, female; FcεRI, High Affinity Immunoglobulin E (IgE) Receptor; FGF, Fibroblast Growth Factor; GM-CSF, Granulocyte-Macrophage Colony-Stimulating Factor; IL, Interleukin; INF-γ, Interferon-γ; m, male; Mas-TRECK, Mast Cell-Specific Enhancer Mediated Toxin Receptor Mediated Conditional Cell Knockout; MCs, Mast Cells; Mcl-1, Myeloid Cell Leukemia Sequence-1; MCP-1, Monocyte Chemoattractant Protein-1; MCps, Mast Cell Progenitors; Mcpt, Mast Cell Protease; M-CSF, Macrophage Colony-Stimulating Factor; MIP-1α, Macrophage Inflammatory Protein-1α; MMCs, Mucosal Mast Cells; MMPs, Matrix Metalloproteinases; MSCs, Mesenchymal Stem Cells; NO, Nitric Oxide; NSAID, Non-Steroidal Anti-Inflammatory Drugs; OA, Osteoarthritis; OVX, Ovariectomy; PAF, Platelet Activating Factor; RA, Rheumatoid Arthritis; RANKL, Receptor Activator Of Nuclear Factor Kappa B Ligand; RFP, Red Fluorescent Protein; RMB, Red Mast Cell And Basophil Mouse; rPTH, Teriparatide; SC, Sodium Cromolyn; SCF, Stem Cell Factor; SM, Systemic Mastocytosis; tdT, td-Tomato; TGF-β, Transforming Growth Factor-β; TLR, Toll-Like Receptor; TNF, Tumor Necrosis Factor; TRAP, Tartrate Resistant Acid Phosphatase; VEGF, Vascular Endothelial Growth Factor; YFP, Yellow Fluorescent Protein; ↓, Decreased; ↑, Increased.

alarmins). Activation results in the release of preformed and newly synthesized mediators via degranulation. Furthermore, depending on the stimulus, MCs can also release the mediators selectively without degranulation (25). The most important and well known mechanism of MC activation is the crosslinking of the FcεRI via IgE and multivalent antigen complexes (26). FcεRI crosslinking triggers a cascade of intracellular signaling events, comprising protein phosphorylation, intracellular calcium mobilization, and transcription factor activation, and culminates in MC degranulation (27). Because MCs are present at the tissue boundaries, they are the first immune cells encountering invading endogenous and exogenous pathogens. Thereby, MCs can be activated directly by pathogens as well as by many pathogen-derived soluble products, including lipopolysaccharide (derived from gram-negative bacteria) and peptidoglycan (derived from gram-positive bacteria). They directly activate MCs via toll-like receptors (TLRs) or indirectly by activating the complement system through its receptors on MCs. Activation through TLRs induces selective cytokine synthesis and release depending on the stimuli, allowing specific responses to certain immunological insults (21, 25, 28, 29). For example, whereas TLR1 stimulation results in degranulation and additional IL-1 production, TLR2 activation induces the synthesis of cytokines and leukotrienes without degranulation (30). MCs can directly kill the pathogens by phagocytosis or extracellular traps similar to neutrophils. Additionally, they enhance the mucus production of epithelial cells to immobilize pathogens and modulate vascular permeability and blood flow to initiate rapid immune cell recruitment of effector cells, including neutrophils, eosinophils, and natural killer cells. Therefore, MCs play an important role in initiating the immune response. MCs and their products are also involved in the regulation of adaptive immune responses. For example, they modulate the migration, maturation, and activation of dendritic cells, present antigens to cytotoxic T cells, and attract effector T cells through their mediators (2, 21, 27, 31).

Beyond the host defense, MCs have many physiological functions. Several studies demonstrated that MCs enhance angiogenesis by secreting pro-angiogenic factors, including VEGF, basic FGF, TNF-α, heparin, histamine, IL-8, and various proteases (32, 33). Furthermore, MCs are considered important for tissue homeostasis, because many of their mediators, including FGF, histamine, and tryptase, induce epithelial cell and fibroblast proliferation. In addition, MCs are the main source of proteases, including tryptases, chymases, and cathepsin G, which activate matrix metalloproteinases (MMPs), thus initiating tissue remodeling (28, 34). MCs also appear to be critical for wound healing. They are present in the connective tissue of the skin in large numbers and are activated by injuries caused by trauma, heat, irradiation, or chemical agents. Thereby, MCs influence the inflammatory response, revascularization, and tissue formation and remodeling (35, 36). However, experimental studies are contradictory as to whether or not MCs promote skin wound healing. These contradictions might depend on the type and size of the wound and the mouse models used (37–39).

THE ROLE OF MAST CELLS IN PHYSIOLOGICAL BONE TURNOVER

A role for MCs in bone metabolism was long suspected (40). Whereas MCs are located in low numbers in the bone marrow at the epiphysis and diaphysis, they are numerous in the metaphyseal bone marrow, where bone remodeling mainly occurs (41). They are preferentially located adjacent to bone surfaces undergoing bone growth or turnover (**Figure 1A**). MCs at the endocortical bone surface are more flattened compared to those at a distance from the bone surface, which are typically round shaped (42). Their close proximity to the bone remodeling surface and the wide spectrum of their mediators, including histamine, heparin, proteases, and various cytokines, raise the question of a potential role for MCs in bone physiology. Many of the MC mediators are able to induce or modulate osteocatabolic effects by promoting osteoclastogenesis (e.g., histamine, TNF, IL-6) and/or inhibiting osteoblast activity (e.g., IL-1, TNF) (4, 43). By contrast, other mediators could act in an osteoprotective manner by stimulating osteoblasts [e.g., transforming growth factor-β (TGF-β)] or reducing osteoclastogenesis [e.g., IL-12, interferon-γ (IFN-γ)] under certain circumstances (4). **Table 1** summarizes the proposed or proven roles of MC mediators in bone formation and resorption.

To investigate the role of MCs and MC-derived products, ideally MCs would be selectively inhibited with a compound or depleted by genetic modification. Because there are no human conditions with reduced numbers or a complete absence of MCs, most data concerning the physiological role of MCs in bone development and turnover were gained either *in vitro* or in MC-deficient mouse models. To date, MC-deficient mice with mutations in the c-Kit receptor ($Kit^{W/W-v}$ and $Kit^{W-sh/W-sh}$ mice) or its ligand SCF ($Kitl^{Sl/Sl-d}$ mice) have been widely used. Whereas the point mutation KitW prevents cell surface c-Kit expression, the KitW-v mutation reduces the receptor kinase activity. KitW-sh is an inversion mutation and affects the transcriptional regulatory elements at the c-Kit transcription site. Furthermore, several mutations of the SCF ligand, including KitlSl and KitlSl-d, lead to a complete or partial deletion of the SCF gene. Because SCF/c-Kit signaling is essential for MC growth and survival, mice with alterations in this signaling lack MCs (109, 110).

Silberstein et al. using $Kit^{W/W-v}$ mice were the first to suggest that MCs might play a role in physiological bone turnover. They found that bone remodeling is delayed in this mouse model because of reduced osteoclast recruitment and osteoblast activity (111). Other studies in $Kit^{W-sh/W-sh}$ mice reported an osteopenic bone phenotype with high bone turnover because osteoclast activity exceeds osteoblast activity (112–114). However, c-Kit-dependent MC-deficient mouse models have many other abnormalities, because c-Kit is expressed not only by MCs but also by numerous other cells, including hematopoietic progenitor cells. Importantly, c-Kit is essential for osteoclast development and also regulates osteoblast activity (113, 115). Therefore, it is difficult to distinguish the effect of MCs on bone physiology from pleiotropic c-Kit effects in these mouse models.

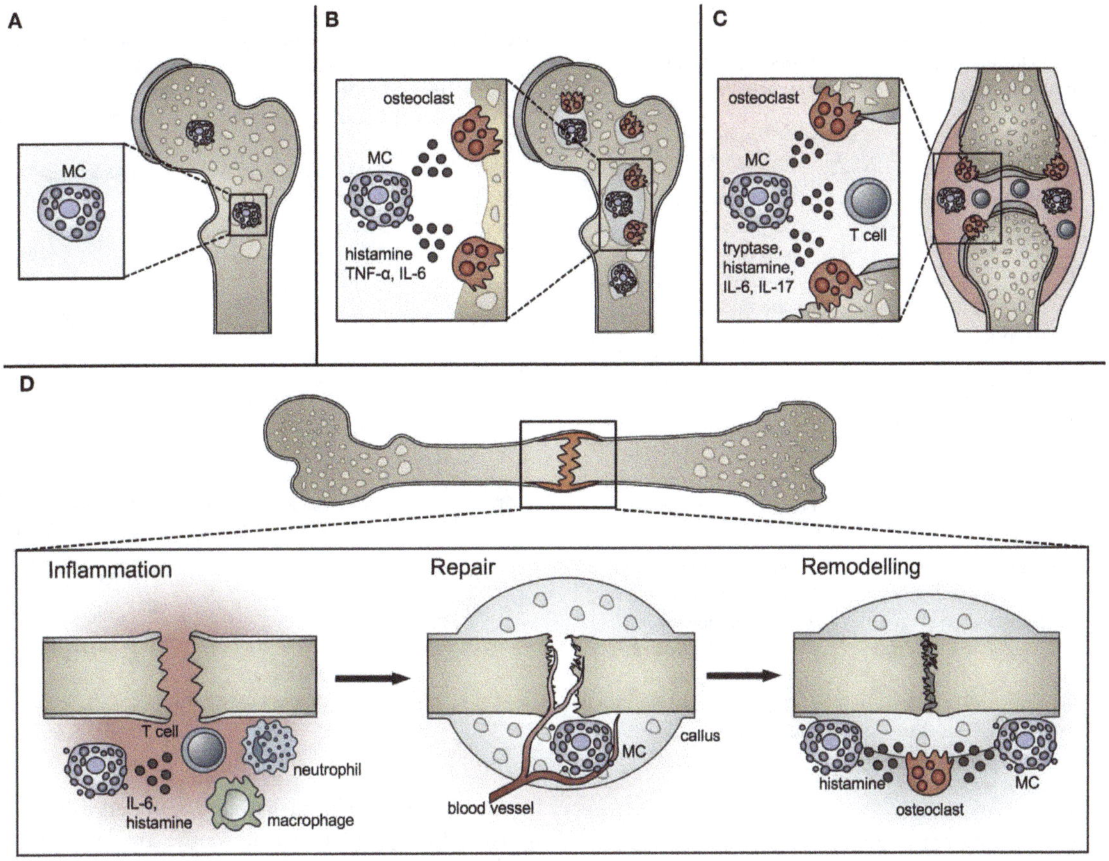

FIGURE 1 | Role of MCs in physiological bone turnover and bone disease. **(A)** In physiological bone turnover, few MCs are located in the bone marrow of the metaphysis, preferentially adjacent to bone surfaces. **(B)** In osteoporotic bone, more MCs are found in the bone marrow which are frequently co-localized with osteoclasts and influence their resorption activity by releasing mediators including histamine, TNF-α and IL-6. **(C)** In rheumatoid arthritis, increased MC numbers and concentrations of MC-mediators including histamine, tryptase, IL-6, and IL-17 are found in the inflamed joint, inducing osteoclastic bone resorption and T-cell driven inflammation. **(D)** In fracture healing, MCs regulate bone-fracture induced inflammation by releasing inflammatory cytokines including IL-6, and influence innate immune cell recruitment. During the repair phase, few MCs are located in the fracture callus mainly near blood vessels; MC numbers increase during callus remodeling, where MCs are found in close proximity to osteoclasts and regulate bone resorption by releasing osteocatabolic mediators including histamine.

In contrast to the above-mentioned studies, our group proposed that MCs do not affect bone formation and turnover under physiological conditions (10). We used the Mcpt-5 Cre R-DTA mouse line, a c-Kit-independent model of MC deficiency expressing diphtheria toxin (DT) under the control of the Mcpt-5 chymase promoter, which is specific for CTMCs and drives Cre-specific ablation of these cells (116). It has been previously proven that these mice specifically lack CTMCs, whereas other immune cell populations are unaffected. Mcpt-5 Cre R-DTA mice have been demonstrated to be useful in elucidating the function of MCs in immune disorders, including contact allergy and RA (9, 116, 117). Therefore, our study may more reliably reflect the role of MCs in bone metabolism than previous investigations (10). We analyzed the bone phenotype in young and adult female and male Mcpt-5 Cre R-DTA mice and compared it to MC-competent mice. The size and shape of the skeleton were not different. We could not detect significant alterations in bone microstructure or osteoblast and osteoclast numbers or activities in MC-deficient mice compared to age- and sex-matched wildtype mice. Bone mass decreased with aging, particularly in the trabecular compartment, both in MC-competent and -deficient mice. These results suggest that MCs might be redundant for physiological bone turnover as well as in age-induced bone loss (**Figure 1A**) (10). However, further studies are needed to elucidate the function of MCs in bone homeostasis. Thereby, other c-Kit-independent mouse models could be used, which were developed to overcome the abnormalities related to c-Kit structure or expression. Feyerabend et al. generated $Cpa3^{Cre/+}$ "Cre-Master" mice by using a knock-in strategy to induce Cre expression under the control of the MC Cpa3 promoter, which yielded deletion of CTMCs and MMCs by a genotoxic Trp53-dependent mechanism. However, Cpa3 is also expressed in basophils, therefore, Cre-Master mice had slightly altered basophil numbers (118). Likewise, another constitutive MC-deficient mouse model Cpa3-Cre; $Mcl\text{-}1^{fl/fl}$ was generated by crossing Cpa3-Cre transgenic mice with mice having a floxed allele of myeloid cell leukemia sequence 1 (Mcl-1). Cpa3-Cre; $Mcl\text{-}1^{fl/fl}$ mice are deficient in both CTMCs and MMCs,

TABLE 1 | Selected MC mediators with effects on bone formation and bone resorption.

Mediators	Bone formation by osteoblasts	Bone resorption by osteoclasts
PRE-FORMED		
Amines		
Histamine	↑ Bone formation after depleting the histamine-producing enzyme (44)	↑ Osteoclast formation and bone resorption (43, 45) ↓ Osteoclast activity and recruitment after histamine blocking (46, 47)
Serotonin	↓ Osteoblast formation (48)	
Enzymes		
Chymase	↑ Bone formation in Mcpt4-deficient mice (49)	
Proteoglycans		
Heparin	↓ Osteoblast formation (50, 51)	↑ Osteoclast formation and bone resorption (52)
Chemokines		
IL-8	↑ Bone formation (53)	↑ Osteoclast formation and bone resorption (54, 55)
MCP-1	↓ Bone formation in MCP-1-deficient mice (56)	↓ Osteoclast formation in MCP-1-deficient mice (57)
Polypeptide		
Renin		↓ Bone resorption after renin inhibition (58)
Substance P	↑ Osteoblast and bone formation (59–61) ↓ Bone formation in the absence of substance P (62)	
Glycoproteins		
Osteopontin		↓ Osteoclast formation and bone resorption in osteopontin-deficient mice (63, 64)
De novo		
Cytokines		
IL-1		↑ Osteoclast formation and bone resorption (65, 66)
IL-1β	↑ Osteoblast formation (67)	↓ Osteoclast formation (68)
IL-4		↓ Osteoclast formation and bone resorption (69–71)
IL-6	↓ Bone formation in IL-6-deficient mice (72) ↑ Bone formation (73, 74)	↑ Osteoclast formation and bone resorption (75, 76)
IL-10	↓ Bone formation in IL-10-deficient mice (77)	↓ Bone resorption (78)
IL-11		↑ Osteoclast formation (79, 80)
IL-13		↓ Osteoclast formation and bone resorption (69)
IL-15	↓ Osteoblast apoptosis (81)	↑ Osteoclast formation (82)
IL-18	↑ Bone formation (83)	↑ Osteoclast formation (84) ↓ Bone resorption (85)
IFN-γ		↑ Osteoclast formation and bone resorption (86) ↓ Osteoclast formation (87–89)
MIP-1α		↑ Osteoclast formation (90)
TNF-α	↓ Osteoblast formation (91)	↑ osteoclast formation and bone resorption (92–94)
TGF-β	↑ Osteoblast and bone formation (95, 96)	↓ Osteoclast formation (97)
Phospholipid metabolites		
Prostaglandin E2	↑ Osteoclast formation and bone resorption (98)	
PAF		↓ Bone resorption in PAF receptor-deficient mice (99)
Growth factors		
FGF	↓ Bone formation in FGF-2-deficient and -overexpressing mice (100, 101)	
GM-CSF	↑ Osteoblast formation (102)	↑ Osteoclast formation (103) ↓ Osteoclast formation (104)
M-CSF		↑ Osteoclast formation (105, 106)
SCF		↑ Osteoclast formation (107)
Nitric oxide		
NO	↓ Bone formation in NO synthase-deficient mice (108)	

but also exhibit reduced basophil numbers (119). In addition to constitutive MC-deficient mouse models, some inducible models are also available. Transgenic Mas-TRECK mice (for Mast cell-specific enhancer mediated Toxin Receptor mediated Conditional cell Knock out) express the human DT receptor (DTR) under the control of an intronic enhancer element of the IL-4 gene, which is essential for IL-4 expression in MCs but not in other immune cells. Repeated intraperitoneal DT injection results in complete MC deletion accompanied by transient blood basophil depletion (120, 121). Recently, Dahdah et al. generated a knock-in mouse model called RMB (Red Mast Cell and Basophil) mice (122). The FcεRI β chain of these mice includes a cassette composed of a sequence coding for the bright red td-Tomato (tdT) fluorescent protein and human DTR, allowing both visualization and conditional ablation of MCs and basophils. Although both basophils and MCs were deleted after DT injections, the authors reported that basophils were fully reconstituted 12 days after DT treatment, whereas MCs remained absent (122). However, to the best of our knowledge, in none of these mouse models have to date the skeletal phenotype or bone turnover been analyzed.

In conclusion, the experimental data regarding a possible regulatory role for MCs in physiological bone turnover are contradictory and dependent on the mouse model used. Therefore, further translational studies on human MCs with respect to their role in bone metabolism are needed. There are no human MC-deficient conditions. However, patients with mastocytosis who display abnormal high MC numbers often suffer from bone disorders (see section Osteoporosis). Analyses of the bone turnover of these patients over their course of treatment (mainly anti-histamine treatment) could provide further insights into MC functions in human bone. Complementary, *in vitro* studies including co-culture models of human MCs derived from healthy individuals and mastocytosis patients and human osteoblasts and osteoclasts could provide deeper mechanistic insights into the interaction of MCs and bone cells in humans.

THE ROLE OF MAST CELLS IN BONE DISORDERS

Osteoporosis

Osteoporosis is a major bone disorder, which is characterized by the deterioration of bone microarchitecture and bone mass reduction. This results from an imbalanced activity of osteoblasts and osteoclasts and leads to an increased fracture risk (123). In Europe, ~20 million people suffer from osteoporosis with an annual incidence of 2.7 million fragility fractures (124). Osteoporosis is categorized into primary and secondary forms. Primary osteoporosis is the most common form, including postmenopausal osteoporosis, which results from a decline in sex hormone levels, and age-related osteoporosis, which gradually develops during aging. Secondary osteoporosis is caused, for example, by drugs (e.g., corticosteroids, barbiturates), comorbidities (e.g., kidney diseases, diabetes, hyperparathyroidism, mastocytosis), and adverse lifestyle and nutrition (e.g., cigarette smoking, alcohol abuse, immobilization, malnutrition) (123, 125). Despite extensive research during recent decades, the pathomechanisms of osteoporosis are still not completely understood. There is evidence that MCs contribute to this multifactorial disease, because increased MC numbers have been found in individuals with bone loss (**Figure 1B**) (5, 6, 40, 126, 127).

Postmenopausal osteoporosis is driven by the decline of estrogen after menopause, which induces increased bone resorption by osteoclasts (128). In 1983, Fallon et al. reported increased numbers of MCs in iliac crest biopsies of females with postmenopausal osteoporosis compared to non-osteoporotic males and females, indicating an involvement of MCs in bone loss (5). Confirming this, other authors similarly observed MC accumulation in bone biopsies of osteoporotic patients compared to healthy controls (6). Interestingly, treatment of postmenopausal females with calcium and promethazine, a blocker of the histamine H1 receptor, significantly increased bone mineral density compared to calcium treatment alone (129). This indicates that histamine, one of the main preformed components in MC granules, could be involved in osteoporotic bone loss (**Figure 1B**). Experimental studies in ovariectomized (OVX) rodents, a common experimental model for postmenopausal bone loss, confirmed the clinical observations. Lesclous and Saffar demonstrated that after OVX-induced estrogen decline the MC numbers in the rat bone marrow were significantly increased (130). The authors further showed that the accumulation of MCs started early and was associated with the increase in osteoclast numbers induced by OVX (131). Confirming this, our group showed that Mcpt-5 Cre R-DTA mice, which lack CTMCs, were protected from OVX-induced bone loss and no increase in osteoclast numbers or activity occurred after OVX (10). Using Mcpt-5 Cre tdRFP MC reporter mice, we further found that after OVX the MCs, and osteoclasts were not only enhanced in number but also frequently co-localized (10). These results are strong indications that MCs may promote osteoclast formation under estrogen-deficient conditions (**Figure 1B**). Confirming this, further *in vitro* studies investigating osteoclast formation under the influence of MC supernatants revealed that estrogen strongly affects MCs and their mediator release (10). When estrogen was present, supernatants derived from MCs that were stimulated with the complement anaphylatoxin C5a, an inducer of MC degranulation, did not enhance osteoclast formation *in vitro* in a preosteoclastic cell line (RAW 264.7 cells) nor in primary bone marrow-derived osteoclast precursors. By contrast, when estrogen was absent, osteoclast formation was induced, suggesting that estrogen has an inhibitory effect on the osteoclast-inducing potential of MCs (10). Indeed, estrogen receptors (ER) are expressed in MCs of various tissues (132, 133) and several groups reported that estrogen influences MC migration, degranulation, and cytokine release (133–138). However, the observed effects are not always consistent. Some authors found that estrogen induces MC degranulation (134, 135), whereas others reported inhibitory effects on the mediator release (136, 137). For example, estrogen did not stimulate the degranulation of MCs derived from ERα knockout mice (134), indicating that estrogen is involved in MC activation via ERα signaling. In agreement with this, estrogen treatment of the human MC line HMC-1 induced the de novo production of tryptase β1 and MC degranulation (135). By contrast, OVX-induced estrogen deficiency reduced MC degranulation in the rat mammary gland (137), and Kim et al. showed that estrogen treatment diminished the *in vitro* release of MC cytokines, including TNF-α and IL-6 (136). Therefore, the effects of estrogen on MC degranulation and mediator release appear to depend on the tissue investigated and the experimental model used.

MCs may also play a role in the development of age-related osteoporosis, the second type of primary osteoporosis, because Frame and Nixon already in 1968 described that MC numbers were increased in bone marrow aspirates of aged female and male patients with reduced bone mineral density compared to healthy controls (126). Because both males and females are affected by age-related osteoporosis, MCs appear to also provoke estrogen-independent osteoclastogenic effects. This is supported by the observation that MCs also play a role in secondary forms of osteoporosis. Most of these indications arise from mastocytosis, a disease characterized by abnormally high MC numbers in one or more organ (139). The clinical picture is categorized into cutaneous mastocytosis, which is restricted to the skin, and systemic mastocytosis (SM), where high MC numbers infiltrate the skin and/or one internal organ, for example, the gastrointestinal tract, bone marrow, lymph nodes, liver, and spleen (139). Mastocytosis is caused by gain-of-function point mutations within the SCF/c-Kit signaling axis, most prominently D816V (140), resulting in a constitutively active c-Kit receptor. This leads to increased MC proliferation, maturation, survival, and activity (141). The boost of released mediators, mainly of histamine and pro-inflammatory cytokines, and excessive MC infiltration cause mild to severe organ-specific symptoms, including flushing, syncope, anaphylactic shock, diarrhea, vomiting, ascites, and hypertension. The clinical picture of SM is very heterogeneous, ranging from indolent to aggressive forms with severe organ dysfunctions (139). Of note, ~50% of patients display a skeletal involvement (142). Several case studies and small clinical trials described a reduced bone mass and an increased fracture occurrence in patients with MC accumulation in the bone marrow (143–146). Larger cohort studies confirmed the high prevalence of osteoporosis (up to ~60%), and fragility fractures (up to ~40%) in SM patients (147–150), as recently reviewed in more detail by Greene et al. (151). The pathomechanisms of MC-induced bone loss are not yet fully understood. Seitz et al. found increased osteoblast and osteoclast numbers in patients with indolent SM, indicating a high bone turnover status (152). Confirming this, bone formation and resorption markers were found to be increased in SM patients (153). However, other authors reported increased serum levels of dickkopf 1 and sclerostin, both inhibitors of the osteoanabolic Wnt signaling pathway, indicating reduced bone formation (154, 155). IL-6 levels are also increased in SM, and correlate with the severity of the symptoms and bone loss (155, 156). The existing data on tryptase levels, a marker for MC activity, in SM are inconsistent. Many authors describe increased concentrations, which correlate with reduced bone mass, whereas others report normal levels despite bone loss (148, 150, 155).

MCs appear also to be involved in secondary bone loss induced by malnutrition or immobilization. Urist et al. observed an accumulation of MCs in osteoporotic bones of rats fed a calcium-deficient diet (40). Additionally, in bone loss caused by the unloading of the hind-limbs in rats, MC numbers were significantly increased (127). These results indicate that MCs may regulate osteoclast activity independently from endocrine dysregulation or inflammatory stimuli. Confirming this, male patients suffering from idiopathic osteoporosis also displayed higher numbers of MCs that were highly organized in clusters in biopsies of the bone marrow. In these patients, the urine N-methylhistamine concentration, a marker for increased MC activity, correlated with the reduced bone mineral density (157).

The above-mentioned clinical and experimental studies suggest that MCs may be involved in osteoporosis development by promoting osteoclast formation (**Figure 1B**). The question arises as to which MC mediators are mainly responsible for the observed osteoclast-stimulating effects. There are many possible candidates, including histamine, heparin, TNF, IL-6, and receptor activator of nuclear factor kappa B ligand (RANKL), as listed in **Table 1**. One of the main components in preformed MC granules is histamine, which was already shown to be associated with bone resorption in RA (158). Furthermore, in patients with SM, histamine levels were reported to predict osteoporotic manifestations (144, 147). Confirming this, histamine-deficient mice displayed an increased bone mass because of reduced osteoclast numbers and were also completely protected from OVX-induced bone loss (44). Lesclous et al. injected histamine receptor blockers in OVX rats, which prevented the OVX-induced bone loss by reducing osteoclast numbers (45, 159). In the above-mentioned study of our group (10), osteoclast formation and activity were studied *in vitro* in the presence of supernatants harvested from MC cultures stimulated with C5a (induces the release of preformed granule-stored mediators). Notably, the blockade of the histamine H1 receptor abolished osteoclast formation by MC supernatants, indicating that histamine may play a crucial role in MC-mediated osteoclast activity (10). This is confirmed by the already above-mentioned clinical study, which demonstrated that the blockade of the histamine H1 receptor with promethazine significantly increased bone mineral density in postmenopausal women (129). However, our experimental data also showed that histamine alone supported osteoclast formation but not their resorption activity (10). This indicates that histamine is not the only MC-derived factor involved in osteoclast activation and that MC-osteoclast interaction might be much more complex.

Rheumatoid Arthritis

RA is a systemic autoimmune disease affecting around 1% of the population, which is associated with a chronic joint inflammation (160, 161). The inflamed joint is characterized by a massive infiltration of immune cells, extensive hyperplasia of synovial macrophages and fibroblasts and thickening of the synovial membrane. The unrestrained inflammatory response leads to the formation of an invasive structure, calles synovial pannus, which finally causes cartilage destruction and bone erosions. The clinical picture is characterized by swelling, pain, and stiffness of the affected joints (160). The pathogenesis of RA is complex and still not entirely known. In addition to other immune cell populations, MCs have been suggested to play a crucial role, because MCs are abundant in inflamed synovial joints of RA patients, especially around blood vessels in the synovial sub-lining, at the cartilage-pannus junction at sites of cartilage erosions, and in joint fluid (**Figure 1C**) [comprehensively reviewed by Rivellese et al. (162)]. Importantly, some of the clinical studies observed a correlation of MC numbers with joint inflammation and disease activity (163–167). In addition, the levels of MC mediators, including histamine and tryptase, were significantly increased in the synovial tissue of RA patients (**Figure 1C**) (8, 168, 169). Therefore, these studies support MC involvement in the pathogenesis of RA.

In agreement with this, MCs are highly responsive to the inflammatory milieu in the synovial joint. For example, they are stimulated by IL-33 and IL-6 (170, 171). Moreover, it has been shown that synovial MCs can be activated by immune complexes, auto-antibodies and complement factors as well as by direct cross-linking of Fc-receptors (172–175). MCs might contribute to the pathogenesis of RA by different mechanisms, which were reviewed in detail by other authors (12–14). Briefly, synovial MCs can rapidly release and produce inflammatory cytokines and chemokines and thus contribute to joint inflammation and immune cell recruitment. For example, MC-derived IL-1 is involved in the initiation of autoantibody-mediated arthritis (176), and activated MCs in human synovial tissue produce TNF-α, IL-1β, and IL-1 receptor antagonist (177). Additionally, MC-derived proteases may play important roles in cartilage and bone breakdown. Histological analysis of inflamed joint specimens showed abundant MC tryptase present in areas of cartilage destruction (178). Supporting these findings, mice deficient in Mcpt-6 or Mcpt-7 displayed an attenuated disease activity and reduced bone and cartilage destruction (179). Similarly, mice lacking the MC chymase Mcpt-4, showed a reduced joint inflammation and pannus formation, diminished cartilage destruction probably due to a reduction in MMP-2 and MMP-9 (180). Of note, the joints of Mcpt-4 deficient mice displayed less infiltrates of MCs and mononuclear cells implicating a crucial role of this MC chymase in disease progression (180). Importantly, some MC mediators, including histamine, TNF-α, IL-6, IL-11, and IFN-γ, have the capacity to increase osteoclast activity (see **Table 1**), and thus may contribute to bone erosion in RA. Indeed, increased levels of RANKL, which is also secreted by MCs, were found in the synovial tissue of RA patients (181, 182).

The specific role of MCs in RA was investigated in different mouse models of MC deficiency. However, these studies revealed contradictory results, depending on the MC-deficient mouse strain and the respective model of RA induction. Rivellese et al. recently reviewed these animal studies in detail (183). Briefly, $Kit^{W/W-v}$ mice were protected from K/BxN serum-induced arthritis (serum from K/BxN mice contains autoantibodies against glucose-6-phosphate isomerase) (184, 185). However, $Kit^{W/Wv}$ mice are fully susceptible to collagen-induced arthritis (CIA), which is induced by the injection of type II collagen in Freund's adjuvant (186). By contrast, another MC-deficient $Kit^{W-sh/W-sh}$ mouse line developed arthritis induced by K/BxN serum as well as CIA (187, 188). However, as already mentioned, Kit-mutant mice exhibit severe alterations of the immune system beyond the MC-deficiency, which may possibly account for the inconsistent outcomes of these studies. Furthermore, the arthritis models used differ in their mechanisms of disease induction. In the CIA model, joint inflammation is induced by autoreactive effector T cells, while in the K/BxN model, immune cell infiltrations and activation is stimulated by the transferred autoantibodies thereby bypassing the T cell response (183).

c-Kit-independent MC-deficient $Cpa3^{Cre/+}$ and Mcpt-5 Cre iDTR mice were not protected from K/BxN serum-induced arthritis (9, 118). However, Mcpt-5 Cre iDTR mice displayed reduced arthritis severity in CIA, indicating that MCs contribute to arthritis induction or progression by affecting the T cell arm of adaptive immunity (9, 118). Interestingly, in CIA, Mcpt-5 Cre iDTR mice showed reduced CD4+ and CD8+ T cell numbers in the lymph nodes draining the site of immunization accompanied by reduced IFN-γ and IL-17 production (**Figure 1C**). These results indicate that MCs may regulate T cell expansion and polarization to Thl and Th17 effector cells in T cell-driven RA (9). Supporting these findings, the depletion of MCs during the early preclinical phase of CIA decreased joint inflammation in another model of c-Kit-independent inducible MC-deficiency, the RMB mouse. Similarly, numbers of CD4+ T cells, in particular IL-17 producing T cells, and serum levels of IL-6 and IL-17 were reduced also here (189). Additionally, in a pharmacological approach in wildtype mice, in which MCs were inhibited using salbutamol and cromolyn, RA development was diminished as indicated by reduced ankle swelling, joint inflammation, and bone destruction (185). Collectively, data of the CIA model demonstrate an important pro-inflammatory role of MCs in the onset of RA by promoting the expansion of autoreactive T cells and the T cell-driven inflammation (**Figure 1C**), whereas in the later disease phase, MCs may have redundant functions as implicated by most of the K/BxN studies. However, more studies are required to further decipher the specific role of MCs in RA-associated joint inflammation and bone resorption.

Interestingly, it has been shown that MCs may also play a role in OA, in which joint destruction is mainly caused by degeneration, abnormal high loads, or traumatic injuries (190), and driven by an increased inflammatory response (191). Several clinical studies reported increased MC numbers in the synovial tissue of OA patients and/or elevated histamine or tryptase levels in the synovial fluid (7, 192–196). Gene cluster analysis revealed increased expression of genes involved in MC differentiation and activity (*c-KIT*, tryptase genes *TPSAB1*, and *TPSAB2)* in the synovial membranes of OA patients (196). Interestingly, two different MC-deficient mouse lines, the c-Kit-dependent $Kit^{W-sh/W-sh}$ line and the Kit-independent $Cpa3^{Cre}$; $Mcl\text{-}1^{fl/fl}$ mice, were protected from OA as demonstrated by reduced inflammation and cartilage destruction, while MC engraftment reversed the protective effects in both mouse lines (196). Furthermore, the inhibition of tryptase activity in wildtype mice prevented OA and reduced the concentrations of the pro-inflammatory and proteolytic mediators, e.g., IL-6, IL-1β, IL-8, and MMP-3. The authors further showed that in OA, MCs are activated via the IgE/FcεRI receptor axis (196). Another study showed that synovial MCs from OA patients produce TNF-α upon stimulation via the high-affinity receptor for IgG (174). These results indicate an important role of MCs in OA development. In support of these findings, a cross-sectional cohort study showed that the usage of Hlanti-histamine treatment correlated with decreased OA prevalence (197), suggesting that MCs could potentially be a therapeutic target in OA, but this needs to be clarified in further studies.

Bone Fracture Healing

The immune system plays a major role in bone repair, because the healing process begins with an acute immune response locally at the fracture site (207, 208). In addition, conditions of acute orresults indicate that MCs may regul chronic inflammation, including poly-trauma, osteoporosis, and RA, negatively impact the fracture healing outcome (207). Bone fracture leads to the rupture of blood vessels and to tissue and cell damage, resulting in the formation of a hematoma, which is characterized by hypoxia, low pH, high lactate levels, as well as high concentrations of inflammatory mediators that attract cells of the innate immune response. First, neutrophils invade the fracture hematoma. They secrete further cytokines, including chemokine (C-X-C motif) ligand 1 (CXCL1) and IL-1β, which attract other immune cells, mainly macrophages. These cells further phagocytize cell and tissue debris and pathogens. Subsequently, T and B cells arrive and initiate adaptive immune responses. Consequently, angiogenesis starts, ensuring debris removal, nutrient and oxygen supply, and the recruitment of mesenchymal stem cells (MSCs). Recruited MCSs initiate the repair phase, where in the process of endochondral healing, first a cartilaginous soft callus is generated that is converted into a hard bony trabecular callus. The bony

TABLE 2 | Experimental studies investigating MC appearance and function in fracture healing.

References	Model	Treatment	Main results
Lindholm et al. (198)	White rats (m/f), tibia fracture	–	Progressive MC accumulation in the periosteal callus; MCs decreased during callus remodeling
Lindholm et al. (199)	White rats (m/f), tibia fracture	17-hydroxy-corticosterone	Progressive MC accumulation in the periosteal callus; delayed healing due to treatment affected MC morphology in size, granulation, and staining
Lindholm et al. (200)	White rats (m/f), tibia fracture	Somatotropin and thyrotropin	Progressive MC accumulation in the periostal callus; improved healing due to treatment led to earlier MC accumulation
Lindholm and Lindholm (201)	Rabbits (m/f), forearm fracture	–	MCs more abundant in the periosteal callus compared to the endosteal callus
Taniguchi (41)	Wistar rats (m), bilateral tibia fracture	–	Few MCs near blood vessels and in the marrow of the early endosteal callus; MCs increase in the late periosteal callus and peak during remodeling
Banovac et al. (202)	Sprague-Dawley rats (f), femur fracture	NSAIDs	Few MCs near blood vessels and cartilage of the early endosteal callus; MC accumulation near osteoclastic bone resorption during late remodeling; NSAIDs delayed healing and MC appearance
Meyer et al. (203)	Sprague-Dawley rats (f), femur fracture	–	Microarray analysis revealed increased MC marker activity from weeks 2 to 4 after fracture in all age groups
Behrends et al. (11)	MC-deficient $Kit^{W-sh/W-sh}$, C57BL/6J mice, femoral cortical window defect	–	Disturbed healing in MC-deficient mice: ↓ Cortical bridging, bone content, endothelial cells, macrophages; ↑ TRAP+ cells
Ramirez-GarciaLuna et al. (204)	MC-deficient $Cpa3^{Cre/+}$ and C57BL/6J mice (m/f), femoral cortical window defect	–	MCs appeared in the connective tissue and marrow of the defect; Disturbed healing in MC-deficient mice: ↓ Cortical bridging, bone content, vascularization, bone mineralization, osteoclasts
Kroner et al. (10)	MC-deficient Mcpt-5 Cre+/− R-DTA mice (m), femur fracture	–	MCs increase in the periostal callus near newly formed bony trabeculae and osteoclastic bone resorption sites; Disturbed healing in MC-deficient mice: ↓ Local and systemic inflammation (cytokine release, immune cell recruitment); ↑ bone content; ↓ osteoclastic remodeling
Zhang et al. (205)	C57BL/6J, Mcpt-5 Cre YFP, Mcpt-5 Cre iDTR mice (m/f), cranial window defect	rPTH, SC	MC inhibition (SC) and deficiency (Mcpt-5 Cre iDTR): ↑ Healing, ↓ arteriogenesis; rPTH: ↓ MCs in the inflammatory phase by acting on osteoblasts releasing anti-MC factors
Hebb et al. (206)	C57BL/6 (m/f), bilateral tibia fracture	–	Microarray analysis revealed increased MC prevalence in younger compared to older mice

callus is finally remodeled to the original bone shape (207, 209). Studies have shown that certain immune cell populations, including neutrophils, macrophages, but also B and T cells, essentially contribute to successful bone repair, because their absence or disturbed function resulted in disrupted fracture healing (210–212). This might also be true for MCs. Indeed, some older phenomenological studies described MC appearance in bone repair, while more recent studies using different MC-deficient models also revealed some specific MC functions. The few existing studies that explored MCs in fracture healing are summarized in **Table 2**.

The presence of MCs during fracture healing was already described in 1967 by the group of Lindholm using a rat tibial fracture model. The authors showed that MC numbers progressively increase in the periostal fracture callus, followed by a decline during callus remodeling (198). In further investigations of experimentally delayed or accelerated fracture healing, the same group observed alterations in MC accumulation, morphology, and degranulation (199, 200). On the basis of these results, the authors concluded that MC invasion and degranulation are essential for endochondral bone formation and mineralization. The presence of MCs in the periostal callus was further confirmed in a rabbit fracture model (201). Two later studies confirmed MC accumulation during fracture healing and both described only a few MCs during the early healing phase, mainly around blood vessels and in the bone marrow cavity of the endosteal callus (41, 202). In the later healing phases, increasing MC numbers were observed in the marrow of the newly formed periostal callus, particularly next to newly formed bony trabeculae. Both studies found the highest numbers of MCs in close proximity to osteoclasts and bone resorption sites during the callus-remodeling phase and suggested that MCs might contribute to callus remodeling by influencing osteoclast activity (41, 202). Furthermore, microarray analysis of a rat femoral fracture callus found increased MC marker gene expression, including the MC *tryptase* $\beta 1$ and *Cpa3* from weeks 2 to 4 after fracture (203). In addition, a recent microarray analysis of a tibial fracture callus of young and old C57Bl/6 mice found a higher MC occurrence in younger mice compared to old mice evaluated by cell type enrichment analysis, showing higher MC *IgE* gene expression in young mice (206). On the basis of the above-mentioned studies, the presence and accumulation of MC is the fracture callus is clear (**Figure 1D**).

To elucidate MC functions, Behrends et al. investigated bone repair in an uni-cortical window defect of MC-deficient $Kit^{W-sh/W-sh}$ mice (11). Interestingly, MC-deficient $Kit^{W-sh/W-sh}$ mice displayed a delayed healing with reduced bone quality because of an impaired transformation of woven into lamellar bone. The authors further observed diminished endothelial cell numbers, but increased numbers of osteoclasts, and suggested that healing was impaired because of disturbed revascularization and increased osteocatabolic activity (11). However, these results were obtained in a c-Kit-dependent mouse model, from which it is known that also osteoclasts and other immune cells are affected (113, 115). This could have influenced the outcome. Investigations of bone repair in a cortical window defect in a c-Kit-independent $Cpa3^{Cre/+}$ mouse model found impaired bone regeneration, as confirmed by reduced cortical bridging, vascularization, and bone mineralization. The authors further observed diminished osteoclast activity at earlier stages, but increased osteoclast activity in the late healing phase (204). Therefore, MC functions in bone repair may comprise blood vessel formation as well as anabolic and catabolic processes during fracture repair and remodeling (**Figure 1D**). However, it was shown that Cpa3 is also expressed in basophils and some T cells (109), which needs to be considered when interpreting these results. Overcoming these drawbacks, our group recently investigated the functions of MCs in bone repair in MC-deficient Mcpt-5 Cre R-DTA mice, which lack CTMCs without affecting other immune cell populations (116, 213). Interestingly, we found reduced levels of pro-inflammatory cytokines, including IL-6, IL-1β, and CXCL1, locally in the early fracture callus, but also systemically, and a reduced recruitment of neutrophils and macrophages to the fracture site in the absence of MCs (10). These results indicate a strong contribution of MCs to fracture-induced systemic inflammation and to the inflammatory mediator and cell milieu at the fracture site (**Figure 1D**). MC-mediated neutrophil recruitment was already described during acute inflammation, including bacteria-induced pneumonia and ischemic-induced gut injury, as well as in inflammatory diseases such as meningitis and periodontitis, contributing to the disease onset and progression (214, 215). During the later healing stage, we found an increased bone content of the fracture callus in MC-deficient Mcpt-5 Cre R-DTA mice (10). Further histomorphometric analysis revealed no changes in osteoblast parameters, however, osteoclast numbers and activity were significantly reduced in the fracture callus of Mcpt-5 Cre R-DTA mice (10). These results indicate that MCs may mediate callus remodeling by regulating osteoclast activity (**Figure 1D**). As indicated earlier in the osteoporosis chapter, MC-derived histamine might be one mechanism contributing to increased osteoclastic bone resorption. Supporting our experimental outcomes, Zhang et al. investigated bone repair in a cranial window defect model in MC-deficient Mcpt-5 Cre iDTA mice, and found accelerated defect closure and impaired angiogenesis in the absence of MCs (205). They observed the same effects by inhibiting MCs in wildtype mice using cromolyn, and suggested that MCs may be negative regulators of bone repair (205).

Concluding, several studies demonstrated MC accumulation in the periostal fracture callus during the healing process. More recent experimental studies also revealed possible functions of MCs in fracture healing, including the regulation of the immune response toward fracture and of angiogenesis as well as anabolic and catabolic effects during the repair and remodeling processes (**Figure 1D**).

CONCLUSION

The important role of MCs in allergic reactions has been known for several decades. However, the involvement of MCs in physiological bone turnover and bone disorders has been described only recently in more detail. As reviewed here, MCs secrete several mediators that are known to regulate bone formation and resorption, including histamine, IL-6, and TNF. Experimental data on the role of MCs in physiological bone turnover are contradictory and depend on the mouse model used. However, the involvement of MCs in various pathological skeletal conditions is clear, particularly in osteoporosis and RA. MCs may also regulate the fracture healing process by influencing the inflammatory response, angiogenesis, bone formation, and osteoclastogenesis (**Figure 1**). Osteoclastogenesis might be mainly, but not solely, regulated by MC-derived histamine. Further mechanistic investigations are required to elucidate MC functions in physiological and pathological conditions in bone. In consequence of the involvement of MCs in bone disorders, MC targeting drugs such as histamine H1 receptor blockers should be further tested for their therapeutic potential to treat osteoporosis, inflammatory bone disorders or disturbed bone repair.

AUTHOR CONTRIBUTIONS

All authors listed have made a substantial, direct and intellectual contribution to the work, and approved it for publication.

FUNDING

The cited work of the authors' own groups was supported by the German Research Foundation (Collaborative Research Center CRC1149, INST 40/491-2, and by the Priority Program SPP1468, DU1172/4-1), and by the Elsbeth-Bonhof-Foundation (P186).

ACKNOWLEDGMENTS

We acknowledge the help of Robert Blakytny in correcting the English language.

REFERENCES

1. Galli SJ, Tsai M. IgE and mast cells in allergic disease. *Nat Med.* (2012) 18:693–704. doi: 10.1038/nm.2755
2. Krystel-Whittemore M, Dileepan KN, Wood JG. Mast cell: a multi-functional master cell. *Front Immunol.* (2015) 6:620. doi: 10.3389/fimmu.2015.00620
3. Wernersson S, Pejler G. Mast cell secretory granules: armed for battle. *Nat Rev Immunol.* (2014) 14:478–94. doi: 10.1038/nri3690
4. Pietschmann P, Mechtcheriakova D, Meshcheryakova A, Foger-Samwald U, Ellinger I. Immunology of osteoporosis: a mini-review. *Gerontology.* (2016) 62:128–37. doi: 10.1159/000431091
5. Fallon MD, Whyte MP, Craig RB Jr, Teitelbaum SL. Mast-cell proliferation in postmenopausal osteoporosis. *Calcif Tissue Int.* (1983) 35:29–31. doi: 10.1007/BF02405002
6. McKenna MJ. Histomorphometric study of mast cells in normal bone, osteoporosis and mastocytosis using a new stain. *Calcif Tissue Int.* (1994) 55:257–9. doi: 10.1007/BF00310402
7. Bridges AJ, Malone DG, Jicinsky J, Chen M, Ory P, Engber W, et al. Human synovial mast cell involvement in rheumatoid arthritis and osteoarthritis. Relationship to disease type, clinical activity, and antirheumatic therapy. *Arthritis Rheum.* (1991) 34:1116–24. doi: 10.1002/art.1780340907
8. Buckley MG, Walters C, Wong WM, Cawley MI, Ren S, Schwartz LB, et al. Mast cell activation in arthritis: detection of alpha- and beta-tryptase, histamine and eosinophil cationic protein in synovial fluid. *Clin Sci.* (1997) 93:363–70. doi: 10.1042/cs0930363
9. Schubert N, Dudeck J, Liu P, Karutz A, Speier S, Maurer M, et al. Mast cell promotion of T cell-driven antigen-induced arthritis despite being dispensable for antibody-induced arthritis in which T cells are bypassed. *Arthritis Rheumatol.* (2015) 67:903–13. doi: 10.1002/art.38996
10. Kroner J, Kovtun A, Kemmler J, Messmann JJ, Strauss G, Seitz S, et al. Mast cells are critical regulators of bone fracture-induced inflammation and osteoclast formation and activity. *J Bone Miner Res.* (2017) 32:2431–44. doi: 10.1002/jbmr.3234
11. Behrends DA, Cheng L, Sullivan MB, Wang MH, Roby GB, Zayed N, et al. Defective bone repair in mast cell deficient mice with c-Kit loss of function. *Eur Cell Mater.* (2014) 28, 209–21; discussion 221–02. doi: 10.22203/eCM.v028a14
12. Nigrovic PA, Lee DM. Mast cells in inflammatory arthritis. *Arthritis Res Ther.* (2005) 7:1–11. doi: 10.1186/ar1446
13. Eklund KK. Mast cells in the pathogenesis of rheumatic diseases and as potential targets for anti-rheumatic therapy. *Immunol Rev.* (2007) 217:38–52. doi: 10.1111/j.1600-065X.2007.00504.x
14. Suurmond J, van der Velden D, Kuiper J, Bot I, Toes RE. Mast cells in rheumatic disease. *Eur J Pharmacol.* (2016) 778:116–24. doi: 10.1016/j.ejphar.2015.03.085
15. Dahlin JS, Hallgren J. Mast cell progenitors: origin, development and migration to tissues. *Mol Immunol.* (2015) 63:9–17. doi: 10.1016/j.molimm.2014.01.018
16. Gurish MF, Austen KF. Developmental origin and functional specialization of mast cell subsets. *Immunity.* (2012) 37:25–33. doi: 10.1016/j.immuni.2012.07.003
17. Okayama Y, Kawakami T. Development, migration, and survival of mast cells. *Immunol Res.* (2006) 34:97–115. doi: 10.1385/IR:34:2:97
18. Yong LC. The mast cell: origin, morphology, distribution, and function. *Exp Toxicol Pathol.* (1997) 49:409–24. doi: 10.1016/S0940-2993(97)80129-7
19. Caughey GH. Mast cell tryptases and chymases in inflammation and host defense. *Immunol Rev.* (2007) 217:141–54. doi: 10.1111/j.1600-065X.2007.00509.x
20. Dai H, Korthuis RJ. Mast cell proteases and inflammation. *Drug Discov Today Dis Models.* (2011) 8:47–55. doi: 10.1016/j.ddmod.2011.06.004
21. Marshall JS, Jawdat DM. Mast cells in innate immunity. *J Allergy Clin Immunol.* (2004) 114:21–7. doi: 10.1016/j.jaci.2004.04.045
22. Metcalfe DD, Baram D, Mekori YA. Mast cells. *Physiol Rev.* (1997) 77:1033–79. doi: 10.1152/physrev.1997.77.4.1033
23. Reber LL, Sibilano R, Mukai K, Galli SJ. Potential effector and immunoregulatory functions of mast cells in mucosal immunity. *Mucosal Immunol.* (2015) 8:444–63. doi: 10.1038/mi.2014.131
24. Pejler G, Ronnberg E, Waern I, Wernersson S. Mast cell proteases: multifaceted regulators of inflammatory disease. *Blood.* (2010) 115:4981–90. doi: 10.1182/blood-2010-01-257287
25. Theoharides TC, Alysandratos KD, Angelidou A, Delivanis DA, Sismanopoulos N, Zhang B, et al. Mast cells and inflammation. *Biochim Biophys Acta.* (2012) 1822:21–33. doi: 10.1016/j.bbadis.2010.12.014
26. Saito H, Ishizaka T, Ishizaka K. Mast cells and IgE: from history to today. *Allergol Int.* (2013) 62:3–12. doi: 10.2332/allergolint.13-RAI-0537
27. da Silva EZ, Jamur MC, Oliver C. Mast cell function: a new vision of an old cell. *J Histochem Cytochem.* (2014) 62:698–738. doi: 10.1369/0022155414545334
28. Galli SJ, Tsai M. Mast cells: versatile regulators of inflammation, tissue remodeling, host defense and homeostasis. *J Dermatol Sci.* (2008) 49:7–19. doi: 10.1016/j.jdermsci.2007.09.009
29. St. John AL, Abraham SN. Innate immunity and its regulation by mast cells. *J Immunol.* (2013) 190:4458–63. doi: 10.4049/jimmunol.1203420
30. McCurdy JD, Olynych TJ, Maher LH, Marshall JS. Cutting edge: distinct Toll-like receptor 2 activators selectively induce different classes of mediator production from human mast cells. *J Immunol.* (2003) 170:1625–9. doi: 10.4049/jimmunol.170.4.1625
31. Urb M, Sheppard DC. The role of mast cells in the defence against pathogens. *PLoS Pathog.* (2012) 8:e1002619. doi: 10.1371/journal.ppat.1002619
32. Maltby S, Khazaie K, McNagny KM. Mast cells in tumor growth: angiogenesis, tissue remodelling and immune-modulation. *Biochim Biophys Acta.* (2009) 1796:19–26. doi: 10.1016/j.bbcan.2009.02.001
33. Norrby K. Mast cells and angiogenesis. *APMIS.* (2002) 110:355–71. doi: 10.1034/j.1600-0463.2002.100501.x
34. Rauter I, Krauth MT, Westritschnig K, Horak F, Flicker S, Gieras A, et al. Mast cell-derived proteases control allergic inflammation through cleavage of IgE. *J Allergy Clin Immunol.* (2008) 121:197–202. doi: 10.1016/j.jaci.2007.08.015
35. Noli C, Miolo A. The mast cell in wound healing. *Vet Dermatol.* (2001) 12:303–13. doi: 10.1046/j.0959-4493.2001.00272.x
36. Ng MF. The role of mast cells in wound healing. *Int Wound J.* (2010) 7:55–61. doi: 10.1111/j.1742-481X.2009.00651.x
37. Wulff BC, Wilgus TA. Mast cell activity in the healing wound: more than meets the eye? *Exp Dermatol.* (2013) 22:507–10. doi: 10.1111/exd.12169
38. Wulff BC, Parent AE, Meleski MA, DiPietro LA, Schrementi ME, Wilgus TA. Mast cells contribute to scar formation during fetal wound healing. *J Invest Dermatol.* (2012) 132:458–65. doi: 10.1038/jid.2011.324
39. Weller K, Foitzik K, Paus R, Syska W, Maurer M. Mast cells are required for normal healing of skin wounds in mice. *FASEB J.* (2006) 20:2366–8. doi: 10.1096/fj.06-5837fje
40. Urist MR, McLean FC. Accumulation of mast cells in endosteum of bones of calcium-deficient rats. *AMA Arch Pathol.* (1957) 63:239–51.
41. Taniguchi H. Mast cells in fracture healing: an experimental study using rat model. *Nihon Seikeigeka Gakkai Zasshi.* (1990) 64:949–57.
42. Turner RT, Iwaniec UT, Marley K, Sibonga JD. The role of mast cells in parathyroid bone disease. *J Bone Miner Res.* (2010) 25:1637–49. doi: 10.1002/jbmr.49
43. Biosse-Duplan M, Baroukh B, Dy M, de Vernejoul MC, Saffar JL. Histamine promotes osteoclastogenesis through the differential expression of histamine receptors on osteoclasts and osteoblasts. *Am J Pathol.* (2009) 174:1426–34. doi: 10.2353/ajpath.2009.080871
44. Fitzpatrick LA, Buzas E, Gagne TJ, Nagy A, Horvath C, Ferencz V, et al. Targeted deletion of histidine decarboxylase gene in mice increases bone formation and protects against ovariectomy-induced bone loss. *Proc Natl Acad Sci USA.* (2003) 100:6027–32. doi: 10.1073/pnas.0934373100
45. Lesclous P, Schramm F, Gallina S, Baroukh B, Guez D, Saffar JL. Histamine mediates osteoclastic resorption only during the acute phase of bone loss in ovariectomized rats. *Exp Physiol.* (2006) 91:561–70. doi: 10.1113/expphysiol.2006.033217
46. Dobigny C, Saffar JL. H1 and H2 histamine receptors modulate osteoclastic resorption by different pathways: evidence obtained by using receptor antagonists in a rat

synchronized resorption model. *J Cell Physiol.* (1997) 173:10–8. doi: 10.1002/(SICI)1097-4652(199710)173:1<10::AID-JCP2>3.0.CO;2-M

47. Fouilloux I, Duplan MB, Baroukh B, Cherruau M, Saffar JL, Lesclous P. Mast cell activation and degranulation occur early during induction of periosteal bone resorption. *Bone.* (2006) 38:59–66. doi: 10.1016/j.bone.2005.07.026
48. Yadav VK, Ryu JH, Suda N, Tanaka KF, Gingrich JA, Schutz G, et al. Lrp5 controls bone formation by inhibiting serotonin synthesis in the duodenum. *Cell.* (2008) 135:825–37. doi: 10.1016/j.cell.2008.09.059
49. Lind T, Gustafson AM, Calounova G, Hu L, Rasmusson A, Jonsson KB, et al. Increased bone mass in female mice lacking mast cell chymase. *PLoS ONE.* (2016) 11:e0167964. doi: 10.1371/journal.pone.0167964
50. Osip SL, Butcher M, Young E, Yang L, Shaughnessy SG. Differential effects of heparin and low molecular weight heparin on osteoblastogenesis and adipogenesis *in vitro*. *Thromb Haemost.* (2004) 92:803–10. doi: 10.1160/TH04-03-0199
51. Xia J, Sheng W, Pei L, Li N, Zhang Z, Wang J, et al. Effects of unfractionated heparin and rivaroxaban on the expression of heparanase and fibroblast growth factor 2 in human osteoblasts. *Mol Med Rep.* (2017) 16:361–6. doi: 10.3892/mmr.2017.6570
52. Li B, Lu D, Chen Y, Zhao M, Zuo L. Unfractionated heparin promotes osteoclast formation *in vitro* by inhibiting osteoprotegerin activity. *Int J Mol Sci.* (2016) 17:613. doi: 10.3390/ijms17040613
53. Yang A, Lu Y, Xing J, Li Z, Yin X, Dou C, et al. IL-8 enhances therapeutic effects of BMSCs on bone regeneration via CXCR2-mediated PI3k/Akt signaling pathway. *Cell Physiol Biochem.* (2018) 48:361–70. doi: 10.1159/000491742
54. Bendre MS, Montague DC, Peery T, Akel NS, Gaddy D, Suva LJ. Interleukin-8 stimulation of osteoclastogenesis and bone resorption is a mechanism for the increased osteolysis of metastatic bone disease. *Bone.* (2003) 33:28–37. doi: 10.1016/S8756-3282(03)00086-3
55. Kopesky P, Tiedemann K, Alkekhia D, Zechner C, Millard B, Schoeberl B, et al. Autocrine signaling is a key regulatory element during osteoclastogenesis. *Biol Open.* (2014) 3:767–76. doi: 10.1242/bio.20148128
56. Ishikawa M, Ito H, Kitaori T, Murata K, Shibuya H, Furu M, et al. MCP/CCR2 signaling is essential for recruitment of mesenchymal progenitor cells during the early phase of fracture healing. *PLoS ONE.* (2014) 9:e104954. doi: 10.1371/journal.pone.0104954
57. Sul OJ, Ke K, Kim WK, Kim SH, Lee SC, Kim HJ, et al. Absence of MCP-1 leads to elevated bone mass via impaired actin ring formation. *J Cell Physiol.* (2012) 227:1619–27. doi: 10.1002/jcp.22879
58. Zhang FY, Yang FJ, Yang JL, Wang L, Zhang Y. Renin inhibition improves ovariectomy-induced osteoporosis of lumbar vertebra in mice. *Biol Pharm Bull.* (2014) 37:1994–7. doi: 10.1248/bpb.b14-00576
59. Goto T, Nakao K, Gunjigake KK, Kido MA, Kobayashi S, Tanaka T. Substance P stimulates late-stage rat osteoblastic bone formation through neurokinin-1 receptors. *Neuropeptides.* (2007) 41:25–31. doi: 10.1016/j.npep.2006.11.002
60. Kan L, Lounev VY, Pignolo RJ, Duan L, Liu Y, Stock SR, et al. Substance P signaling mediates BMP-dependent heterotopic ossification. *J Cell Biochem.* (2011) 112:2759–72. doi: 10.1002/jcb.23259
61. Fu S, Mei G, Wang Z, Zou ZL, Liu S, Pei GX, et al. Neuropeptide substance P improves osteoblastic and angiogenic differentiation capacity of bone marrow stem cells *in vitro*. *Biomed Res Int.* (2014) 2014:596023. doi: 10.1155/2014/596023
62. Niedermair T, Kuhn V, Doranehgard F, Stange R, Wieskotter B, Beckmann J, et al. Absence of substance P and the sympathetic nervous system impact on bone structure and chondrocyte differentiation in an adult model of endochondral ossification. *Matrix Biol.* (2014) 38:22–35. doi: 10.1016/j.matbio.2014.06.007
63. Yoshitake H, Rittling SR, Denhardt DT, Noda M. Osteopontin-deficient mice are resistant to ovariectomy-induced bone resorption. *Proc Natl Acad Sci USA.* (1999) 96:8156–60. doi: 10.1073/pnas.96.14.8156
64. Ishijima M, Rittling SR, Yamashita T, Tsuji K, Kurosawa H, Nifuji A, et al. Enhancement of osteoclastic bone resorption and suppression of osteoblastic bone formation in response to reduced mechanical stress do not occur in the absence of osteopontin. *J Exp Med.* (2001) 193:399–404. doi: 10.1084/jem.193.3.399
65. Lee YM, Fujikado N, Manaka H, Yasuda H, Iwakura Y. IL-1 plays an important role in the bone metabolism under physiological conditions. *Int Immunol.* (2010) 22:805–16. doi: 10.1093/intimm/dxq431
66. Kim JH, Jin HM, Kim K, Song I, Youn BU, Matsuo K, et al. The mechanism of osteoclast differentiation induced by IL-1. *J Immunol.* (2009) 183:1862–70. doi: 10.4049/jimmunol.0803007
67. Lange J, Sapozhnikova A, Lu C, Hu D, Li X, Miclau T, 3rd, et al. Action of IL-1beta during fracture healing. *J Orthop Res.* (2010) 28:778–84. doi: 10.1002/jor.21061
68. Lee B, Kim TH, Jun JB, Yoo DH, Woo JH, Choi SJ, et al. Direct inhibition of human RANK+ osteoclast precursors identifies a homeostatic function of IL-1beta. *J Immunol.* (2010) 185:5926–34. doi: 10.4049/jimmunol.1001591
69. Onoe Y, Miyaura C, Kaminakayashiki T, Nagai Y, Noguchi K, Chen QR, et al. IL-13 and IL-4 inhibit bone resorption by suppressing cyclooxygenase-2-dependent prostaglandin synthesis in osteoblasts. *J Immunol.* (1996) 156:758–64.
70. Bendixen AC, Shevde NK, Dienger KM, Willson TM, Funk CD, Pike JW. IL-4 inhibits osteoclast formation through a direct action on osteoclast precursors via peroxisome proliferator-activated receptor gamma 1. *Proc Natl Acad Sci USA.* (2001) 98:2443–8. doi: 10.1073/pnas.041493198
71. Hakami Z, Kitaura H, Kimura K, Ishida M, Sugisawa H, Ida H, et al. Effect of interleukin-4 on orthodontic tooth movement and associated root resorption. *Eur J Orthod.* (2015) 37:87–94. doi: 10.1093/ejo/cju016
72. Yang X, Ricciardi BF, Hernandez-Soria A, Shi Y, Pleshko Camacho N, Bostrom MP. Callus mineralization and maturation are delayed during fracture healing in interleukin-6 knockout mice. *Bone.* (2007) 41:928–36. doi: 10.1016/j.bone.2007.07.022
73. Prystaz K, Kaiser K, Kovtun A, Haffner-Luntzer M, Fischer V, Rapp AE, et al. Distinct effects of IL-6 classic and trans-signaling in bone fracture healing. *Am J Pathol.* (2018) 188:474–90. doi: 10.1016/j.ajpath.2017.10.011
74. Erices A, Conget P, Rojas C, Minguell JJ. Gp130 activation by soluble interleukin-6 receptor/interleukin-6 enhances osteoblastic differentiation of human bone marrow-derived mesenchymal stem cells. *Exp Cell Res.* (2002) 280:24–32. doi: 10.1006/excr.2002.5627
75. Palmqvist P, Persson E, Conaway HH, Lerner UH. IL-6, leukemia inhibitory factor, and oncostatin M stimulate bone resorption and regulate the expression of receptor activator of NF-kappa B ligand, osteoprotegerin, and receptor activator of NF-kappa B in mouse calvariae. *J Immunol.* (2002) 169:3353–62. doi: 10.4049/jimmunol.169.6.3353
76. Gorny G, Shaw A, Oursler MJ. IL-6, LIF, and TNF-alpha regulation of GM-CSF inhibition of osteoclastogenesis *in vitro*. *Exp Cell Res.* (2004) 294:149–58. doi: 10.1016/j.yexcr.2003.11.009
77. Dresner-Pollak R, Gelb N, Rachmilewitz D, Karmeli F, Weinreb M. Interleukin 10-deficient mice develop osteopenia, decreased bone formation, and mechanical fragility of long bones. *Gastroenterology.* (2004) 127:792–801. doi: 10.1053/j.gastro.2004.06.013
78. Sasaki H, Hou L, Belani A, Wang CY, Uchiyama T, Muller R, et al. IL-10, but not IL-4, suppresses infection-stimulated bone resorption *in vivo*. *J Immunol.* (2000) 165:3626–30. doi: 10.4049/jimmunol.165.7.3626
79. Kudo O, Sabokbar A, Pocock A, Itonaga I, Fujikawa Y, Athanasou NA. Interleukin-6 and interleukin-11 support human osteoclast formation by a RANKL-independent mechanism. *Bone.* (2003) 32:1–7. doi: 10.1016/S8756-3282(02)00915-8
80. McCoy EM, Hong H, Pruitt HC, Feng X. IL-11 produced by breast cancer cells augments osteoclastogenesis by sustaining the pool of osteoclast progenitor cells. *BMC Cancer.* (2013) 13, 16. doi: 10.1186/1471-2407-13-16
81. Takeda H, Kikuchi T, Soboku K, Okabe I, Mizutani H, Mitani A, et al. Effect of IL-15 and natural killer cells on osteoclasts and osteoblasts in a mouse coculture. *Inflammation.* (2014) 37:657–69. doi: 10.1007/s10753-013-9782-0
82. Okabe I, Kikuchi T, Mogi M, Takeda H, Aino M, Kamiya Y, et al. IL-15 and RANKL play a synergistically important role in osteoclastogenesis. *J Cell Biochem.* (2017) 118:739–47. doi: 10.1002/jcb.25726
83. Raggatt LJ, Qin L, Tamasi J, Jefcoat SC, Jr., Shimizu E, Selvamurugan N, et al. Interleukin-18 is regulated by parathyroid hormone and is required for its bone anabolic actions. *J Biol Chem.* (2008) 283:6790–8. doi: 10.1074/jbc.M709909200

84. Dai SM, Matsuno H, Nakamura H, Nishioka K, Yudoh K. Interleukin-18 enhances monocyte tumor necrosis factor alpha and interleukin-1beta production induced by direct contact with T lymphocytes: implications in rheumatoid arthritis. *Arthritis Rheum.* (2004) 50:432–43. doi: 10.1002/art.20064
85. Yamada N, Niwa S, Tsujimura T, Iwasaki T, Sugihara A, Futani H, et al. Interleukin-18 and interleukin-12 synergistically inhibit osteoclastic bone-resorbing activity. *Bone.* (2002) 30:901–8. doi: 10.1016/S8756-3282(02)00722-6
86. Gao Y, Grassi F, Ryan MR, Terauchi M, Page K, Yang X, et al. IFN-gamma stimulates osteoclast formation and bone loss *in vivo* via antigen-driven T cell activation. *J Clin Invest.* (2007) 117:122–32. doi: 10.1172/JCI30074
87. Takahashi N, Mundy GR, Roodman GD. Recombinant human interferon-gamma inhibits formation of human osteoclast-like cells. *J Immunol.* (1986) 137:3544–9.
88. Takayanagi H, Ogasawara K, Hida S, Chiba T, Murata S, Sato K, et al. T-cell-mediated regulation of osteoclastogenesis by signalling cross-talk between RANKL and IFN-gamma. *Nature.* (2000) 408:600–5. doi: 10.1038/35046102
89. Ji JD, Park-Min KH, Shen Z, Fajardo RJ, Goldring SR, McHugh KP, et al. Inhibition of RANK expression and osteoclastogenesis by TLRs and IFN-gamma in human osteoclast precursors. *J Immunol.* (2009) 183:7223–33. doi: 10.4049/jimmunol.0900072
90. Choi SJ, Cruz JC, Craig F, Chung H, Devlin RD, Roodman GD, et al. Macrophage inflammatory protein 1-alpha is a potential osteoclast stimulatory factor in multiple myeloma. *Blood.* (2000) 96:671–5. doi: 10.1182/blood.V96.2.671
91. Gilbert LC, Rubin J, Nanes MS. The p55 TNF receptor mediates TNF inhibition of osteoblast differentiation independently of apoptosis. *Am J Physiol Endocrinol Metab.* (2005) 288:E1011–8. doi: 10.1152/ajpendo.00534.2004
92. Graves DT, Oskoui M, Volejnikova S, Naguib G, Cai S, Desta T, et al. Tumor necrosis factor modulates fibroblast apoptosis, PMN recruitment, and osteoclast formation in response to *P. gingivalis* infection. *J Dent Res.* (2001) 80:1875–9. doi: 10.1177/002203450108001 00301
93. Azuma Y, Kaji K, Katogi R, Takeshita S, Kudo A. Tumor necrosis factor-alpha induces differentiation of and bone resorption by osteoclasts. *J Biol Chem.* (2000) 275:4858–64. doi: 10.1074/jbc.275.7.4858
94. Kitaura H, Kimura K, Ishida M, Kohara H, Yoshimatsu M, Takano-Yamamoto T. Immunological reaction in TNF-alpha-mediated osteoclast formation and bone resorption *in vitro* and *in vivo*. *Clin Dev Immunol.* (2013) 2013:181849. doi: 10.1155/2013/181849
95. Kassem M, Kveiborg M, Eriksen EF. Production and action of transforming growth factor-beta in human osteoblast cultures: dependence on cell differentiation and modulation by calcitriol. *Eur J Clin Invest.* (2000) 30:429–37. doi: 10.1046/j.1365-2362.2000.00645.x
96. Iwata J, Hosokawa R, Sanchez-Lara PA, Urata M, Slavkin H, Chai Y. Transforming growth factor-beta regulates basal transcriptional regulatory machinery to control cell proliferation and differentiation in cranial neural crest-derived osteoprogenitor cells. *J Biol Chem.* (2010) 285:4975–82. doi: 10.1074/jbc.M109.035105
97. Takai H, Kanematsu M, Yano K, Tsuda E, Higashio K, Ikeda K, et al. Transforming growth factor-beta stimulates the production of osteoprotegerin/osteoclastogenesis inhibitory factor by bone marrow stromal cells. *J Biol Chem.* (1998) 273:27091–6. doi: 10.1074/jbc.273.42. 27091
98. Kawaguchi H, Pilbeam CC, Vargas SJ, Morse EE, Lorenzo JA, Raisz LG. Ovariectomy enhances and estrogen replacement inhibits the activity of bone marrow factors that stimulate prostaglandin production in cultured mouse calvariae. *J Clin Invest.* (1995) 96:539–48. doi: 10.1172/JCI118066
99. Hikiji H, Ishii S, Shindou H, Takato T, Shimizu T. Absence of platelet-activating factor receptor protects mice from osteoporosis following ovariectomy. *J Clin Invest.* (2004) 114:85–93. doi: 10.1172/JCI 20504
100. Montero A, Okada Y, Tomita M, Ito M, Tsurukami H, Nakamura T, et al. Disruption of the fibroblast growth factor-2 gene results in decreased bone mass and bone formation. *J Clin Invest.* (2000) 105:1085–93. doi: 10.1172/JCI8641
101. Sobue T, Naganawa T, Xiao L, Okada Y, Tanaka Y, Ito M, et al. Over-expression of fibroblast growth factor-2 causes defective bone mineralization and osteopenia in transgenic mice. *J Cell Biochem.* (2005) 95:83–94. doi: 10.1002/jcb.20389
102. Modrowski D, Lomri A, Marie PJ. Endogenous GM-CSF is involved as an autocrine growth factor for human osteoblastic cells. *J Cell Physiol.* (1997) 170:35–46. doi: 10.1002/(SICI)1097-4652(199701)170:1<35::AID-JCP5>3.0.CO;2-M
103. Lee MS, Kim HS, Yeon JT, Choi SW, Chun CH, Kwak HB, et al. GM-CSF regulates fusion of mononuclear osteoclasts into bone-resorbing osteoclasts by activating the Ras/ERK pathway. *J Immunol.* (2009) 183:3390–9. doi: 10.4049/jimmunol.0804314
104. Atanga E, Dolder S, Dauwalder T, Wetterwald A, Hofstetter W. TNFalpha inhibits the development of osteoclasts through osteoblast-derived GM-CSF. *Bone.* (2011) 49:1090–100. doi: 10.1016/j.bone.2011. 08.003
105. Tanaka S, Takahashi N, Udagawa N, Tamura T, Akatsu T, Stanley ER, et al. Macrophage colony-stimulating factor is indispensable for both proliferation and differentiation of osteoclast progenitors. *J Clin Invest.* (1993) 91:257–63. doi: 10.1172/JCI116179
106. Fujikawa Y, Sabokbar A, Neale SD, Itonaga I, Torisu T, Athanasou NA. The effect of macrophage-colony stimulating factor and other humoral factors (interleukin-1,–3,–6, and–11, tumor necrosis factor-alpha, and granulocyte macrophage-colony stimulating factor) on human osteoclast formation from circulating cells. *Bone.* (2001) 28:261–7. doi: 10.1016/S8756-3282(00)00453-1
107. Chae HJ, Park RK, Kang JS, Shin HS, Kim SC, Chung HT, et al. Effect of stem cell factor, interleukin-6, nitric oxide and transforming growth factor-beta on the osteoclast differentiation induced by 1 alpha,25-(OH)2D3 in primary murine bone marrow cultures. *Pharmacol Toxicol.* (1998) 82:223–9. doi: 10.1111/j.1600-0773.1998.tb01429.x
108. Armour KE, Armour KJ, Gallagher ME, Godecke A, Helfrich MH, Reid DM, et al. Defective bone formation and anabolic response to exogenous estrogen in mice with targeted disruption of endothelial nitric oxide synthase. *Endocrinology.* (2001) 142:760–6. doi: 10.1210/endo.142.2.7977
109. Reber LL, Marichal T, Galli SJ. New models for analyzing mast cell functions *in vivo*. *Trends Immunol.* (2012) 33:613–25. doi: 10.1016/j.it.2012.09.008
110. Jonsson F, Daeron M. Mast cells and company. *Front Immunol.* (2012) 3:16. doi: 10.3389/fimmu.2012.00016
111. Silberstein R, Melnick M, Greenberg G, Minkin C. Bone remodeling in W/Wv mast cell deficient mice. *Bone.* (1991) 12:227–36. doi: 10.1016/8756-3282(91)90068-T
112. Cindik ED, Maurer M, Hannan MK, Muller R, Hayes WC, Hovy L, et al. Phenotypical characterization of c-kit receptor deficient mouse femora using non-destructive high-resolution imaging techniques and biomechanical testing. *Technol Health Care.* (2000) 8:267–75. doi: 10.3233/THC-20 00-8502
113. Lotinun S, Krishnamra N. Disruption of c-Kit signaling in Kit(W-sh/W-sh) growing mice increases bone turnover. *Sci Rep.* (2016) 6:31515. doi: 10.1038/srep31515
114. Iwaniec UT, Turner RT. Failure to generate bone marrow adipocytes does not protect mice from ovariectomy-induced osteopenia. *Bone.* (2013) 53:145–53. doi: 10.1016/j.bone.2012.11.034
115. Katz HR, Austen KF. Mast cell deficiency, a game of kit and mouse. *Immunity.* (2011) 35:668–70. doi: 10.1016/j.immuni.2011.11.004
116. Dudeck A, Dudeck J, Scholten J, Petzold A, Surianarayanan S, Kohler A, et al. Mast cells are key promoters of contact allergy that mediate the adjuvant effects of haptens. *Immunity.* (2011) 34:973–84. doi: 10.1016/j.immuni.2011.03.028
117. De Filippo K, Dudeck A, Hasenberg M, Nye E, van Rooijen N, Hartmann K, et al. Mast cell and macrophage chemokines CXCL1/CXCL2 control the early stage of neutrophil recruitment during tissue inflammation. *Blood.* (2013) 121:4930–7. doi: 10.1182/blood-2013-02-486217
118. Feyerabend TB, Weiser A, Tietz A, Stassen M, Harris N, Kopf M, et al. Cre-mediated cell ablation contests mast cell contribution in models of antibody- and T cell-mediated autoimmunity. *Immunity.* (2011) 35:832–44. doi: 10.1016/j.immuni.2011.09.015
119. Lilla JN, Chen CC, Mukai K, BenBarak MJ, Franco CB, Kalesnikoff J, et al. Reduced mast cell and basophil numbers and function in Cpa3-Cre;

Mcl-1fl/fl mice. *Blood.* (2011) 118:6930–8. doi: 10.1182/blood-2011-03-343962
120. Sawaguchi M, Tanaka S, Nakatani Y, Harada Y, Mukai K, Matsunaga Y, et al. Role of mast cells and basophils in IgE responses and in allergic airway hyperresponsiveness. *J Immunol.* (2012) 188:1809–18. doi: 10.4049/jimmunol.1101746
121. Otsuka A, Kubo M, Honda T, Egawa G, Nakajima S, Tanizaki H, et al. Requirement of interaction between mast cells and skin dendritic cells to establish contact hypersensitivity. *PLoS ONE.* (2011) 6:e25538. doi: 10.1371/journal.pone.0025538
122. Dahdah A, Gautier G, Attout T, Fiore F, Lebourdais E, Msallam R, et al. Mast cells aggravate sepsis by inhibiting peritoneal macrophage phagocytosis. *J Clin Invest.* (2014) 124:4577–89. doi: 10.1172/JCI75212
123. Rachner TD, Khosla S, Hofbauer LC. Osteoporosis: now and the future. *Lancet.* (2011) 377:1276–87. doi: 10.1016/S0140-6736(10)62349-5
124. IOF. *Broken Bones, Broken Lives: A roadmap to solve the fragility fracture crisis in Europe.* Available online at: http://share.iofbonehealth.org/EU-6-Material/Reports/IOF%20Report_EU.pdf (accessed July 8, 2019).
125. Cosman F, de Beur SJ, LeBoff MS, Lewiecki EM, Tanner B, Randall S, et al. Clinician's guide to prevention and treatment of osteoporosis. *Osteoporos Int.* (2014) 25:2359–81. doi: 10.1007/s00198-014-2794-2
126. Frame B, Nixon RK. Bone-marrow mast cells in osteoporosis of aging. *N Engl J Med.* (1968) 279:626–30. doi: 10.1056/NEJM196809192791203
127. Chan BC, Lee HY, Siu WS, Yip KH, Ko CH, Lau CB, et al. Suppression of mast cell activity contributes to the osteoprotective effect of an herbal formula containing Herba Epimedii, Fructus Ligustri Lucidi and Fructus Psoraleae. *J Pharm Pharmacol.* (2014) 66:437–44. doi: 10.1111/jphp.12166
128. Faienza MF, Ventura A, Marzano F, Cavallo L. Postmenopausal osteoporosis: the role of immune system cells. *Clin Dev Immunol.* (2013) 2013:575936. doi: 10.1155/2013/575936
129. Tyan ML. Effect of promethazine on lumbar vertebral bone mass in postmenopausal women. *J Intern Med.* (1993) 234:143–8. doi: 10.1111/j.1365-2796.1993.tb00723.x
130. Lesclous P, Saffar JL. Mast cells accumulate in rat bone marrow after ovariectomy. *Cells Tissues Organs.* (1999) 164:23–9. doi: 10.1159/000016639
131. Lesclous P, Guez D, Llorens A, Saffar JL. Time-course of mast cell accumulation in rat bone marrow after ovariectomy. *Calcif Tissue Int.* (2001) 68:297–303. doi: 10.1007/BF02390837
132. Pang X, Cotreau-Bibbo MM, Sant GR, Theoharides TC. Bladder mast cell expression of high affinity oestrogen receptors in patients with interstitial cystitis. *Br J Urol.* (1995) 75:154–61. doi: 10.1111/j.1464-410X.1995.tb07303.x
133. Jiang YA, Zhang YY, Luo HS, Xing SF. Mast cell density and the context of clinicopathological parameters and expression of p185, estrogen receptor, and proliferating cell nuclear antigen in gastric carcinoma. *World J Gastroenterol.* (2002) 8:1005–8. doi: 10.3748/wjg.v8.i6.1005
134. Zaitsu M, Narita S, Lambert KC, Grady JJ, Estes DM, Curran EM, et al. Estradiol activates mast cells via a non-genomic estrogen receptor-alpha and calcium influx. *Mol Immunol.* (2007) 44:1977–85. doi: 10.1016/j.molimm.2006.09.030
135. Jensen F, Woudwyk M, Teles A, Woidacki K, Taran F, Costa S, et al. Estradiol and progesterone regulate the migration of mast cells from the periphery to the uterus and induce their maturation and degranulation. *PLoS ONE.* (2010) 5:e14409. doi: 10.1371/journal.pone.0014409
136. Kim MS, Chae HJ, Shin TY, Kim HM, Kim HR. Estrogen regulates cytokine release in human mast cells. *Immunopharmacol Immunotoxicol.* (2001) 23:495–504. doi: 10.1081/IPH-100108596
137. Jing H, Wang Z, Chen Y. Effect of oestradiol on mast cell number and histamine level in the mammary glands of rat. *Anat Histol Embryol.* (2012) 41:170–6. doi: 10.1111/j.1439-0264.2011.01120.x
138. Padilla L, Reinicke K, Montesino H, Villena F, Asencio H, Cruz M, et al. Histamine content and mast cells distribution in mouse uterus: the effect of sexual hormones, gestation and labor. *Cell Mol Biol.* (1990) 36:93–100.
139. Renke J, Kedzierska-Mieszkowska S, Lange M, Nedoszytko B, Wasilewska E, Liberek A, et al. Mast cells in mastocytosis and allergy - Important player in metabolic and immunological homeostasis. *Adv Med Sci.* (2019) 64:124–30. doi: 10.1016/j.advms.2018.08.013
140. Lim KH, Tefferi A, Lasho TL, Finke C, Patnaik M, Butterfield JH, et al. Systemic mastocytosis in 342 consecutive adults: survival studies and prognostic factors. *Blood.* (2009) 113:5727–36. doi: 10.1182/blood-2009-02-205237
141. Cruse G, Metcalfe DD, Olivera A. Functional deregulation of KIT: link to mast cell proliferative diseases and other neoplasms. *Immunol Allergy Clin North Am.* (2014) 34:219–37. doi: 10.1016/j.iac.2014.01.002
142. Arock M, Akin C, Hermine O, Valent P. Current treatment options in patients with mastocytosis: status in 2015 and future perspectives. *Eur J Haematol.* (2015) 94:474–90. doi: 10.1111/ejh.12544
143. Chines A, Pacifici R, Avioli LV, Teitelbaum SL, Korenblat PE. Systemic mastocytosis presenting as osteoporosis: a clinical and histomorphometric study. *J Clin Endocrinol Metab.* (1991) 72:140–4. doi: 10.1210/jcem-72-1-140
144. Johansson C, Roupe G, Lindstedt G, Mellstrom D. Bone density, bone markers and bone radiological features in mastocytosis. *Age Ageing.* (1996) 25:1–7. doi: 10.1093/ageing/25.1.1
145. Mathew R, Dhillon V, Shepherd P. Systemic mastocytosis presenting as osteoporosis–a case report. *Clin Rheumatol.* (2009) 28:865–6. doi: 10.1007/s10067-009-1165-4
146. Manara M, Varenna M, Cantoni S, Parafioriti A, Gallazzi MB, Sinigaglia L. Osteoporosis with vertebral fractures in young males, due to bone marrow mastocytosis: a report of two cases. *Clin Exp Rheumatol.* (2010) 28:97–100.
147. van der Veer E, van der Goot W, de Monchy JG, Kluin-Nelemans HC, van Doormaal JJ. High prevalence of fractures and osteoporosis in patients with indolent systemic mastocytosis. *Allergy.* (2012) 67:431–8. doi: 10.1111/j.1398-9995.2011.02780.x
148. Rossini M, Zanotti R, Bonadonna P, Artuso A, Caruso B, Schena D, et al. Bone mineral density, bone turnover markers and fractures in patients with indolent systemic mastocytosis. *Bone.* (2011) 49:880–5. doi: 10.1016/j.bone.2011.07.004
149. Hermans MAW, Rietveld MJA, van Laar JAM, Dalm V, Verburg M, Pasmans S, et al. Systemic mastocytosis: a cohort study on clinical characteristics of 136 patients in a large tertiary centre. *Eur J Intern Med.* (2016) 30:25–30. doi: 10.1016/j.ejim.2016.01.005
150. Degboe Y, Eischen M, Nigon D, Apoil PA, Mailhol C, Tournier E, et al. Prevalence and risk factors for fragility fracture in systemic mastocytosis. *Bone.* (2017) 105:219–25. doi: 10.1016/j.bone.2017.09.005
151. Greene LW, Asadipooya K, Corradi PF, Akin C. Endocrine manifestations of systemic mastocytosis in bone. *Rev Endocr Metab Disord.* (2016) 17:419–31. doi: 10.1007/s11154-016-9362-3
152. Seitz S, Barvencik F, Koehne T, Priemel M, Pogoda P, Semler J, et al. Increased osteoblast and osteoclast indices in individuals with systemic mastocytosis. *Osteoporos Int.* (2013) 24:2325–34. doi: 10.1007/s00198-013-2305-x
153. Guillaume N, Desoutter J, Chandesris O, Merlusca L, Henry I, Georgin-Lavialle S, et al. Bone complications of mastocytosis: a link between clinical and biological characteristics. *Am J Med.* (2013) 126:75.e71–7. doi: 10.1016/j.amjmed.2012.07.018
154. Rossini M, Viapiana O, Zanotti R, Tripi G, Perbellini O, Idolazzi L, et al. Dickkopf-1 and sclerostin serum levels in patients with systemic mastocytosis. *Calcif Tissue Int.* (2015) 96:410–6. doi: 10.1007/s00223-015-9969-5
155. Rabenhorst A, Christopeit B, Leja S, Gerbaulet A, Kleiner S, Forster A, et al. Serum levels of bone cytokines are increased in indolent systemic mastocytosis associated with osteopenia or osteoporosis. *J Allergy Clin Immunol.* (2013) 132:1234–7.e7. doi: 10.1016/j.jaci.2013.06.019
156. Theoharides TC, Boucher W, Spear K. Serum interleukin-6 reflects disease severity and osteoporosis in mastocytosis patients. *Int Arch Allergy Immunol.* (2002) 128:344–50. doi: 10.1159/000063858
157. Brumsen C, Papapoulos SE, Lentjes EG, Kluin PM, Hamdy NA. A potential role for the mast cell in the pathogenesis of idiopathic osteoporosis in men. *Bone.* (2002) 31:556–61. doi: 10.1016/S8756-3282(02)00875-X
158. Kim KW, Kim BM, Lee KA, Lee SH, Firestein GS, Kim HR. Histamine and Histamine H4 Receptor Promotes Osteoclastogenesis in Rheumatoid Arthritis. *Sci Rep.* (2017) 7:1197. doi: 10.1038/s41598-017-01101-y
159. Lesclous P, Guez D, Baroukh B, Vignery A, Saffar JL. Histamine participates in the early phase of trabecular bone loss in ovariectomized rats. *Bone.* (2004) 34:91–9. doi: 10.1016/j.bone.2003.08.007

160. Guo Q, Wang Y, Xu D, Nossent J, Pavlos NJ, Xu J. Rheumatoid arthritis: pathological mechanisms and modern pharmacologic therapies. *Bone Res.* (2018) 6:15. doi: 10.1038/s41413-018-0016-9
161. Silman AJ, Pearson JE. Epidemiology and genetics of rheumatoid arthritis. *Arthritis Res.* (2002) 4(Suppl. 3):S265–72. doi: 10.1186/ar578
162. Rivellese F, Rossi FW, Galdiero MR, Pitzalis C, de Paulis A. Mast cells in early rheumatoid arthritis. *Int J Mol Sci.* (2019) 20:2040. doi: 10.3390/ijms20082040
163. Crisp AJ. Mast cells in rheumatoid arthritis. *J R Soc Med.* (1984) 77:450–1.
164. Godfrey HP, Ilardi C, Engber W, Graziano FM. Quantitation of human synovial mast cells in rheumatoid arthritis and other rheumatic diseases. *Arthritis Rheum.* (1984) 27:852–6. doi: 10.1002/art.1780270803
165. Gotis-Graham I, McNeil HP. Mast cell responses in rheumatoid synovium. Association of the MCTC subset with matrix turnover and clinical progression. *Arthritis Rheum.* (1997) 40:479–89. doi: 10.1002/art.1780400314
166. Ramirez J, Celis R, Usategui A, Ruiz-Esquide V, Fare R, Cuervo A, et al. Immunopathologic characterization of ultrasound-defined synovitis in rheumatoid arthritis patients in clinical remission. *Arthritis Res Ther.* (2016) 18:74. doi: 10.1186/s13075-016-0970-9
167. Rivellese F, Mauro D, Nerviani A, Pagani S, Fossati-Jimack L, Messemaker T, et al. Mast cells in early rheumatoid arthritis associate with disease severity and support B cell autoantibody production. *Ann Rheum Dis.* (2018) 77:1773–81. doi: 10.1136/annrheumdis-2018-213418
168. Malone DG, Irani AM, Schwartz LB, Barrett KE, Metcalfe DD. Mast cell numbers and histamine levels in synovial fluids from patients with diverse arthritides. *Arthritis Rheum.* (1986) 29:956–63. doi: 10.1002/art.1780290803
169. Frewin DB, Cleland LG, Jonsson JR, Robertson PW. Histamine levels in human synovial fluid. *J Rheumatol.* (1986) 13:13–4.
170. Xu D, Jiang HR, Kewin P, Li Y, Mu R, Fraser AR, et al. IL-33 exacerbates antigen-induced arthritis by activating mast cells. *Proc Natl Acad Sci USA.* (2008) 105:10913–8. doi: 10.1073/pnas.0801898105
171. Desai A, Jung MY, Olivera A, Gilfillan AM, Prussin C, Kirshenbaum AS, et al. IL-6 promotes an increase in human mast cell numbers and reactivity through suppression of suppressor of cytokine signaling 3. *J Allergy Clin Immunol.* (2016) 137:1863–71.e1866. doi: 10.1016/j.jaci.2015.09.059
172. Suurmond J, Rivellese F, Dorjee AL, Bakker AM, Rombouts YJ, Rispens T, et al. Toll-like receptor triggering augments activation of human mast cells by anti-citrullinated protein antibodies. *Ann Rheum Dis.* (2015) 74:1915–23. doi: 10.1136/annrheumdis-2014-205562
173. Nigrovic PA, Malbec O, Lu B, Markiewski MM, Kepley C, Gerard N, et al. C5a receptor enables participation of mast cells in immune complex arthritis independently of Fcgamma receptor modulation. *Arthritis Rheum.* (2010) 62:3322–33. doi: 10.1002/art.27659
174. Lee H, Kashiwakura J, Matsuda A, Watanabe Y, Sakamoto-Sasaki T, Matsumoto K, et al. Activation of human synovial mast cells from rheumatoid arthritis or osteoarthritis patients in response to aggregated IgG through Fcgamma receptor I and Fcgamma receptor II. *Arthritis Rheum.* (2013) 65:109–19. doi: 10.1002/art.37741
175. Suurmond J, Stoop JN, Rivellese F, Bakker AM, Huizinga TW, Toes RE. Activation of human basophils by combined toll-like receptor- and FcepsilonRI-triggering can promote Th2 skewing of naive T helper cells. *Eur J Immunol.* (2014) 44:386–96. doi: 10.1002/eji.201343617
176. Nigrovic PA, Binstadt BA, Monach PA, Johnsen A, Gurish M, Iwakura Y, et al. Mast cells contribute to initiation of autoantibody-mediated arthritis via IL-1. *Proc Natl Acad Sci USA.* (2007) 104:2325–30. doi: 10.1073/pnas.0610852103
177. Sandler C, Lindstedt KA, Joutsiniemi S, Lappalainen J, Juutilainen T, Kolah J, et al. Selective activation of mast cells in rheumatoid synovial tissue results in production of TNF-alpha, IL-1beta and IL-1Ra. *Inflamm Res.* (2007) 56:230–9. doi: 10.1007/s00011-007-6135-1
178. Tetlow LC, Woolley DE. Mast cells, cytokines, and metalloproteinases at the rheumatoid lesion: dual immunolocalisation studies. *Ann Rheum Dis.* (1995) 54:896–903. doi: 10.1136/ard.54.11.896
179. Shin K, Nigrovic PA, Crish J, Boilard E, McNeil HP, Larabee KS, et al. Mast cells contribute to autoimmune inflammatory arthritis via their tryptase/heparin complexes. *J Immunol.* (2009) 182:647–56. doi: 10.4049/jimmunol.182.1.647
180. Magnusson SE, Pejler G, Kleinau S, Abrink M. Mast cell chymase contributes to the antibody response and the severity of autoimmune arthritis. *FASEB J.* (2009) 23:875–82. doi: 10.1096/fj.08-120394
181. Haynes DR, Crotti TN, Potter AE, Loric M, Atkins GJ, Howie DW, et al. The osteoclastogenic molecules RANKL and RANK are associated with periprosthetic osteolysis. *J Bone Joint Surg Br.* (2001) 83:902–11. doi: 10.1302/0301-620X.83B6.0830902
182. Crotti TN, Smith MD, Weedon H, Ahern MJ, Findlay DM, Kraan M, et al. Receptor activator NF-kappaB ligand (RANKL) expression in synovial tissue from patients with rheumatoid arthritis, spondyloarthropathy, osteoarthritis, and from normal patients: semiquantitative and quantitative analysis. *Ann Rheum Dis.* (2002) 61:1047–54. doi: 10.1136/ard.61.12.1047
183. Rivellese F, Nerviani A, Rossi FW, Marone G, Matucci-Cerinic M, de Paulis A, et al. Mast cells in rheumatoid arthritis: friends or foes? *Autoimmun Rev.* (2017) 16:557–63. doi: 10.1016/j.autrev.2017.04.001
184. Lee DM, Friend DS, Gurish MF, Benoist C, Mathis D, Brenner MB. Mast cells: a cellular link between autoantibodies and inflammatory arthritis. *Science.* (2002) 297:1689–92. doi: 10.1126/science.1073176
185. Kneilling M, Hultner L, Pichler BJ, Mailhammer R, Morawietz L, Solomon S, et al. Targeted mast cell silencing protects against joint destruction and angiogenesis in experimental arthritis in mice. *Arthritis Rheum.* (2007) 56:1806–16. doi: 10.1002/art.22602
186. Pitman N, Asquith DL, Murphy G, Liew FY, McInnes IB. Collagen-induced arthritis is not impaired in mast cell-deficient mice. *Ann Rheum Dis.* (2011) 70:1170–71. doi: 10.1136/ard.2010.134528
187. Zhou JS, Xing W, Friend DS, Austen KF, Katz HR. Mast cell deficiency in Kit(W-sh) mice does not impair antibody-mediated arthritis. *J Exp Med.* (2007) 204:2797–802. doi: 10.1084/jem.20071391
188. Elliott ER, Van Ziffle JA, Scapini P, Sullivan BM, Locksley RM, Lowell CA. Deletion of Syk in neutrophils prevents immune complex arthritis. *J Immunol.* (2011) 187:4319–30. doi: 10.4049/jimmunol.1100341
189. van der Velden D, Lagraauw HM, Wezel A, Launay P, Kuiper J, Huizinga TW, et al. Mast cell depletion in the preclinical phase of collagen-induced arthritis reduces clinical outcome by lowering the inflammatory cytokine profile. *Arthritis Res Ther.* (2016) 18:138. doi: 10.1186/s13075-016-1036-8
190. Mican JM, Metcalfe DD. Arthritis and mast cell activation. *J Allergy Clin Immunol.* (1990) 86(4 Pt 2):677–83. doi: 10.1016/S0091-6749(05)80240-4
191. Chen D, Shen J, Zhao W, Wang T, Han L, Hamilton JL, et al. Osteoarthritis: toward a comprehensive understanding of pathological mechanism. *Bone Res.* (2017) 5:16044. doi: 10.1038/boneres.2016.44
192. de Lange-Brokaar BJ, Kloppenburg M, Andersen SN, Dorjee AL, Yusuf E, Herb-van Toorn L, et al. Characterization of synovial mast cells in knee osteoarthritis: association with clinical parameters. *Osteoarthr Cartil.* (2016) 24:664–71. doi: 10.1016/j.joca.2015.11.011
193. Uchida K, Takano S, Inoue G, Iwase D, Aikawa J, Takata K, et al. Increase in mast cell marker expression in the synovium of obese patients with osteoarthritis of the knee. *Diabetes Metab Syndr Obes.* (2019) 12:377–82. doi: 10.2147/DMSO.S201523
194. Renoux M, Hilliquin P, Galoppin L, Florentin I, Menkes CJ. Release of mast cell mediators and nitrites into knee joint fluid in osteoarthritis–comparison with articular chondrocalcinosis and rheumatoid arthritis. *Osteoarthr Cartil.* (1996) 4:175–9. doi: 10.1016/S1063-4584(96)80013-6
195. Nakano S, Mishiro T, Takahara S, Yokoi H, Hamada D, Yukata K, et al. Distinct expression of mast cell tryptase and protease activated receptor-2 in synovia of rheumatoid arthritis and osteoarthritis. *Clin Rheumatol.* (2007) 26:1284–92. doi: 10.1007/s10067-006-0495-8
196. Wang Q, Lepus CM, Raghu H, Reber LL, Tsai MM, Wong HH, et al. IgE-mediated mast cell activation promotes inflammation and cartilage destruction in osteoarthritis. *Elife.* (2019) 8:e39905. doi: 10.7554/eLife.39905
197. Shirinsky I, Shirinsky V. H1-antihistamines are associated with lower prevalence of radiographic knee osteoarthritis: a cross-sectional analysis of the Osteoarthritis Initiative data. *Arthritis Res Ther.* (2018) 20:116. doi: 10.1186/s13075-018-1619-7
198. Lindholm R, Lindholm S, Liukko P. Fracture healing and mast cells. I. The periosteal callus in rats. *Acta Orthop Scand.* (1967) 38:115–22. doi: 10.3109/17453676708989624

199. Lindholm S, Lindholm R, Liukko P. Fracture healing and mast cells. II. Influence of 17-hydroxy-corticosterone. *Acta Orthop Scand.* (1967) 38:123–8. doi: 10.3109/17453676708989625
200. Lindholm R, Lindholm S, Paasimaki J. Fracture healing and mast cells. 3. Action of combined growth hormone and thyrotropin. *Acta Orthop Scand.* (1967) 38:129–32. doi: 10.3109/17453676708989626
201. Lindholm RV, Lindholm TS. Mast cells in endosteal and periosteal bone repair. A quantitative study on callus tissue of healing fractures in rabbits. *Acta Orthop Scand.* (1970) 41:129–33. doi: 10.3109/17453677008991500
202. Banovac K, Renfree K, Makowski AL, Latta LL, Altman RD. Fracture healing and mast cells. *J Orthop Trauma.* (1995) 9:482–90. doi: 10.1097/00005131-199509060-00005
203. Meyer RA, Jr., Desai BR, Heiner DE, Fiechtl J, Porter S, Meyer MH. Young, adult, and old rats have similar changes in mRNA expression of many skeletal genes after fracture despite delayed healing with age. *J Orthop Res.* (2006) 24:1933–44. doi: 10.1002/jor.20124
204. Ramirez-GarciaLuna JL, Chan D, Samberg R, Abou-Rjeili M, Wong TH, Li A, et al. Defective bone repair in mast cell-deficient Cpa3Cre/+ mice. *PLoS ONE.* (2017) 12:e0174396. doi: 10.1371/journal.pone.0174396
205. Zhang L, Wang T, Chang M, Kaiser C, Kim JD, Wu T, et al. Teriparatide treatment improves bone defect healing via anabolic effects on new bone formation and non-anabolic effects on inhibition of mast cells in a murine cranial window model. *J Bone Miner Res.* (2017) 32:1870–83. doi: 10.1002/jbmr.3178
206. Hebb JH, Ashley JW, McDaniel L, Lopas LA, Tobias J, Hankenson KD, et al. Bone healing in an aged murine fracture model is characterized by sustained callus inflammation and decreased cell proliferation. *J Orthop Res.* (2018) 36:149–58. doi: 10.1002/jor.23652
207. Claes L, Recknagel S, Ignatius A. Fracture healing under healthy and inflammatory conditions. *Nat Rev Rheumatol.* (2012) 8:133–43. doi: 10.1038/nrrheum.2012.1
208. Bahney CS, Zondervan RL, Allison P, Theologis A, Ashley JW, Ahn J, et al. Cellular biology of fracture healing. *J Orthop Res.* (2019) 37:35–50. doi: 10.1002/jor.24170
209. Einhorn TA, Gerstenfeld LC. Fracture healing: mechanisms and interventions. *Nat Rev Rheumatol.* (2015) 11:45–54. doi: 10.1038/nrrheum.2014.164
210. Kovtun A, Bergdolt S, Wiegner R, Radermacher P, Huber-Lang M, Ignatius A. The crucial role of neutrophil granulocytes in bone fracture healing. *Eur Cell Mater.* (2016) 32:152–62. doi: 10.22203/eCM.v032a10
211. Alexander KA, Chang MK, Maylin ER, Kohler T, Muller R, Wu AC, et al. Osteal macrophages promote *in vivo* intramembranous bone healing in a mouse tibial injury model. *J Bone Miner Res.* (2011) 26:1517–32. doi: 10.1002/jbmr.354
212. Toben D, Schroeder I, El Khassawna T, Mehta M, Hoffmann JE, Frisch JT, et al. Fracture healing is accelerated in the absence of the adaptive immune system. *J Bone Miner Res.* (2011) 26:113–24. doi: 10.1002/jbmr.185
213. Peschke K, Dudeck A, Rabenhorst A, Hartmann K, Roers A. Cre/loxP-based mouse models of mast cell deficiency and mast cell-specific gene inactivation. *Methods Mol Biol.* (2015) 1220:403–21. doi: 10.1007/978-1-4939-1568-2_25
214. Schramm R, Thorlacius H. Neutrophil recruitment in mast cell-dependent inflammation: inhibitory mechanisms of glucocorticoids. *Inflamm Res.* (2004) 53:644–52. doi: 10.1007/s00011-004-1307-8
215. Christy AL, Walker ME, Hessner MJ, Brown MA. Mast cell activation and neutrophil recruitment promotes early and robust inflammation in the meninges in EAE. *J Autoimmun.* (2013) 42:50–61. doi: 10.1016/j.jaut.2012.11.003

4

Foxp3$^+$ Regulatory T Cells in Bone and Hematopoietic Homeostasis

Luise Fischer[1,2], Caroline Herkner[1], Reni Kitte[1], Sebastian Dohnke[1,2], Julia Riewaldt[2†], Karsten Kretschmer[2] and Annette I. Garbe[1]*

[1] Osteoimmunology, DFG-Center for Regenerative Therapies Dresden (CRTD), Technische Universität Dresden, Dresden, Germany, [2] Molecular and Cellular Immunology/Immune Regulation, DFG-Center for Regenerative Therapies Dresden (CRTD), Technische Universität Dresden, Dresden, Germany

***Correspondence:**
Annette I. Garbe
annette.garbe@tu-dresden.de

The bone represents surprisingly dynamic structures that are subject to constant remodeling by the concerted action of bone-forming osteoblasts and bone-resorbing osteoclasts - two cell subsets of distinct developmental origin that are key in maintaining skeletal integrity throughout life. In general, abnormal bone remodeling due to dysregulated bone resorption and formation is an early event in the manifestation of various human bone diseases, such as osteopetrosis/osteoporosis and arthritis. But bone remodeling is also closely interrelated with lympho-hematopoietic homeostasis, as the bone marrow niche is formed by solid and trabecular bone structures that provide a framework for the long-term maintenance and differentiation of HSCs (>blood lineage cells and osteoclasts) and MSCs (>osteoblasts). Numerous studies in mice and humans have implicated innate and adaptive immune cells in the dynamic regulation of bone homeostasis, but despite considerable clinical relevance, the exact mechanisms of such immuno-bone interplay have remained incompletely understood. This holds particularly true for CD4$^+$ regulatory T (Treg) cells expressing the lineage specification factor Foxp3: Foxp3$^+$ Treg cells have been shown to play an indispensable role in maintaining immune homeostasis, but may also exert critical non-immune functions, which includes the control of metabolic and regenerative processes, as well as the differentiation of HSCs and function of osteoclasts. Here, we summarize our current knowledge on the T cell/bone interplay, with a particular emphasis on our own efforts to dissect the role of Foxp3$^+$ Treg cells in bone and hematopoietic homeostasis, employing experimental settings of gain- and loss-of-Treg cell function. These data make a strong case that Foxp3$^+$ Treg cells impinge on lympho-hematopoiesis through indirect mechanisms, i.e., by acting on osteoclast development and function, which translates into changes in niche size. Furthermore, we propose that, besides disorders that involve inflammatory bone loss, the modulation of Foxp3$^+$ Treg cell function *in vivo* may represent a suitable approach to reinstate bone homeostasis in non-autoimmune settings of aberrant bone remodeling.

Keywords: bone disorders, bone microenvironment, lympho-hematopoiesis, osteoclasts, Foxp3$^+$ Treg cells

INTRODUCTION

In adult mammals, the bone marrow (BM) is the primary site of hematopoiesis. Hematopoietic stem cells (HSCs) reside within specific niches, which are specialized microenvironments within the BM cavity, providing HSCs with regulatory signals essential for their maintenance, proliferation and differentiation into blood and immune cells. HSCs dynamically regulate their numbers by undergoing asymmetric, self-renewing divisions depending upon cell-intrinsic and cell-extrinsic mechanisms, thereby sustaining hematopoiesis over lifetime (1, 2). Homeostasis of the bone microenvironment critically depends on bone remodeling, a tightly regulated process involving three major cell types: bone-resorbing osteoclasts, bone-forming osteoblasts and osteocytes. Osteocytes originate from mature osteoblasts, residing within the lacuna of the mineralized bone matrix, and act as orchestrators of bone remodeling (3). Under physiological conditions, resorption of damaged bone by osteoclasts is followed by the recruitment of osteoblasts and the formation of new bone, a concerted action critical for the maintenance of skeletal integrity and bone homeostasis. Defects in osteoclastic activity cause osteopetrosis, a disease associated with high bone mass, whereas enhanced osteoclastic bone resorption results in low bone mass and osteoporosis (4). While the direct impact of osteoclasts on maintenance and BM retention of HSCs remains controversial (5–7), there is accumulating evidence that osteoblast lineage cells play a crucial role in the regulation of hematopoiesis (8–10). Since the majority of the cells in the BM are hematopoietic cells, it appears likely that, in addition to stromal niche components, HSCs are regulated by their own progeny. In this context, megakaryocytes have recently been identified as direct regulators of homeostatic HSC quiescence using several mechanisms, including secretion of CXCL4 and TGF-β (11–13), while direct cell-cell interaction of megakaryocytes and bone cells have been described to affect skeletal homeostasis (14–16). Similarly, it has been suggested that the function of osteoblasts in maintaining the HSC niche is controlled by macrophages, whereas "HSC niche macrophages" have been described to govern maintenance of hematopoiesis directly (17–20). However, due to the heterogeneity of macrophages, and since the bone- and BM-residing macrophage populations, including osteoclasts, are primarily defined by their histological location, the precise identity and role of the different macrophage subpopulations in bone remodeling, regeneration, and shaping the HSC niche still need to be defined (21–23).

The impact of cells of the adaptive immune system — B and T lymphocytes — on bone remodeling under physiological conditions is still a matter of debate: while some studies using lymphocyte-deficient mouse models such as $Rag^{-/-}$, μMT or nude mice described low bone mass phenotypes, others did not (24–27). Given the fact that several populations of mature lymphocytes, such as long-lived memory T and B cells reside in the BM (28, 29) and share common niches with HSCs, it is reasonable to assume that these mature cells impinge on bone and hematopoietic homeostasis. In this context, it has been shown, that after allogeneic BM stem cell transplantation, T cells act as a double-edged sword as they can on the one hand promote graft-versus-host-disease (GvHD), but on the other hand can also provide beneficial effects on the engraftment (30). High-resolution imaging over time in an experimental setup of allogeneic HSC transplantation provided evidence that HSCs preferentially co-localize with CD4$^+$ regulatory T (Treg) cells, expressing the lineage specification factor Foxp3, that accumulate on the endosteal surface of the bones of non-irradiated recipient mice, enabling transplanted stem cells to evade from allogeneic rejection (31, 32). The essential role of Foxp3$^+$ Treg cells in maintaining immune homeostasis is firmly established (33, 34), but additional, non-immunological functions of Treg cells, such as controlling (i) the metabolic function in adipose tissue, (ii) regeneration of muscle cells, (iii) lympho-hematopoiesis, and (iv) osteoclast and osteoblast development and function, become increasingly apparent (35–41).

While much less is known about the interplay between Treg cells and osteoclasts/osteoblasts in bone remodeling and the formation of the HSC niche, a large body of experimental evidence focused on the immuno-bone crosstalk in rheumatoid arthritis (RA), one of the most common human autoimmune diseases. Osteoclasts play a central role in the pathogenesis of RA, where bone destruction is characterized by inflammatory osteolysis, caused by aberrant activation of the immune system, eventually leading to the destruction of surface cartilage and subchondral bone (42, 43). It has been proposed that the onset and pathogenesis of RA critically depends on the balance between two distinct CD4$^+$ T cell subsets: type 17 helper T (TH17) cells, a pathogenic subset of CD4$^+$ T cells that produces IL-17, and thereby promoting osteoclastogenesis, and Treg cells, crucial for the prevention of autoimmune diseases driven by TH17 cells (34, 44). The role of Treg cells in animal models for autoimmune arthritis has been demonstrated by amelioration of the disease following adoptive transfer of Treg cells and induction of an accelerated and more severe form of arthritis after depletion of Treg cells (45–48). Moreover, it has been described that under certain conditions of experimental arthritis a subpopulation of Foxp3$^+$ Treg cells can convert into autoreactive Foxp3$^-$ TH17 cells (49).

There is also evidence that Treg cells interact with osteoblasts. For example, studies on intermittent PTH-induced bone anabolism propose that Treg cells are involved in the up-regulation of the expression of the osteogenic factor Wnt10b by CD8$^+$ T cells, which was also suggested to be the main mechanism in the promotion of bone formation by oral supplementation with the probiotic *Lactobacillus rhamnosus* GG (50–53). On the other hand, Treg cells have been implicated to play a role in bone formation by promoting the differentiation of osteoblasts directly (54).

Although the close relationship between the bone and the immune system has long been recognized (55), the spatial relationship and the interaction between the different cell types within the bone microenvironment as well as the identity of their communication factors, in particular under physiological conditions, is still incompletely understood.

Studies on the interplay between osteoclasts/osteoblasts and Treg cells in the BM microenvironment are hampered by several unresolved issues: (a) osteoclasts are difficult to study due to the lack of reliable methods for their *ex vivo* purification, owing to their low abundance, large size, and lack of specific surface marker expression. Furthermore, the phenotypic definition of "true" osteoclast precursors and their developmental stages vary considerably; (b) constitutive Treg cell deficiency inevitably results in secondary effects due to systemic autoimmunity and increased systemic levels of inflammatory factors. Mice with constitutive Treg cell deficiency suffer from severe morbidity leading to premature death prior to completion of bone development; (c) due to the unique properties and structure of bone, it is technically challenging to assess and visualize interactions between cells in the BM niche. Thus, it will be essential to develop experimental systems and more advanced imaging that keep these limitations to a minimum.

In this review we discuss the impact of BM-residing Treg cells on the bone microenvironment, central to the development of therapeutic strategies for the treatment of bone diseases and to promote tolerance after stem cell transplantation.

LYMPHO-HEMATOPOIETIC NICHE AND FOXP3$^+$ TREG CELLS

For a long time, HSCs were considered as dormant cells but increasing evidence suggests HSCs as direct targets of inflammatory signals. Earlier studies have identified HSCs as "first responders" during inflammatory responses, e.g., during infections, later it became clear that pro-inflammatory cytokines such as interleukin (IL)-1, IL-6, IL-8, tumor necrosis factor (TNF) and type I and type II interferons (IFNs), G-CSF, and Toll-like receptor (TLR) ligands regulate HSCs not only in response to stress but also under homeostatic conditions. Together with BM niche signals such as CXCL12, basal levels of inflammatory cytokines provided by T cells, NK cells, neutrophils and macrophages control the balance between HSC dormancy and lineage fate decision under homeostatic conditions, while inflammatory conditions promote HSC proliferation and differentiation at the expense of self-renewal, emphasizing the interdependency of the distinct BM niche components in health and disease (56–60). However, increasing evidence is pointing towards regulation of HSC maintenance by distal/systemic factors: in addition to the nervous system (e.g., by oscillation of CXCL12 production) and hormones such as PTH or estrogen that have been described to regulate HSCs from the outside, two recent studies demonstrate that also the liver and the intestine contribute to HSC maintenance under steady-state conditions (61–65). Given that bone remodeling is also highly regulated by systemic factors, further studies are required to dissect direct and indirect contributions of distal organs on hematopoietic and skeletal homeostasis.

In both mouse and man, the T cell compartment in the BM, which constitutes only about 5% of mononuclear BM cells, is characterized by a lower CD4/CD8 T cell ratio and notably, by substantially elevated frequencies of Foxp3$^+$ Treg cells within the CD4$^+$ T cell population compared to peripheral lymphoid organs (66, 67). Like other BM T cells, BM Treg cells exhibit a more activated/memory phenotype. Transcriptional characterization of BM Treg cells revealed a signature distinct from Treg cells in the periphery. The differential expression of cytokine/chemokine receptors such as *Il9r*, *Ccr2,* and *Cxcr3* and effector molecules such as *Il10* and *Ctla4* suggests increased suppressive capacity of BM resident Treg cells (68). The transcriptional signature is consistent with the idea that these niche-associated Treg cells contribute to the maintenance of the BM microenvironment as an immune privilege site, crucial for HSC survival (31, 32).

Interestingly, and reminiscent of the above-described observations, our temporal analysis of Treg cells in the BM of wildtype mice revealed that the proportion of Foxp3$^+$ Treg cells among CD4$^+$ T cells further increases with age. While in juvenile mice, Foxp3$^+$ Treg cells account for approximately 20% of the CD4$^+$ T cell population, their frequency has almost doubled in aged mice (**Figure 1A**). This can be recapitulated by adoptive Treg cell transfers into Treg cell-deficient mice: here we found Foxp3^{GFP+} Treg cells, which initially comprised about 10–15% of the adoptively transferred splenic bulk CD4$^+$ T cell population, to be selectively enriched in the BM of Foxp3-deficient recipient mice [up to 90% of transferred CD4$^+$ T cells (69)] and in the BM of T and B cell-deficient *Rag1*$^{-/-}$ recipient mice (up to 40% of transferred CD4$^+$ T cells; **Figure 1B**), indicating the physiological relevance of the enrichment. Overall, these observations raise the question whether this accumulation of Foxp3$^+$ Treg cells within the BM is due to preferential *de novo* induction of initially Foxp3-negative CD4$^+$ T cells or preferential recruitment of preformed cells to the bone microenvironment (70, 71).

Since CD4$^+$ Treg cells were originally identified exclusively by the constitutive expression of the IL-2 receptor alpha chain CD25, employing depleting antibodies directed against CD25 still represents the most widely used loss-of-function approach to characterize Treg cell function *in vivo* (72, 73). Whether the *in vivo* administration of anti-CD25 monoclonal antibodies (mAbs) leads to depletion or to functional inactivation of CD25-expressing Treg cells has been controversially discussed (74–77). In mouse models for RA, administration of anti-CD25 mAbs exacerbates the disease (45, 78, 79). However, interpretation of results from studies using this approach to assess the direct impact of Treg cells on bone cells is hampered due to the upregulation of CD25 expression on activated CD4 and CD8 T cells and in addition, due to the existence of CD25-negative Treg cells in particular in peripheral tissues and the BM. Consistently, anti-CD25 treatment spares Foxp3$^+$ Treg cells with a CD25$^{low/-}$ phenotype (80).

Only the identification of Foxp3 as the Treg cell lineage specification factor, necessary and sufficient for their development and function (81–83) allowed specific *in vivo* targeting of Foxp3$^+$ Treg cells and with this the generation of mouse models with abrogated or enhanced Foxp3$^+$ Treg cell activity.

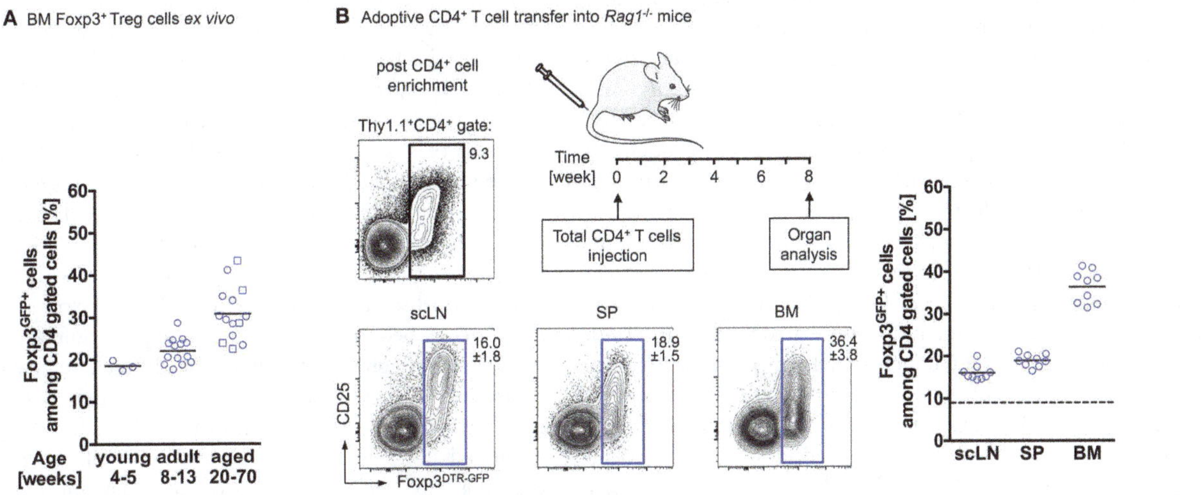

FIGURE 1 | Accumulation of Foxp3$^+$ Treg cells in the BM. **(A)** Age-related accumulation of BM-resident Foxp3$^+$ Treg cells. Flow cytometry analysis of Foxp3^{GFP+} cells within the CD4$^+$ T cell population in the BM of wildtype mice of different age groups. Each experiment was performed with at least 3 mice and symbols and lines indicate individual mice and mean values, respectively (young: 4–5 weeks; adult: 8–13 weeks; aged: circles: 20–22 weeks; and squares: 50–70 weeks). **(B)** Schematic overview of the experimental design. Four-week-old *Rag1*$^{-/-}$ mice were adoptively transferred with bulk CD4$^+$ T cells (upper plot: Foxp3$^+$ Treg cell proportion among total CD4$^+$ T cells before adoptively transferred). The distributions of gated Foxp3$^{DTR-GFP+}$ cells in various organs of the recipient mice (scLN, subcutaneous lymph nodes; SP, spleen, and BM, bone marrow) were analyzed by flow cytometry 8 weeks after transfer. Numbers in plots indicate the mean percentages ± SD of gated cells within the respective gate. Graph illustrates the accumulation of Foxp3$^+$ Treg cells in the BM. Data are collected from two independent experiments with 4–5 mice; symbols and lines denote individual mice and mean values, respectively.

Lympho-Hematopoiesis in Mice With Constitutive Treg Cell Deficiency

Scurfy mice exhibit a spontaneous loss-of-function mutation in the gene encoding Foxp3, resulting in complete absence of Foxp3 protein and functional CD4$^+$Foxp3$^+$ Treg cells. In addition to systemic autoimmunity targeting several organs such as skin, lung, stomach and liver, severe lympho-hyperproliferation represents another hallmark of the scurfy phenotype, resulting in massively increased secondary lymphoid organs and peripheral immune effector compartments (82, 84).

In initial studies in 3 to 4-week-old scurfy mice, we unexpectedly noticed that the immature B cell compartment in the spleen was essentially completely absent, which appeared to be at odds with the existing mature B cell compartments at the same anatomical site. A more systematic analysis of peripheral B cell compartments revealed even higher numbers of mature B cells in lymph nodes of scurfy mice as compared to wildtype control mice (69). These observations raised several important questions, including the origin of mature B cells in scurfy mice and the possibility that scurfy mice exhibit a heretofore-unappreciated defect in B cell development in the BM, in addition to the well-known hematopoietic bias in scurfy mice towards macrophages (85, 86). When we extended our analysis to lympho-hematopoiesis, it became clear that adolescent scurfy mice exhibit severe B cell developmental defects with near-complete absence of B lymphopoiesis in the BM. Pre-B-II and immature B cell stages were found consistently below the detection level. Several lines of evidence such as the indistinguishability of the BM microenvironment of scurfy and Foxp3-proficient mice within the first week of life with regard to the capacity to support B cell development *in vivo* argue against a constitutive lympho-hematopoietic defect, but support the assumption of an ontogenetic acquisition of B cell developmental defects in scurfy mice. The apparent inconsistency between previously described significant residual B lymphopoietic activity in the BM of 28-day-old scurfy mice (39) and the almost entire block of B cell development observed in mice of the same age in our study is most likely due to differences in the kinetics of autoimmune manifestations, perhaps due to microbial flora variations between independent colonies of Foxp3-deficient mice.

Overall, our results were further corroborated by other recent studies showing that the constitutive absence of Foxp3$^+$ Treg cells impinges on lympho-hematopoiesis in the BM although significant differences between those studies exist. In conjunction with aberrant B lymphopoiesis and in line with other reports, we detected aberrantly increased proportions and numbers of Lin$^-$Sca-1$^+$c-Kit^{hi} (LSK) cells early during ontogeny, suggesting that HSCs might be directly affected by inflammatory cytokines such as type I and type II IFNs. Analysis of *in vivo* reconstitution capacities of scurfy-derived HSCs in BM irradiation chimeras provided inconsistent results, with either substantially reduced or efficient although delayed reconstitution of lymphoid and myeloid lineages (38, 39, 87–89). Moreover, the underlying mechanism and in particular the direct and/or indirect roles of Treg cells remain a matter of debate. While it has been suggested that an altered cytokine milieu in scurfy mice promotes the differentiation of myeloid lineage cells at the expense of lymphopoiesis (87, 89, 90), indicating that the hematopoietic changes are not directly caused by the lack of Treg cells, additional mechanisms such as significantly increased cell death of developing B cells may affect B lymphopoiesis (88).

Nevertheless, our data indicate that the observed defects may not be exclusively mediated by systemic autoimmunity that negatively feeds back to BM hematopoiesis, as neonatal adoptive Treg cell therapy suppressed exacerbated production of inflammatory cytokines such as IL-17 and IL-6, but not IFN-γ and restored defective thymopoiesis, but was ineffective in recovering defective hematopoiesis and B lymphopoiesis. One possible explanation for this might be the failure to re-establish efficient production of CXCL12 and IL-7, which was consistently decreased in the BM of untreated scurfy mice (69). Thus, it appears likely that the aberrant B lymphopoiesis in scurfy mice is a consequence of the diversion of lymphoid progenitors from the B lymphoid lineage in favor of increased myelopoiesis (85–87, 89, 90) and the corporate action of the enhanced systemic production of helper T cell cytokines and locally reduced expression of B lymphopoiesis-promoting factors in the BM (69).

Overall, our observations indicate that re-establishment of immune homeostasis is not sufficient to reinstate hematopoietic homeostasis. We speculate that the adult BM niche might be irreversibly affected by constitutive Treg cell deficiency, which is in line with the severe bone loss afflicted with pronounced autoimmune pathologies, we and others (87) detected in scurfy mice.

Lympho-Hematopoiesis in Mice With Acute Treg Cell Ablation

In contrast to the above described conventional mouse models and depletion strategies, the diphtheria toxin (DT)-mediated deletion of Foxp3$^+$ Treg cells allows for efficient, selective and temporally controlled depletion of Foxp3$^+$ Treg cells without affecting CD25$^+$ effector T cells (91, 92) and thus has provided essential information on Foxp3$^+$ Treg cell biology in health and disease.

However, striking differences exist with regard to depletion efficiency and severity of clinical symptoms after Treg cell ablation (93, 94). Two independent mouse models with an insertion of a DT receptor (DTR) into either the endogenous Foxp3 locus (91) or a Foxp3 promoter-encoding bacterial artificial chromosome [BAC; these mice were termed "depletion of regulatory T cells" (DEREG) mice, (92)] were generated in parallel. In both models, expression of the DTR under the control of the Foxp3 promoter and administration of DT leads to the induction of apoptotic cell death due to blockage of protein synthesis (95), specifically in Foxp3$^+$ Treg cells. When DT was applied to neonatal mice, both, the BAC-transgenic and the knock-in approach resulted in an autoimmune disease similar in severity to that of Foxp3-deficient scurfy mice (91, 92). However, while DT-induced Treg cell ablation in adult mice did not induce scurfy-like disease in DEREG mice (92), Foxp3^{DTR} knock-in mice succumbed to a severe lympho-hyperproliferative disorder (91), which might be explained by different efficiencies with regard to transgene expression (93). Another study assessed BAC transgenic Foxp3DTR lines (Foxp3.LuciDTR, specifically generated for bioluminescence imaging of Treg cells) for depletion efficiencies and signs of pathology and demonstrated that lines with depletion efficiencies of >95% succumbed to a wasting disease, whereas lines with depleting efficiencies <95% lacked the onset of autoimmunity (96).

To deplete Foxp3$^+$ Treg cells in adult steady-state mice, we therefore took advantage of the well-characterized DEREG mouse model (92–94, 97).

Our results show that upon administration of consecutive doses of DT, Foxp3^{GFP+} Treg cells in primary (thymus, BM) and secondary (spleen, lymph nodes, peritoneum) lymphoid organs of NOD.Foxp3$^{DTR-GFP}$ mice were highly efficiently depleted with minimal systemic effects due to rapid recovery of the depleted Treg cell compartment. In contrast to DT-treated C57BL/6 and Balb/c mice, NOD control mice did not show any DT side effects. As a read-out for the impact of Treg cell activity on the generation of adaptive immune cells from HSCs, we assessed the developmental B lymphopoietic activity in the absence and presence of Foxp3$^+$ Treg cells. Our comprehensive analysis of the BM niche revealed that acute Foxp3$^+$ Treg cell ablation in Foxp3$^{DTR-GFP}$ mice results in rapid dysregulation of lympho-hematopoiesis, as evidenced by a strongly increased HSC compartment size (**Figure 2A**) and a strong reduction of BM-residing mature B cells (**Figure 2B**). Of note, and in contrast to our results obtained in mice with constitutive Treg cell deficiency showing that B cell development was almost

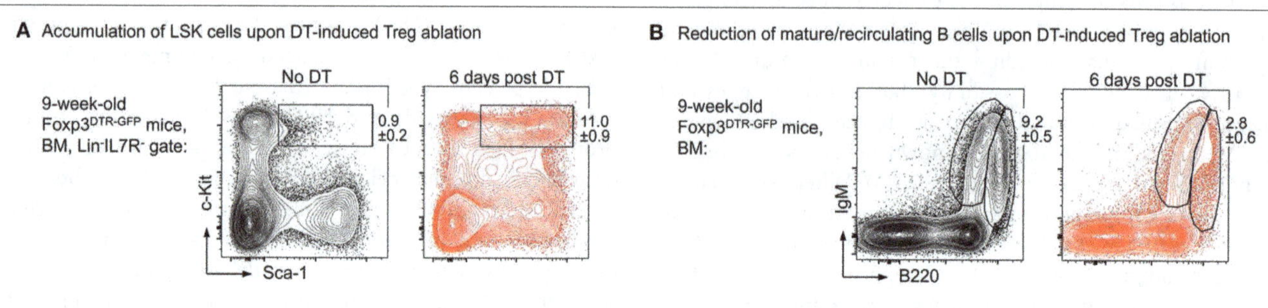

FIGURE 2 | Impact of Foxp3$^+$ Treg cell ablation on the BM niche. Foxp3$^{DTR-GFP}$ mice were *i.p.* injected with DT on 3 consecutive days and the BM was analyzed at day 6 after the first DT dose by flow cytometry. Representative plots of **(A)** LSK (Lineage$^-$IL7R$^-$Sca-1$^+$c-Kit$^+$) cells and **(B)** mature/recirculating B cells (B220^{high}IgM$^+$) in the BM of 9-week-old untreated (left) and DT-treated (right) mice.

completely abrogated (69), we observed that acute Treg cell ablation in adolescent NOD.Foxp3$^{DTR-GFP}$ mice induced only a slight reduction in B cell development. In contrast to scurfy mice, where already the earliest c-Kit^{+} Pro/Pre-B-I cell precursors were significantly reduced, this compartment remained unaffected by the DT-mediated Treg cell depletion, emphasizing that the effects observed in scurfy mice are not directly caused by Treg cell deficiency.

The apparent discrepancy between the recently reported almost complete block in B cell development observed in C57BL/6 Foxp3^{DTR} knock-in mice (98) and the only partial block in early B cell development we observed in NOD.Foxp3$^{DTR-GFP}$ mice, could most likely be attributed to scurfy-like lethal autoimmunity and unwanted DT side effects that have been described for the former mouse model but not for the latter (91, 92, 94, 99, 100).

Overall, the prompt alteration of B lymphopoiesis in the BM upon DT-mediated Treg cell ablation in the absence of overt autoimmunity further support a potential direct role of Treg cells in hematopoiesis.

BONE HOMEOSTASIS AND FOXP3^{+} TREG CELLS

Osteoclast Development and Treg Cells

Osteoclasts, exclusive bone-resorbing cells of hematopoietic origin, are giant multinucleated cells derived from fused precursor cells of the myeloid lineage. The development of mature osteoclasts from early myeloid progenitors is a tightly controlled process involving multiple mediators within the bone microenvironment. Osteoclastogenesis is controlled by ligation of macrophage colony-stimulating factor (c-Fms; M-CSF) and membrane receptors for receptor activator of NF-kB ligand (RANK; RANKL). Under physiological conditions, osteoblast lineage cells, which are of mesenchymal origin, seem to be the main source for M-CSF and RANKL. The central role of M-CSF in survival and proliferation of osteoclast precursors was already revealed decades ago, by studying osteopetrotic op/op mice that bear a natural mutation in the *Csf1* gene coding for M-CSF (101, 102). The discovery of the RANK/RANKL/osteoprotegerin (OPG) signaling axis represents another milestone in bone biology: the finding that RANKL-deficient mice develop severe osteoclast-deficient osteopetrosis, whereas overexpression of RANKL or the lack of the decoy receptor for RANKL, OPG, result in osteoporosis, due to excessive osteoclast formation (103–105), emphasize the critical role of these pathways in osteoclastogenesis.

RANKL promotes the differentiation of committed osteoclast precursor cells by inducing the expression of several genes, such as *cathepsin K*, *tartrate-resistant acid phosphatase* (*TRAP*) and *calcitonin receptor*, as well as transcription factors, such as NF-κB, c-Fos, and the master transcription regulator of osteoclast differentiation NFATc1 (106). Important signals downstream of c-Fms include the PI3K/Akt pathway, crucial for cell survival and the MAPK/ERK pathway essential for survival and proliferation of precursor cells (4).

The discovery that activated T cells express RANKL along with the identification of RANKL as a key differentiation factor for osteoclasts represented one of the first links between the immune and the bone system (107–109). To date, the impact of numerous inflammatory cytokines on the fate of bone cells has been investigated *in vitro* and *in vivo*, and it has been shown that for example IL-1, TNF-α, IL-17, and IL-6 promote osteoclastogenesis by either inducing RANKL expression or directly acting on osteoclast precursor cells, whereas IL-10, IL-4, IFN-γ, and GM-CSF have inhibitory effects on osteoclast differentiation and function, illustrating the tight relationship of osteoclast precursor cells with other cells in the bone microenvironment such as innate and adaptive immune cells (9).

Despite extensive research efforts, osteoclast developmental stages as well as the precise identity of bona fide osteoclast precursors have remained poorly defined and thus there is still fundamental lack of reliable methods for *ex vivo* purification of osteoclasts and their precursors. For this reason, most studies are based on *in vitro* differentiated osteoclasts derived either from macrophages expanded *in vitro* in the presence of M-CSF or from unfractionated whole BM cells cultured under osteoclastogenic conditions, i.e., in the presence of M-CSF and RANKL. However, both methods have their drawbacks since interpretation of data obtained from these cultures is hampered by the heterogeneity of the starting population of which only a minor faction represents osteoclast progenitor cells that differ in their growth kinetics and differentiation potential. Moreover, isolation of primary cells from their *in vivo* microenvironment and subsequent *in vitro* culture results in altered phenotypic and functional characteristics of these cells.

To characterize and isolate osteoclast precursor cells, we combined complex state-of-the-art experimental approaches such as osteoclast differentiation and functional assessment (110, 111) with high-end flow cytometry and cell sorting of very rare cell populations employing a comprehensive array of hematopoietic cell surface markers suggested in varying combinations in the literature (112–116). Multicolor flow cytometry allowed for identification and prospective isolation of these infrequent cell subsets, which — in some cases — account for <0.1% of total BM cells in wildtype mice. To determine the osteoclastogenic potential of the identified populations, FACS-purified cells were cultured in the presence of M-CSF and RANKL. Differentiated osteoclasts were detected as giant, multinucleated, and TRAP-positive cells.

With regard to CD11b expression on potential progenitor cells earlier studies have yielded contradictory results: while some groups described CD11b^{+} precursor cells to exhibit high osteoclastogenic potential, others reported on CD11b$^{-/low}$ cells being more potent (114–118). In our hands, B220^{-}CD3^{-}Ter119^{-}CD11b^{+} BM cells did not have a high osteoclastogenic potential, independent of the expression of Ly6C, whereas the B220^{-}CD3^{-}Ter119^{-}CD11b$^{-/low}$Ly6C^{hi} cell population contained the majority of osteoclast progenitors (**Figure 3**, left), which is in accordance with recent findings by Nakamura and colleagues (116). Since that study detected heterogeneous CD115 (c-Fms) and CD117 (c-Kit) expression on B220^{-}CD3^{-}Ter119^{-}CD11b$^{-/low}$Ly6C^{hi}

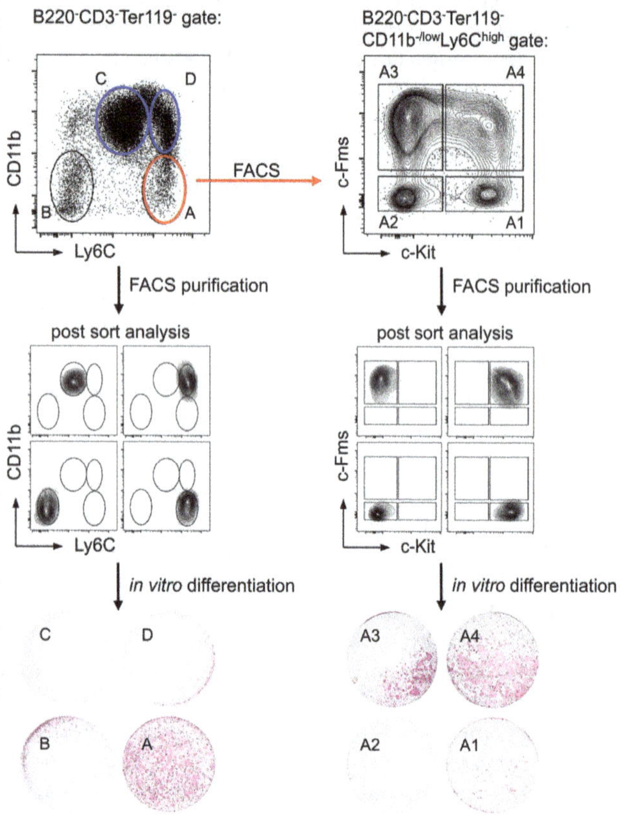

FIGURE 3 | Identification of a cell population with high *in vitro* osteoclast differentiation potential. Ly6C and CD11b expression of bead-enriched $B220^{-}CD3^{-}Ter119^{-}$ BM cells was detected by flow cytometry. Four distinct populations (A: $Ly6C^{high}CD11b^{-/low}$; B: $Ly6C^{-}CD11b^{-}$; C: $Ly6C^{low}CD11b^{+}$; D: $Ly6C^{+}CD11b^{+}$) were FACS-purified and after post-sort analysis *in vitro* differentiated under osteoclast-forming conditions (cytokines: M-CSF and RANKL). The differentiated cultures were fixed and a TRAP staining was performed to identify mature osteoclasts. Additionally, population A was further subdivided by the expression of c-Kit and c-Fms (A1: $c\text{-}Kit^{+}c\text{-}Fms^{-}$; A2: $c\text{-}Kit^{-}c\text{-}Fms^{-}$; A3: $c\text{-}Kit^{-}c\text{-}Fms^{+}$; A4: $c\text{-}Kit^{+}c\text{-}Fms^{+}$). After FACS-purification and post-sort analysis, the populations were cultured and analyzed for their osteoclastogenic potential.

osteoclast progenitor cells (116) and others identified $CD115^{+}CD117^{+}$ double positive cells as highly osteoclastogenic (113, 115), we applied in our study a combination of the surface markers used in these studies. Our results show that $B220^{-}CD3^{-}Ter119^{-}CD11b^{-/low}Ly6C^{hi}CD115^{+}CD117^{+}$ BM cells efficiently differentiate into mature TRAP-expressing osteoclasts *in vitro* (**Figure 3**, right). Initial analyses of the BM niche of $Foxp3^{DTR-GFP}$ mice provided first evidence that acute $Foxp3^{+}$ Treg cell ablation results in substantial changes in osteoclast precursors in the BM.

The sorting of low-abundance prospective primary osteoclast precursors to high purity allow for detailed *ex vivo* analysis without contamination by unwanted cells and hence represents a powerful method to evaluate how Treg cells are affecting the formation of osteoclast precursors in mouse models with abrogated or enhanced Treg cell activity.

Osteoclast Function and Treg Cells

$Foxp3^{+}$ Treg cells control adaptive and innate immune responses by the suppression of activation, proliferation and function of various immune cell types, as for example $CD4^{+}$ helper T cells, $CD8^{+}$ cytotoxic T cells, B cells, NKT cells, macrophages, and dendritic cells (DCs). Multiple mechanisms of $Foxp3^{+}$ Treg cell-mediated suppression have been proposed, involving cell contact-dependent and cell contact-independent mechanisms. The basic mechanisms used by Treg cells include (a) secretion of inhibitory cytokines, such as TGF-β, IL-10, and IL-35, (b) induction of cytolysis by for example granzymes, (c) metabolic disruption by e.g., IL-2-deprivation-mediated apoptosis, and (d) functional modification of antigen presenting cells (APCs) such as DCs. Expression of the cytotoxic T-lymphocyte antigen 4 (CTLA-4) enables Treg cells to interact with CD80/CD86 on DCs outcompeting CD28-mediated co-stimulation and thereby indirectly preventing differentiation of effector T cells (119).

In this context, it has been suggested that Treg cells have the ability to suppress osteoclastogenesis *in vitro*, but the mechanisms of suppression remain incompletely understood and controversial: while some studies identified inhibitory cytokines as key players in Treg cell-mediated suppression of osteoclasts, other reports suggested cell-cell-contact dependent mechanisms (40, 47, 48, 120–122). Most studies addressing the impact of $Foxp3^{+}$ Treg cells on bone homeostasis *in vivo* employed mouse models with either constitutive Foxp3 deficiency or constitutive Foxp3 overexpression (48, 87, 123). As mice with constitutive Foxp3 deficiency suffer from a massive autoimmune lymphoproliferative disease and die approximately at 3 weeks of age (84) and overexpression of Foxp3 in $CD4^{+}$ T cells *in vivo* results in reduced total numbers and functional impairment of T cells (124, 125) potential direct effects of gain and loss of $Foxp3^{+}$ Treg cells are difficult to dissect from the impact of systemic immune dysregulation.

To our knowledge, the impact of temporally controlled, transient $Foxp3^{+}$ Treg cell ablation (91, 92) on skeletal homeostasis under physiological conditions has not been addressed so far.

Osteoclasts and DCs share several features (126, 127). In this context, a recent study proposed that osteoclasts express the co-stimulatory molecules CD80 and CD86 and that Treg cells can regulate osteoclast differentiation via CTLA-4 (128). Moreover, it has been described that BM-residing Treg cells express higher levels of CTLA-4 than peripheral Treg cells (68). Therefore, we hypothesize that this direct cell-cell interaction may indeed play a central role in the crosstalk of osteoclasts and Treg cells.

To investigate the direct interaction of osteoclasts and Treg cells, we performed *in vitro* co-cultures of Treg cells and BM-derived precursor cells. These experiments revealed that the expression of co-stimulatory molecules on the surface of osteoclasts is down-regulated in the presence of Treg cells which leads to the suppression of osteoclast differentiation and function. To directly study cell-cell interactions, cells harvested from these cultures were subjected to simultaneous analysis by multi-parameter flow cytometry and fluorescence microscopy. Imaging flow cytometry showed the direct cell-cell interaction between individual $CD11b^{+}$ late osteoclast precursors and $Foxp3^{GFP+}$

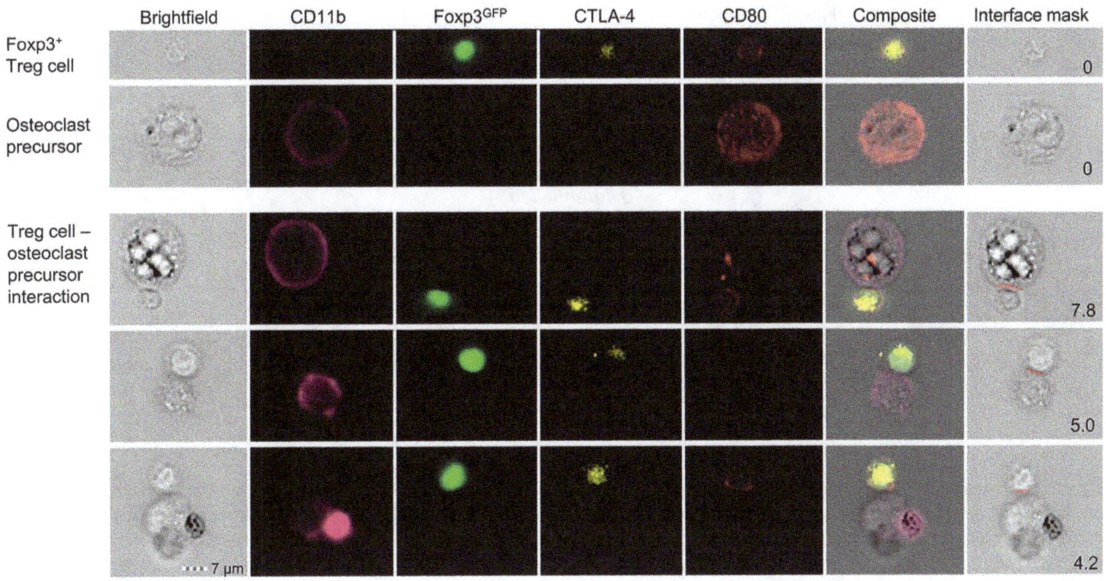

FIGURE 4 | Detailed characterization of *in vitro* Foxp3$^+$ Treg cell-osteoclast precursor interaction. Representative single cell (upper panels) and cluster (lower panels) analysis by imaging flow cytometry. Stimulated FACS-purified CD4$^+$CD25$^+$Foxp3^{GFP+} Treg cells and freshly isolated irradiated T-cell-depleted splenocytes were added to the BM culture and cultured under osteoclastogenic conditions. After 48 h, Foxp3$^+$ Treg cells and CD11b$^+$ osteoclast precursors were analyzed for intracellular expression of CD80 and CTLA-4 by imaging flow cytometry. Cell clusters depict physical interaction of CTLA-4$^+$Foxp3^{GFP+} Treg cells and CD11b$^+$ osteoclast precursors. Co-localization of CD80 in Treg cells indicates trans-endocytosis from CD11b$^+$ osteoclast precursors. Numbers indicate the interface area and illustrate the overlapping fluorescence of Foxp3 and CD11b.

Treg cells which additionally exhibited intracellular red puncta (**Figure 4**), providing first direct evidence that Treg cells can remove CD80/CD86 from the surface of osteoclast precursors by CTLA-4 mediated trans-endocytosis, potentially leading to reduced co-stimulation by osteoclasts — a mechanism which has been described for the interaction of Treg cells and APCs such as DCs (129).

In sum, available data suggest that Treg cells can interfere with bone resorption by affecting osteoclast development and function at multiple stages. However, the mechanism of action is still controversial, emphasizing the complexity of this relationship.

Whether or not T cell regulation of bone and hematopoietic homeostasis requires APCs within the bone microenvironment, is still unknown, but based on the notion that osteoclasts are derived from hematopoietic precursors of the myeloid lineage, express a number of immune receptors and are regulated similarly to macrophages and DCs (130), it is a legitimate question, whether osteoclasts play a role in the active regulation of the immune system, can act e.g., as APCs. Indeed, albeit critically discussed (131), it has been suggested that, in addition to their ability to resorb bone, *in vitro* differentiated osteoclasts can function as APCs and activate CD4$^+$ and CD8$^+$ cells (132). In this context, it was reported that osteoclasts are capable to cross-present antigens to CD8$^+$ T cells, thereby inducing Foxp3 in these cells, which were characterized as osteoclast-induced regulatory CD8$^+$ T cells (133–135).

In addition, recent data suggest that osteoclasts can on the one hand participate in immunogenic T cell responses under chronic inflammatory diseases (136) and on the other hand exhibit immune suppressive functions in multiple myeloma (137, 138). Whether these proposed immune-modulating functions of osteoclasts play a role under physiological conditions or depend on the pathological conditions still needs to be defined. Data from our own group propose the concomitant up-regulation of c-Fms, RANK, and the ligand for the immune checkpoint molecule programmed death 1 protein (PD-1; PD-L1) on the surface of murine CD11b$^+$ osteoclast precursors cultured under osteoclastogenic conditions, which complements the findings on human osteoclast precursor cells (137).

Overall, these observations open additional new prospects for the role of osteoclast in the intercellular interaction of bone cells and immune cells in health and disease (**Figure 5**).

CONCLUSION

The clinical relevance of the BM niche is reflected by its function as (a) the primary hematopoietic site in the adult, (b) a reservoir for memory cells, and (c) in the support of HSC transplantation. The nature of the HSC niche in the BM is defined by various components of the BM microenvironment. Several independent lines of evidence are pointing towards specialized local functions of BM-residing Treg cells in settings of unwanted (autoimmunity, transplant rejection, GvHD) and insufficient immunity (cancer, chronic infections). Modulation of Treg cell activity *in vivo* can be achieved by means such as application of IL-2/anti-IL-2 immune complexes to enhance Treg cell function, whereas depletion or other means of interference with Treg cell function promotes immune responses. This raises the question whether comparable strategies may also be suitable to modulate bone remodeling to manipulate lympho-hematopoiesis in the adult

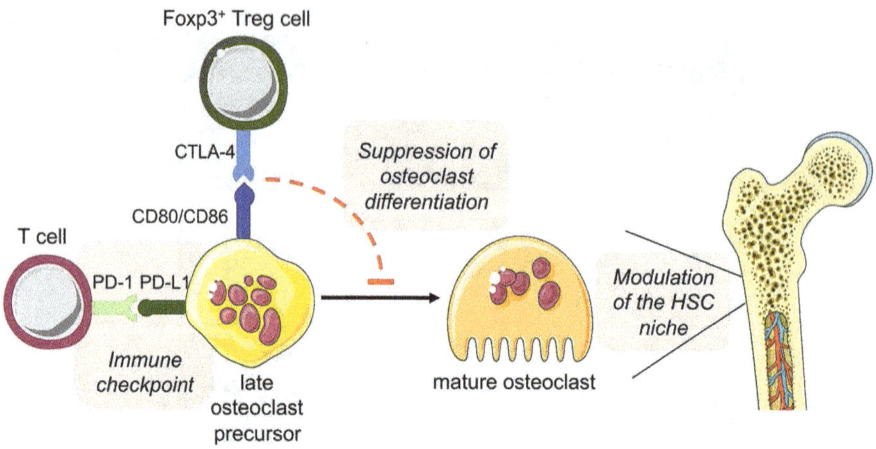

FIGURE 5 | Hypothesized direct cross-talk between osteoclast precursors and T cells and the indirect effect on hematopoiesis. The expression of the costimulatory molecules CD80 and CD86 on osteoclast precursors has been implicated in the interplay with Foxp3+ Treg cells (via the inhibitory molecule CTLA-4), leading to the suppression of the differentiation of osteoclast precursors into mature functional osteoclasts. As a consequence, disturbed bone remodeling results in modulation of the HSC niche. On the other hand, osteoclast precursors are able to upregulate the expression of PD-L1, whose interaction with PD-1 on T cells has immune modulatory functions, thus representing a crucial immune checkpoint. This figure was in part created with modified Servier Medical Art templates, licensed under a Creative Commons Attribution 3.0 Unported license: http://smart.servier.com.

BM. Are there niche-associated Treg cell subsets that specifically interact with bone cells such as osteoclasts? Overall, future studies are warranted to further define the molecular pathways involved in the complex intercellular communication between BM-residing Treg cells, hematopoietic stem and progenitor cells, mature immune cells, and the skeletal system. Understanding the immune regulatory mechanisms in the BM microenvironment is central for the development of effective therapeutic strategies for the treatment of bone diseases and to improve current protocols for HSC transplantation and peripheral immune reconstitution.

AUTHOR CONTRIBUTIONS

LF, CH, RK, SD, and JR designed, performed, and analyzed the experiments. KK and AG conceived the research, guided its design, analysis, and interpretation and wrote the manuscript. All authors contributed to discussions and writing of the manuscript.

FUNDING

AG was supported by a DFG grant (GA1576/1-2) within the SPP1468 IMMUNOBONE. In addition, AG and KK received funds from the FZT 111 (DFG, Center for Regenerative Therapies Dresden, Cluster of Excellence).

ACKNOWLEDGMENTS

The authors would like to thank Tim Sparwasser (University Medical Center of the Johannes Gutenberg University, Mainz, Germany) for providing DEREG mice.

REFERENCES

1. Morrison SJ, Scadden DT. The bone marrow niche for haematopoietic stem cells. *Nature.* (2014) 505:327–34. doi: 10.1038/nature12984
2. Baryawno N, Severe N, Scadden DT. Hematopoiesis: reconciling historic controversies about the Niche. *Cell Stem Cell.* (2017) 20:590–2. doi: 10.1016/j.stem.2017.03.025
3. Bonewald LF. Osteocytes as dynamic multifunctional cells. *Ann N Y Acad Sci.* (2007) 1116:281–90. doi: 10.1196/annals.1402.018
4. Novack DV, Teitelbaum SL. The osteoclast: friend or foe? *Annu Rev Pathol.* (2008) 3:457–84. doi: 10.1146/annurev.pathmechdis.3.121806.151431
5. Kollet O, Dar A, Shivtiel S, Kalinkovich A, Lapid K, Sztainberg Y, et al. Osteoclasts degrade endosteal components and promote mobilization of hematopoietic progenitor cells. *Nat Med.* (2006) 12:657–64. doi: 10.1038/nm1417
6. Mansour A, Abou-Ezzi G, Sitnicka E, Jacobsen SE, Wakkach A, Blin-Wakkach C. Osteoclasts promote the formation of hematopoietic stem cell niches in the bone marrow. *J Exp Med.* (2012) 209:537–49. doi: 10.1084/jem.20110994
7. Miyamoto K, Yoshida S, Kawasumi M, Hashimoto K, Kimura T, Sato Y, et al. Osteoclasts are dispensable for hematopoietic stem cell maintenance and mobilization. *J Exp Med.* (2011) 208:2175–81. doi: 10.1084/jem.20101890
8. Calvi LM, Adams GB, Weibrecht KW, Weber JM, Olson DP, Knight MC, et al. Osteoblastic cells regulate the haematopoietic stem cell niche. *Nature.* (2003) 425:841–6. doi: 10.1038/nature02040
9. Okamoto K, Nakashima T, Shinohara M, Negishi-Koga T, Komatsu N, Terashima A, et al. Osteoimmunology: the conceptual framework unifying the immune and skeletal systems. *Physiol Rev.* (2017) 97:1295–349. doi: 10.1152/physrev.00036.2016
10. Walsh MC, Takegahara N, Kim H, Choi Y. Updating osteoimmunology: regulation of bone cells by innate and adaptive immunity. *Nat Rev Rheumatol.* (2018) 14:146–56. doi: 10.1038/nrrheum.2017.213
11. Bruns I, Lucas D, Pinho S, Ahmed J, Lambert MP, Kunisaki Y, et al. Megakaryocytes regulate hematopoietic stem cell quiescence through CXCL4 secretion. *Nat Med.* (2014) 20:1315–20. doi: 10.1038/nm.3707

12. Zhao M, Perry JM, Marshall H, Venkatraman A, Qian P, He XC, et al. Megakaryocytes maintain homeostatic quiescence and promote post-injury regeneration of hematopoietic stem cells. *Nat Med.* (2014) 20:1321–6. doi: 10.1038/nm.3706
13. Jiang L, Han X, Wang J, Wang C, Sun X, Xie J, et al. SHP-1 regulates hematopoietic stem cell quiescence by coordinating TGF-beta signaling. *J Exp Med.* (2018) 215:1337–47. doi: 10.1084/jem.20171477
14. Kacena MA, Shivdasani RA, Wilson K, Xi Y, Troiano N, Nazarian A, et al. Megakaryocyte-osteoblast interaction revealed in mice deficient in transcription factors GATA-1 and NF-E2. *J Bone Miner Res.* (2004) 19:652–60. doi: 10.1359/JBMR.0301254
15. Kacena MA, Gundberg CM, Horowitz MC. A reciprocal regulatory interaction between megakaryocytes, bone cells, and hematopoietic stem cells. *Bone.* (2006) 39:978–84. doi: 10.1016/j.bone.2006.05.019
16. Kacena MA, Nelson T, Clough ME, Lee SK, Lorenzo JA, Gundberg CM, et al. Megakaryocyte-mediated inhibition of osteoclast development. *Bone.* (2006) 39:991–9. doi: 10.1016/j.bone.2006.05.004
17. Winkler IG, Sims NA, Pettit AR, Barbier V, Nowlan B, Helwani F, et al. Bone marrow macrophages maintain hematopoietic stem cell (HSC) niches and their depletion mobilizes HSCs. *Blood.* (2010) 116:4815–28. doi: 10.1182/blood-2009-11-253534
18. Chow A, Lucas D, Hidalgo A, Mendez-Ferrer S, Hashimoto D, Scheiermann C, et al. Bone marrow CD169+ macrophages promote the retention of hematopoietic stem and progenitor cells in the mesenchymal stem cell niche. *J Exp Med.* (2011) 208:261–71. doi: 10.1084/jem.20101688
19. Christopher MJ, Rao M, Liu F, Woloszynek JR, Link DC. Expression of the G-CSF receptor in monocytic cells is sufficient to mediate hematopoietic progenitor mobilization by G-CSF in mice. *J Exp Med.* (2011) 208:251–60. doi: 10.1084/jem.20101700
20. Hur J, Choi JI, Lee H, Nham P, Kim TW, Chae CW, et al. CD82/KAI1 Maintains the dormancy of long-term hematopoietic stem cells through interaction with DARC-expressing macrophages. *Cell Stem Cell.* (2016) 18:508–21. doi: 10.1016/j.stem.2016.01.013
21. Szade K, Gulati GS, Chan CKF, Kao KS, Miyanishi M, Marjon KD, et al. Where hematopoietic stem cells live: the bone marrow niche. *Antioxid Redox Signal.* (2018) 29:191–204. doi: 10.1089/ars.2017.7419
22. Pinho S, Frenette PS. Haematopoietic stem cell activity and interactions with the niche. *Nat Rev Mol Cell Biol.* (2019) 20:303–20. doi: 10.1038/s41580-019-0103-9
23. Michalski MN, McCauley LK. Macrophages and skeletal health. *Pharmacol Ther.* (2017) 174:43–54. doi: 10.1016/j.pharmthera.2017.02.017
24. Li Y, Toraldo G, Li A, Yang X, Zhang H, Qian WP, et al. B cells and T cells are critical for the preservation of bone homeostasis and attainment of peak bone mass *in vivo*. *Blood.* (2007) 109:3839–48. doi: 10.1182/blood-2006-07-037994
25. Lee SK, Kadono Y, Okada F, Jacquin C, Koczon-Jaremko B, Gronowicz G, et al. T lymphocyte-deficient mice lose trabecular bone mass with ovariectomy. *J Bone Miner Res.* (2006) 21:1704–12. doi: 10.1359/jbmr.060726
26. Horowitz MC, Xi Y, Pflugh DL, Hesslein DG, Schatz DG, Lorenzo JA, et al. Pax5-deficient mice exhibit early onset osteopenia with increased osteoclast progenitors. *J Immunol.* (2004) 173:6583–91. doi: 10.4049/jimmunol.173.11.6583
27. Sauer AV, Mrak E, Hernandez RJ, Zacchi E, Cavani F, Casiraghi M, et al. ADA-deficient SCID is associated with a specific microenvironment and bone phenotype characterized by RANKL/OPG imbalance and osteoblast insufficiency. *Blood.* (2009) 114:3216–26. doi: 10.1182/blood-2009-03-209221
28. Di Rosa F. Two Niches in the bone marrow: a hypothesis on life-long T cell memory. *Trends Immunol.* (2016) 37:503–12. doi: 10.1016/j.it.2016.05.004
29. Manz RA, Thiel A, Radbruch A. Lifetime of plasma cells in the bone marrow. *Nature.* (1997) 388:133–4. doi: 10.1038/40540
30. Geerman S, Nolte MA. Impact of T cells on hematopoietic stem and progenitor cell function: Good guys or bad guys? *World J Stem Cells.* (2017) 9:37–44. doi: 10.4252/wjsc.v9.i2.37
31. Fujisaki J, Wu J, Carlson AL, Silberstein L, Putheti P, Larocca R, et al. *In vivo* imaging of Treg cells providing immune privilege to the haematopoietic stem-cell niche. *Nature.* (2011) 474:216–9. doi: 10.1038/nature10160
32. Hirata Y, Furuhashi K, Ishii H, Li HW, Pinho S, Ding L, et al. CD150(high) bone marrow tregs maintain hematopoietic stem cell quiescence and immune privilege via adenosine. *Cell Stem Cell.* (2018) 22:445–53.e5. doi: 10.1016/j.stem.2018.01.017
33. Sakaguchi S. Naturally arising Foxp3-expressing CD25+CD4+ regulatory T cells in immunological tolerance to self and non-self. *Nat Immunol.* (2005) 6:345–52. doi: 10.1038/ni1178
34. Sakaguchi S, Yamaguchi T, Nomura T, Ono M. Regulatory T cells and immune tolerance. *Cell.* (2008) 133:775–87. doi: 10.1016/j.cell.2008.05.009
35. Feuerer M, Herrero L, Cipolletta D, Naaz A, Wong J, Nayer A, et al. Lean, but not obese, fat is enriched for a unique population of regulatory T cells that affect metabolic parameters. *Nat Med.* (2009) 15:930–9. doi: 10.1038/nm.2002
36. Burzyn D, Kuswanto W, Kolodin D, Shadrach JL, Cerletti M, Jang Y, et al. A special population of regulatory T cells potentiates muscle repair. *Cell.* (2013) 155:1282–95. doi: 10.1016/j.cell.2013.10.054
37. Burzyn D, Benoist C, Mathis D. Regulatory T cells in nonlymphoid tissues. *Nat Immunol.* (2013) 14:1007–13. doi: 10.1038/ni.2683
38. Chen C, Liu Y, Liu Y, Zheng P. Mammalian target of rapamycin activation underlies HSC defects in autoimmune disease and inflammation in mice. *J Clin Invest.* (2010) 120:4091–101. doi: 10.1172/JCI43873
39. Leonardo SM, Josephson JA, Hartog NL, Gauld SB. Altered B cell development and anergy in the absence of Foxp3. *J Immunol.* (2010) 185:2147–56. doi: 10.4049/jimmunol.1000136
40. Zaiss MM, Axmann R, Zwerina J, Polzer K, Guckel E, Skapenko A, et al. Treg cells suppress osteoclast formation: a new link between the immune system and bone. *Arthritis Rheum.* (2007) 56:4104–12. doi: 10.1002/art.23138
41. Wang T, Qiao H, Zhai Z, Zhang J, Tu J, Zheng X, et al. Plumbagin ameliorates collagen-induced arthritis by regulating Treg/Th17 cell imbalances and suppressing osteoclastogenesis. *Front Immunol.* (2018) 9:3102. doi: 10.3389/fimmu.2018.03102
42. McInnes IB, Schett G. Cytokines in the pathogenesis of rheumatoid arthritis. *Nat Rev Immunol.* (2007) 7:429–42. doi: 10.1038/nri2094
43. Gravallese EM. Bone destruction in arthritis. *Ann Rheum Dis.* (2002) 61(Suppl. 2):ii84–6. doi: 10.1136/ard.61.suppl_2.ii84
44. Sato K, Suematsu A, Okamoto K, Yamaguchi A, Morishita Y, Kadono Y, et al. Th17 functions as an osteoclastogenic helper T cell subset that links T cell activation and bone destruction. *J Exp Med.* (2006) 203:2673–82. doi: 10.1084/jem.20061775
45. Morgan ME, Sutmuller RP, Witteveen HJ, van Duivenvoorde LM, Zanelli F, Melief CJ, et al. CD25+ cell depletion hastens the onset of severe disease in collagen-induced arthritis. *Arthritis Rheum.* (2003) 48:1452–60. doi: 10.1002/art.11063
46. Morgan ME, Flierman R, van Duivenvoorde LM, Witteveen HJ, van Ewijk W, van Laar JM, et al. Effective treatment of collagen-induced arthritis by adoptive transfer of CD25+ regulatory T cells. *Arthritis Rheum.* (2005) 52:2212–21. doi: 10.1002/art.21195
47. Kelchtermans H, Geboes L, Mitera T, Huskens D, Leclercq G, Matthys P. Activated CD4+CD25+ regulatory T cells inhibit osteoclastogenesis and collagen-induced arthritis. *Ann Rheum Dis.* (2009) 68:744–50. doi: 10.1136/ard.2007.086066
48. Zaiss MM, Frey B, Hess A, Zwerina J, Luther J, Nimmerjahn F, et al. Regulatory T cells protect from local and systemic bone destruction in arthritis. *J Immunol.* (2010) 184:7238–46. doi: 10.4049/jimmunol.0903841
49. Komatsu N, Okamoto K, Sawa S, Nakashima T, Oh-hora M, Kodama T, et al. Pathogenic conversion of Foxp3+ T cells into TH17 cells in autoimmune arthritis. *Nat Med.* (2014) 20:62–8. doi: 10.1038/nm.3432
50. Terauchi M, Li JY, Bedi B, Baek KH, Tawfeek H, Galley S, et al. T lymphocytes amplify the anabolic activity of parathyroid hormone through Wnt10b signaling. *Cell Metab.* (2009) 10:229–40. doi: 10.1016/j.cmet.2009.07.010
51. Li JY, Walker LD, Tyagi AM, Adams J, Weitzmann MN, Pacifici R. The sclerostin-independent bone anabolic activity of intermittent PTH treatment is mediated by T-cell-produced Wnt10b. *J Bone Miner Res.* (2014) 29:43–54. doi: 10.1002/jbmr.2044
52. Tyagi AM, Yu M, Darby TM, Vaccaro C, Li JY, Owens JA, et al. The microbial metabolite butyrate stimulates bone formation via T regulatory

cell-mediated regulation of WNT10B expression. *Immunity.* (2018) 49:1116–31.e7. doi: 10.1016/j.immuni.2018.10.013
53. Yu M, D'Amelio P, Tyagi AM, Vaccaro C, Li JY, Hsu E, et al. Regulatory T cells are expanded by Teriparatide treatment in humans and mediate intermittent PTH-induced bone anabolism in mice. *EMBO Rep.* (2018) 19:156–71. doi: 10.15252/embr.201744421
54. Lei H, Schmidt-Bleek K, Dienelt A, Reinke P, Volk HD. Regulatory T cell-mediated anti-inflammatory effects promote successful tissue repair in both indirect and direct manners. *Front Pharmacol.* (2015) 6:184. doi: 10.3389/fphar.2015.00184
55. Arron JR, Choi Y. Bone versus immune system. *Nature.* (2000) 408:535–6. doi: 10.1038/35046196
56. King KY, Goodell MA. Inflammatory modulation of HSCs: viewing the HSC as a foundation for the immune response. *Nat Rev Immunol.* (2011) 11:685–92. doi: 10.1038/nri3062
57. Pietras EM. Inflammation: a key regulator of hematopoietic stem cell fate in health and disease. *Blood.* (2017) 130:1693–8. doi: 10.1182/blood-2017-06-780882
58. Christopher MJ, Liu F, Hilton MJ, Long F, Link DC. Suppression of CXCL12 production by bone marrow osteoblasts is a common and critical pathway for cytokine-induced mobilization. *Blood.* (2009) 114:1331–9. doi: 10.1182/blood-2008-10-184754
59. Sato N, Takahashi N, Suda K, Nakamura M, Yamaki M, Ninomiya T, et al. MyD88 but not TRIF is essential for osteoclastogenesis induced by lipopolysaccharide, diacyl lipopeptide, and IL-1alpha. *J Exp Med.* (2004) 200:601–11. doi: 10.1084/jem.20040689
60. Hayashi S, Yamada T, Tsuneto M, Yamane T, Takahashi M, Shultz LD, et al. Distinct osteoclast precursors in the bone marrow and extramedullary organs characterized by responsiveness to Toll-like receptor ligands and TNF-alpha. *J Immunol.* (2003) 171:5130–9. doi: 10.4049/jimmunol.171.10.5130
61. Katayama Y, Battista M, Kao WM, Hidalgo A, Peired AJ, Thomas SA, et al. Signals from the sympathetic nervous system regulate hematopoietic stem cell egress from bone marrow. *Cell.* (2006) 124:407–21. doi: 10.1016/j.cell.2005.10.041
62. Mendez-Ferrer S, Lucas D, Battista M, Frenette PS. Haematopoietic stem cell release is regulated by circadian oscillations. *Nature.* (2008) 452:442–7. doi: 10.1038/nature06685
63. Lucas D. Leukocyte trafficking and regulation of murine hematopoietic stem cells and their niches. *Front Immunol.* (2019) 10:387. doi: 10.3389/fimmu.2019.00387
64. Decker M, Leslie J, Liu Q, Ding L. Hepatic thrombopoietin is required for bone marrow hematopoietic stem cell maintenance. *Science.* (2018) 360:106–10. doi: 10.1126/science.aap8861
65. Casanova-Acebes M, Nicolas-Avila JA, Li JL, Garcia-Silva S, Balachander A, Rubio-Ponce A, et al. Neutrophils instruct homeostatic and pathological states in naive tissues. *J Exp Med.* (2018) 215:2778–95. doi: 10.1084/jem.20181468
66. Di Rosa F, Pabst R. The bone marrow: a nest for migratory memory T cells. *Trends Immunol.* (2005) 26:360–6. doi: 10.1016/j.it.2005.04.011
67. Zou L, Barnett B, Safah H, Larussa VF, Evdemon-Hogan M, Mottram P, et al. Bone marrow is a reservoir for CD4+CD25+ regulatory T cells that traffic through CXCL12/CXCR4 signals. *Cancer Res.* (2004) 64:8451–5. doi: 10.1158/0008-5472.CAN-04-1987
68. Glatman Zaretsky A, Konradt C, Depis F, Wing JB, Goenka R, Atria DG, et al. T regulatory cells support plasma cell populations in the bone marrow. *Cell Rep.* (2017) 18:1906–16. doi: 10.1016/j.celrep.2017.01.067
69. Riewaldt J, Duber S, Boernert M, Krey M, Dembinski M, Weiss S, et al. Severe developmental B lymphopoietic defects in foxp3-deficient mice are refractory to adoptive regulatory T cell therapy. *Front Immunol.* (2012) 3:141. doi: 10.3389/fimmu.2012.00141
70. Kretschmer K, Apostolou I, Hawiger D, Khazaie K, Nussenzweig MC, von Boehmer H. Inducing and expanding regulatory T cell populations by foreign antigen. *Nat Immunol.* (2005) 6:1219–27. doi: 10.1038/ni1265
71. Kretschmer K, Apostolou I, Jaeckel E, Khazaie K, von Boehmer H. Making regulatory T cells with defined antigen specificity: role in autoimmunity and cancer. *Immunol Rev.* (2006) 212:163–9. doi: 10.1111/j.0105-2896.2006.00411.x
72. Taguchi O, Takahashi T. Administration of anti-interleukin-2 receptor alpha antibody *in vivo* induces localized autoimmune disease. *Eur J Immunol.* (1996) 26:1608–12. doi: 10.1002/eji.1830260730
73. McHugh RS, Shevach EM. Cutting edge: depletion of CD4+CD25+ regulatory T cells is necessary, but not sufficient, for induction of organ-specific autoimmune disease. *J Immunol.* (2002) 168:5979–83. doi: 10.1023/A:1020665614139
74. Kohm AP, McMahon JS, Podojil JR, Begolka WS, DeGutes M, Kasprowicz DJ, et al. Cutting Edge: Anti-CD25 monoclonal antibody injection results in the functional inactivation, not depletion, of CD4+CD25+ T regulatory cells. *J Immunol.* (2006) 176:3301–5. doi: 10.4049/jimmunol.176.6.3301
75. Stephens LA, Anderton SM. Comment on "cutting edge: anti-CD25 monoclonal antibody injection results in the functional inactivation, not depletion, of CD4+CD25+ T regulatory cells". *J Immunol.* (2006) 177:2036; author reply 7–8. doi: 10.4049/jimmunol.177.4.2036
76. Zelenay S, Demengeot J. Comment on "cutting edge: anti-CD25 monoclonal antibody injection results in the functional inactivation, not depletion, of CD4+CD25+ T regulatory cells". *J Immunol.* (2006) 177:2036–7; author reply 7–8. doi: 10.4049/jimmunol.177.4.2036-a
77. Huss DJ, Pellerin AF, Collette BP, Kannan AK, Peng L, Datta A, et al. Anti-CD25 monoclonal antibody Fc variants differentially impact regulatory T cells and immune homeostasis. *Immunology.* (2016) 148:276–86. doi: 10.1111/imm.12609
78. Kelchtermans H, De Klerck B, Mitera T, Van Balen M, Bullens D, Billiau A, et al. Defective CD4+CD25+ regulatory T cell functioning in collagen-induced arthritis: an important factor in pathogenesis, counter-regulated by endogenous IFN-gamma. *Arthritis Res Ther.* (2005) 7:R402–15. doi: 10.1186/ar1500
79. Frey O, Petrow PK, Gajda M, Siegmund K, Huehn J, Scheffold A, et al. The role of regulatory T cells in antigen-induced arthritis: aggravation of arthritis after depletion and amelioration after transfer of CD4+CD25+ T cells. *Arthritis Res Ther.* (2005) 7:R291–301. doi: 10.1186/ar1484
80. Couper KN, Blount DG, de Souza JB, Suffia I, Belkaid Y, Riley EM. Incomplete depletion and rapid regeneration of Foxp3+ regulatory T cells following anti-CD25 treatment in malaria-infected mice. *J Immunol.* (2007) 178:4136–46. doi: 10.4049/jimmunol.178.7.4136
81. Hori S, Nomura T, Sakaguchi S. Control of regulatory T cell development by the transcription factor Foxp3. *Science.* (2003) 299:1057–61. doi: 10.1126/science.1079490
82. Fontenot JD, Gavin MA, Rudensky AY. Foxp3 programs the development and function of CD4+CD25+ regulatory T cells. *Nat Immunol.* (2003) 4:330–6. doi: 10.1038/ni904
83. Khattri R, Cox T, Yasayko SA, Ramsdell F. An essential role for Scurfin in CD4+CD25+ T regulatory cells. *Nat Immunol.* (2003) 4:337–42. doi: 10.1038/ni909
84. Brunkow ME, Jeffery EW, Hjerrild KA, Paeper B, Clark LB, Yasayko SA, et al. Disruption of a new forkhead/winged-helix protein, scurfin, results in the fatal lymphoproliferative disorder of the scurfy mouse. *Nat Genet.* (2001) 27:68–73. doi: 10.1038/83784
85. Clark LB, Appleby MW, Brunkow ME, Wilkinson JE, Ziegler SF, Ramsdell F. Cellular and molecular characterization of the scurfy mouse mutant. *J Immunol.* (1999) 162:2546–54.
86. Lee JH, Wang C, Kim CH. FoxP3+ regulatory T cells restrain splenic extramedullary myelopoiesis via suppression of hemopoietic cytokine-producing T cells. *J Immunol.* (2009) 183:6377–86. doi: 10.4049/jimmunol.0901268
87. Chen TH, Swarnkar G, Mbalaviele G, Abu-Amer Y. Myeloid lineage skewing due to exacerbated NF-kappaB signaling facilitates osteopenia in Scurfy mice. *Cell Death Dis.* (2015) 6:e1723. doi: 10.1038/cddis.2015.87
88. Chang SE, Guo L, Tian J, Liu Y, Guo Z, Zheng B, et al. Autoimmune bone marrow environment severely inhibits B cell development by inducing extensive cell death and inhibiting proliferation. *Autoimmunity.* (2012) 45:210–7. doi: 10.3109/08916934.2011.632455
89. Skuljec J, Cabanski M, Surdziel E, Lachmann N, Brennig S, Pul R, et al. Monocyte/macrophage lineage commitment and distribution are affected by the lack of regulatory T cells in scurfy mice. *Eur J Immunol.* (2016) 46:1656–68. doi: 10.1002/eji.201546200

90. Kim S, Park K, Choi J, Jang E, Paik DJ, Seong RH, et al. Foxp3+ regulatory T cells ensure B lymphopoiesis by inhibiting the granulopoietic activity of effector T cells in mouse bone marrow. *Eur J Immunol.* (2015) 45:167-79. doi: 10.1002/eji.201444532
91. Kim JM, Rasmussen JP, Rudensky AY. Regulatory T cells prevent catastrophic autoimmunity throughout the lifespan of mice. *Nat Immunol.* (2007) 8:191-7. doi: 10.1038/ni1428
92. Lahl K, Loddenkemper C, Drouin C, Freyer J, Arnason J, Eberl G, et al. Selective depletion of Foxp3+ regulatory T cells induces a scurfy-like disease. *J Exp Med.* (2007) 204:57-63. doi: 10.1084/jem.20061852
93. Lahl K, Sparwasser T. *In vivo* depletion of FoxP3+ Tregs using the DEREG mouse model. *Methods Mol Biol.* (2011) 707:157-72. doi: 10.1007/978-1-61737-979-6_10
94. Mayer CT, Lahl K, Milanez-Almeida P, Watts D, Dittmer U, Fyhrquist N, et al. Advantages of Foxp3(+) regulatory T cell depletion using DEREG mice. *Immun Inflamm Dis.* (2014) 2:162-5. doi: 10.1002/iid3.33
95. Saito M, Iwawaki T, Taya C, Yonekawa H, Noda M, Inui Y, et al. Diphtheria toxin receptor-mediated conditional and targeted cell ablation in transgenic mice. *Nat Biotechnol.* (2001) 19:746-50. doi: 10.1038/90795
96. Suffner J, Hochweller K, Kuhnle MC, Li X, Kroczek RA, Garbi N, et al. Dendritic cells support homeostatic expansion of Foxp3+ regulatory T cells in Foxp3.LuciDTR mice. *J Immunol.* (2010) 184:1810-20. doi: 10.4049/jimmunol.0902420
97. Kim J, Lahl K, Hori S, Loddenkemper C, Chaudhry A, deRoos P, et al. Cutting edge: depletion of Foxp3+ cells leads to induction of autoimmunity by specific ablation of regulatory T cells in genetically targeted mice. *J Immunol.* (2009) 183:7631-4. doi: 10.4049/jimmunol.0804308
98. Pierini A, Nishikii H, Baker J, Kimura T, Kwon HS, Pan Y, et al. Foxp3(+) regulatory T cells maintain the bone marrow microenvironment for B cell lymphopoiesis. *Nat Commun.* (2017) 8:15068. doi: 10.1038/ncomms15068
99. Lahl K, Mayer CT, Bopp T, Huehn J, Loddenkemper C, Eberl G, et al. Nonfunctional regulatory T cells and defective control of Th2 cytokine production in natural scurfy mutant mice. *J Immunol.* (2009) 183:5662-72. doi: 10.4049/jimmunol.0803762
100. Mayer CT, Ghorbani P, Kuhl AA, Stuve P, Hegemann M, Berod L, et al. Few Foxp3(+) regulatory T cells are sufficient to protect adult mice from lethal autoimmunity. *Eur J Immunol.* (2014) 44:2990-3002. doi: 10.1002/eji.201344315
101. Wiktor-Jedrzejczak WW, Ahmed A, Szczylik C, Skelly RR. Hematological characterization of congenital osteopetrosis in op/op mouse. Possible mechanism for abnormal macrophage differentiation. *J Exp Med.* (1982) 156:1516-27. doi: 10.1084/jem.156.5.1516
102. Felix R, Cecchini MG, Hofstetter W, Elford PR, Stutzer A, Fleisch H. Impairment of macrophage colony-stimulating factor production and lack of resident bone marrow macrophages in the osteopetrotic op/op mouse. *J Bone Miner Res.* (1990) 5:781-9. doi: 10.1002/jbmr.5650050716
103. Kong YY, Feige U, Sarosi I, Bolon B, Tafuri A, Morony S, et al. Activated T cells regulate bone loss and joint destruction in adjuvant arthritis through osteoprotegerin ligand. *Nature.* (1999) 402:304-9. doi: 10.1038/35005552
104. Kong YY, Yoshida H, Sarosi I, Tan HL, Timms E, Capparelli C, et al. OPGL is a key regulator of osteoclastogenesis, lymphocyte development and lymph-node organogenesis. *Nature.* (1999) 397:315-23. doi: 10.1038/16852
105. Bucay N, Sarosi I, Dunstan CR, Morony S, Tarpley J, Capparelli C, et al. osteoprotegerin-deficient mice develop early onset osteoporosis and arterial calcification. *Genes Dev.* (1998) 12:1260-8. doi: 10.1101/gad.12.9.1260
106. Novack DV, Mbalaviele G. Osteoclasts-key players in skeletal health and disease. *Microbiol Spectr.* (2016) 4:1-19. doi: 10.1128/microbiolspec.MCHD-0011-2015
107. Wong BR, Rho J, Arron J, Robinson E, Orlinick J, Chao M, et al. TRANCE is a novel ligand of the tumor necrosis factor receptor family that activates c-Jun N-terminal kinase in T cells. *J Biol Chem.* (1997) 272:25190-4. doi: 10.1074/jbc.272.40.25190
108. Lacey DL, Timms E, Tan HL, Kelley MJ, Dunstan CR, Burgess T, et al. Osteoprotegerin ligand is a cytokine that regulates osteoclast differentiation and activation. *Cell.* (1998) 93:165-76. doi: 10.1016/S0092-8674(00)81569-X
109. Yasuda H, Shima N, Nakagawa N, Yamaguchi K, Kinosaki M, Mochizuki S, et al. Osteoclast differentiation factor is a ligand for osteoprotegerin/osteoclastogenesis-inhibitory factor and is identical to TRANCE/RANKL. *Proc Natl Acad Sci USA.* (1998) 95:3597-602. doi: 10.1073/pnas.95.7.3597
110. Lutter AH, Hempel U, Wolf-Brandstetter C, Garbe AI, Goettsch C, Hofbauer LC, et al. A novel resorption assay for osteoclast functionality based on an osteoblast-derived native extracellular matrix. *J Cell Biochem.* (2010) 109:1025-32. doi: 10.1002/jcb.22485
111. Garbe AI, Roscher A, Schuler C, Lutter AH, Glosmann M, Bernhardt R, et al. Regulation of bone mass and osteoclast function depend on the F-actin modulator SWAP-70. *J Bone Miner Res.* (2012) 27:2085-96. doi: 10.1002/jbmr.1670
112. Muguruma Y, Lee MY. Isolation and characterization of murine clonogenic osteoclast progenitors by cell surface phenotype analysis. *Blood.* (1998) 91:1272-9.
113. Arai F, Miyamoto T, Ohneda O, Inada T, Sudo T, Brasel K, et al. Commitment and differentiation of osteoclast precursor cells by the sequential expression of c-Fms and receptor activator of nuclear factor kappaB (RANK) receptors. *J Exp Med.* (1999) 190:1741-54. doi: 10.1084/jem.190.12.1741
114. Jacome-Galarza CE, Lee SK, Lorenzo JA, Aguila HL. Identification, characterization, and isolation of a common progenitor for osteoclasts, macrophages, and dendritic cells from murine bone marrow and periphery. *J Bone Miner Res.* (2013) 28:1203-13. doi: 10.1002/jbmr.1822
115. Jacquin C, Gran DE, Lee SK, Lorenzo JA, Aguila HL. Identification of multiple osteoclast precursor populations in murine bone marrow. *J Bone Miner Res.* (2006) 21:67-77. doi: 10.1359/JBMR.051007
116. Charles JF, Hsu LY, Niemi EC, Weiss A, Aliprantis AO, Nakamura MC. Inflammatory arthritis increases mouse osteoclast precursors with myeloid suppressor function. *J Clin Invest.* (2012) 122:4592-605. doi: 10.1172/JCI60920
117. Li P, Schwarz EM, O'Keefe RJ, Ma L, Looney RJ, Ritchlin CT, et al. Systemic tumor necrosis factor alpha mediates an increase in peripheral CD11bhigh osteoclast precursors in tumor necrosis factor alpha-transgenic mice. *Arthritis Rheum.* (2004) 50:265-76. doi: 10.1002/art.11419
118. Yao Z, Li P, Zhang Q, Schwarz EM, Keng P, Arbini A, et al. Tumor necrosis factor-alpha increases circulating osteoclast precursor numbers by promoting their proliferation and differentiation in the bone marrow through up-regulation of c-Fms expression. *J Biol Chem.* (2006) 281:11846-55. doi: 10.1074/jbc.M512624200
119. Vignali DA, Collison LW, Workman CJ. How regulatory T cells work. *Nat Rev Immunol.* (2008) 8:523-32. doi: 10.1038/nri2343
120. Kim YG, Lee CK, Nah SS, Mun SH, Yoo B, Moon HB. Human CD4+CD25+ regulatory T cells inhibit the differentiation of osteoclasts from peripheral blood mononuclear cells. *Biochem Biophys Res Commun.* (2007) 357:1046-52. doi: 10.1016/j.bbrc.2007.04.042
121. Axmann R, Herman S, Zaiss M, Franz S, Polzer K, Zwerina J, et al. CTLA-4 directly inhibits osteoclast formation. *Ann Rheum Dis.* (2008) 67:1603-9. doi: 10.1136/ard.2007.080713
122. Luo CY, Wang L, Sun C, Li DJ. Estrogen enhances the functions of CD4(+)CD25(+)Foxp3(+) regulatory T cells that suppress osteoclast differentiation and bone resorption *in vitro*. *Cell Mol Immunol.* (2011) 8:50-8. doi: 10.1038/cmi.2010.54
123. Zaiss MM, Sarter K, Hess A, Engelke K, Bohm C, Nimmerjahn F, et al. Increased bone density and resistance to ovariectomy-induced bone loss in FoxP3-transgenic mice based on impaired osteoclast differentiation. *Arthritis Rheum.* (2010) 62:2328-38. doi: 10.1002/art.27535
124. Khattri R, Kasprowicz D, Cox T, Mortrud M, Appleby MW, Brunkow ME, et al. The amount of scurfin protein determines peripheral T cell number and responsiveness. *J Immunol.* (2001) 167:6312-20. doi: 10.4049/jimmunol.167.11.6312
125. Kasprowicz DJ, Droin N, Soper DM, Ramsdell F, Green DR, Ziegler SF. Dynamic regulation of FoxP3 expression controls the balance between CD4+ T cell activation and cell death. *Eur J Immunol.* (2005) 35:3424-32. doi: 10.1002/eji.200526339
126. Xiao Y, Zijl S, Wang L, de Groot DC, van Tol MJ, Lankester AC, et al. Identification of the common origins of osteoclasts, macrophages, and dendritic cells in human hematopoiesis. *Stem Cell Reports.* (2015) 4:984-94. doi: 10.1016/j.stemcr.2015.04.012

127. Laperine O, Blin-Wakkach C, Guicheux J, Beck-Cormier S, Lesclous P. Dendritic-cell-derived osteoclasts: a new game changer in bone-resorption-associated diseases. *Drug Discov Today.* (2016) 21:1345–54. doi: 10.1016/j.drudis.2016.04.022
128. Bozec A, Zaiss MM, Kagwiria R, Voll R, Rauh M, Chen Z, et al. T cell costimulation molecules CD80/86 inhibit osteoclast differentiation by inducing the IDO/tryptophan pathway. *Sci Transl Med.* (2014) 6:235ra60. doi: 10.1126/scitranslmed.3007764
129. Qureshi OS, Zheng Y, Nakamura K, Attridge K, Manzotti C, Schmidt EM, et al. Trans-endocytosis of CD80 and CD86: a molecular basis for the cell-extrinsic function of CTLA-4. *Science.* (2011) 332:600–3. doi: 10.1126/science.1202947
130. Wu Y, Humphrey MB, Nakamura MC. Osteoclasts - the innate immune cells of the bone. *Autoimmunity.* (2008) 41:183–94. doi: 10.1080/08916930701693180
131. Lorenzo JA. Do osteoclasts have dual roles: bone resorption and antigen presentation? *IBMS BoneKEy.* (2011) 8:37–40. doi: 10.1138/20110488
132. Li H, Hong S, Qian J, Zheng Y, Yang J, Yi Q. Cross talk between the bone and immune systems: osteoclasts function as antigen-presenting cells and activate CD4+ and CD8+ T cells. *Blood.* (2010) 116:210–7. doi: 10.1182/blood-2009-11-255026
133. Kiesel JR, Buchwald ZS, Aurora R. Cross-presentation by osteoclasts induces FoxP3 in CD8+ T cells. *J Immunol.* (2009) 182:5477–87. doi: 10.4049/jimmunol.0803897
134. Buchwald ZS, Kiesel JR, DiPaolo R, Pagadala MS, Aurora R. Osteoclast activated FoxP3+ CD8+ T-cells suppress bone resorption *in vitro*. *PLoS ONE.* (2012) 7:e38199. doi: 10.1371/journal.pone.0038199
135. Buchwald ZS, Kiesel JR, Yang C, DiPaolo R, Novack DV, Aurora R. Osteoclast-induced Foxp3+ CD8 T-cells limit bone loss in mice. *Bone.* (2013) 56:163–73. doi: 10.1016/j.bone.2013.05.024
136. Ibanez L, Abou-Ezzi G, Ciucci T, Amiot V, Belaid N, Obino D, et al. Inflammatory osteoclasts prime TNFalpha-producing CD4(+) T cells and express CX3 CR1. *J Bone Miner Res.* (2016) 31:1899–908. doi: 10.1002/jbmr.2868
137. An G, Acharya C, Feng X, Wen K, Zhong M, Zhang L, et al. Osteoclasts promote immune suppressive microenvironment in multiple myeloma: therapeutic implication. *Blood.* (2016) 128:1590–603. doi: 10.1182/blood-2016-03-707547
138. Mansour A, Wakkach A, Blin-Wakkach C. Emerging roles of osteoclasts in the modulation of bone microenvironment and immune suppression in multiple myeloma. *Front Immunol.* (2017) 8:954. doi: 10.3389/fimmu.2017.00954

5

Immune Modulation by Transplanted Calcium Phosphate Biomaterials and Human Mesenchymal Stromal Cells in Bone Regeneration

Paul Humbert[1], *Meadhbh Á. Brennan*[1,2], *Noel Davison*[3,4], *Philippe Rosset*[1,5], *Valérie Trichet*[1], *Frédéric Blanchard*[1*] *and Pierre Layrolle*[1]

[1] Laboratory Phy-Os, Inserm UMR1238, University of Nantes, Nantes, France, [2] Harvard School of Engineering and Applied Sciences, Harvard University, Cambridge, MA, United States, [3] MERLN Institute for Technology-Inspired Regenerative Medicine, Maastricht University, Maastricht, Netherlands, [4] Instructure Labs, B.V., The Hague, Netherlands, [5] Centre Hospitalier Universitaire de Tours, Tours, France

***Correspondence:**
Frédéric Blanchard
frederic.blanchard@univ-nantes.fr

A wide variety of biomaterials have been developed as both stabilizing structures for the injured bone and inducers of bone neoformation. They differ in chemical composition, shape, porosity, and mechanical properties. The most extensively employed and studied subset of bioceramics are calcium phosphate materials (CaPs). These materials, when transplanted alongside mesenchymal stem cells (MSCs), lead to ectopic (intramuscular and subcutaneous) and orthotopic bone formation in preclinical studies, and effective fracture healing in clinical trials. Human MSC transplantation in pre-clinical and clinical trials reveals very low engraftment in spite of successful clinical outcomes and their therapeutic actions are thought to be primarily through paracrine mechanisms. The beneficial role of transplanted MSC could rely on their strong immunomodulatory effect since, even without long-term engraftment, they have the ability to alter both the innate and adaptive immune response which is critical to facilitate new bone formation. This study presents the current knowledge of the immune response to the implantation of CaP biomaterials alone or in combination with MSC. In particular the central role of monocyte-derived cells, both macrophages and osteoclasts, in MSC-CaP mediated bone formation is emphasized. Biomaterial properties, such as macroporosity and surface microstructure, dictate the host response, and the ultimate bone healing cascade. Understanding intercellular communications throughout the inflammation, its resolution and the bone regeneration phase, is crucial to improve the current therapeutic strategies or develop new approaches.

Keywords: osteoimmunology, mesenchymal stromal cell, calcium phosphate biomaterial, bone regeneration, osteoclast, immune modulation

INTRODUCTION

Bone regeneration strategies remain a critical challenge in the treatment of delayed union and non-union fractures (1), bone loss due to tumor resection (2), metabolic bone diseases, or to heritable skeletal dysplasia such as *osteogenesis imperfecta.* Autologous bone grafting is the current clinical gold standard to repair large bone defects. This entails harvesting the patient's own bone fragments, and transplanting them to the site of injury (3). There are ~2.2 million bone graft procedures performed annually worldwide, including 1 million procedures in Europe (4). Indeed, after blood, bone is the most frequently transplanted tissue. The significant disadvantages of bone grafting, including the severe pain and morbidity endured by patients as a consequence of the bone harvest site, have prompted advances in the development of synthetic biomaterials targeting bone repair. Human bone comprises ~70% of calcium phosphate (CaP) mineral; therefore CaPs are the biomaterials of choice to heal injured bone. They were first introduced in the 1920s as materials to facilitate bone repair (5) and have since undergone intense chemical and physical developments aimed at optimizing porosity, surface architecture, resorption rates, and mechanical strength in order to improve their bone healing capacities. Despite these advances in biomaterial design, CaPs still lack adequate osteogenecity to heal large, critical sized bone defects, and thus cell therapy has been employed for bone defect treatment with biomaterial bone substitutes such as CaPs to increase bone regeneration efficiency. Mesenchymal stromal stem cells (MSCs), derived primarily from the bone marrow and isolated by adherence to plastic, show great capacity for bone healing in unison with CaPs (6, 7). Although it is yet to be adopted into standard clinical practice, this state-of-the-art cell therapy is currently the most promising regenerative medicine strategy and has demonstrated successful bone healing in patients in clinical trials (8). The initial premise that MSCs, through cellular differentiation, regenerated damaged tissue was largely disregarded following observations that very few transplanted cells survive and engraft (9–11). Few children with severe *osteogenesis imperfecta* have received allogenic bone marrow transplant or allogenic MSC and showed faster growth, higher bone mineral content and less bone fracture than before transplant (12–16). Such growth and mineralization improvements were associated with <5% of donor cell engraftment. Consequently, it is proposed that the therapeutic benefit of transplanted MSCs is largely through a paracrine mechanism that stimulates recruitment of host cells, which ultimately form the new bone tissue. The underlying mechanisms involved have yet to be delineated, however evidence to date reveals that roles of MSCs and their secretions such as modulating immune responses (17), attenuating inflammation, and promoting angiogenesis (18), together act to ultimately ameliorate healing and restore function. The host immune-modulatory response to both CaPs and MSCs, encompassing both innate and adaptive immunity, and how this contributes to bone healing in the context of tissue engineered implants is the focus of the current review.

OSTEOIMMUNOLOGY OF CALCIUM PHOSPHATE CERAMICS IN BONE REGENERATION

A wide variety of CaP biomaterials have been developed to fill bone defects as alternatives to autologous bone grafting. Synthetically synthesized ceramics mainly comprise sintered CaPs in order to achieve higher mechanical strength, including β-tricalcium phosphate (β -TCP), hydroxyapatite (HA), or their mixtures (biphasic calcium phosphate: BCP). These CaPs are therefore widely described in terms of their interactions with cells and tissues following implantation, as well as in relation to their bone forming abilities. Synthetic CaPs bioceramics are used successfully to fill bone defects in various clinical indications since they are considered biocompatible, bioactive and osteoconductive, thereby permitting guidance of the bone healing process (19). *In vivo*, the chemical and physical properties of the biomaterial dictate the host response and the ultimate bone healing cascade and osteoinduction has been achieved by various CaP ceramics, which demonstrate ectopic bone formation when implanted in the muscles or subcutaneously in animals [reviewed in (13)].While the interactions of these CaP materials with body fluids, cells, and tissues have been investigated at both the microscopic and ultrastructural levels, there is still a lack of understanding of the potential mechanisms leading to osteoinduction. Early on, the dissolution and precipitation of an apatite layer on CaP materials was identified as a potential major trigger for bone formation (20). It was further proposed that concentration of bone growth factors from body fluids, especially BMPs onto the biomaterial surface, attracts circulating stem cells to form bone tissue (21). The geometry of the biomaterial is certainly a critical parameter for bone induction. Studies demonstrate that in order for CaPs to exhibit osteoinductive properties, both a macroporous structure and surface microporosity are prerequisites. Micro- and macro-porous BCP biomaterials demonstrated the ability to induce mature lamellar bone tissue after 6 months without the addition of osteogenic cells or bone growth factors when implanted ectopically in sheep (22). Macro pores are introduced into CaPs by the addition of pore makers during the fabrication process. The importance of macrostructure in efficient osteoinduction is highlighted as bone formation occurs primarily in concavities (23). Microporosity is controlled by the sintering temperature, with lower sintering temperatures resulting in higher surface microporosity. Interestingly, the microporous CaPs bioceramics exhibited higher bone growth in critical size bone defects in goats compared with autologous bone grafts or the same CaPs bearing larger surface micropores and lower specific surface area (higher sintering temperature) (24). Increasing the microporosity increases the surface area thus possibly enhancing the dissolution/reprecipitation phenomenon (21). Further to biomaterial geometry, it has been speculated that low oxygen tension in the central region of the implants might provoke dedifferentiation of pericytes from blood vessels into osteoblasts (25). Most recently, Bohner and Miron added the idea that depletion of calcium and/or phosphate ions in the center of an implanted material could induce bone formation *via* the calcium-sensing of immune and bone cells (26).

In early reports, bone induction by CaPs ceramics was thought to be limited to the muscles of large animals such as rabbits, sheep, goats, dogs, and baboon, until Barradas et al. screened various different mouse strains and found osteoinduction by CaPs ceramics in FVB/NCrl mice (27). This study was a major step for further understanding the biological mechanisms of osteoinduction by these ceramics because there are abundant immunohistochemistry protocols available for mice compared to large animals, not to mention their ease of handling and low cost.

Innate Immune Response to Calcium Phosphate Biomaterials

Various innate immune cells participate in the host-cell response to the implantation of CaP materials including mast cells, neutrophils, monocytes, macrophages, and multinucleated giant cells (MNGCs) (28). In addition to their role in the innate immune response, macrophages have tissue-specific functions. Osteal macrophages (so called OsteoMacs), a specific type of specialized macrophages residing in the periosteum and endosteum, are an important cell type for the regulation of bone healing (29) but less is known about their relationship with implanted biomaterials (30). Depletion of OsteoMacs in mice demonstrates their key role in regulating bone regeneration in normal bone healing in a bone injury model (31, 32), suggesting that resident macrophages may also possess the phenotypic capability to instruct bone regeneration upon implantation of biomaterials used for bone repair. Previous studies have documented that resident or infiltrating monocyte-derived macrophages present at early time points after tissue trauma or the implantation of a biomaterial are characterized as pro-inflammatory (M1 macrophages), typified by their secretion of inflammatory cytokines such as TNFα, IL-1, IL-6, and IL-12, while macrophages present at later time points exhibit a predominantly anti-inflammatory profile (M2 subtype) and promote healing by secretion of cytokines such as IL-10 and TGF-β, stimulating angiogenesis, and recruiting cells for tissue repair (33–36). Importantly, macrophage polarization can be switched between M1 and M2, rendering them highly sensitive and adaptive to their environment. Moreover, mounting evidence suggests that macrophage polarization occurs over a continuous spectrum, rendering the M1/M2 classification paradigm too simple to accurately characterize their dynamic phenotypic changes and plasticity *in vivo*. In any case, macrophages are among the first cells present at the site of CaP implantation and play an integral role in MSC migration and bone formation (**Table 1**). The infiltration of macrophages and the subsequent homing of MSCs and ectopic bone formation was observed after CaP implantation in mice (44). Interestingly, MSCs migration and osteogenic differentiation was significantly enhanced by conditioned media (CM) from macrophages cultured on BCP, compared to CM from macrophages cultured on tissue culture plastic (43, 44). Furthermore, it was shown that macrophage-secreted MCP-1 and MIP-1α were the effectors of enhanced MSC migration.

Osteoclasts, which originate from the same hematopoietic precursor as macrophages, are multi-nucleated cells capable of efficiently degrading both the organic and inorganic fractions of bone. Activated osteoclasts have a characteristic morphology including a ruffle border by which they secrete proteases, such as cathepsin K and matrix metalloproteinases, and release hydrogen ions by proton pumps to acidify the resorptive pit. Histologically, osteoclasts can be identified by intensely positive tartrate-resistant acid phosphatase (TRAP) activity, which relates to their functional activity in resorbing bone or mineralized substrates such as CaPs (45). Osteoclastogenesis is essentially regulated, both *in vivo* and *in vitro*, by the macrophage colony-stimulating factor (M-CSF) and the tripartite system constituted by the receptor activator of nuclear factor κB (RANK), its ligand (RANKL) and osteoprotegerin (OPG). M-CSF permits survival and proliferation of osteoclast-precursors, also allowing them to respond efficiently to RANKL stimulation. RANKL triggers differentiation into osteoclasts by binding RANK, while OPG can prevent the interaction as a decoy receptor for RANKL (46). Osteoclasts are important players in the bone healing cascade. Several studies have documented that osteoclast presence at the site of CaP implantation precedes new bone formation (39). Evidence to demonstrate the crucial interplay between osteoclasts and osteoblasts, in association with CaPs, was highlighted by several studies (**Table 1**). Bisphosphonates are a class of drug employed to inhibit bone resorption by induced osteoclast apoptosis (47). The first-line medical management for *osteogenesis imperfecta* is based on bisphosphonates to inhibit osteoclasts, while the disease relies on osteoblast dysfunction. Bisphosphonates allow an increase of bone mineral density and a 20% decrease of fractures in long-bone in the pediatric *osteogenesis imperfecta* population (48, 49). However, in CaP-mediated bone formation, several osteoclast depletion strategies including the administration of bisphosphonates highlight the important role of osteoclasts, suggesting that coupling mechanisms linking osteoclast resorption to osteogenesis may be involved (50). Of note, Takeshita et al. convincingly showed that osteoclasts in association with CaP or bone secrete CTHRC1, which enhances osteoblastogenesis, thereby coupling bone resorption to formation. CTHRC1-triggered bone turnover was attenuated when resorption was inhibited by bisphosphonate (alendronate) treatment, and OC-specific CTHRC1 KO mice led to reduced bone formation and lower bone mass (37). This concurs with findings by other groups that bisphosphonates inhibited osteoclasts and osteoinduction by CaPs in baboons (38) or rabbits (41). Furthermore, depletion of osteoclasts by local injection of liposome-encapsulated clodronate impeded heterotopic bone formation by intrinsically osteoinductive microstructured CaPs after subcutaneous implantation in mice (42). Surface microstructure stimulates osteoclastogenesis and therefore may be a primary trigger for subsequent *de novo* bone formation for certain CaPs which do not require the addition of MSCs or growth factors to induce bone formation (40). The biological mechanism by which osteoclasts stimulate subsequent osteogenesis in response to these microstructured CaPs is still not understood. Even more interesting, non-microstructured CaPs, which possess no intrinsic osteoinduction potential, have been show to induce heterotopic bone formation when first seeded with osteoclasts prior to implantation. Taken together, OC depletion and enrichment strategies combined with implanted CaPs points to an essential role of this cell type in inducing new bone formation

Distinct from osteoclasts, MNGCs are observed in human histological samples around various CaP bone substitutes and their presence correlates with a higher maintenance of bone

TABLE 1 | Implication of macrophages and osteoclasts in the bone formation induced by calcium phosphate biomaterials.

CaP biomaterial	*In vitro* and *in vivo* models	Outcome	References
Hydroxyapatite (HA)	*In vitro:* Osteoclasts (OCs) were differentiated from bone marrow monocytes from C57BL/6 mice. Primary osteoblasts (OBs) were derived from the calvaria. *Ex vivo:* Organ culture of explanted calvaria. *In vivo model:* C57BL/6mice	CTHRC1 protein is secreted by mature OCs. CTHRC1 mRNA expression is elevated in OCs cultured on HA compared to tissue culture plastic (TCP). CTHRC1 stimulates osteoblastogenesis (gene expression and mineralized matrix deposition). CTHRC1 expression and bone turnover *in vivo* was increased by RANKL injections and conversely decreased by alendronate treatment. OC-specific CTHRC1 KO mice led to reduced bone formation and lower bone mass.	(37)
Coral derived calcium carbonate (CC)/ HA constructs	*In vivo model:* Intramuscular implantation in Chacma baboons	Osteoinduction of biomaterials was inhibited by preloading constructs with the bisphosphonate zoledronate.	(38)
β-TCP	*In vivo model:* Intramuscular implantation in female beagle dogs	CaP induces the formation of TRAP and Cathepsin K positive, multinucleated cells on the biomaterial, and their presence precedes ectopic bone formation	(39)
β-TCP with different surface microstructures	*In vitro:* Osteoclasts were differentiated from a murine macrophage cell line RAW264.7 Human MSCs were isolated from bone marrow harvested from femoral heads. *In vivo model:* Intramuscular implantation in male mongrel dogs	*In vitro*, CaPs with submicron-scale surfaces lead to increased differentiation of OCs and higher secretions of factors that induced osteogenic differentiation of MSCs. *In vivo*, submicro-structured CaPs formed bone and OCs presence was significant, whereas micro-structured CaPs formed no bone and OC presence was spare.	(40)
β-TCP	*In vivo model:* Rabbit femoral condyles	Loading of Alendronate (bisphosphonate) onto β-TCP inhibited the presence of TRAP-positive cells on the surface of the biomaterial and abrogated the CaP-mediated bone formation.	(41)
β-TCP	*In vivo model:* FVB/NCrl strain mice	CaPs induced osteoclastogenesis and ectopic bone formation. Depletion of osteoclasts by local injection of liposome-encapsulated clodronate impeded bone formation by CaPs.	(42)
Biphasic calcium phosphate (BCP) HA/ β-TCP composite	*In vitro:* Mouse macrophage cell line RAW264.7. Mouse bone marrow-derived MSCs.	Macrophages upregulated gene expression of inflammatory factors (IL-1, IL-6, MCP-1) and growth factors (EGF, PDGF, and VEGF) as a consequence of their CaP substrate. This macrophage conditioned media (CM) increased MSC migration and osteogenic differentiation (osteogenic gene expression and mineralized matrix deposition).	(43)
BCP (HA/ β-TCP)	*In vitro:* Mouse macrophage cell line RAW264.7. Mouse bone marrow-derived MSCs. *In vivo model:* Implantation into thigh muscle of male BALB/c mice.	BCP implantation *in vivo* caused infiltration of macrophages to the site, followed by homing of MSCs and subsequent ectopic bone formation. BMSCs migrated significantly faster under stimulation by CM from macrophages cultured on BCP, compared to CM from macrophages cultured on TCP. Secretion of MCP-1 and MIP- 1α by macrophages was increased by culture on BCP and were shown to be the effectors of enhanced migration since blocking these in macrophage CM had inhibited MSC migration.	(44)

mass in grafted sites (51). Such MNGCs are formed by fusion of monocytes/macrophages on various bone substitutes not surrounded by bone. Histologically, they are slightly TRAP positive and occasionally associated with small resorption lacunae, indicating a potential osteoclast-like activity. *In vitro*, they can be obtained by stimulation of monocytes with IL-4 and IL-13 (52, 53). These *in vitro* generated MNGCs can dissolve hydroxyapatite, although not as efficiently as osteoclasts, but they cannot digest the bone matrix (54). The case *in vivo* may however be more complex, particularly since mononucleated and fused macrophages found at the surface of implanted biomaterials or wounds may express a variety of markers spanning both classical M1 and alternatively activated M2 phenotypes.

Dendritic cells (DC) have been described as the scavenging sentinel cells also responsible for identifying foreign materials and organisms in the host. Although 25% of monocytes present at the site of injury or inflammation differentiate into DCs, the current knowledge of how DCs interact with biomaterials is incomplete—particularly whether they interact with the foreign body distinctly or in concert with macrophages and MNGCs (55). This is compounded by the heterogeneity of DC subsets, similar to macrophages (56). Still, it is clear that DCs also possess phagocytic ability and can readily internalize CaP particles or polymeric beads. Such particle internalization causes DCs to secrete inflammatory cytokines as well as migrate back to the lymph nodes and instruct the adaptive immune response through T cell priming (55, 57). Because these cells interrogate and recognize foreign bodies as well as prolifically express surface antigens, DCs represent an important bridge between the innate and adaptive immune system and may mediate the polarization or transition between inflammatory or anti-inflammatory adaptive immunity. Illustrating this immune-modulatory role, DCs have been implicated with suppression of a chronic inflammatory response to implanted biomaterials and thus may play a key role in mediating the transition from fibrous encapsulation to functional tissue regeneration, and as the case may be with CaPs implanted in bony locations, the regeneration of bone tissue. Similar to macrophages, DCs have been shown to distinctly respond to biomaterial surface chemistry, hydrophobicity, and topography which direct activated vs. suppressive states of DCs (58). Some work has been conducted to explore the role of DCs in mediating the innate and adaptive immune response to subcutaneously implanted polymeric materials *in vivo* (59), but less is known about how DCs may interact with resorbable biomaterials such as calcium phosphates, particularly those that are too large to phagocytose.

These studies emphasize the crucial role of the innate immune system and osteoclastogenesis in modulating and facilitating bone healing and how CaP biomaterial properties such as surface microporosity significantly affect such responses. It should be noted that the combination of CaP biomaterial and natural (collagen, fibrinogen etc.) or synthetic polymers are also developed to influence the osteoinductive capacities of the implant (60) and could therefore influence the immune response. In spite of the significant improvements in CaPs, yielding well tolerated, osteoconductive biomaterials with some osteoinductive capability, most CaPs still lack adequate osteoinduction capacity for regenerating large bone defects. Therefore, they are generally employed for treating small bone defects, to supplement autologous bone grafting, or, increasingly, as scaffolds to deliver cells or growth factors targeting bone repair (61, 62).

OSTEOIMMUNOMODULATION AND OSTEOINDUCTION BY MSC/CaP COMBINATIONS

Bone marrow derived mesenchymal stromal cells may overcome the challenges of autologous bone grafting for the regeneration of large defects. Transplanted in unison with CaP bioceramics, MSCs achieve ectopic (intramuscular and subcutaneous) (7, 9, 63) and orthotopic bone formation and critical-sized defect healing in preclinical studies, and efficient fracture healing and bone augmentation in clinical trials (64, 65). The key role of implanted MSCs was initially thought to be their differentiation into bone forming osteoblast cells and studies observing transplanted MSCs within osteocyte lacunae of newly formed bone support this hypothesis (6, 66–68). However, in general, cell engraftment of transplanted MSCs is very low or completely absent, in spite of successful outcomes (10, 11, 69), leading to the contention that the therapeutic benefit of transplanted MSCs is largely through a paracrine mechanism. These conflicting observations of the fate of transplanted MSCs is present throughout the literature and could be caused by a multitude of reasons such as initial cell dosage, biomaterial scaffold employed, implantation site, and host immune response. In our own hands, we have observed instances of some, albeit a small proportion, transplanted MSCs present in newly formed bone (9), and others where cell engraftment was not detected (10), while both resulted in ectopic bone formation. Although not quantified, it appears the transplanted MSCs persisted in outcomes of abundant bone formation and interestingly human MSCs resided in osteocyte lacunae in the vicinity of host (mice) osteocytes, with host osteocytes representing the larger proportion (9). MSCs secrete a vast array of paracrine factors into their conditioned media (MSC-CM) *in vitro* and interestingly, administration of MSC-CM *in vivo*, induces healing in many tissues including bone (70–72) providing evidence that the MSC secretome can initiate the bone tissue regeneration cascade. The MSC secretome comprises all factors secreted by MSCs, including soluble secretions (cytokines, growth factors, chemokines, and hormones) as well as vesicular secretions, or extracellular vesicles (EVs), which encompass exosomes, microvesicles, and apoptotic bodies. EVs are nanoparticles (ranging in size from 30 to 1,000 nm) that are secreted by all cells and carry bioactive cargo from the parental cells including lipids, proteins, RNA, and DNA (73, 74). It was recently reported that EVs secreted by MSCs have therapeutic potential in preclinical studies targeting bone repair (75–78). While not yet investigated in the context of bone regeneration, it has been observed in other settings that EVs secreted from MSCs mimic the immune-regulatory function of MSCs (79).

The Immune System Influences MSC-Based Bone Regeneration

Several studies have observed that MSCs enhance bone repair by modulating the foreign body response to CaPs. Macrophages are an important innate immune cell population for the regulation of MSC-based bone regeneration. Interestingly, it was observed that the mobilization of macrophages to the site of CaP implantation was significantly enhanced by MSC transplantation prior to MSC-mediated ectopic bone formation (10, 17). Early studies indicated that inflammatory macrophages suppressed osteoblastogenesis, through secretion of TNFα and IL1b [reviewed in (50)]. However, in contrast to this, both Tour et al. (17) and Gamblin et al. (10) independently observed that transplanted MSCs led to a M1 dominant macrophage phenotype, which was followed by bone formation. In line with these *in vivo* studies, several *in vitro* studies have demonstrated the impact of M1 macrophages on enhancing the osteogenic differentiation of MSCs. We previously demonstrated that inflammatory M1 macrophages secrete Oncostatin M (OSM) to improve osteoblastogenesis *in vitro* (80). In addition, OSM production by macrophages sustained bone regeneration in a mouse model of tibia injury (81). Furthermore, MSCs treated with conditioned media (CM) from lipopolysaccharide (LPS) stimulated monocytes exhibited increased osteogenic differentiation (82), an effect partially imparted by extracellular vesicles secreted by the activated monocytes (83). Conversely, other *in vitro* studies have reported that M2, and not M1 macrophages, enhanced osteogenic differentiation of MSCs (84). The exact role of resident vs. monocyte-derived macrophages or of M1 vs. M2 alternatively activated macrophages in response to transplanted MSCs are still not clear. The M1/M2 paradigm is certainly a key for successful bone regeneration, since resolution of inflammation and tissue repair are tightly linked (85). Interestingly, M1 and M2 macrophages were both recently demonstrated to modulate MSC osteogenic differentiation but in disparate manners, whereby M1 macrophages enhanced early osteogenic differentiation without any effect on matrix mineralization, which was subsequently enhanced by M2 macrophages (86). In addition, it was demonstrated that macrophages preferentially recruit fibroblasts over MSCs. Pre-incubation of macrophages with immunomodulatory MSCs impairs fibroblast recruitment (87). Taken together, these studies indicate that macrophage polarization is important for distinct roles in the bone healing cascade by MSCs in association with CaPs, much like how normal tissue repair encompasses a transition from a pro-inflammatory status to a pro-reparative status.

Osteoclasts also play a central role in the regulation of MSC-based bone regeneration. It was demonstrated *in vitro* that osteoclasts secrete factors (S1P, BMPs, WNTs etc.) which induce MSC migration and osteogenic differentiation (88, 89). Interestingly, MSCs transplanted with BCP were shown to positively influence the foreign body reaction by attracting circulating monocytes and inducing their differentiation into osteoclasts, thus favoring bone formation. Importantly, depletion of osteoclasts by local injection of clodronate or injection of neutralizing anti-RANKL antibodies impeded bone formation, highlighting the imperative role of osteoclasts in MSC-mediated bone formation (10).

The adaptive immune system also plays an important role in MSC-modulated bone regeneration, which was elegantly shown by Liu et al. (90) and is discussed in detail in **Table 2**. Briefly, MSCs together with CaP particles induced ectopic bone formation in immuno-deficient mice but failed to do so in immune competent C57BL/6 mice (90). Moreover, infusion of CD4+ T cells in nude mice blocked ectopic bone formation through secretion of TNFα and IFNγ, which inhibited MSC differentiation and induced MSC apoptosis (90, 92). Interestingly, infusion of CD4+ CD25+ Treg abolished TNFα and IFNγ production and improved MSC-mediated bone regeneration in critical-sized calvarial bone defects in C57BL/6 mice (90). These observations were corroborated by findings that MSC from immune-competent mice formed ectopic bone in immune deficient mice, but much less in syngenic mice with the initiation of an inflammatory reaction involving Th1, Th2, and cytotoxic T-cell responses (91). Collectively these data demonstrate that modulation of both the innate and adaptive host immune response facilitates MSC-based bone regeneration.

IMPACT OF MSC STRESS ON IMMUNOMODULATION

As indicated above, implantation of MSCs with CaP results in the local recruitment of various innate immune cells including mast cells, neutrophils, monocytes, macrophages, and several types of multinucleated giant cells. An exhaustive overview of how MSC influence the innate and adaptive immune system is outside the scope of this review. Rather, we focus on how transplanted MSCs in association with CaPs may modulate the immune system by focusing on the conditions that MSCs encounter following transplantation and the potential impact that these cell stresses can have on MSCs immunomodulation.

MSC Influence the Innate and Adaptive Immune System

Since MSCs express low levels of MHC-II and costimulatory molecules (CD40, CD80, CD86), but substantial amount of the tolerogenic HLA-G molecule, they are considered as immunoprivileged cells, and thus would be ideal for tissue repair even in allogeneic transplantation (92, 93). Moreover, the discovery of the immunomodulatory roles of MSCs fostered their therapeutic use to suppress inflammation and limit pathogenic immune responses in graft-vs-host and auto-immune diseases such as multiple sclerosis, diabetes, and rheumatoid arthritis. Indeed, MSCs tend to limit macrophage polarization to M1, favoring M2 polarization. They also favor the generation of regulatory dendritic cells. They inhibit mast cells degranulation and NK cell effector functions (**Figure 1**). MSC production of PGE2, IL-6, TGFβ, and IDO for example has a key role in these suppressive effects on innate immune cells (93, 94). With regard to adaptive immune cells, MSCs favor the development of Th2 and Treg cells, with suppression of CD4+ T cells proliferation and polarization toward Th1 and Th17 cells. They also inhibit B cell activation, proliferation, and differentiation into plasma cells. These suppressive effects depend on MSCs production of NO, TGFβ, PGE2, IL-10, and ligation of PD-1/PD-L1 for example (93, 94). Interestingly, culture of MSC on BCP did not impair their suppressive effect toward T, B, and Natural Killer (NK) cells (95). Extracellular vesicles produced by MSC are also implicated in immunomodulation (96). It is important to note that the immunosuppressive effect of MSCs when delivered systemically is well documented, but the possible role of MSCs in regulating the innate and adaptive immune responses when delivered locally to regenerate bone remains elusive.

Impact of Stressful Conditions on MSCs Phenotype/Secretome

Because MSCs disappear shortly after implantation with CaP, it is important to consider the impact of cell stress or cell death on MSCs immunomodulation activity. The primary factors responsible for the large cell death of transplanted BMSCs include the ischemic environment and the lack of glucose that the BMSCs encounter (97–100). It is unclear the exact means of MSCs death after implantation with CaP

TABLE 2 | Osteoimmunology of mesenchymal stem cells transplantation with calcium phosphate biomaterials.

CaP Biomaterial	MSC origin	*In vitro* and *In vivo* models	Outcome	References
BCP (HA/ β-TCP)	Human bone marrow derived MSCs	*In vivo model:* Intramuscular implantation in immunocompromised nude NMRI Nu/Nu female mice	Both macrophage and osteoclast presence at the CaP site was significantly enhanced by MSC transplantation. Their presence preceded MSC-mediated ectopic bone formation. Depletion of osteoclasts by local injection of clodronate impeded bone formation, highlighting the imperative role of osteoclasts in MSC-mediated bone formation	(10)
HA	Rat (Lewis) bone marrow derived MSCs	*In vivo model:* Rat calvaria critical-sized defects	MSCs increase bone formation by modulating (both up- and down-regulation) the foreign body reaction. MSCs increased macrophage presence at the CaP implantation site and enhanced bone healing. However, MSCs reduced the immune cell presence (macrophages and eosinophils at the site when the scaffold was delivered with extracellular matrix produced by fibroblasts (dermis of Sprague-Dawley rats), indicating that MSCs modulate the host immune response depending on the environment with the aim of positively influencing the tissue healing cascade.	(17)
BCP (HA/ β-TCP)	Bone marrow MSCs C57BL/6-Tg (CAG-EGFP)1Osb/J mice	*In vivo model:* Subcutaneous and calvaria implants. Female C3H/HeJ, C57BL6J, B6.129S7-Ifng^{tm1Ts}/J, C57BL/6-Tg(CAG-EGFP)1Osb/J, B6.MRL-Fas^{lpr}/J, immunocompromised nude mice (Beige nude/nudeXIDIII).	Firstly, MSC transplantation with CaP formed ectopic bone in nude mice but not in C57BL/6 mice. Interestingly CD8+ T cells, and CD4+ T cell infusion into nude mice partially and totally blocked bone formation, respectively. Inhibition of MSC-mediated bone formation in C57BL/6 was caused by interferon (IFN)-γ induced down-regulation of the runt-related transcription factor 2 (Runx-2) pathway and tumor necrosis factor (TNF)-α-induced MSC apoptosis. Treatment with IFN-γ and TNF-α also inhibited MSC-mediated bone formation in nude mice and interestingly antibodies to neutralize IFN-γ and TNF-α, as well as infusion of Treg cells rescued bone formation by transplanted MSCs in C57BL/6 mice. Together, this reveals that pro-inflammatory T cells inhibit transplanted MSC-mediated bone repair.	(90)
BCP (HA/ β-TCP)	Bone marrow MSCs from C57BL/6 mice	*In vivo model:* Subcutaneous implantation in C57BL/6 and immunocompromised nude mice (NMRI Nu/Nu)	MSC transplantation into nude mice led to abundant ectopic bone and bone marrow formation, whereas MSC transplantation into syngenic C57BL/6 mice resulted in only minor quantities of ectopic bone formation and significant quantities of multinucleated giant cells (MNGCs). MSCs survived for a shorter duration in immune-competent mice and the implant site was characterized by Th1, Th2, and cytotoxic T-lymphocyte activation, highlighting the benefit T-lymphocyte absence in nude mice for bone formation.	(91)

but senescence, apoptosis, necrosis, or other types of cell death could presumably be implicated which can have a profound effect on MSC-mediated immunomodulation. MSCs are considered relatively resistant to programmed apoptosis and prefer senescent growth arrest or autophagy to cell death (101). In general, necrotic (necroptotic, pyroptotic) cell death is associated with inflammation and exacerbated immune responses, whereas apoptosis avoids an inflammatory response and rather contributes to its resolution. For example, Laing et al. demonstrated that systemic injection of H_2O_2-induced apoptotic MSCs is more efficient than injection of live MSCs to induce a robust immune suppressive reaction in an ovalbumin induced model of allergic airway inflammation (102). Similarly, Galleu et al. showed that after infusion of apoptotic MSCs in a murine model of graft-vs-host disease, recipient phagocytes engulf apoptotic MSCs and produce IDO, which is ultimately necessary for effecting immunosuppression (103). The authors also observed that cytotoxic cells, such as CD8+ T lymphocytes and NK cells, induce MSCs apoptosis through perforin, granzyme B, and FasL, and that PBMCs from patients that responded to MSC therapy had more cytotoxic activity against MSCs. Another level of complexity is that when apoptotic cells are not cleared in an efficient and timely manner, they progress to secondary necrosis and lose their membrane integrity. This results in a leakage of immunostimulatory, danger associated molecular patterns (DAMPs) such as HMGB1 and nucleosomes (104, 105). They induce an inflammatory response which can become chronic and even induce an adaptive immune response, a situation that would

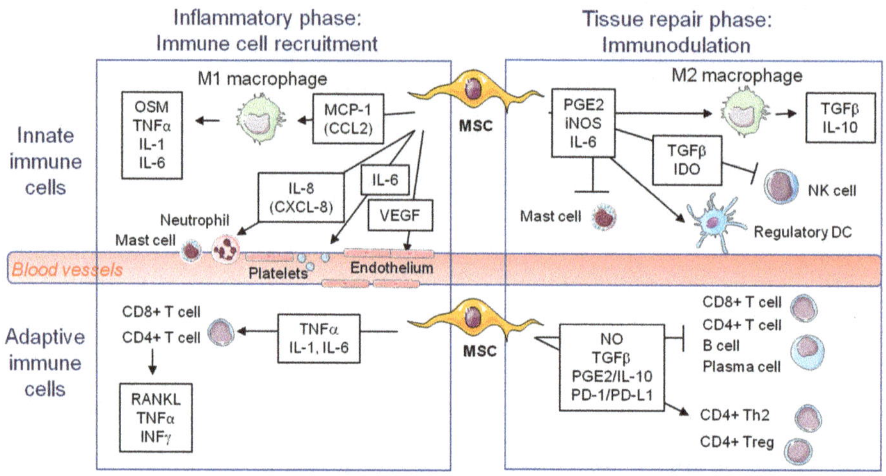

FIGURE 1 | Known immunomodulatory secretions from mesenchymal stem cells favoring (↑) or inhibiting (-) various cells potentially involved in bone formation on a biomaterial during early inflammation or the later stage of tissue repair. MSC, mesenchymal stem cell; M1, pro-inflammatory macrophages; M2, alternatively activated macrophages; NK, natural killer; DC, dendritic cell; OSM, oncostatin M; TNFα, tumor necrosis factor alpha; IL, interleukin; VEGF, vascular endothelial growth factor; PGE2, prostaglandin E2; iNOS, inducible nitric oxide synthase; TGFβ, transforming growth factor beta; IDO, indoleamine 2,3-dioxygenase; RANKL, receptor activator of nuclear factor kappa-B ligand; IFNγ, interferon gamma; NO, nitric oxide; PD-1/PD-L1, programmed cell death protein 1/programmed cell death-ligand 1.

presumably preclude local bone formation. Additional studies are mandatory in the context of bone regeneration induced by MSC-CaP combination.

Upon aging and in age-related deficiencies, compromised MSC-mediated immunological responses have been observed and attributed to MSC senescence. Senescence by replicative exhaustion or genotoxic stress during *ex vivo* culturing was also demonstrated (69). Acute, transient senescence induced by cell stresses such as hypoxia is presumably beneficial, because senescent cells secrete a plethora of molecules as part of the senescence-associated secretory phenotype (SASP), leading to rapid MSC clearance by immune cells, modulation of innate and adaptive immune cells, followed by tissue healing and regeneration (106). However, when chronic senescence occurs, for example upon aging, it impacts on the SASP, the local microenvironment and causes local and/or systemic inflammation.

The modifications of the secretome of MSCs induced by various stimuli, either mimicking physiological situations such as hypoxia and inflammatory stress or specific *in vitro* culture conditions to enhance the immunomodulatory properties of the cells, were previously widely reviewed (107–109). Those stresses could also alter the production and composition of EVs (110–112). Hypoxia is a main characteristic of the natural environment of MSCs and a major difference with *in vitro* culture. Overall, culture under low-oxygen atmosphere results in higher proliferation rate, survival, differentiation potential, and immune modulating secretions (113). For example, Paquet et al. (114) reported an upregulation of proangiogenic and chemotactic mediators (VEGF-A/-C, IL-8, MCP-1, and RANTES) and a downregulation of inflammatory mediators (IL-1b, IL-6, IL-15, IL-1Ra) with close to anoxic conditions (0.1% O_2). An artificial overexpression of the hypoxia-inducible factor 1 (HIF-1) in dental stem cells leads to an improved resistance to NK cells, an upregulation of CXCL12, CCL5, and IL-6 as well as a downregulation of CXCL10 (115).

Inflammatory stress is also characteristic of an implantation site and is mimicked *in vitro* by exogenous addition of LPS, TNFα, and/or IFNγ, usually termed MSC priming. When primed with inflammatory cytokines, MSCs increase their suppressive capacities (95). MSCs express constitutively many mitogenic growth factors, chemokines and matrix metalloproteinases at various levels. They are sensors and modulators of their microenvironment; i.e., MSC response to TNFα by increasing expression of some growth factor receptors, growth factors, chemokines, and matrix metalloproteases (116). Just as hypoxia, MSCs stimulated with LPS or TNFα produced more VEGF and FGF2 but also more HGF and IGF-1 via the activation of NFκB (117). Stimulation with IFNγ increases the expression of anti-inflammatory and regenerative molecules such as IDO, TGFβ or PGE2 for example (60). The addition of hypoxia to a TNFα and IFNγ stimulation on adipose-derived stem cells did not impair their higher secretion of immunomodulatory molecules IDO and PD-L1 (118).

PROPOSED MECHANISM OF BONE FORMATION AFTER MSC-CAP IMPLANTATION

It has been shown in many studies that only the combination of CaP and MSCs has the ability to induce abundant bone formation. MSCs have numerous, complex, and sometimes antagonist effects on the immune system depending on the physiological context. Their role in bone regeneration on CaP biomaterials remains unclear but evidence indicate that their immunomodulatory properties are involved. We previously highlighted the crucial role that osteoclasts seem to play and

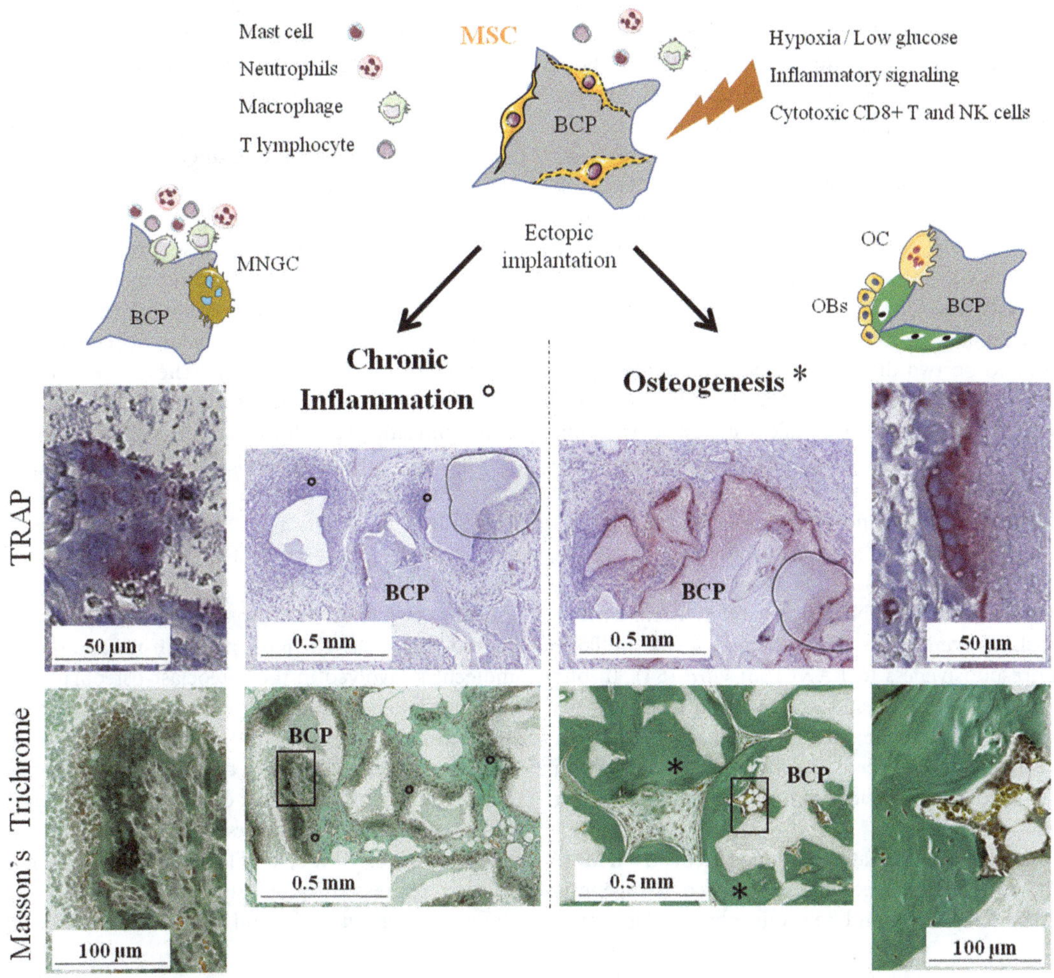

FIGURE 2 | The two possible outcomes of subcutaneous implantation of mesenchymal stem cells on calcium phosphate ceramic in mice. Histology of the implants: TRAP staining for osteoclasts detection after 4 weeks and Masson's trichrome to evaluate bone formation after 8 weeks. On the left, chronic inflammation (o) with formation of TRAP negative MNGCs followed by fibrous encapsulation and no sign of bone formation. On the right, osteoclastogenesis on the biomaterial followed by abundant bone formation (*). NK, natural killer; BCP, biphasic calcium phosphate; MNGC, multi-nucleated giant cell; OC, osteoclast; OBs, osteoblasts; TRAP, tartrate-resistant acid phosphatase.

the rapid disappearance of implanted MSCs before new bone is formed. Therefore, we hypothesize that MSCs, through their dialogue with various cells of the immune system, favor osteoclastogenesis on lieu of MNGCs formation, i.e., inducing a switch from chronic inflammation and fibrous encapsulation to bone formation via the recruitment and differentiation of new MSCs or skeletal stem cells in the bone remodeling process (**Figure 2**).

In detail, the environment just after implantation consists of the biomaterial exhibiting specific properties (chemical composition, micro-/macro-porosity, topography) and the MSCs adhering and reacting to it. Neutrophils, mast cells and macrophages are the first immune cells in contact with the implant, the latter mostly polarizing toward the inflammatory M1 phenotype (28). Therefore, inflammatory cytokines, ions released by the biomaterial, lack of O_2 (98), and nutrients (97), presence of cytotoxic CD8+ T and NK cells are all environmental factors influencing MSCs' behavior in the early stages of implantation. Most of those stresses were individually found to increase the production of pro- or anti-inflammatory molecules by MSCs (107–109). Given the osteogenic effect of the biomaterial (119) and the M1 population of macrophages (86), implanted MSCs might also express some markers of early osteoblast precursors. Eventually, MSCs will disappear by senescence, apoptosis and/or necrosis, releasing novel pro- and anti-inflammatory signals. Clearance of dead MSC by immune cells would also modulate the innate and adaptive immune system.

We believe that the secretions from those highly stimulated MSCs directly or indirectly (through modulation of innate and adaptive immune cells) favor the formation of osteoclasts at the expense of MNGCs. Indeed, MSC-based bone formation was significantly altered by anti-RANKL mAB (10) or clodronate (42) administration. While clodronate also affects MNGCs, the anti-RANKL mAB is specifically restricting osteoclastogenesis. Due to their common origin and similar morphology, osteoclasts, and MNGCs are difficult to distinguish. Theoretically, both osteoclasts and MNGCs can arise from the fusion of circulating monocytes, M1/M2 macrophages or even of dendritic cells. An in depth description of the known differences between osteoclasts and MNGCs have already been well reviewed (120). Both cell types share a lot of markers but they can be differentiated by expression of the calcitonin receptor and RANK only in osteoclasts, or CD86 (B7-2), CD206, and HLA-DR only present in MNGCs. Interestingly, MNGCs are able to express low levels of TRAP a few days after formation (both *in vitro* and *in vivo*) while there seem to be two distinct populations expressing or not Cathepsin K (121, 122). Miron et al. also discussed the polarization potential of MNGCs, in parallel with the polarization of macrophages, with a proposed distinction between pro-inflammatory M1-MNGCs that were also called foreign body giant cells (FBGCs) and wound-healing M2-MNGCs. It is impossible to state whether the suggested M2-MNGCs are the MNGCs observed in close contact to the CaP materials leading to bone formation or if M2-MNGCs can differentiate further into true osteoclasts even if this last statement seems unlikely due to their unresponsiveness to RANKL *in vitro* (54). In our hypothesis, M2-MNGCs are likely to be involved in late stages of chronic inflammation, leading to fibrous encapsulation. In any case, there is an urgent need to better characterize those MNGCs and to discover the cell communications involved in their formation.

Preliminary results showed that conditioned media from MSC culture could have a positive direct impact on osteoclastogenesis (123). This effect of MSCs could rely on enhanced secretion or membrane expression of RANKL. Activated T cells were also reported to increase osteoclastogenesis *in vitro* (124) but they cannot be the main source of RANKL in MSC-based bone formation as many successful experiments were carried out in Nude mice. Also, a number of factors are known to influence osteoclastogenesis, primarily by modifying RANKL/RANK signaling (125). *In vitro*, TGFβ (a known product of MSC but also Treg) promote osteoclast formation from RANKL stimulated precursors but also decreases RANKL expression in osteoblasts resulting in fewer osteoclasts in co-culture (126). In mice, activation of the non-canonical Wnt pathway by Wnt5a in osteoclast precursors increases the production of RANK (127). These are only few examples of molecules that could be implicated in the MSC-osteoclast communications and future studies will certainly better delineate this key step toward MSC-CaP induced bone formation.

As the newly formed bone comes mostly from host osteoblasts, it entails recruitment and differentiation of new MSCs or the newly characterized subset of skeletal stem cells [SSC, (128)]. We hypothesize that osteoclasts might be the essential attractor for those cells, setting off a local bone remodeling cycle. The basic mechanisms and the major signaling molecules involved in the osteoclast-osteoblast crosstalk during the physiological coupling of bone resorption and formation are well described (129, 130). Osteoclasts are known to release growth factors from the degradation of bone matrix and, most importantly in our case, to express chemotactic and osteogenic coupling factors toward cell of the osteoblastic lineage such as BMP6, WNT10b, and S1P (131). The CTHRC1 protein, expressed by mature osteoclasts, promote osteoblastic differentiation *in vitro* and an osteoclast-specific KO induce

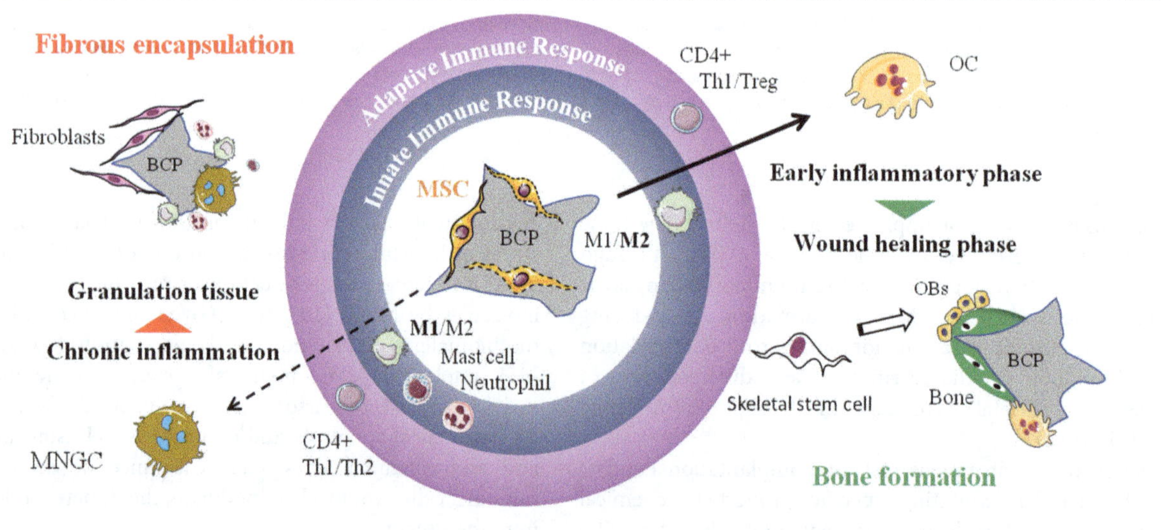

FIGURE 3 | Proposed mechanism of MSC-CaP immune modulation leading to bone formation. The local innate and adaptive immune response will determine the fate of the implanted biomaterial (central part of the drawing). On the left, is displayed the classical foreign body reaction characterized by activation of M1 macrophages, mast cells, neutrophils, Th1, and Th2 CD4+ lymphocytes. It leads to the formation of MNGCs, chronic inflammation and subsequent fibrous encapsulation of the implant. On the right, adjunction of MSCs to the biomaterial favor M2 macrophages, Th1, Treg, and osteoclastogenesis followed by recruitment of new stem cells, likely from the skeletal subtype, that differentiate into bone forming osteoblasts. MSC, mesenchymal stem cell; BCP, biphasic calcium phosphate; M1, pro-inflammatory macrophages; M2, alternatively activated macrophages; Th1/Th2/Treg, type 1 helper/type 2 helper/regulatory T cells; MNGC, multi-nucleated giant cell; OC, osteoclast; OBs, osteoblasts.

a low bone mass phenotype in mice (37). More recently, an important study unveiled a reverse signaling mechanism whereby osteoclasts secrete extracellular vesicles expressing RANK which are able to stimulate membrane RANKL on the surface of osteoblasts to induce bone formation (132). Also, as osteoclasts can degrade the biomaterial, they modulate the local calcium and phosphate concentrations, thus influencing the deposition of the apatite layer and the calcium sensing of other cell types (26, 133).

Simultaneously to this main phenomenon, MSCs are likely to induce a switch from M1 macrophages to the M2 phenotype, the formation of regulatory dendritic cells and the suppression of B, NK, CD4+, and CD8+ T cells while promoting Th2 and Treg cells. The timing of activation of the various cells is critical as the initial acute inflammation is necessary to recruit all the immune cells but is detrimental if it becomes chronic and favors the formation of MNGCs. The M1/M2 balance of macrophages phenotype has a key role in this switch to resolve inflammation and move on to bone formation (85, 134). Moreover, the M2 phenotype favored by MSCs is thought to help in late stages of osteoblastic differentiation and mineralization (86). The stressful conditions and, eventually, the apoptosis of implanted MSCs might increase their inherent immunomodulatory properties.

CONCLUSION

The implantation of CaP biomaterials in combination with MSCs emphasizes the central role of the host immune system in bone regeneration. It is important to consider that the cellular events hypothesized here may only occur on an osteoconductive CaP material. The implanted MSCs potentiate the effect of the biomaterial allowing ectopic bone formation by creating a bone-like microenvironment. We highlighted here the pivotal role that macrophages and osteoclasts play in the multistep process of bone formation induced by MSC-CaP implantation (**Figure 3**) but this complex mechanism is just beginning to be explored. Over the course of several weeks, multiples cells types and molecules appear implicated in a coordinated manner before bone is formed. Any dysregulation would lead to unwanted chronic inflammation and fibrosis. A better comprehension of these spatiotemporal cell communications is mandatory to reach more efficient bone healing and develop better cell-free approaches.

AUTHOR CONTRIBUTIONS

All authors participated in the literature search, organization, writing, reviewing, and proofreading of the manuscript. PH, ND, VT, and FB designed the figures. MB and PL created the tables.

FUNDING

This work is financially supported by the European Commission through the H2020 project ORTHOUNION (Grant Agreement: 733288). PH receives a PhD fellowship from the Regional Council Pays de la Loire and the ORTHOUNION project. MB benefits from a Marie Skłodowska-Curie Individual Fellowships from the European Commission through the H2020 project PARAGEN (Project ID: 708711).

REFERENCES

1. Stanovici J, Le Nail L-R, Brennan MA, Vidal L, Trichet V, Rosset P, et al. Bone regeneration strategies with bone marrow stromal cells in orthopaedic surgery. *Curr Res Transl Med.* (2016) 64:83–90. doi: 10.1016/j.retram.2016.04.006
2. Abe K, Yamamoto N, Hayashi K, Takeuchi A, Miwa S, Igarashi K, et al. The usefulness of wide excision assisted by a computer navigation system and reconstruction using a frozen bone autograft for malignant acetabular bone tumors: a report of two cases. *BMC Cancer.* (2018) 18:1036. doi: 10.1186/s12885-018-4971-8
3. Ahlmann E, Patzakis M, Roidis N, Shepherd L, Holtom P. Comparison of anterior and posterior iliac crest bone grafts in terms of harvest-site morbidity and functional outcomes. *J Bone Joint Surg Am.* (2002) 84-A:716–20. doi: 10.2106/00004623-200205000-00003
4. Giannoudis PV, Dinopoulos H, Tsiridis E. Bone substitutes: an update. *Injury.* (2005) 36:S20–7. doi: 10.1016/j.injury.2005.07.029
5. Albee FH. Studies in bone growth triple calcium phosphate as a stimulus to osteogenesis. *Ann Surg.* (1920) 71:32–9.
6. Mankani MH, Kuznetsov SA, Wolfe RM, Marshall GW, Robey PG. *In vivo* bone formation by human bone marrow stromal cells: reconstruction of the mouse calvarium and mandible. *Stem Cells.* (2006) 24:2140–9. doi: 10.1634/stemcells.2005-0567
7. Mankani MH, Kuznetsov SA, Robey PG. Formation of hematopoietic territories and bone by transplanted human bone marrow stromal cells requires a critical cell density. *Exp Hematol.* (2007) 35:995–1004. doi: 10.1016/J.EXPHEM.2007.01.051
8. Granchi D, Gómez-Barrena E, Rojewski M, Rosset P, Layrolle P, Spazzoli B, et al. Changes of bone turnover markers in long bone nonunions treated with a regenerative approach. *Stem Cells Int.* (2017) 2017:1–11. doi: 10.1155/2017/3674045
9. Brennan MÁ, Renaud A, Amiaud J, Rojewski MT, Schrezenmeier H, Heymann D, et al. Pre-clinical studies of bone regeneration with human bone marrow stromal cells and biphasic calcium phosphate. *Stem Cell Res Ther.* (2014) 5:114. doi: 10.1186/scrt504
10. Gamblin A-L, Brennan MA, Renaud A, Yagita H, Lézot F, Heymann D, et al. Bone tissue formation with human mesenchymal stem cells and biphasic calcium phosphate ceramics: the local implication of osteoclasts and macrophages. *Biomaterials.* (2014) 35:9660–7. doi: 10.1016/j.biomaterials.2014.08.018
11. Giannoni P, Scaglione S, Daga A, Ilengo C, Cilli M, Quarto R. Short-time survival and engraftment of bone marrow stromal cells in an ectopic model of bone regeneration. *Tissue Eng Part A.* (2010) 16:489–99. doi: 10.1089/ten.tea.2009.0041
12. Otsuru S, Gordon PL, Shimono K, Jethva R, Marino R, Phillips CL, et al. Transplanted bone marrow mononuclear cells and MSCs impart clinical benefit to children with osteogenesis imperfecta through different mechanisms. *Blood.* (2012) 120:1933–41. doi: 10.1182/blood-2011-12-400085
13. Götherström C, Westgren M, Shaw SWS, Åström E, Biswas A, Byers PH, et al. Pre- and postnatal transplantation of fetal mesenchymal stem cells in osteogenesis imperfecta: a two-center experience. *Stem Cells Transl Med.* (2014) 3:255–64. doi: 10.5966/sctm.2013-0090
14. Le Blanc K, Götherström C, Ringdén O, Hassan M, McMahon R, Horwitz E, et al. Fetal mesenchymal stem-cell engraftment in bone after *in utero* transplantation in a patient with severe osteogenesis imperfecta. *Transplantation.* (2005) 79:1607–14. doi: 10.1097/01.TP.0000159029.48678.93

15. Horwitz EM, Gordon PL, Koo WKK, Marx JC, Neel MD, McNall RY, et al. Isolated allogeneic bone marrow-derived mesenchymal cells engraft and stimulate growth in children with osteogenesis imperfecta: implications for cell therapy of bone. *Proc Natl Acad Sci USA.* (2002) 99:8932–7. doi: 10.1073/pnas.132252399
16. Horwitz EM, Prockop DJ, Fitzpatrick LA, Koo WWK, Gordon PL, Neel M, et al. Transplantability and therapeutic effects of bone marrow-derived mesenchymal cells in children with osteogenesis imperfecta. *Nat Med.* (1999) 5:309–13. doi: 10.1038/6529
17. Tour G, Wendel M, Tcacencu I. Bone marrow stromal cells enhance the osteogenic properties of hydroxyapatite scaffolds by modulating the foreign body reaction. *J Tissue Eng Regen Med.* (2014) 8:841–9. doi: 10.1002/term.1574
18. Qi X, Zhang J, Yuan H, Xu Z, Li Q, Niu X, et al. Exosomes secreted by human-induced pluripotent stem cell-derived mesenchymal stem cells repair critical-sized bone defects through enhanced angiogenesis and osteogenesis in osteoporotic rats. *Int J Biol Sci.* (2016) 12:836–49. doi: 10.7150/ijbs.14809
19. Barradas AMCA, Yuan H, van Blitterswijk CAC, Habibovic P. Osteoinductive biomaterials: current knowledge of properties, experimental models and biological mechanisms. *Eur Cells Mater.* (2011) 21:407–29. doi: 10.22203/eCM.v021a31
20. Daculsi G, Legeros RZ, Nery E, Lynch K, Kerebel B. Transformation of biphasic calcium phosphate ceramics *in vivo*: ultrastructural and physicochemical characterization. *J Biomed Mater Res.* (1989) 23:883–94. doi: 10.1002/jbm.820230806
21. Habibovic P, Yuan H, van der Valk CM, Meijer G, van Blitterswijk CA, de Groot K. 3D microenvironment as essential element for osteoinduction by biomaterials. *Biomaterials.* (2005) 26:3565–75. doi: 10.1016/j.biomaterials.2004.09.056
22. Le Nihouannen D, Daculsi G, Saffarzadeh A, Gauthier O, Delplace S, Pilet P, et al. Ectopic bone formation by microporous calcium phosphate ceramic particles in sheep muscles. *Bone.* (2005) 36:1086–93. doi: 10.1016/j.bone.2005.02.017
23. Ripamonti U, Roden LC, Ferretti C, Klar RM. Biomimetic matrices self-initiating the induction of bone formation. *J Craniofac Surg.* (2011) 22:1859–70. doi: 10.1097/SCS.0b013e31822e83fe
24. Fellah BH, Gauthier O, Weiss P, Chappard D, Layrolle P. Osteogenicity of biphasic calcium phosphate ceramics and bone autograft in a goat model. *Biomaterials.* (2008) 29:1177–88. doi: 10.1016/j.biomaterials.2007.11.034
25. Diaz-Flores L, Gutierrez R, Lopez-Alonso A, Gonzalez R, Varela H. Pericytes as a supplementary source of osteoblasts in periosteal osteogenesis. *Clin Orthop Relat Res.* (1992)280–6.
26. Bohner M, Miron RJ. A proposed mechanism for material-induced heterotopic ossification. *Mater Today.* (2018) 22:132–41. doi: 10.1016/j.mattod.2018.10.036
27. Barradas AMC, Yuan H, van der Stok J, Le Quang B, Fernandes H, Chaterjea A, et al. The influence of genetic factors on the osteoinductive potential of calcium phosphate ceramics in mice. *Biomaterials.* (2012) 33:5696–705. doi: 10.1016/j.biomaterials.2012.04.021
28. Anderson JM, Rodriguez A, Chang DT. Foreign body reaction to biomaterials. *Semin Immunol.* (2008) 20:86–100. doi: 10.1016/j.smim.2007.11.004
29. Batoon L, Millard SM, Raggatt LJ, Pettit AR. Osteomacs and bone regeneration. *Curr Osteoporos Rep.* (2017) 15:385–95. doi: 10.1007/s11914-017-0384-x
30. Miron RJ, Bosshardt DD. OsteoMacs: key players around bone biomaterials. *Biomaterials.* (2016) 82:1–19. doi: 10.1016/j.biomaterials.2015.12.017
31. Alexander KA, Chang MK, Maylin ER, Kohler T, Müller R, Wu AC, et al. Osteal macrophages promote *in vivo* intramembranous bone healing in a mouse tibial injury model. *J Bone Miner Res.* (2011) 26:1517–32. doi: 10.1002/jbmr.354
32. Batoon L, Millard SM, Wullschleger ME, Preda C, Wu AC-K, Kaur S, et al. CD169 + macrophages are critical for osteoblast maintenance and promote intramembranous and endochondral ossification during bone repair. *Biomaterials.* (2017) 2017:33. doi: 10.1016/j.biomaterials.201 7.10.033
33. Mantovani A, Sica A, Sozzani S, Allavena P, Vecchi A, Locati M. The chemokine system in diverse forms of macrophage activation and polarization. *Trends Immunol.* (2004) 25:677–86. doi: 10.1016/j.it.2004.09.015
34. Mantovani A, Sozzani S, Locati M, Allavena P, Sica A. Macrophage polarization: tumor-associated macrophages as a paradigm for polarized M2 mononuclear phagocytes. *Trends Immunol.* (2002) 23:549–55. doi: 10.1016/S1471-4906(02)02302-5
35. Jones JA, Chang DT, Meyerson H, Colton E, Kwon IK, Matsuda T, et al. Proteomic analysis and quantification of cytokines and chemokines from biomaterial surface-adherent macrophages and foreign body giant cells. *J Biomed Mater Res Part A.* (2007) 83A:585–96. doi: 10.1002/jbm.a.31221
36. Badylak SF, Valentin JE, Ravindra AK, McCabe GP, Stewart-Akers AM. Macrophage phenotype as a determinant of biologic scaffold remodeling. *Tissue Eng Part A.* (2008) 14:1835–42. doi: 10.1089/ten.tea.2007.0264
37. Takeshita S, Fumoto T, Matsuoka K, Park K, Aburatani H, Kato S, et al. Osteoclast-secreted CTHRC1 in the coupling of bone resorption to formation. *J Clin Invest.* (2013) 123:3914–24. doi: 10.1172/JCI69493
38. Ripamonti U, Klar RM, Renton LF, Ferretti C. Synergistic induction of bone formation by hOP-1, hTGF-β3 and inhibition by zoledronate in macroporous coral-derived hydroxyapatites. *Biomaterials.* (2010) 31:6400–10. doi: 10.1016/j.biomaterials.2010.04.037
39. Kondo N, Ogose A, Tokunaga K, Umezu H, Arai K, Kudo N, et al. Osteoinduction with highly purified β-tricalcium phosphate in dog dorsal muscles and the proliferation of osteoclasts before heterotopic bone formation. *Biomaterials.* (2006) 27:4419–27. doi: 10.1016/j.biomaterials.2006.04.016
40. Barrère-de Groot F, de Bruijn, Everts V, Davison N, Yuan H, Luo X, et al. Submicron-scale surface architecture of tricalcium phosphate directs osteogenesis *in vitro* and *in vivo*. *Eur Cells Mater.* (2016) 27:281–97. doi: 10.22203/ecm.v027a20
41. Tanaka T, Saito M, Chazono M, Kumagae Y, Kikuchi T, Kitasato S, et al. Effects of alendronate on bone formation and osteoclastic resorption after implantation of beta-tricalcium phosphate. *J Biomed Mater Res A.* (2010) 93:469–74. doi: 10.1002/jbm.a.32560
42. Davison NL, Gamblin A-L, Layrolle P, Yuan H, de Bruijn JD, Barrère-de Groot F. Liposomal clodronate inhibition of osteoclastogenesis and osteoinduction by submicrostructured beta-tricalcium phosphate. *Biomaterials.* (2014) 35:5088–97. doi: 10.1016/j.biomaterials.2014.03.013
43. Wang J, Liu D, Guo B, Yang X, Chen X, Zhu X, et al. Role of biphasic calcium phosphate ceramic-mediated secretion of signaling molecules by macrophages in migration and osteoblastic differentiation of MSCs. *Acta Biomater.* (2017) 51:447–60. doi: 10.1016/j.actbio.2017.01.059
44. Wang M, Chen F, Wang J, Chen X, Liang J, Yang X, et al. Calcium phosphate altered the cytokine secretion of macrophages and influenced the homing of mesenchymal stem cells. *J Mater Chem B.* (2018) 6:4765–74. doi: 10.1039/C8TB01201F
45. Hayman AR. Tartrate-resistant acid phosphatase (TRAP) and the osteoclast/immune cell dichotomy. *Autoimmunity.* (2008) 41:218–23. doi: 10.1080/08916930701694667
46. Feng W. Osteoclastogenesis and osteoimmunology. *Front Biosci.* (2014) 19:758. doi: 10.2741/4242
47. Drake MT, Clarke BL, Khosla S. Bisphosphonates: mechanism of action and role in clinical practice. *Mayo Clin Proc.* (2008) 83:1032–45. doi: 10.4065/83.9.1032
48. Shi CG, Zhang Y, Yuan W. Efficacy of bisphosphonates on bone mineral density and fracture rate in patients with osteogenesis imperfecta: a systematic review and meta-analysis. *Am J Ther.* (2016) 23:e894-904. doi: 10.1097/MJT.0000000000000236
49. Biggin A, Munns CF. Long-term bisphosphonate therapy in osteogenesis imperfecta. *Curr Osteoporos Rep.* (2017) 15:412–8. doi: 10.1007/s11914-017-0401-0
50. Sims NA, Martin TJ, Quinn JMW. Coupling: the influences of immune and bone cells. In: Lorenzo J, Horowitz MC, Choi Y, Takayanagi H, Schett G, editors. *Osteoimmunology: Interactions of the Immune and Skeletal Systems.* London: Academic Press. p. 169–85. Available online at: https://www.sciencedirect.com/science/article/pii/B9780128005712000219 doi: 10.1016/B978-0-12-800571-2.00010-4
51. Jensen SS, Gruber R, Buser D, Bosshardt DD. Osteoclast-like cells on deproteinized bovine bone mineral and biphasic calcium phosphate: light

and transmission electron microscopical observations. *Clin Oral Implants Res.* (2015) 26:859–64. doi: 10.1111/clr.12376

52. DeFife KM, Jenney CR, McNally AK, Colton E, Anderson JM. Interleukin-13 induces human monocyte/macrophage fusion and macrophage mannose receptor expression. *J Immunol.* (1997) 158:3385–90.
53. McNally AK, Jones JA, MacEwan SR, Colton E, Anderson JM. Vitronectin is a critical protein adhesion substrate for IL-4-induced foreign body giant cell formation. *J Biomed Mater Res Part A.* (2008) 86A:535–43. doi: 10.1002/jbm.a.31658
54. ten Harkel B, Schoenmaker T, Picavet DI, Davison NL, de Vries TJ, Everts V. The foreign body giant cell cannot resorb bone, but dissolves hydroxyapatite like osteoclasts. *PLoS ONE.* (2015) 10:e0139564. doi: 10.1371/journal.pone.0139564
55. Randolph GJ, Inaba K, Robbiani DF, Steinman RM, Muller WA. Differentiation of phagocytic monocytes into lymph node dendritic cells *in vivo*. *Immunity.* (1999) 11:753–61. doi: 10.1016/S1074-7613(00)80149-1
56. Merad M, Sathe P, Helft J, Miller J, Mortha A. The dendritic cell lineage: ontogeny and function of dendritic cells and their subsets in the steady state and the inflamed setting. *Annu Rev Immunol.* (2013) 31:563–604. doi: 10.1146/annurev-immunol-020711-074950
57. Sokolova V, Knuschke T, Kovtun A, Buer J, Epple M, Westendorf AM. The use of calcium phosphate nanoparticles encapsulating Toll-like receptor ligands and the antigen hemagglutinin to induce dendritic cell maturation and T cell activation. *Biomaterials.* (2010) 31:5627–33. doi: 10.1016/j.biomaterials.2010.03.067
58. Keselowsky BG, Lewis JS. Dendritic cells in the host response to implanted materials. *Semin Immunol.* (2017) 29:33–40. doi: 10.1016/j.smim.2017.04.002
59. Vasilijić S, Savić D, Vasilev S, Vučević D, Gašić S, Majstorović I, et al. Dendritic cells acquire tolerogenic properties at the site of sterile granulomatous inflammation. *Cell Immunol.* (2005) 233:148–57. doi: 10.1016/J.CELLIMM.2005.04.007
60. Michel J, Penna M, Kochen J, Cheung H. Recent advances in hydroxyapatite scaffolds containing mesenchymal stem cells. *Stem Cells Int.* (2015) 2015:305217. doi: 10.1155/2015/305217
61. Miron RJ, Zhang YF. Osteoinduction. *J Dent Res.* (2012) 91:736–44. doi: 10.1177/0022034511435260
62. García-Gareta E, Coathup MJ, Blunn GW. Osteoinduction of bone grafting materials for bone repair and regeneration. *Bone.* (2015) 81:112–21. doi: 10.1016/J.BONE.2015.07.007
63. Brennan MA, Renaud A, Guilloton F, Mebarki M, Trichet V, Sensebé L, et al. Inferior *in vivo* osteogenesis and superior angiogeneis of human adipose-derived stem cells compared with bone marrow-derived stem cells cultured in xeno-free conditions. *Stem Cells Transl Med.* (2017) 6:2160–72. doi: 10.1002/sctm.17-0133
64. Gjerde C, Mustafa K, Hellem S, Rojewski M, Gjengedal H, Yassin MA, et al. Cell therapy induced regeneration of severely atrophied mandibular bone in a clinical trial. *Stem Cell Res Ther.* (2018) 9:213. doi: 10.1186/s13287-018-0951-9
65. Gómez-Barrena E, Rosset P, Gebhard F, Hernigou P, Baldini N, Rouard H, et al. Feasibility and safety of treating non-unions in tibia, femur and humerus with autologous, expanded, bone marrow-derived mesenchymal stromal cells associated with biphasic calcium phosphate biomaterials in a multicentric, non-comparative trial. *Biomaterials.* (2018) 196:100–8. doi: 10.1016/j.biomaterials.2018.03.033
66. Fang D, Seo B-M, Liu Y, Sonoyama W, Yamaza T, Zhang C, et al. Transplantation of mesenchymal stem cells is an optimal approach for plastic surgery. *Stem Cells.* (2007) 25:1021–8. doi: 10.1634/stemcells.2006-0576
67. Hasegawa N, Kawaguchi H, Hirachi A, Takeda K, Mizuno N, Nishimura M, et al. Behavior of transplanted bone marrow–derived mesenchymal stem cells in periodontal defects. *J Periodontol.* (2006) 77:1003–7. doi: 10.1902/jop.2006.050341
68. Oshima Y, Watanabe N, Matsuda K, Takai S, Kawata M, Kubo T. Behavior of transplanted bone marrow-derived GFP mesenchymal cells in osteochondral defect as a simulation of autologous transplantation. *J Histochem Cytochem.* (2005) 53:207–16. doi: 10.1369/jhc.4A6280.2005
69. Tasso R, Augello A, Boccardo S, Salvi S, Caridà M, Postiglione F, et al. Recruitment of a host's osteoprogenitor cells using exogenous mesenchymal stem cells seeded on porous ceramic. *Tissue Eng Part A.* (2009) 15:2203–12. doi: 10.1089/ten.tea.2008.0269
70. Ando Y, Matsubara K, Ishikawa J, Fujio M, Shohara R, Hibi H, et al. Stem cell-conditioned medium accelerates distraction osteogenesis through multiple regenerative mechanisms. *Bone.* (2014) 61:82–90. doi: 10.1016/j.bone.2013.12.029
71. Xu J, Wang B, Sun Y, Wu T, Liu Y, Zhang J, et al. Human fetal mesenchymal stem cell secretome enhances bone consolidation in distraction osteogenesis. *Stem Cell Res Ther.* (2016) 7:134. doi: 10.1186/s13287-016-0392-2
72. Osugi M, Katagiri W, Yoshimi R, Inukai T, Hibi H, Ueda M. Conditioned media from mesenchymal stem cells enhanced bone regeneration in rat calvarial bone defects. *Tissue Eng Part A.* (2012) 18:1479–89. doi: 10.1089/ten.tea.2011.0325
73. Skog J, Würdinger T, van Rijn S, Meijer DH, Gainche L, Curry WT, et al. Glioblastoma microvesicles transport RNA and proteins that promote tumour growth and provide diagnostic biomarkers. *Nat Cell Biol.* (2008) 10:1470–6. doi: 10.1038/ncb1800
74. Valadi H, Ekström K, Bossios A, Sjöstrand M, Lee JJ, Lötvall JO. Exosome-mediated transfer of mRNAs and microRNAs is a novel mechanism of genetic exchange between cells. *Nat Cell Biol.* (2007) 9:654–9. doi: 10.1038/ncb1596
75. Furuta T, Miyaki S, Ishitobi H, Ogura T, Kato Y, Kamei N, et al. Mesenchymal stem cell-derived exosomes promote fracture healing in a mouse model. *Stem Cells Transl Med.* (2016) 5:1620–30. doi: 10.5966/sctm.2015-0285
76. Xie H, Wang Z, Zhang L, Lei Q, Zhao A, Wang H, et al. Extracellular vesicle-functionalized decalcified bone matrix scaffolds with enhanced pro-angiogenic and pro-bone regeneration activities. *Sci Rep.* (2017) 7:45622. doi: 10.1038/srep45622
77. Zhang J, Liu X, Li H, Chen C, Hu B, Niu X, et al. Exosomes/tricalcium phosphate combination scaffolds can enhance bone regeneration by activating the PI3K/Akt signaling pathway. *Stem Cell Res Ther.* (2016) 7:136. doi: 10.1186/s13287-016-0391-3
78. Otsuru S, Desbourdes L, Guess AJ, Hofmann TJ, Relation T, Kaito T, et al. Extracellular vesicles released from mesenchymal stromal cells stimulate bone growth in osteogenesis imperfecta. *Cytotherapy.* (2018) 20:62–73. doi: 10.1016/j.jcyt.2017.09.012
79. Burrello J, Monticone S, Gai C, Gomez Y, Kholia S, Camussi G. Stem cell-derived extracellular vesicles and immune-modulation. *Front Cell Dev Biol.* (2016) 4:83. doi: 10.3389/fcell.2016.00083
80. Guihard P, Danger Y, Brounais B, David E, Brion R, Delecrin J, et al. Induction of osteogenesis in mesenchymal stem cells by activated monocytes/macrophages depends on oncostatin M signaling. *Stem Cells.* (2012) 30:762–72. doi: 10.1002/stem.1040
81. Guihard P, Boutet M-A, Brounais-Le Royer B, Gamblin A-L, Amiaud J, Renaud A, et al. Oncostatin M, an inflammatory cytokine produced by macrophages, supports intramembranous bone healing in a mouse model of tibia injury. *Am J Pathol.* (2015) 185:765–75. doi: 10.1016/J.AJPATH.2014.11.008
82. Omar OM, Granéli C, Ekström K, Karlsson C, Johansson A, Lausmaa J, et al. The stimulation of an osteogenic response by classical monocyte activation. *Biomaterials.* (2011) 32:8190–204. doi: 10.1016/j.biomaterials.2011.07.055
83. Ekström K, Omar O, Granéli C, Wang X, Vazirisani F, Thomsen P. Monocyte exosomes stimulate the osteogenic gene expression of mesenchymal stem cells. *PLoS ONE.* (2013) 8:e75227. doi: 10.1371/journal.pone.0075227
84. Gong L, Zhao Y, Zhang Y, Ruan Z. The macrophage polarization regulates MSC osteoblast differentiation *in vitro*. *Ann Clin Lab Sci.* (2016) 46:65–71.
85. Pajarinen J, Lin T, Gibon E, Kohno Y, Maruyama M, Nathan K, et al. Mesenchymal stem cell-macrophage crosstalk and bone healing. *Biomaterials.* (2018) 196:80–9. doi: 10.1016/j.biomaterials.2017.12.025
86. Zhang Y, Böse T, Unger RE, Jansen JA, Kirkpatrick CJ, van den Beucken JJJP. Macrophage type modulates osteogenic differentiation of adipose tissue MSCs. *Cell Tissue Res.* (2017) 369:273–86. doi: 10.1007/s00441-017-2598-8
87. Caires HR, Barros da Silva P, Barbosa MA, Almeida CR. A co-culture system with three different primary human cell populations reveals that biomaterials and MSC modulate macrophage-driven fibroblast recruitment. *J Tissue Eng Regen Med.* (2018) 12:e1433–40. doi: 10.1002/term.2560

88. Quint P, Ruan M, Pederson L, Kassem M, Westendorf JJ, Khosla S, et al. Sphingosine 1-phosphate (S1P) receptors 1 and 2 coordinately induce mesenchymal cell migration through S1P activation of complementary kinase pathways. *J Biol Chem.* (2013) 288:5398–406. doi: 10.1074/jbc.M112.413583
89. Pederson L, Ruan M, Westendorf JJ, Khosla S, Oursler MJ. Regulation of bone formation by osteoclasts involves Wnt/BMP signaling and the chemokine sphingosine-1-phosphate. *Proc Natl Acad Sci.* (2008) 105:20764–9. doi: 10.1073/pnas.0805133106
90. Liu Y, Wang L, Kikuiri T, Akiyama K, Chen C, Xu X, et al. Mesenchymal stem cell-based tissue regeneration is governed by recipient T lymphocytes via IFN-γ and TNF-α. *Nat Med.* (2011) 17:1594–601. doi: 10.1038/nm.2542
91. Bouvet-Gerbettaz S, Boukhechba F, Balaguer T, Schmid-Antomarchi H, Michiels J-F, Scimeca J-C, et al. Adaptive immune response inhibits ectopic mature bone formation induced by BMSCs/BCP/plasma composite in immune-competent mice. *Tissue Eng Part A.* (2014) 20:2950–62. doi: 10.1089/ten.tea.2013.0633
92. Su Y, Shi S, Liu Y. Immunomodulation regulates mesenchymal stem cell-based bone regeneration. *Oral Dis.* (2014) 20:633–6. doi: 10.1111/odi.12248
93. Najar M, Raicevic G, Crompot E, Fayyad-Kazan H, Bron D, Toungouz M, et al. The immunomodulatory potential of mesenchymal stromal cells. *J Immunother.* (2016) 39:45–59. doi: 10.1097/CJI.0000000000000108
94. Glenn JD. Mesenchymal stem cells: emerging mechanisms of immunomodulation and therapy. *World J Stem Cells.* (2014) 6:526. doi: 10.4252/wjsc.v6.i5.526
95. Bassi G, Guilloton F, Menard C, Di Trapani M, Deschaseaux F, Sensebé L, Schrezenmeier H, et al. Effects of a ceramic biomaterial on immune modulatory properties and differentiation potential of human mesenchymal stromal cells of different origin. *Tissue Eng Part A.* (2015) 21:767–81. doi: 10.1089/ten.tea.2014.0269
96. Giebel B, Kordelas L, Börger V. Clinical potential of mesenchymal stem/stromal cell-derived extracellular vesicles. *Stem Cell Investig.* (2017) 4:84. doi: 10.21037/sci.2017.09.06
97. Deschepper M, Manassero M, Oudina K, Paquet J, Monfoulet L-E, Bensidhoum M, et al. Proangiogenic and prosurvival functions of glucose in human mesenchymal stem cells upon transplantation. *Stem Cells.* (2013) 31:526–35. doi: 10.1002/stem.1299
98. Becquart P, Cambon-Binder A, Monfoulet L-E, Bourguignon M, Vandamme K, Bensidhoum M, et al. Ischemia is the prime but not the only cause of human multipotent stromal cell death in tissue-engineered constructs *in vivo*. *Tissue Eng Part A.* (2012) 18:2084–94. doi: 10.1089/ten.tea.2011.0690
99. Potier E, Ferreira E, Meunier A, Sedel L, Logeart-Avramoglou D, Petite H. Prolonged hypoxia concomitant with serum deprivation induces massive human mesenchymal stem cell death. *Tissue Eng.* (2007) 13:1325–31. doi: 10.1089/ten.2006.0325
100. Moya A, Paquet J, Deschepper M, Larochette N, Oudina K, Denoeud C, et al. Human mesenchymal stem cell failure to adapt to glucose shortage and rapidly use intracellular energy reserves through glycolysis explains poor cell survival after implantation. *Stem Cells.* (2018) 36:363–76. doi: 10.1002/stem.2763
101. Nicolay NH, Perez RL, Saffrich R, Huber PE, Nicolay NH, Perez RL, et al. Radio-resistant mesenchymal stem cells: mechanisms of resistance and potential implications for the clinic. *Oncotarget.* (2015) 6:19366–80. doi: 10.18632/oncotarget.4358
102. Laing AG, Riffo-Vasquez Y, Sharif-Paghaleh E, Lombardi G, Sharpe PT. Immune modulation by apoptotic dental pulp stem cells *in vivo*. *Immunotherapy.* (2018) 10:201–11. doi: 10.2217/imt-2017-0117
103. Galleu A, Riffo-Vasquez Y, Trento C, Lomas C, Dolcetti L, Cheung TS, et al. Apoptosis in mesenchymal stromal cells induces *in vivo* recipient-mediated immunomodulation. *Sci Transl Med.* (2017) 9:eaam7828. doi: 10.1126/scitranslmed.aam7828
104. Sachet M, Liang YY, Oehler R. The immune response to secondary necrotic cells. *Apoptosis.* (2017) 22:1189–204. doi: 10.1007/s10495-017-1413-z
105. Bianchi ME, Crippa MP, Manfredi AA, Mezzapelle R, Rovere Querini P, Venereau E. High-mobility group box 1 protein orchestrates responses to tissue damage via inflammation, innate and adaptive immunity, and tissue repair. *Immunol Rev.* (2017) 280:74–82. doi: 10.1111/imr.12601
106. Lunyak VV, Amaro-Ortiz A, Gaur M. Mesenchymal stem cells secretory responses: senescence messaging secretome and immunomodulation perspective. *Front Genet.* (2017) 8:1–21. doi: 10.3389/fgene.2017.00220
107. Madrigal M, Rao KS, Riordan NH. A review of therapeutic effects of mesenchymal stem cell secretions and induction of secretory modification by different culture methods. *J Transl Med.* (2014) 12:260. doi: 10.1186/s12967-014-0260-8
108. Sisakhtnezhad S, Alimoradi E, Akrami H. External factors influencing mesenchymal stem cell fate *in vitro*. *Eur J Cell Biol.* (2017) 96:13–33. doi: 10.1016/j.ejcb.2016.11.003
109. Silva LHA, Antunes MA, Dos Santos CC, Weiss DJ, Cruz FF, Rocco PRM. Strategies to improve the therapeutic effects of mesenchymal stromal cells in respiratory diseases. *Stem Cell Res Ther.* (2018) 9:45. doi: 10.1186/s13287-018-0802-8
110. Xue C, Shen Y, Li X, Li B, Zhao S, Gu J, et al. Exosomes derived from hypoxia-treated human adipose mesenchymal stem cells enhance angiogenesis through the PKA signaling pathway. *Stem Cells Dev.* (2018) 27:456–65. doi: 10.1089/scd.2017.0296
111. Ban J-J, Lee M, Im W, Kim M. Low pH increases the yield of exosome isolation. *Biochem Biophys Res Commun.* (2015) 461:76–9. doi: 10.1016/j.bbrc.2015.03.172
112. Eldh M, Ekström K, Valadi H, Sjöstrand M, Olsson B, Jernås M, et al. Exosomes communicate protective messages during oxidative stress; possible role of exosomal shuttle RNA. *PLoS ONE.* (2010) 5:e15353. doi: 10.1371/journal.pone.0015353
113. Ejtehadifar M, Shamsasenjan K, Movassaghpour A, Akbarzadehlaleh P, Dehdilani N, Abbasi P, et al. The effect of hypoxia on mesenchymal stem cell biology. *Adv Pharm Bull.* (2015) 5:141–9. doi: 10.15171/apb.2015.021
114. Paquet J, Deschepper M, Moya A, Logeart-Avramoglou D, Boisson-Vidal C, Petite H. Oxygen tension regulates human mesenchymal stem cell paracrine functions. *Stem Cells Transl Med.* (2015) 4:809–21. doi: 10.5966/sctm.2014-0180
115. Martinez VG, Ontoria-Oviedo I, Ricardo CP, Harding SE, Sacedon R, Varas A, et al. Overexpression of hypoxia-inducible factor 1 alpha improves immunomodulation by dental mesenchymal stem cells. *Stem Cell Res Ther.* (2017) 8:208. doi: 10.1186/s13287-017-0659-2
116. Ponte AL, Marais E, Gallay N, Langonné A, Delorme B, Hérault O, et al. The *in vitro* migration capacity of human bone marrow mesenchymal stem cells: comparison of chemokine and growth factor chemotactic activities. *Stem Cells.* (2007) 25:1737–45. doi: 10.1634/stemcells.2007-0054
117. Crisostomo PR, Wang Y, Markel TA, Wang M, Lahm T, Meldrum DR. Human mesenchymal stem cells stimulated by TNF-α, LPS, or hypoxia produce growth factors by an NFκB- but not JNK-dependent mechanism. *Am J Physiol Physiol.* (2008) 294:C675–82. doi: 10.1152/ajpcell.00437.2007
118. Roemeling-van Rhijn M, Mensah FKF, Korevaar SS, Leijs MJ, van Osch GJVM, IJzermans JNM, et al. Effects of hypoxia on the immunomodulatory properties of adipose tissue-derived mesenchymal stem cells. *Front Immunol.* (2013) 4:1–8. doi: 10.3389/fimmu.2013.00203
119. Cordonnier T, Layrolle P, Gaillard J, Langonné A, Sensebé L, Rosset P, et al. 3D environment on human mesenchymal stem cells differentiation for bone tissue engineering. *J Mater Sci Mater Med.* (2010) 21:981–7. doi: 10.1007/s10856-009-3916-9
120. Miron RJ, Zohdi H, Fujioka-Kobayashi M, Bosshardt DD. Giant cells around bone biomaterials: osteoclasts or multi-nucleated giant cells? *Acta Biomater.* (2016) 46:15–28. doi: 10.1016/j.actbio.2016.09.029
121. Ahmed GJ, Tatsukawa E, Morishita K, Shibata Y, Suehiro F, Kamitakahara M, et al. Regulation and biological significance of formation of osteoclasts and foreign body giant cells in an extraskeletal implantation model. *Acta Histochem Cytochem.* (2016) 49:97–107. doi: 10.1267/ahc.16007
122. Khan UA, Hashimi SM, Bakr MM, Forwood MR, Morrison NA. Foreign body giant cells and osteoclasts are TRAP positive, have podosome-belts and both require OC-STAMP for cell fusion. *J Cell Biochem.* (2013) 114:1772–8. doi: 10.1002/jcb.24518
123. Ogata K, Katagiri W, Hibi H. Secretomes from mesenchymal stem cells participate in the regulation of osteoclastogenesis *in vitro*. *Clin Oral Investig.* (2017) 21:1979–88. doi: 10.1007/s00784-016-1986-x

124. Horwood NJ, Kartsogiannis V, Quinn JMW, Romas E, Martin TJ, Gillespie MT. Activated T lymphocytes support osteoclast formation *in vitro*. *Biochem Biophys Res Commun.* (1999) 265:144–50. doi: 10.1006/bbrc.1999.1623
125. Martin TJ, Sims NA. RANKL/OPG; critical role in bone physiology. *Rev Endocr Metab Disord.* (2015) 16:131–9. doi: 10.1007/s11154-014-9308-6
126. Quinn JMW, Itoh K, Udagawa N, Häusler K, Yasuda H, Shima N, et al. Transforming growth factor β affects osteoclast differentiation via direct and indirect actions. *J Bone Miner Res.* (2001) 16:1787–94. doi: 10.1359/jbmr.2001.16.10.1787
127. Maeda K, Kobayashi Y, Udagawa N, Uehara S, Ishihara A, Mizoguchi T, et al. Wnt5a-Ror2 signaling between osteoblast-lineage cells and osteoclast precursors enhances osteoclastogenesis. *Nat Med.* (2012) 18:405–12. doi: 10.1038/nm.2653
128. Chan CKF, Gulati GS, Sinha R, Tompkins JV, Lopez M, Carter AC, et al. Identification of the human skeletal stem cell. *Cell.* (2018) 175:43–56.e21. doi: 10.1016/J.CELL.2018.07.029
129. Sims NA, Martin TJ. Coupling the activities of bone formation and resorption: a multitude of signals within the basic multicellular unit. *Bonekey Rep.* (2014) 3:1–10. doi: 10.1038/bonekey.2013.215
130. Matsuo K, Irie N. Osteoclast–osteoblast communication. *Arch Biochem Biophys.* (2008) 473:201–9. doi: 10.1016/j.abb.2008.03.027
131. Henriksen K, Karsdal MA, John Martin T. Osteoclast-derived coupling factors in bone remodeling. *Calcif Tissue Int.* (2014) 94:88–97. doi: 10.1007/s00223-013-9741-7
132. Ikebuchi Y, Aoki S, Honma M, Hayashi M, Sugamori Y, Khan M, et al. Coupling of bone resorption and formation by RANKL reverse signalling. *Nature.* (2018) 561:195–200. doi: 10.1038/s41586-018-0482-7
133. Cianferotti L, Gomes AR, Fabbri S, Tanini A, Brandi ML. The calcium-sensing receptor in bone metabolism: from bench to bedside and back. *Osteoporos Int.* (2015) 26:2055–71. doi: 10.1007/s00198-015-3203-1
134. Chen Z, Klein T, Murray RZ, Crawford R, Chang J, Wu C, et al. Osteoimmunomodulation for the development of advanced bone biomaterials. *Mater Today.* (2016) 19:304–21. doi: 10.1016/j.mattod.2015.11.004

6

A Jack of All Trades: Impact of Glucocorticoids on Cellular Cross-Talk in Osteoimmunology

Mubashir Ahmad[1†], *Yasmine Hachemi*[1†], *Kevin Paxian*[1], *Florian Mengele*[1,2], *Mascha Koenen*[1,3] *and Jan Tuckermann*[1*]

[1] *Institute of Comparative Molecular Endocrinology (CME), University of Ulm, Ulm, Germany,* [2] *Praxisklinik für Orthopädie, Unfall- und Neurochirurgie Prof. Bischoff/ Dr. Spies/ Dr. Mengele, Neu-Ulm, Germany,* [3] *Department of Immunobiology, Yale School of Medicine, New Haven, CT, United States*

Correspondence:
Jan Tuckermann
jan.tuckermann@uni-ulm.de

[†] *These authors have contributed equally to this work*

Glucocorticoids (GCs) are known to have a strong impact on the immune system, metabolism, and bone homeostasis. While these functions have been long investigated separately in immunology, metabolism, or bone biology, the understanding of how GCs regulate the cellular cross-talk between innate immune cells, mesenchymal cells, and other stromal cells has been garnering attention rather recently. Here we review the recent findings of GC action in osteoporosis, inflammatory bone diseases (rheumatoid and osteoarthritis), and bone regeneration during fracture healing. We focus on studies of pre-clinical animal models that enable dissecting the role of GC actions in innate immune cells, stromal cells, and bone cells using conditional and function-selective mutant mice of the GC receptor (GR), or mice with impaired GC signaling. Importantly, GCs do not only directly affect cellular functions, but also influence the cross-talk between mesenchymal and immune cells, contributing to both beneficial and adverse effects of GCs. Given the importance of endogenous GCs as stress hormones and the wide prescription of pharmaceutical GCs, an improved understanding of GC action is decisive for tackling inflammatory bone diseases, osteoporosis, and aging.

Keywords: glucocorticoids, glucocorticoid receptor, osteoporosis, arthritis, inflammation, fracture healing, conditional knockout mice

INTRODUCTION

Glucocorticoids (GCs) form one major axis of the stress response (1) and are used as immunosuppressive therapeutics in a variety of inflammatory bone diseases (2, 3). Strong impact on innate immune cells, namely macrophages, dendritic cells, and mast cells, contribute to the inhibition of inflammation. On the other hand, GCs are known to cause the most frequent secondary osteoporosis at conditions of high GC exposure. In this process myeloid cells, osteoclasts, and mesenchymal cells and their derivatives, chondrocytes, osteoblasts, and osteocytes are affected. Whereas, the cell-autonomous roles of GCs acting via the nuclear glucocorticoid receptor (GR) had been investigated intensively, the knowledge about the influence of GCs on cross-talk between innate immune cells, mesenchymal cells, and bone cells is scarce. How GCs act on cellular interactions in the osteo-immunological network is currently unraveled and is subject to this review.

GLUCOCORTICOIDS (GCs), STRESS HORMONES AND ANTI-INFLAMMATORY AGENTS

Two different axes initiate the human physiological reaction to stress. While the activation of sympathetic-adrenal medulla (SAM)-axis starts a short-term stress reactions, long-term stress responses are mediated by the hypothalamus-pituitary-adrenal (HPA)-axis. Stress exposure results in the releases of corticotrophin-releasing hormone (CRH) from the hypothalamus, causing the synthesis of adrenocorticotropic hormone (ACTH) in the anterior pituitary gland, which activates the production of GCs in the adrenal cortex via induction of key enzymes of steroid synthesis (4).

Under long-term stress conditions GC release from the adrenal cortex also results in diverse physiological adaptations. Cortisol activates gluconeogenesis in the liver, decreases pancreatic insulin secretion, and promotes the release of glucagon. Furthermore, blood pressure elevates, the effect of catecholamines is potentiated, and a mild sodium/water-retention induced (5).

Since the first successful treatment of arthritis (6), GCs have been in frequent use and approximately 3% of the elderly population are being treated with GCs (7, 8), to reduce inflammatory symptoms in acute and chronic inflammatory diseases, including rheumatoid and osteoarthritis.

Adverse side effects of GCs on the human body have been observed upon extended treatment with daily prednisolone-doses of 7.5 mg and above. Besides the Cushingoid phenotype and osteoporosis, metabolic side effects as peripheral insulin resistance, type 2 diabetes and dyslipidemia are predominant (1). In addition, atrophy of skin and impact on the central nervous system can occur. To a similar extent, long-term GC treatment affects the cardiovascular system, resulting in hypertension, thrombotic stroke or myocardial infarction (9). These well-known side effects often preclude long-term treatment and cause occasional severe long lasting damage to the patient. Given the strong acute action of GCs to reduce inflammation, however, side effects are accepted to a certain extent in clinical praxis.

At the molecular level, intracellular GC-activity depends on the enzymes 11β-hydroxysteroid dehydrogenase type 1 and 2 (11β-HSD1 and 11β-HSD2). 11β-HSD1 catalyzes the conversion of cortisone into active cortisol, 11β-HSD2 mainly induces the reverse reaction by inactivating cortisol (10). A specific ratio of both isozymes is given in different tissue types, for example 11β-HSD1 being predominant in liver and adipose tissue (11). Molecular actions of GCs are initiated by binding to the mineralocorticoid receptor (MR) and the GC receptor (GR). Due to the wide expression of GR compared to MR and the inactivation of GCs by 11β-HSD2 in MR high expressing tissues, most of the GC effects are mediated by the GR as evident from knockout studies. However, the role of MR in inflammation is becoming more recognized and is reviewed elsewhere (12). The GR belongs to the nuclear receptor superfamily and acts as a ligand-induced transcription factor, resulting in transactivation or transrepression of genes (10). The GR structure is constituted by four domains: the transactivation domain AF1/2 (docking station for co-regulators and regulative enzymes), the DNA-binding-domain, the ligand-binding domain (binding locus for GCs) and the hinge-region (involved in translocation of GR) (10). When located in the cytoplasm GR, is in a state of high affinity to GCs and captured in a complex with immunophilins (FKBP51), heat-shock-proteins (Hsp90) and p23 (13). GC binding leads to an exchange of FKBP51 into FKBP52, resulting in translocation of the protein complex via interaction with the microtubules (10, 13). In case of nuclear transactivation, the GR tends to dimerize and bind to specific motives on target DNA, the GC response element (GRE). The ability of GCs to downregulate genes is mediated in part by GR-binding to negative GREs and consecutive recruitment of corepressors; all leading to deacetylation of histones and decrease of gene transcription [reviewed in (10, 14)]. A "tethering mode" whereby a GR-monomer interacts with DNA-bound inflammatory transcription factors (NF-κB, AP-1, STAT3, IRF3) instead of directly binding to DNA was observed for the repression of genes encoding pro-inflammatory mediators, such as cytokines and matrix metalloproteases (15). This way of cytokine-transrepression eventually leads to immunosuppression. Furthermore, crosstalk exists between DNA-bound GRs and NF-κB or AP-1 bound to transcription-factor binding-sites in the vicinity. However, both mechanisms—transactivation via dimerized GRs and transrepression via tethering of monomeric GR—are obligatory for complete anti-inflammatory GC actions (16). Non-genomic GR-effects can be observed under high-dose GC-application and modulated by GR-interaction with membranes or mitochondria (3).

Short term rise in physiological levels of GCs can stimulate the immune function, whereas immunosuppression resulting from chronic stress, favors infections or tumorigenesis (17). The immunomodulatory actions of GCs are amongst other functions achieved by priming of innate immunity. Under physiological stress conditions macrophage phagocytosis, natural killer-cell activity and cytokine production are increased (17). Furthermore, a wide range of stress-effects on leukocytes is observed: ranging from enhanced proliferation and distribution in the lymphatic system or better endothelial adhesion, to leukocyte margination and transmigration into the inflamed tissue (17). In contrast, chronically elevated GCs levels impair leukocyte proliferation and redistribution and cytokine and prostaglandin synthesis (17).

Accordingly Frank et al. (18) showed that GCs play an important role as an alarmin in neuroinflammatory priming. Stress induced high GC levels result in NLRP3 inflammasome priming, whereby the innate immune system (e.g., microglia) switches into activation mode (18). Frank et al. describe this paradox GC-induced neuroimmune activation under neuroinflammatory conditions to be an adaptive way of preparing against potential neuronal injuries or infections (18).

Thus, GCs via the GR suppress inflammatory reactions, but may also stimulate them, depending on pharmacological conditions. Whereas, for immune suppression several molecular mechanisms of the GR, transactivation of anti-inflammatory acting genes and repression of pro-inflammatory acting genes is required, the mode of action for immune priming remains elusive.

How the different modes of action of the GR impact osteoimmunological cross-talk by influencing bone and immune cells is discussed in this review.

GLUCOCORTICOID (GC) ACTION ON BONE: DIRECT EFFECTS AND THE MODULATION OF THE CROSSTALK OF BONE CELLS

Cell Autonomous Effects of GCs on Bone Cells

Previous research focused on cell-autonomous effects of GC and GR action within bone cells toward bone homeostasis and insights were provided by the use of cell type specific mutant mouse strains compromising GC signaling.

Intriguingly, GCs at the physiological levels have anabolic effects on bone. They promote the formation of osteoblasts from mesenchymal progenitor cells and are essential for maintaining bone homeostasis (19). This is evident from patients (20), since fracture risk is increased during adrenal insufficiency (21) and was shown experimentally through the use of mice that have either impaired GC metabolism in the osteoblast lineage or a selective deletion of the GR. Overexpression of the GC inactivating enzyme 11β-HSD2 in mice in early differentiated osteoblasts (22–24), but not at late differentiation stages (25) led to a reduction of cortical and trabecular bone mass in adult mice. Furthermore, a defective mineralization in the calvaria was observed which was associated with diminished Wnt Signaling (26). A reduced trabecular bone mass was also seen in mice lacking the GR in the osteoblast lineages using the Runx2 as a driver for the cre expression in the cre-loxP system (27). Furthermore, GR deficient cells displayed strongly diminished differentiation potential *in vitro*. Since osteocytes are also mutant in $GR^{Runx2Cre}$ mice, currently it remains unclear how much the GR in osteocytes contributes to the bone mass at physiological conditions. Taken together, endogenous GC signaling via the GR promotes osteoblastogenesis. However, the GR is not essential for osteoblast generation. The embryonic lethal GR knockout mice (27) and mesenchymal specific GR knockout mice (28) displayed no absence of calcification in late stage embryos. Thus, GR is a positive modulator of osteoblastogenesis, but not a crucial factor. In contrast to the GR deletion in mesenchymal cells, deletion of GR in myeloid cells including macrophages, neutrophils, and osteoclasts, does not affect bone in adult mice in the absence of inflammation, indicating that osteo-immunological cross-talk in the absence of inflammation at physiological GC levels plays a minor role in controlling bone mass (27).

This becomes strikingly altered at conditions with high exposure of GCs as it occurs in steroid therapy. GC-induced osteoporosis is among the most common so-called secondary osteoporosis (29), when bone loss is induced as side effects by medication. Here exogenous GCs have contrasting effects to endogenous GCs on osteoblasts, which decreases their proliferation (30), differentiation, and induce apoptosis and modulate autophagy (25, 31–35). Whereas, induction of autophagy seems not to be decisive for inhibition of osteoblast and osteocyte function *in vivo* (36), an impaired differentiation and induction of apoptosis likely lead to decreased bone formation rate (27, 33). The molecular mechanisms of the pharmacological effects on osteoblast function are partially understood. The inhibition of proliferation and differentiation is supposed to be due to inhibition of growth factors (IGF-1, WNT proteins, BMPs), expression and inhibiting the activity of their downstream signaling pathways [reviewed in (10, 19)]. The molecular mechanisms of this inhibition involves in part the induction of inhibitory molecules such as DKK1, Sclerostin, secreted frizzled and WIF1, all antagonizing Wnt signaling (19, 37). Furthermore, negative interference of the activity of the transcription factors AP-1 and Notch had been proposed (27, 38). Recently, the involvement of miRNAs was suggested (39, 40). This was challenged by a study showing that the abrogation of dicer dependent processing of miRNAs did not inhibit decreased bone formation by GCs in osteoblast specific mutant Dicer mice (41). The induction of osteoblast and osteocyte apoptosis, another cellular phenotype associated with decreased bone formation was attributed to suppression of the pro-survival gene Bcl-XL and increase of pro-apoptotic genes BIM and BAK (42–44). Additionally the generation of reactive oxygen species by rapid activation of pro-active kinases Pyk2, and JNK were suggested (45) (**Figure 1**).

GCs also directly act on osteoclasts stimulating initial resorption after high GC exposure (46), which then declines with prolonged GC exposures. These effects are known to be mediated through the stimulatory actions of GCs on proliferation and differentiation of osteoclast precursors as well as by prolongation of their longevity (47–49). In contrast, early progenitors are attenuated by GCs (48, 49). This latter effect might explain the decline of resorption at very long GC treatments. Nonetheless, once the osteoclasts had been formed GCs lead to enhanced longevity (46, 50), apoptosis could be suppressed, and the effects of receptor activator of nuclear factor kappa-B ligand (RANKL) potentiated. Importantly, this was abrogated in osteoclasts from GRA485T (GR^{dim}) knock-in mice, with impaired GR dimerization (50, 51). This indicates that in contrast to GC-mediated suppression of bone formation for the increase of resorption, GR dimer dependent genetic programs are required.

GCs Affecting Cellular Cross-Talk of Bone Cells

Since the observation that bone formation and bone resorption are functionally coupled at the bone remodeling unit (52), cross-talk of cells in bone was considered as a hall mark of bone metabolism. This observation was supported by the discovery that osteoblasts and osteocytes are regulating bone resorption by triggering osteoclastogenesis via the induction of the pro-osteoclastogenic factor RANKL (53, 54) following exposure to M-CSF. This occurs in response to systemic hormones, such as PTH. RANKL on the other hand is counteracted by OPG. GCs seem to affect this cross-talk in part as well,

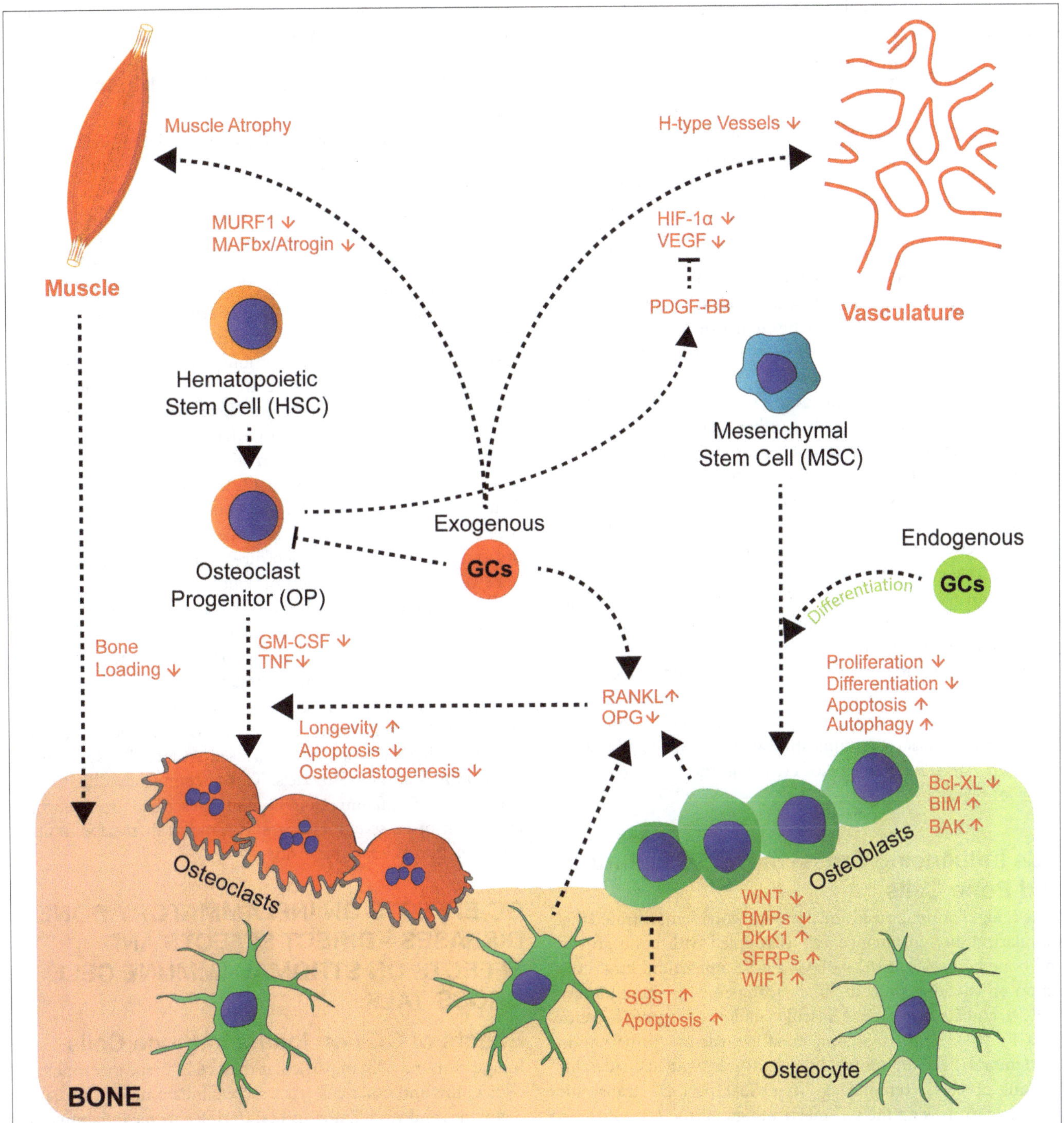

FIGURE 1 | GCs affect cross-talk of bone cells and their communication with muscle, vasculature and myeloid cell-derived osteoclasts. GCs act directly and indirectly on bone, hematopoietic and mesenchymal cells and tissues that affect bone integrity. Endogenous GCs (green) rather favour differentiation of osteoblasts, whereas exogenous (red) rather decrease proliferation, differentiation and enhance apoptosis and autophagy of osteoblasts and osteocytes by differential regulation of signalling molecules of the Wnt and BMP pathway and pro- and anti-apoptotic molecules. Direct effects on osteoclasts are differential concerning longevity, apoptosis, osteoclastogenesis (for details see text) and indirect by altering RANKL/OPG ratio. GCs regulate cross-talk of vasculature toward bone and muscle toward bone by exerting modulatory effects on both systems (muscle atrophy) and likely impairing H-type vessels, since respective signalling molecules (VEGF and PDGF-BB are regulated by GCs).

since GCs induce RANKL and suppress OPG in osteoblastic cells, affecting bone resorption (27, 55–57) (**Figure 1**). RANKL inhibition by Denosumab in humanized mice improved some, but not all parameters of bone loss to GC effects (57). For the increase of osteoclasts in cortical bone, RANKL expression in osteocytes is decisive as shown by Piemontese et al. using mice with a conditional deletion of RANKL using *Rankl*^{Dmp1Cre} mice (58).

Besides, the crucial soluble factors RANKL and M-CSF, TNF and TREM2 ligands play a decisive role in commitment, fusion and maturation of osteoclasts (59). Of these, TNF expression is strongly reduced by GCs at a transcriptional and post-transcriptional level. GM-CSF itself is reduced by the GR via interaction with NF-AT/AP-1 binding sites in the enhancer of the GM-CSF gene (60) (**Figure 1**). This is consistent with the observation that the onset of osteoclastogenesis is inhibited by GCs, which depends on cell autonomous effects (48, 49) and the down regulation of extracellular mediators. The latter was shown by coculture experiments where GCs strongly suppressed osteoclastogenesis dependent on the GR in osteoblasts despite the GR deficiency in osteoclast progenitors (27). This might play in particular a role during inflammation, where osteoclastogenesis and resorption is usually enhanced, and might be beneficially counteracted by GCs. Whether other osteoclast regulatory extracellular factors are under the control of GCs and whether this matters for osteoclastogenesis and activity is still unexplored.

Even less is understood, whether GCs affect osteoclast signals toward osteoblasts or osteocytes. This is still due to the paucity of knowledge of osteoclast-derived factors influencing osteoblasts and osteocytes. Among these identified are ephrinB2, the D2 isoforms of vacuolar (H+) ATPase (v-ATPase) V0 domain (Atp6v0d2), the complement component 3a, semaphorin 4D and microRNAs [reviewed in (61)]. It is not known whether any of these are regulated by GCs to our knowledge. Regulation of microRNAs had been shown for cell-autonomous effects in osteoblasts and osteoclasts, respectively, but whether the osteoclast-osteoblast communication or *vice versa* is affected is unknown. Thus, for this type of cross talk there is tremendous scope for research.

GCs Influencing Cross-Talk of Vasculature and Bone Cells

Bone is highly vascularized and previous work demonstrated that vascularization and angiogenesis is coupled with bone growth and bone homeostasis (62–64). GCs have a profound inhibitory action on vasculogenesis in bone accompanied by inhibition of HIF-1α and its target gene vascular endothelial growth factor (VEGF) (65). This is accompanied by edema formation in the femoral head in mouse bone, an area with considerable amount of vessel remodeling. In OG2-11β-HSD2 transgenic mice, overexpressing the GC inactivating enzyme 11β-HSD2 in osteocalcin expressing cells, the decrease of vasculature volume was in part prevented (62, 65). Recent studies identified the presence of a subtype of vessels, so-called H-Type vessels, positive for CD31 and endocmucin being associated with bone formation (63). These H-Type vessels were found to be reduced by GC excess, a process that could be prevented by addition of platelet-derived growth factor-BB (PDGF-BB) (66). Since PDGF-BB is in part derived from osteoclast progenitors (67), PDGF-BB could be a factor targeted by GCs.

Taken together, the precise contribution of GC signaling in cells of the vasculature vs. osteoclasts, osteoblasts and osteocytes remain to be determined, which will be of importance to decipher the effects of GC excess on bone integrity.

GCs Influencing Cross-Talk of Muscle and Bone

Since GC excess does not only influence bone strength, but also leads to muscle atrophy, this increases the risks of falls and reduces load on bone, thus accelerating bone loss and increasing fracture risk (68). GCs induce protein degradation in muscles associated with induced FoxO-dependent expression of E3 ubiquitin ligases atrophy F-Box [MAFbx/atrogin and muscle RING finger 1 (MURF1)], which is mediated in part through the GR in muscle (69–71). Surprisingly, some of these genes are also regulated in bone by excessive GC amounts (68), suggesting that some deleterious pathways might be shared between bone and muscle. The cross-talk between muscle and bone exist beyond the mechanical load. Kim et al., discovered that the muscle derived hormone Irisin binds to alphaV class of integrins in osteocytes and might stimulate resorption and increased sclerostin expression (72). Whether further soluble factors participate in this muscle bone cross-talk and whether they or Irisin signaling itself, are a target of GCs remains to be investigated. Nonetheless, both direct effects on muscle and on bone cells accelerate weakness of bone.

Interestingly, in the absence of inflammation, models of GC induced osteoporosis so far provide no clear evidence of regulation of the cross-talk between bone cells such as osteoblast/osteocytes with innate immune cells, except osteoclasts and their progenitors. This does not mean that GC mediated regulation of this cross-talk does not exist. However, this has not been addressed so far with appropriate cell conditional mouse models. This is completely different for conditions of inflammation in bone described below, where regulation of cross-talk emerges as a major theme for limiting inflammation at least in arthritis.

GC EFFECTS ON INFLAMMATORY BONE DISEASES—DIRECT EFFECTS AND EFFECTS ON STROMAL-IMMUNE CELL CROSS-TALK

Effects of GCs on Innate Immune Cells

Innate immune cells, in particular mast cells, tissue macrophages, neutrophils and other cell types secrete inflammatory mediators (cytokines and vasodilator agents) during chronic inflammation, as it occurs e.g., during tissue damage. GCs are known to suppress the production of inflammatory mediators partially by acting on Toll-like receptor (TLR) signaling (73, 74). They also act on macrophages to inhibit the production of eicosanoids, which are lipid mediators that promote vascular dilation and permeability (75, 76). GCs also reduce the blood flow to inflammatory sites by sensitizing endothelial cells to vasoconstrictors and by inhibiting the production of vasodilators (77). In addition, GCs attenuate leukocyte extravasation by inhibiting transcription of integrins and their ligands, intercellular adhesion molecule 1 (ICAM1) as an example (78, 79). Finally, GCs inhibit the expression of many pro-inflammatory cytokines and chemokines. Mice with conditional GR ablation in macrophages or dendritic cells (DCs), produced higher levels of IL-1β, IL-6, TNF, and IL-12, and exhibited greater mortality during experimentally induced sepsis (80–82). Whereas, downregulation of chemokines, such as CC-chemokine ligand 2 (CCL2), CCL3, CCL5, restrains leukocyte migration, and deficiency of macrophage-recruiting molecule MCP-1 in mice (also known as C-C motif chemokine receptor 2 [CCR-2]), led to compromised fracture healing (83).

Interestingly, GCs reduce mast cell number, maturation and activation (84–87) and stabilize mast cells dose-dependently by inhibiting their exocytotic process. This effect is ascribed to the non-genomic actions of GCs, acting via the GR present in the plasma membrane of mast cells, and directly influencing the intracellular Ca^{2+} signaling pathway (88). In a mouse model of 11β-HSD1 deficiency, reduced intracellular GC action in mast cells correlated with increased activation demonstrating a clear influence of 11β-HSD1 on mast cell degranulation (89).

Despite suppressing inflammatory activity of immune cells, the concept emerges that GCs terminate inflammation by polarizing cells toward an anti-inflammatory phenotype. This has been thoroughly investigated in macrophages. Several studies demonstrated that GCs induce specific differentiation of monocytes with an anti-inflammatory phenotype and promote their survival, contributing majorly to the resolution of inflammation (90–93).

The induction of anti-inflammatory acting immune cells is decisive for resolution of inflammation during fracture healing and arthritis and is subject to GC action.

GLUCOCORTICOIDS (GCs) AND FRACTURE HEALING

Cells Involved in Fracture Healing

The role of GCs during fracture healing, a process that requires multiple communication steps between different cell types, is not well-understood. Fracture healing involves close interaction between bone cells and immune cells. Bone injury causes the onset of inflammation. A fracture hematoma is formed containing DAMPs and PAMPs (danger/pathogen-associated molecular patterns), erythrocytes, inflammatory cytokines and cells of the innate immunity. The inflammatory phase is followed by the repair phase where a cartilaginous callus is formed and then remodeled by osteoblast and osteoclasts (94).

Several innate immune cells are present in the early fracture hematoma such as neutrophils, macrophages and mast cells (95–98). Activated mast cells release inflammatory mediators, including histamine, KC, IL-1β, TNF, and IL-6, as well as various chemokines attracting other immune cells (99, 100). Neutrophils and macrophages migrate to the injury site in response to inflammatory mediators to phagocytose debris and pathogens (96, 97, 101, 102) (**Figure 2**).

Depletion of neutrophils, leads to impairment of fracture healing in mice (95, 103), and a reduction of mesenchymal tissue repair in a rat model of growth plate injury (104). Macrophages persist during all phases of fracture repair (96, 97), where they are important for bone healing (105). In a mouse model of femoral fracture, Raggatt et al. showed that inflammatory macrophages were required for the initiation of the fracture repair, while both inflammatory and osteomacs, specialized resident bone macrophages, promoted anabolic processes during endochondral callus formation (106). Mast cell deficiency in mice, however, causes a reduction of the inflammatory response after fracture and disturbed callus remodeling. In the same study, *in vitro* investigation suggested histamine as a major mediator of mast cells action on osteoclastogenesis (98) (**Figure 2**).

During the repair phase, mesenchymal precursors, close to the site of the fracture, differentiate into chondrocytes and start the process of endochondral ossification. A cartilaginous soft callus is formed in order to stabilize the fracture (107). Under stable mechanical conditions the vascularization of the callus is initiated and subsequently followed by its mineralization and its conversion into bone (108). Finally, the callus is remodeled by osteoclasts and osteoblasts and the original bone architecture is restored (109).

Cells of the immune system influence the process of endochondral ossification. Tissue resident and infiltrating macrophages, in particular M2 macrophages enhance vascularization by secreting VEGF at the fracture site (97). They also release TGF-β that plays a pivotal role in chondrogenic differentiation of mesenchymal stem cells for callus formation (110). Monocytes, neutrophils, DC, and B and T lymphocytes produce RANKL and subsequently influence osteoclast and osteoblast activity (111, 112) (**Figure 2**).

Effects of GCs on Fracture Healing

The injury represents a stress stimulus that triggers endogenous GC release to control the inflammation. We have previously shown, in a mouse model of fracture, that mice with an induced global deletion of the GR, including bone and immune cells, had an impaired fracture healing. The presence of the GR had a protective role in our model partially by shaping the inflammatory response (113).

Few studies investigated the effects of synthetic GCs on fracture healing. It was shown that short-term treatment with GCs had minor effects on bone repair (114) while long-term treatments significantly impaired the healing process (115, 116). In a medaka fish fracture model, although both chronic and acute GC treatment affected osteoclast recruitment and osteoblast accumulation, only chronic GC treatment significantly delayed the healing (117).

The role of GCs on endochondral ossification in fracture healing hasn't been widely investigated. In a model of glucocorticoid-induced osteoporosis, endochondral ossification was impaired after fracture as chondrocyte hypertrophy was delayed (118). In a tibial metaphyseal fracture model, GR deletion in chondrocytes attenuated endochondral bone healing by momentarily increasing the cartilage content of the callus, but didn't impact negatively on the healing outcome (119). In contrast, treatment with dexamethasone had an inhibitory effect on healing in the femur shaft fracture in comparison to metaphyseal fracture, suggesting a more important role of GCs in endochondral rather than intramembranous ossification (120).

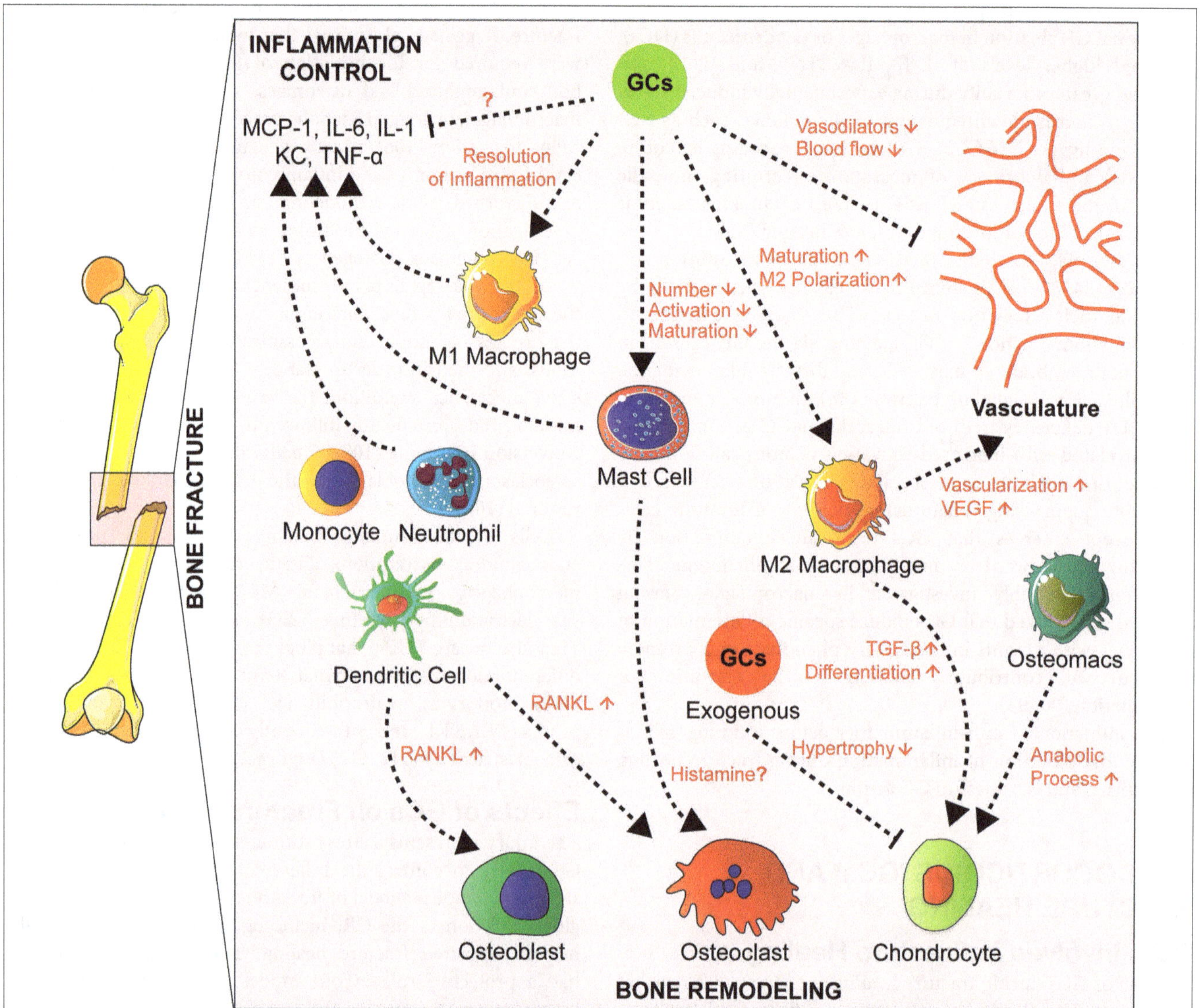

FIGURE 2 | Effects of GCs on the cross-talk between cells of the innate immunity, bone cells, and vascularization during fracture healing. During fracture healing, cells of the innate immunity such as neutrophils, macrophages and mast cells produce pro-inflammatory cytokines and attract other phagocytes to remove debris. GCs act on these cell types to control the inflammation and resolve it partially by polarizing macrophages toward an anti-inflammatory phenotype that will in turn promote tissue repair by increasing vascularization. Presumably GCs also inhibit M1 macrophages and cytokine expression, which is not proven yet. On the other hand, GCs have counterbalancing effects by inhibiting the production of vasodilators in order to control the inflammation. Innate immune cells act on bone cells by secreting factors such as RANKL affecting then osteoblast and osteoclast activity. Also, tissue resident and infiltrating macrophages play a role in endochondral ossification by promoting chondrocyte differentiation for callus formation. Chronic GCs treatment delays chondrocyte hypertrophy and attenuates endochondral bone healing.

Given the distinct roles of GCs on cross-talk of immune, bone and stromal cells, and on vasculature and muscle during osteoporosis and arthritis, it is very likely that GCs shape different aspects of fracture healing positively and negatively. The exact interplay requires intensive investigations.

GLUCOCORTICOIDS (GCs) IN OSTEOARTHRITIS

GC Effects on Osteoarthritis

Osteoarthritis (OA) is the most common form of arthritis and the leading cause of pain and disability in elder people (121). The clinical picture includes not only a process of "wear and tear" but also an unbalanced remodeling of the joint associated with inflammatory processes (122). Among the main risk factors for OA are obesity, gender and age (123).

Degeneration of joints occurs as damage in articular cartilage and subchondral bone, accompanied by ectopic bone formation, so-called osteophytes. The slow turnover of extracellular matrix is dramatically enhanced in OA due to secretion of degrading proteinases and consequent loss of proteoglycans and collagen (124). This process is likely triggered by a vicious cycle of cross-talk of inflammatory cells and stromal cells, such as chondrocytes and synovial cells.

The role of endogenous GCs in this process is obscure, a recent study of Tu et al., however, showed that overexpression of the GC inactivating enzyme 11β-HSD2 in osteoblasts in transgenic mice attenuates OA in a model of destabilization of the medial meniscus (DMM) in older mice (125). This indicates that in bone cells GCs might trigger the inflammatory and erosive process (**Figure 3**).

Administered GCs are accepted as short term, but not as long term agents for intra-articular injections of knee OA with few side effects [reviewed in (10)]. In the literature, the mechanisms are attributed to effects on stromal cells, by increasing the expression of ECM molecules and reduction of degradative proteases. This had been investigated in OA models, cartilage explant cultures and in cartilage cell lines [reviewed in (10, 126)] (**Figure 3**).

Macrophages are part of the inflammatory infiltrate in OA (127). Interestingly, a depletion of synovial macrophages led to the augmentation of OA in a model of destabilization of the medial meniscus (DMM) combined with high fat diet (128). The absence of macrophages caused intriguingly an increased numbers of T cells indicated a hyperinflammation. This indicates that anti-inflammatory polarized macrophages are essential to prevent aberrant progression of OA.

The precise contribution of GR in immune cells for GC effects on OA has not been addressed mechanistically so far. Furthermore, the suppression of VEGF by GCs (129), strongly suggests that effects on the vasculature, could be beneficial to facilitate repair processes during acute GC exposure. Long term effects on the vasculature could also be non-favorably and trigger further OA progression.

Overall, the GC action in OA is not completely understood and requires further elucidation given that GCs are frequently used for treatment, and that obesity, stress and age are known risk factors for the development of this pathology.

GC Effects on Osteophytes in Arthritis

Beside the effects of GCs on joint erosion, not much is known about their protective effects against ectopically grown bone, so-called osteophytes. In both, inflammatory and osteoarthritis, osteophytes can be observed (130, 131) and result in pain and loss of function of joints (132). Osteophytes arise from periosteal mesenchymal stem cells (MSCs) that undergo chondrogenic differentiation, mature and produce a cartilaginous scaffold that is replaced by bone in the end-stage of osteophyte formation (133), a process closely related to endochondral ossification (130, 134–137). GCs are shown to suppress osteophyte formation (138–140), as well as endochondral ossification (141), however, it is uncertain whether the same mechanisms are involved. Interestingly, besides MSCs and chondrocytes, cross-talk with components of the innate immunity are shown to play an important role in the initiation of osteophytes (142–144). Osteophytes often develop in close proximity to synovial lining (144) and synovial inflammation is considered a key contributor to osteophyte formation (145). In this regard, it was shown that a single low-dose of avidin-conjugated dexamethasone (Dex) suppress synovial infiltration and osteophyte formation in post-traumatic OA (138). Especially, synovial macrophages, as part of the synovial infiltrate, are considered key players in osteophyte formation as their depletion significantly suppress osteophytes in two different mouse models of OA (142, 144) and GC-mediated inhibition of synovial macrophages might be beneficial to prevent osteophyte formation. Interestingly, inhibition of TNF does not result in the reduction of osteophytes in patients with psoriatic arthritis or mouse models of inflammatory arthritis (146, 147). Thus, GC-mediated suppression of pro-inflammatory cytokines alone might not be sufficient to suppress osteophyte formation. On the other hand, damage-associated molecules derived from degrading cartilage (142) can also activate synovial macrophages and depending on dosage and duration, GC treatment can protect against this cartilage degradation in OA (140, 148) and inflammatory arthritis (149). In this regard, experimental reduction of cartilage degradation reduces formation of osteophytes in mouse models of OA (150, 151).

The most prominent pathways involved in synovial macrophage activation and osteophyte growth are transforming growth factor β (TGFβ) and bone morphogenetic proteins (BMP-2/-4) (142, 144, 152, 153). TGFβ and BMPs initiate chondrogenic differentiation from periosteal MSCs and co-cultures of MSCs and macrophages enhanced spheroid formation after TGFβ treatment when compared to MSCs alone (144). Interestingly, macrophage-specific delivery of liposomal packed prednisolone results in down regulation of TGFβ in inflammatory arthritis (154) and Dex treatment was shown to suppress BMP-signaling and induce BMP-antagonists at least in osteoblast cell lines (155, 156). In addition, blockage of the hedgehog-signaling pathway also resulted in the suppression of TGFβ and BMPs and completely prevented osteophyte formation without affecting synovial inflammation (157). Thereby, GC-mediated control of TGFβ and BMPs might counteract osteophyte formation. Surprisingly, intra-articular injections of triamcinonone acetonide (TA, another GC) were associated with a higher macrophage activity, using folate-based radiotracers, but also resulted in a significant reduction of osteophytes (158). *In vitro* results of Siebelt et al. (158) suggested that the induction of CD163, folate receptor-β and interleukin-10 by TA might play a role in osteophyte suppression (158), however, this needs to be validated *in vivo*. Besides TGFβ and BMPs, dickkopf-1 (Dkk1), a master regulator of bone remodeling is strongly regulated by GCs (159) and is involved in osteophyte formation (160). Inhibition of Dkk1 results in osteophyte formation in an inflammatory mouse model that does not initially develop osteophytes (160). In addition, patients with spondylarthritis (SpA) arthritis that do develop osteophytes, show lower levels of Dkk1 (161), whereas rheumatoid arthritis (RA) patients that do not develop osteophytes have higher levels of Dkk1 (162). GCs, however, strongly induce Dkk1 expression and thereby inhibiting osteoblast differentiation and bone formation (163, 164), which might be beneficial to suppress osteophyte growth. Accordingly, overexpression of Dkk1 in the osteoblast-lineage significantly reduces osteophyte size in OA (165).

In contrast to exogenous GCs, disruption of endogenous GC signaling in the osteoblast-lineage reduces osteophyte formation in an age-related OA mouse model suggesting an osteophyte-promoting role of endogenous GC (125). Further experimental work is needed to discriminate the endogenous vs. the exogenous

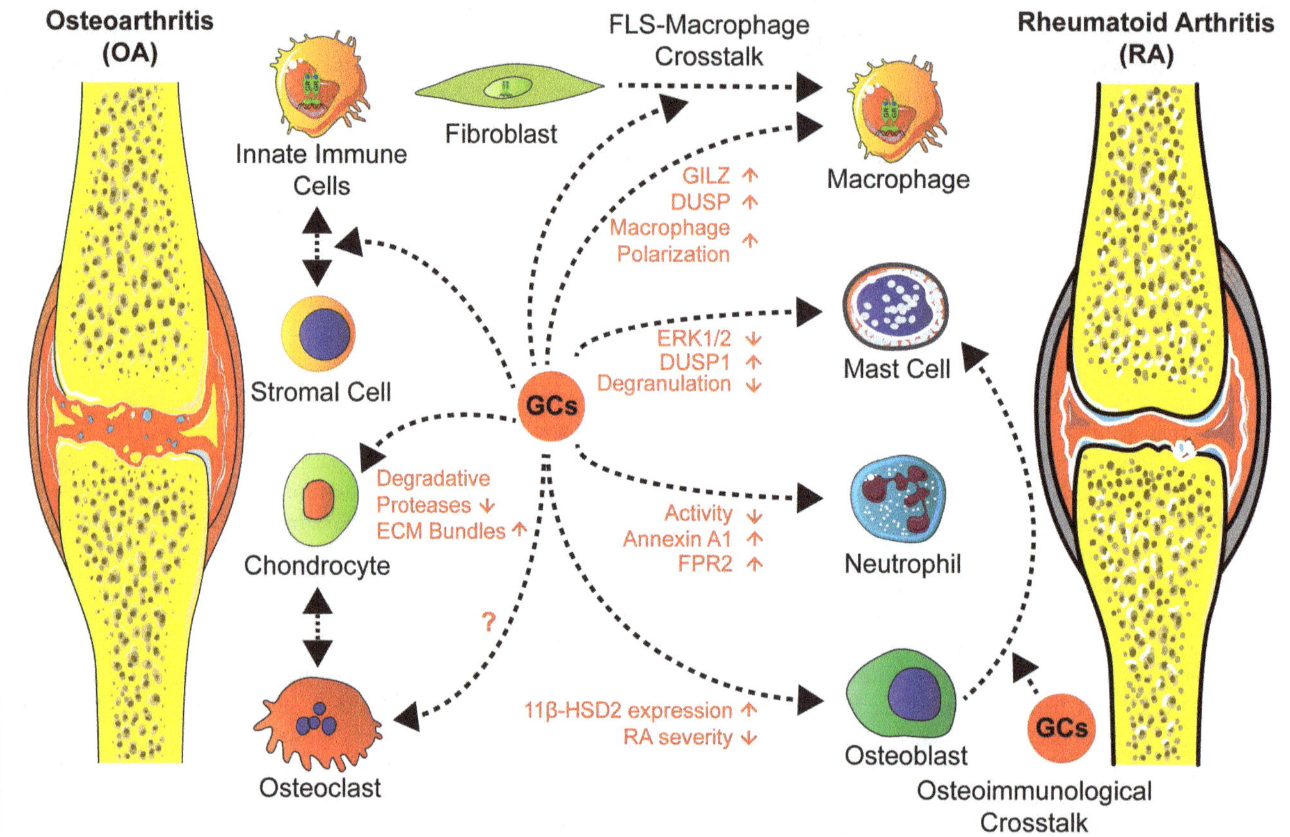

FIGURE 3 | GCs administration in the treatment of OA and RA exert direct effects on different cell types and influence stromal-immune cell crosstalk. Actions of GCs on neutrophils and mast cells lead to an attenuated inflammation and an induction of anti-inflammatory mediators. GCs operate on macrophages either directly, causing increased levels of GILZ and decreased inflammation, or indirectly via FLS through a cross-talk between both, leading to a shift of macrophage polarization toward an anti-inflammatory phenotype and an increased efferocytosis activity. Further effects on stromal cells, in particular chondrocytes are a reduction of degradative protease levels and an increase of ECM molecules. Concerning cross-talk between osteoclasts and chondrocytes in OA or in RA the influence of GCs are unknown. Strikingly, in RA osteoblasts GC effects might lead to inflammatory and erosive processes, since the overexpression of the GC inactivating enzyme 11β-HSD2 in osteoblasts, results in an attenuated disease severity by a non defined cross-talk.

effects of GCs on osteophyte formation and to validate potential pathways involved in GC-mediated suppression of osteophytes to better understand the crosstalk of bone and immune cells involved in this process.

RHEUMATOID ARTHRITIS (RA)

Rheumatoid arthritis (RA) is a chronic, autoimmune disease with a worldwide prevalence of 0.5–1% (166). It affects all types of patients with the highest occurrence in elderly women and a female to male ratio of 3:1 (167). RA is associated with several contributing factors, such as genetics, smoking, obesity and the environment (168). A hallmark of RA is synovial inflammation and the destruction of cartilage and bone, which makes RA a bona-fide disease of osteo-immunological interactions. The etiology is still to a certain extend unclear, but involves rheumatoid factor and anti-citrullinated peptide antibodies (ACPAs), which are at least predictive for the development of RA. The expression of pro-inflammatory mediators, like TNF and IL-6 activating the innate immune system concomitant with aberrant T- and B-Cell regulation finally leads to the development of autoantibodies (169). In the joints, osteoclasts activated by citrullinated autoantibodies, lead to bone damage. This further results in cytokine release by local cells and activation of synovial fibroblasts and macrophages (170, 171), exaggerating the inflammatory and destructive response.

Since the discovery of their anti-inflammatory action 70 years ago, GCs are still one of the most frequently used medications to treat the acute inflammatory response in RA.

Our knowledge of the mechanisms of action of GCs rely on different animal models that comply with certain aspects of the inflammatory phase in arthritis, such as collagen-induced arthritis (involving aspects of T-cells, mast cells and macrophage functions), antigen-induced arthritis (strictly T cell dependent), serum transfer-induced arthritis (T-cell independent) and TNFα transgenic mice (involving multiple cell types).

In the serum transfer-induced arthritis (STIA) and TNF-transgenic model of arthritis, it could be shown that a deficiency of 11β-HSD1 leads to an increase of inflammation, suggesting attenuation of endogenous GC action (172, 173). However, in another model of collagen-induced arthritis (CIA), 11β-HSD1 deletion caused an attenuation of inflammation indicating a pro-inflammatory role of GC activation in this model.

A clear anti-inflammatory role for the GR could be demonstrated in these models (**Figure 3**). For this, the capacity of the GR for dimerization seems to be required for suppression of inflammation in all arthritis models tested so far. GRA458T (GR^{dim}) knock-in mice with attenuated GR dimerization (51), but intact monomer activity, were found refractory in arthritis models of antigen-induced arthritis, glucose-6 phosphate isomerase (G6PI)-induced arthritis and STIA (174, 175). Thus, GR dimerization-induced gene regulation seems to be a general mechanism and is in accordance with animal models with disturbed GR dimer-dependent target genes of the GR such as mitogen-activated protein kinase phosphatase 1 (MKP1), Glucocorticoid-induced leucine zipper (GILZ), and Annexin A1 (**Figure 3**).

GILZ interacts with several crucial signaling pathways, such as NF-κB signaling and T-cell activation (176). GILZ is constantly produced in macrophages and is stimulated by GCs and IL-10, thereby mediating the deactivation of macrophages and thus a decrease of macrophage infiltration (177). This regulation affects the balance between intensified immune reactions and immune tolerance. In mice with CIA and in human patients with RA, it could be shown that GILZ was upregulated in the synovium after the administration of GCs. Furthermore, in cultured RA synovial fibroblasts, an overexpression of GILZ inhibited the release of IL-6 and IL-8 (178).

DUSP1/MKP1 is induced by the GR dimer (179), and an important mediator of anti-inflammatory actions of the GR (81, 180, 181). It inhibits MAP Kinase signaling and DUSP-1 knockout mice have an earlier onset and higher score in CIA (182).

Annexin A1 is associated with the adaptive and the innate immunity. The anti-inflammatory effects of GCs are partly regulated by the release of Annexin A1 and the activation of its receptor formyl peptide receptor 2 (FPR2, also known as ALXR) in neutrophils and macrophages (183). Annexin A1 deficient animals render resistant to GCs in STIA (184), indicating a pivotal role for inhibition of inflammation.

Cell Type Specific GC Action and Crosstalk Between Immune— and Stromal Cells

Depending on the model used different cell type specific requirements for GC signaling and the GR were suggested to attenuate arthritis. For the T-cell dependent antigen-induced arthritis indeed the GR in T cells is absolutely essential for GC-mediated immune suppression in part by suppressing the generation of IL-17 producing T-cells (174). In contrast in the STIA model the deletion of GR in T-cells does not attenuate the response toward GCs (175). Strikingly, in both models GR deletion in macrophages in $GR^{LysMCre}$ mice hardly affected the efficiency of suppression of inflammation (174, 175). This is surprising, since there is multiple evidence for macrophages to respond to GCs during inflammation in general and the requirement of the GR in models of systemic inflammation, contact allergy and acute lung injury (80, 81, 185). In addition in STIA the presence of alternative activating macrophages is decisive for resolution of inflammation (186).

Despite other immune cells, such as type 2 innate lymphoid (ILC2) cells or others, have not been exploited yet for their functional relevance of anti-inflammatory efficacy, a new theme is emerging demonstrating the role of GR in non-immune cells.

Genetic inhibition of GC signaling in osteoblasts by overexpression of 11β-HSD2 lead surprisingly to an attenuated STIA (187). The mechanism is not clear yet, but maybe in accordance to the global 11β-HSD1 deletion in CIA.

In contrast, deletion of GR in chondrocytes in GR $Col2a1CreER^{T2}$ mice leads to an accelerated inflammation in both CIA and STIA model (188). This was accompanied by an increased CXCR2 expression in the joint suggesting that GR controls chondrocyte-immune cell cross-talk on the level of CXL2/5 CXCR2 chemokine axis involved in leukocyte recruitment.

A recent study showed that GC actions in stromal cells are decisive and GR expression in immune cells alone is not sufficient to suppress inflammation in STIA (175) (**Figure 3**). Experiments in bone marrow chimeric mice lacking the GR in the hematopoietic compartment showed no differences in the onset or progression of STIA, nor the responsiveness to GC treatment compared to chimeric mice with a functional GR in immune cells. Furthermore, a reverse approach with chimeric mice lacking the GR globally except for the hematopoietic system revealed that GR expression in stromal cells is essential for the anti-inflammatory actions of GCs. More precisely, the study showed that for these anti-inflammatory actions, the homodimer form of the GR in stromal cells is critical. Interestingly, deficiency of GR dimerization in these cells had no effect on the suppression of inflammatory cytokines upon GC treatment. This indicates that their decrease alone is not sufficient to suppress inflammation. Additionally, GR dimers in stromal cells induce non-classical, anti-inflammatory macrophages while the levels of classical macrophages are not altered. Several anti-inflammatory markers, associated with enhanced phagocytosis and efferocytosis activity, are increased only in wildtype (wt) but not in GR dimer deficient stromal cells. This suggests an insufficient clearance of apoptotic cells after GC treatment, which leads to a persisting inflammatory condition. Finally, the study suggests that the induction of anti-inflammatory macrophages may be indirectly guided by actions of stromal cells, in particular fibroblast-like synoviocytes (FLS), since cocultures of macrophages and FLS showed an elevated efferocytosis competence when compared to cocultures of macrophages and GR dimer-deficient FLS. In addition to that, the levels of macrophage associated chemokines macrophage inflammatory protein−1α and−1β (Mip-1α / Mip-1β) are decreased in wt but not in GR dimer-deficient FLS after GC treatment. Taken together, this indicates a GC-mediated, GR dimer-dependent cross-talk between FLS and macrophages that induces an increase in the anti-inflammatory macrophage population and thereby a suppression of inflammation and STIA itself (175) (**Figure 3**).

OVERALL CONCLUSION/OUTLOOK

Overall GCs and the GR have complex actions in bone diseases. The power of conditional mouse genetics demonstrated that GC signaling and GR action in distinct cell types of the immune system, stromal cells and bone cells have different contributions to the overall effects of GCs. Moreover, going away from this simplistic approach of interpreting cell type specific—cell autonomous effects, the field is now moving toward understanding the impact of GCs on interactions of distinct cell types or even organs.

Other issues that remain unexplored are the interplay of GC triggered immune cells in the normal pathology of postmenopausal and age-related osteoporosis. This is striking since the immune cells from the bone marrow need the bone as a niche, therefore strong interactions of immune and bone cells occur as a normal physiological process.

Given that GCs are part of the neuroendocrine regulatory network that also control inflammation and healthy bone homeostasis, a more holistic view will be needed. With the technologies of high content analysis, single cell sequencing and systemic approaches in combination with organoid models and carefully interpreted animal models, our understanding will substantially increase about the influence of these versatile hormones on the immune-metabolic crosstalk.

AUTHOR CONTRIBUTIONS

MA, YH, FM, KP, MK, and JT wrote individual sections of the article. MA, YH, and KP generated the figures.

FUNDING

This work was funded by the Deutsche Forschungsgemeinschaft (DFG, Collaborative research Centre 1149, C02/InSt 40/492-2, Tu220/13-1, Tu 220/14-1).

REFERENCES

1. McEwen BS. Physiology and neurobiology of stress and adaptation: central role of the brain. *Physiol Rev.* (2007) 87:873–904. doi: 10.1152/physrev.00041.2006
2. Mazziotti G, Giustina A, Canalis E, Bilezikian JP. Treatment of glucocorticoid-induced osteoporsis. *Ther Adv Musculoskelet Dis.* (2009) 1:27–34. doi: 10.1177/1759720X09343222
3. Buttgereit F, Burmester GR, Straub RH, Seibel MJ, Zhou H. Exogenous and endogenous glucocorticoids in rheumatic diseases. *Arthritis Rheum.* (2011) 63:1–9. doi: 10.1002/art.30070
4. Cruz-Topete D, Cidlowski JA. One hormone, two actions: anti- and pro-inflammatory effects of glucocorticoids. *Neuroimmunomodulation.* (2015) 22:20–32. doi: 10.1159/000362724
5. Becker DE. Basic and clinical pharmacology of glucocorticosteroids. *Anaesthesia Prog.* (2013) 60:25–32. doi: 10.2344/0003-3006-60.1.25
6. Hench PS, Kendall EC, Slocumb CH, Polley HF. The effect of a hormone of the adrenal cortex (17-hydroxy-11-dehydrocorticosterone: compound E) and of pituitary adrenocortical hormone in arthritis: preliminary report. *Ann Rheum Dis.* (1949) 8:97–104. doi: 10.1136/ard.8.2.97
7. Van Staa TP, Leufkens HG, Abenhaim L, Zhang B, Cooper C. Use of oral corticosteroids and risk of fractures. *J Bone Miner Res.* (2000) 15:993–1000. doi: 10.1359/jbmr.2000.15.6.993
8. Overman RA, Yeh J-Y, Deal CL. Prevalence of oral glucocorticoid usage in the United States: a general population perspective. *Arthritis Care Res.* (2013) 65:294–8. doi: 10.1002/acr.21796
9. Wilson JC, Sarsour K, Gale S, Pethö-Schramm A, Jick SS, Meier CR. Incidence and risk of glucocorticoid-associated adverse effects in patients with rheumatoid arthritis. *Arthritis Care Res.* (2018) 71:498–511. doi: 10.1002/acr.23611
10. Hartmann K, Koenen M, Schauer S, Wittig-Blaich S, Ahmad M, Baschant U, et al. Molecular actions of glucocorticoids in cartilage and bone during health, disease, and steroid therapy. *Physiol Rev.* (2016) 96:409–47. doi: 10.1152/physrev.00011.2015
11. Hughes KA, Webster SP, Walker BR. 11-Beta-hydroxysteroid dehydrogenase type 1 (11beta-HSD1) inhibitors in type 2 diabetes mellitus and obesity. *Expert Opin Investig Drugs.* (2008) 17:481–96. doi: 10.1517/13543784.17.4.481
12. Muñoz-Durango N, Vecchiola A, Gonzalez-Gomez LM, Simon F, Riedel CA, Fardella CE, et al. Modulation of immunity and inflammation by the mineralocorticoid receptor and aldosterone. *Biomed Res Int.* (2015) 2015:1–14. doi: 10.1155/2015/652738
13. Heitzer MD, Wolf IM, Sanchez ER, Witchel SF, DeFranco DB. Glucocorticoid receptor physiology. *Rev Endocr Metab Disord.* (2007) 8:321–30. doi: 10.1007/s11154-007-9059-8
14. Weikum ER, Knuesel MT, Ortlund EA, Yamamoto KR. Glucocorticoid receptor control of transcription: precision and plasticity via allostery. *Nat Rev Mol Cell Biol.* (2017) 18:159–74. doi: 10.1038/nrm.2016.152
15. Beck IME, Vanden Berghe W, Vermeulen L, Yamamoto KR, Haegeman G, De Bosscher K. Crosstalk in inflammation: the interplay of glucocorticoid receptor-based mechanisms and kinases and phosphatases. *Endocr Rev.* (2009) 30:830–82. doi: 10.1210/er.2009-0013
16. Hübner S, Dejager L, Libert C, Tuckermann JP. The glucocorticoid receptor in inflammatory processes: transrepression is not enough. *Biol Chem.* (2015) 396:93–9. doi: 10.1515/hsz-2015-0106
17. Dhabhar FS, Mcewen BS. Enhancing versus suppressive effects of stress hormones on skin immune function. *Proc Natl Acad Sci USA.* (1999) 96:1059–64. doi: 10.1073/pnas.96.3.1059
18. Frank GF, Weber MD, Watkins LR, Maier SF. Stress sounds the alarmin: the role of the danger-associated molecular pattern HMGB1 in stress-induced neuroinflammatory priming. *Brain Behav Immun.* (2015) 48:1–7. doi: 10.1016/j.bbi.2015.03.010
19. Frenkel B, White W, Tuckermann J. Glucocorticoid-induced osteoporosis. *Adv Exp Med Biol.* (2015) 872:179–215. doi: 10.1007/978-1-4939-2895-8_8
20. Caplan A, Fett N, Rosenbach M, Werth VP, Micheletti RG. Prevention and management of glucocorticoid-induced side effects: a comprehensive review. *J Am Acad Dermatol.* (2017) 76:11–16. doi: 10.1016/j.jaad.2016.02.1239
21. Björnsdottir S, Sääf M, Bensing S, Kämpe O, Michaëlsson K, Ludvigsson JF. Risk of hip fracture in Addison's disease: a population-based cohort study. *J Intern Med.* (2011) 270:187–95. doi: 10.1111/j.1365-2796.2011.02352.x
22. Sher LB, Woitge HW, Adams DJ, Gronowicz GA, Krozowski Z, Harrison JR, et al. Transgenic expression of 11beta-hydroxysteroid dehydrogenase type 2 in osteoblasts reveals an anabolic role for endogenous glucocorticoids in bone. *Endocrinology.* (2004) 145:922–9. doi: 10.1210/en.2003-0655
23. Kalak R, Zhou H, Street J, Day RE, Modzelewski JRK, Spies CM, et al. Endogenous glucocorticoid signalling in osteoblasts is necessary to maintain normal bone structure in mice. *Bone.* (2009) 45:61–7. doi: 10.1016/j.bone.2009.03.673
24. Yang M, Trettel LB, Adams DJ, Harrison JR, Canalis E, Kream BE. Col3.6-HSD2 transgenic mice: a glucocorticoid loss-of-function model spanning early and late osteoblast differentiation. *Bone.* (2010) 47:573–82. doi: 10.1016/j.bone.2010.06.002
25. O'Brien CA, Jia D, Plotkin LI, Bellido T, Powers CC, Stewart SA, et al. Glucocorticoids act directly on osteoblasts and osteocytes to induce their

apoptosis and reduce bone formation and strength. *Endocrinology.* (2004) 145:1835–41. doi: 10.1210/en.2003-0990
26. Zhou H, Mak W, Kalak R, Street J, Fong-Yee C, Zheng Y, et al. Glucocorticoid-dependent Wnt signaling by mature osteoblasts is a key regulator of cranial skeletal development in mice. *Development.* (2009) 136:427–36. doi: 10.1242/dev.027706
27. Rauch A, Seitz S, Baschant U, Schilling AF, Illing A, Stride B, et al. Glucocorticoids suppress bone formation by attenuating osteoblast differentiation via the monomeric glucocorticoid receptor. *Cell Metab.* (2010) 11:517–31. doi: 10.1016/j.cmet.2010.05.005
28. Li A, Hardy R, Stoner S, Tuckermann J, Seibel M, Zhou H. Deletion of mesenchymal glucocorticoid receptor attenuates embryonic lung development and abdominal wall closure. *PLoS ONE.* (2013) 8:e63578. doi: 10.1371/journal.pone.0063578
29. Weinstein RS. Clinical practice. Glucocorticoid-induced bone disease. *N Engl J Med.* (2011) 365:62–70. doi: 10.1056/NEJMcp1012926
30. Reid IR. Glucocorticoid effects on bone. *J Clin Endocrinol Metab.* (1998) 83:1860–2. doi: 10.1210/jc.83.6.1860
31. Weinstein RS. Glucocorticoid-induced osteonecrosis. *Endocrine.* (2012) 41:183–90. doi: 10.1007/s12020-011-9580-0
32. Plotkin LI, Manolagas SC, Bellido T. Glucocorticoids induce osteocyte apoptosis by blocking focal adhesion kinase-mediated survival. Evidence for inside-out signaling leading to anoikis. *J Biol Chem.* (2007) 282:24120–30. doi: 10.1074/jbc.M611435200
33. Weinstein RS, Jilka RL, Parfitt AM, Manolagas SC. Inhibition of osteoblastogenesis and promotion of apoptosis of osteoblasts and osteocytes by glucocorticoids. Potential mechanisms of their deleterious effects on bone. *J Clin Invest.* (1998) 102:274–82. doi: 10.1172/JCI2799
34. Weinstein RS, Nicholas RW, Manolagas SC. Apoptosis of osteocytes in glucocorticoid-induced osteonecrosis of the hip. *J Clin Endocrinol Metab.* (2000) 85:2907–12. doi: 10.1210/jc.85.8.2907
35. Wang L, Heckmann BL, Yang X, Long H. Osteoblast autophagy in glucocorticoid-induced osteoporosis. *J Cell Physiol.* (2019) 234:3207–15. doi: 10.1002/jcp.27335
36. Piemontese M, Onal M, Xiong J, Wang Y, Almeida M, Thostenson JD, et al. Suppression of autophagy in osteocytes does not modify the adverse effects of glucocorticoids on cortical bone. *Bone.* (2015) 75:18–26. doi: 10.1016/j.bone.2015.02.005
37. Morimoto E, Li M, Khalid AB, Krum SA, Chimge N-O, Frenkel B. Glucocorticoids Hijack Runx2 to stimulate Wif1 for suppression of osteoblast growth and differentiation. *J Cell Physiol.* (2017) 232:145–53. doi: 10.1002/jcp.25399
38. Pereira RMR, Delany AM, Durant D, Canalis E. Cortisol regulates the expression of Notch in osteoblasts. *J Cell Biochem.* (2002) 85:252–8. doi: 10.1002/jcb.10125
39. Xu D, Gao Y, Hu N, Wu L, Chen Q. miR-365 ameliorates dexamethasone-induced suppression of osteogenesis in MC3T3-E1 cells by targeting HDAC4. *IJMS.* (2017) 18:977. doi: 10.3390/ijms18050977
40. Li T, Li H, Li T, Fan J, Zhao RC, Weng X. MicroRNA expression profile of dexamethasone-induced human bone marrow-derived mesenchymal stem cells during osteogenic differentiation: microrna expression profile. *J Cell Biochem.* (2014) 115:1683–91. doi: 10.1002/jcb.24831
41. Liu P, Baumgart M, Groth M, Wittmann J, Jäck H-M, Platzer M, et al. Dicer ablation in osteoblasts by Runx2 driven cre-loxP recombination affects bone integrity, but not glucocorticoid-induced suppression of bone formation. *Sci Rep.* (2016) 6:32112. doi: 10.1038/srep32112
42. Espina B, Liang M, Russell RG, Hulley PA. Regulation of bim in glucocorticoid-mediated osteoblast apoptosis. *J Cell Physiol.* (2008) 215:488–96. doi: 10.1002/jcp.21335
43. Chang JK, Li CJ, Liao HJ, Wang CK, Wang GJ, Ho ML. Anti-inflammatory drugs suppress proliferation and induce apoptosis through altering expressions of cell cycle regulators and pro-apoptotic factors in cultured human osteoblasts. *Toxicology.* (2009) 258:148–56. doi: 10.1016/j.tox.2009.01.016
44. Li H, Qian W, Weng X, Wu Z, Li H, Zhuang Q, et al. Glucocorticoid receptor and sequential P53 activation by dexamethasone mediates apoptosis and cell cycle arrest of osteoblastic MC3T3-E1 cells. *PLoS ONE.* (2012) 7:e37030. doi: 10.1371/journal.pone.0037030
45. Almeida M, Han L, Ambrogini E, Weinstein RS, Manolagas SC. Glucocorticoids and tumor necrosis factor α increase oxidative stress and suppress Wnt protein signaling in osteoblasts. *J Biol Chem.* (2011) 286:44326–35. doi: 10.1074/jbc.M111.283481
46. Sivagurunathan S, Muir MM, Brennan TC, Seale JP, Mason RS. Influence of glucocorticoids on human osteoclast generation and activity. *J Bone Miner Res.* (2005) 20:390–8. doi: 10.1359/JBMR.041233
47. Hirayama T, Sabokbar A, Athanasou N. Effect of corticosteroids on human osteoclast formation and activity. *J Endocrinol.* (2002) 175:155–63. doi: 10.1677/joe.0.1750155
48. Kim H-J, Zhao H, Kitaura H, Bhattacharyya S, Brewer JA, Muglia LJ, et al. Glucocorticoids suppress bone formation via the osteoclast. *J Clin Invest.* (2006) 116:2152–60. doi: 10.1172/JCI28084
49. Jia D, O'Brien CA, Stewart SA, Manolagas SC, Weinstein RS. Glucocorticoids act directly on osteoclasts to increase their life span and reduce bone density. *Endocrinology.* (2006) 147:5592–9. doi: 10.1210/en.2006-0459
50. Conaway HH, Henning P, Lie A, Tuckermann J, Lerner UH. Activation of dimeric glucocorticoid receptors in osteoclast progenitors potentiates RANKL induced mature osteoclast bone resorbing activity. *Bone.* (2016) 93:43–54. doi: 10.1016/j.bone.2016.08.024
51. Reichardt HM, Kaestner KH, Tuckermann J, Kretz O, Wessely O, Bock R, et al. DNA binding of the glucocorticoid receptor is not essential for survival. *Cell.* (1998) 93:531–41. doi: 10.1016/S0092-8674(00)81183-6
52. Parfitt AM. The coupling of bone formation to bone resorption: a critical analysis of the concept and of its relevance to the pathogenesis of osteoporosis. *Metab Bone Dis Relat Res.* (1982) 4:1–6. doi: 10.1016/0221-8747(82)90002-9
53. Kong YY, Yoshida H, Sarosi I, Tan HL, Timms E, Capparelli C, et al. OPGL is a key regulator of osteoclastogenesis, lymphocyte development and lymph-node organogenesis. *Nature.* (1999) 397:315–23. doi: 10.1038/16852
54. Yasuda H, Shima N, Nakagawa N, Yamaguchi K, Kinosaki M, Mochizuki SI, et al. Osteoclast differentiation factor is a ligand for osteoprotegerin/osteoclastogenesis-inhibitory factor and is identical to TRANCE/RANKL. *Proc Natl Acad Sci USA.* (1998) 95:3597–602. doi: 10.1073/pnas.95.7.3597
55. Hofbauer LC, Gori F, Riggs BL, Lacey DL, Dunstan CR, Spelsberg TC, et al. Stimulation of osteoprotegerin ligand and inhibition of osteoprotegerin production by glucocorticoids in human osteoblastic lineage cells: potential paracrine mechanisms of glucocorticoid-induced osteoporosis. *Endocrinology.* (1999) 140:4382–9. doi: 10.1210/endo.140.10.7034
56. Rauner M, Goettsch C, Stein N, Thiele S, Bornhaeuser M, De Bosscher K, et al. Dissociation of osteogenic and immunological effects by the selective glucocorticoid receptor agonist, compound A, in human bone marrow stromal cells. *Endocrinology.* (2011) 152:103–12. doi: 10.1210/en.2010-0456
57. Hofbauer LC, Zeitz U, Schoppet M, Skalicky M, Schüler C, Stolina M, et al. Prevention of glucocorticoid-induced bone loss in mice by inhibition of RANKL. *Arthritis Rheum.* (2009) 60:1427–37. doi: 10.1002/art.24445
58. Piemontese M, Xiong J, Fujiwara Y, Thostenson JD, O'Brien CA. Cortical bone loss caused by glucocorticoid excess requires RANKL production by osteocytes and is associated with reduced OPG expression in mice. *Am J Physiol Endocrinol Metab.* (2016) 311:E587–93. doi: 10.1152/ajpendo.00219.2016
59. Pereira M, Petretto E, Gordon S, Bassett JHD, Williams GR, Behmoaras J. Common signalling pathways in macrophage and osteoclast multinucleation. *J Cell Sci.* (2018) 131:cs216267. doi: 10.1242/jcs.216267
60. Smith PJ, Cousins DJ, Jee Y-K, Staynov DZ, Lee TH, Lavender P. Suppression of granulocyte-macrophage colony-stimulating factor expression by glucocorticoids involves inhibition of enhancer function by the glucocorticoid receptor binding to composite NF-AT/activator protein-1 elements. *J Immunol.* (2001) 167:2502–10. doi: 10.4049/jimmunol.167.5.2502
61. Chen X, Wang Z, Duan N, Zhu G, Schwarz EM, Xie C. Osteoblast–osteoclast interactions. *Connect Tissue Res.* (2018) 59:99–107. doi: 10.1080/03008207.2017.1290085
62. Weinstein RS, Wan C, Liu Q, Wang Y, Almeida M, O'Brien CA, et al. Endogenous glucocorticoids decrease skeletal angiogenesis, vascularity, hydration, and strength in 21-month-old mice. *Aging Cell.* (2010) 9:147–61. doi: 10.1111/j.1474-9726.2009.00545.x

63. Kusumbe AP, Ramasamy SK, Adams RH. Coupling of angiogenesis and osteogenesis by a specific vessel subtype in bone. *Nature*. (2014) 507:323–8. doi: 10.1038/nature13145
64. Ramasamy SK, Kusumbe AP, Itkin T, Gur-Cohen S, Lapidot T, Adams RH. Regulation of hematopoiesis and osteogenesis by blood vessel-derived signals. *Annu Rev Cell Dev Biol*. (2016) 32:649–75. doi: 10.1146/annurev-cellbio-111315-124936
65. Weinstein RS, Hogan EA, Borrelli MJ, Liachenko S, O'Brien CA, Manolagas SC. The pathophysiological sequence of glucocorticoid-induced osteonecrosis of the femoral head in male mice. *Endocrinology*. (2017) 158:3817–31. doi: 10.1210/en.2017-00662
66. Yang P, Lv S, Wang Y, Peng Y, Ye Z, Xia Z, et al. Preservation of type H vessels and osteoblasts by enhanced preosteoclast platelet-derived growth factor type BB attenuates glucocorticoid-induced osteoporosis in growing mice. *Bone*. (2018) 114:1–13. doi: 10.1016/j.bone.2018.05.025
67. Xie H, Cui Z, Wang L, Xia Z, Hu Y, Xian L, et al. PDGF-BB secreted by preosteoclasts induces angiogenesis during coupling with osteogenesis. *Nat Med*. (2014) 20:1270–8. doi: 10.1038/nm.3668
68. Sato AY, Peacock M, Bellido T. Glucocorticoid excess in bone and muscle. *Clinic Rev Bone Miner Metab*. (2018) 16:33–47. doi: 10.1007/s12018-018-9242-3
69. Sandri M, Lin J, Handschin C, Yang W, Arany ZP, Lecker SH, et al. PGC-1 protects skeletal muscle from atrophy by suppressing FoxO3 action and atrophy-specific gene transcription. *Proc Natl Acad Sci USA*. (2006) 103:16260–5. doi: 10.1073/pnas.0607795103
70. Bodine SC. Identification of ubiquitin ligases required for skeletal muscle atrophy. *Science*. (2001) 294:1704–8. doi: 10.1126/science.1065874
71. Watson ML, Baehr LM, Reichardt HM, Tuckermann JP, Bodine SC, Furlow JD. A cell-autonomous role for the glucocorticoid receptor in skeletal muscle atrophy induced by systemic glucocorticoid exposure. *Am J Physiol Endocrinol Metab*. (2012) 302:E1210–20. doi: 10.1152/ajpendo.00512.2011
72. Kim H, Wrann CD, Jedrychowski M, Vidoni S, Kitase Y, Nagano K, et al. Irisin mediates effects on bone and fat via αV integrin receptors. *Cell*. (2018) 175:1756–68.e17. doi: 10.1016/j.cell.2018.10.025
73. Miyata M, Lee J-Y, Susuki-Miyata S, Wang WY, Xu H, Kai H, et al. Glucocorticoids suppress inflammation via the upregulation of negative regulator IRAK-M. *Nat Commun*. (2015) 6:6062. doi: 10.1038/ncomms7062
74. Oppong E, Flink N, Cato ACB. Molecular mechanisms of glucocorticoid action in mast cells. *Mol Cell Endocrinol*. (2013) 380:119–26. doi: 10.1016/j.mce.2013.05.014
75. Kim SW, Rhee HJ, Ko J, Kim YJ, Kim HG, Yang JM, et al. Inhibition of cytosolic phospholipase A2 by annexin I. Specific interaction model and mapping of the interaction site. *J Biol Chem*. (2001) 276:15712–19. doi: 10.1074/jbc.M009905200
76. Yang N, Zhang W, Shi X-M. Glucocorticoid-induced leucine zipper (GILZ) mediates glucocorticoid action and inhibits inflammatory cytokine-induced COX-2 expression. *J Cell Biochem*. (2008) 103:1760–71. doi: 10.1002/jcb.21562
77. Perretti M, Ahluwalia A. The microcirculation and inflammation : site of action for glucocorticoids. *Microcirculation*. (2000) 7:147–61. doi: 10.1080/mic.7.3.147.161
78. Cronstein BN, Kimmel SC, Levin RI, Martiniuk F, Weissmann G. A mechanism for the antiinflammatory effects of corticosteroids: the glucocorticoid receptor regulates leukocyte adhesion to endothelial cells and expression of endothelial-leukocyte adhesion molecule 1 and intercellular adhesion molecule 1. *Proc Natl Acad Sci USA*. (1992) 89:9991–5. doi: 10.1073/pnas.89.21.9991
79. Atsuta J, Plitt J, Bochner BS, Schleimer RP. Inhibition of VCAM-1 expression in human bronchial epithelial cells by glucocorticoids. *Am J Respir Cell Mol Biol*. (1999) 20:643–50. doi: 10.1165/ajrcmb.20.4.3265
80. Kleiman A, Hübner S, Rodriguez Parkitna JM, Neumann A, Hofer S, Weigand MA, et al. Glucocorticoid receptor dimerization is required for survival in septic shock via suppression of interleukin-1 in macrophages. *FASEB J*. (2012) 26:722–9. doi: 10.1096/fj.11-192112
81. Bhattacharyya S, Brown DE, Brewer JA, Vogt SK, Muglia LJ. Macrophage glucocorticoid receptors regulate Toll-like receptor 4–mediated inflammatory responses by selective inhibition of p38 MAP kinase. *Blood*. (2007) 109:4313–19. doi: 10.1182/blood-2006-10-048215
82. Li CC, Munitic I, Mittelstadt PR, Castro E, Ashwell JD. Suppression of dendritic cell-derived IL-12 by endogenous glucocorticoids is protective in LPS-induced sepsis. *PLoS Biol*. (2015) 13:e1002269. doi: 10.1371/journal.pbio.1002269
83. Xing Z, Lu C, Hu D, Yu YY, Wang X, Colnot C, et al. Multiple roles for CCR2 during fracture healing. *Dis Models Mech*. (2010) 3:451–8. doi: 10.1242/dmm.003186
84. Heiman AS, Crews FT. Hydrocortisone selectively inhibits IgE-dependent arachidonic acid release from rat peritoneal mast cells. *Prostaglandins*. (1984) 27:335–43. doi: 10.1016/0090-6980(84)90084-4
85. Rider LG, Hirasawa N, Santini F, Beaven MA. Activation of the mitogen-activated protein kinase cascade is suppressed by low concentrations of dexamethasone in mast cells. *J Immunol*. (1996) 157:2374–80.
86. Eklund KK, Humphries DE, Xia Z, Ghildyal N, Friend DS, Gross V, et al. Glucocorticoids inhibit the cytokine-induced proliferation of mast cells, the high affinity IgE receptor-mediated expression of TNF-alpha, and the IL-10-induced expression of chymases. *J Immunol*. (1997) 158:4373–80.
87. Finotto S, Mekori YA, Metcalfe DD. Glucocorticoids decrease tissue mast cell number by reducing the production of the c-kit ligand, stem cell factor, by resident cells: *in vitro* and *in vivo* evidence in murine systems. *J Clin Investig*. (1997) 99:1721–8. doi: 10.1172/JCI119336
88. Mori T, Abe N, Saito K, Toyama H, Endo Y, Ejima Y, et al. Hydrocortisone and dexamethasone dose-dependently stabilize mast cells derived from rat peritoneum. *Pharmacol Rep*. (2016) 68:1358–65. doi: 10.1016/j.pharep.2016.09.005
89. Coutinho AE, Brown JK, Yang F, Brownstein DG, Gray M, Seckl JR, et al. Mast cells express 11beta-hydroxysteroid dehydrogenase type 1: a role in restraining mast cell degranulation. *PloS ONE*. (2013) 8:e54640. doi: 10.1371/journal.pone.0054640
90. Ehrchen J, Steinmüller L, Barczyk K, Tenbrock K, Nacken W, Eisenacher M, et al. Glucocorticoids induce differentiation of a specifically activated, anti-inflammatory subtype of human monocytes. *Blood*. (2007) 109:1265–74. doi: 10.1182/blood-2006-02-001115
91. Yona S, Gordon S. Inflammation: glucocorticoids turn the monocyte switch. *Immunol Cell Biol*. (2007) 85:81–2. doi: 10.1038/sj.icb.7100034
92. Varga G, Ehrchen J, Tsianakas A, Tenbrock K, Rattenholl A, Seeliger S, et al. Glucocorticoids induce an activated, anti-inflammatory monocyte subset in mice that resembles myeloid-derived suppressor cells. *J Leukoc Biol*. (2008) 84:644–50. doi: 10.1189/jlb.1107768
93. Barczyk K, Ehrchen J, Tenbrock K, Ahlmann M, Kneidl J, Viemann D, et al. Glucocorticoids promote survival of anti-inflammatory macrophages via stimulation of adenosine receptor A3. *Blood*. (2010) 116:446–55. doi: 10.1182/blood-2009-10-247106
94. Hachemi Y, Rapp AE, Hachemi Y, Rapp AE, Picke A, Weidinger G, et al. Molecular mechanisms of glucocorticoids on skeleton and bone regeneration after fracture. *J Mol Endocrinol*. (2018) 61:R75–90. doi: 10.1530/JME-18-0024
95. Kovtun A, Bergdolt S, Wiegner R, Radermacher P, Ignatius A. The crucial role of neutrophil granulocytes in bone fracture healing. *Eur Cell Mater*. (2016) 32:152–62. doi: 10.22203/eCM.v032a10
96. Sinder BP, Pettit AR, McCauley LK. Macrophages: their emerging roles in bone. *J Bone Mineral Res*. (2015) 30:2140–9. doi: 10.1002/jbmr.2735
97. Wu AC, Raggatt LJ, Alexander KA, Pettit AR. Unraveling macrophage contributions to bone repair. *Bonekey Rep*. (2013) 2:373. doi: 10.1038/bonekey.2013.107
98. Kroner J, Kovtun A, Kemmler J, Messmann JJ, Strauß G, Seitz S, et al. Mast cells are critical regulators of bone fracture-induced inflammation and osteoclast formation and activity. *J Bone Miner Res*. (2017) 32:2431–44. doi: 10.1002/jbmr.3234
99. Ramirez-Garcialuna JL, Chan D, Samberg R, Abou-Rjeili M, Wong TH, Li A, et al. Defective bone repair in mast cell-deficient Cpa3 Cre/+ mice. *PLoS ONE*. (2017) 12:e0174396. doi: 10.1371/journal.pone.0174396
100. De Filippo K, Dudeck A, Hasenberg M, Nye E, van Rooijen N, Hartmann K, et al. Mast cell and macrophage chemokines CXCL1/CXCL2 control the early stage of neutrophil recruitment during tissue inflammation. *Blood*. (2013) 121:4930–7. doi: 10.1182/blood-2013-02-486217

101. Furze RC, Rankin SM. Neutrophil mobilization and clearance in the bone marrow. *Immunology.* (2008) 125:281–8. doi: 10.1111/j.1365-2567.2008.02950.x
102. Sadik CD, Kim ND, Luster AD. Neutrophils cascading their way to inflammation. *Trends Immunol.* (2011) 32:452–60. doi: 10.1016/j.it.2011.06.008
103. Chan JK, Glass GE, Ersek A, Freidin A, Williams GA, Gowers K, et al. Low-dose TNF augments fracture healing in normal and osteoporotic bone by up-regulating the innate immune response. *EMBO Mol Med.* (2015) 7:547–61. doi: 10.15252/emmm.201404487
104. Chung R, Cool JC, Scherer MA, Foster BK, Xian CJ. Roles of neutrophil-mediated inflammatory response in the bony repair of injured growth plate cartilage in young rats. *J Leukoc Biol.* (2006) 80:1272–80. doi: 10.1189/jlb.0606365
105. Alexander KA, Chang MK, Maylin ER, Kohler T, Müller R, Wu AC, et al. Osteal macrophages promote *in vivo* intramembranous bone healing in a mouse tibial injury model. *J Bone Mineral Res.* (2011) 26:1517–32. doi: 10.1002/jbmr.354
106. Raggatt LJ, Wullschleger ME, Alexander KA, Wu ACK, Millard SM, Kaur S, et al. Fracture healing via periosteal callus formation requires macrophages for both initiation and progression of early endochondral ossification. *Am J Pathol.* (2014) 184:3192–204. doi: 10.1016/j.ajpath.2014.08.017
107. Shapiro F. Bone development and its relation to fracture repair. The role of mesenchymal osteoblasts and surface osteoblasts. *Eur Cells Mater.* (2008) 15:53–76. doi: 10.22203/eCM.v015a05
108. Einhorn TA, Gerstenfeld LC. Fracture healing: mechanisms and interventions. *Nat Rev Rheumatol.* (2015) 11:45–54. doi: 10.1038/nrrheum.2014.164
109. Schindeler A, McDonald MM, Bokko P, Little DG. Bone remodeling during fracture repair: the cellular picture. *Semin Cell Dev Biol.* (2008) 19:459–66. doi: 10.1016/j.semcdb.2008.07.004
110. Schlundt C, El Khassawna T, Serra A, Dienelt A, Wendler S, Schell H, et al. Macrophages in bone fracture healing: their essential role in endochondral ossification. *Bone.* (2018) 106:78–89. doi: 10.1016/j.bone.2015.10.019
111. Caetano-Lopes J, Canhao H, Fonseca JE. Osteoimmunology–the hidden immune regulation of bone. *Autoimmun Rev.* (2009) 8:250–5. doi: 10.1016/j.autrev.2008.07.038
112. Cao X. RANKL-RANK signaling regulates osteoblast differentiation and bone formation. *Bone Res.* (2018) 6:1–2. doi: 10.1038/s41413-018-0040-9
113. Rapp AE, Hachemi Y, Kemmler J, Koenen M, Tuckermann J, Ignatius A. Induced global deletion of glucocorticoid receptor impairs fracture healing. *FASEB J.* (2018) 32:2235–45. doi: 10.1096/fj.201700459RR
114. Aslan M, Simşek G, Yildirim Ü. Effects of short-term treatment with systemic prednisone on bone healing: an experimental study in rats. *Dental Traumatol.* (2005) 21:222–5. doi: 10.1111/j.1600-9657.2005.00300.x
115. Waters RV, Gamradt SC, Asnis P, Vickery BH, Avnur Z, Hill E, et al. Systemic corticosteroids inhibit bone healing in a rabbit ulnar osteotomy model. *Acta Orthopaedica Scand.* (2000) 71:316–21. doi: 10.1080/000164700317411951
116. Liu Y, Akhter MP, Gao X, Wang X, Wang X, Zhao G, et al. Glucocorticoid-induced delayed fracture healing and impaired bone biomechanical properties in mice. *CIA.* (2018) 13:1465–74. doi: 10.2147/CIA.S167431
117. Azetsu Y, Chatani M, Dodo Y, Karakawa A, Sakai N, Negishi-Koga T, et al. Treatment with synthetic glucocorticoid impairs bone metabolism, as revealed by *in vivo* imaging of osteoblasts and osteoclasts in medaka fish. *Biomed Pharmacother.* (2019) 118:109101. doi: 10.1016/j.biopha.2019.109101
118. Zhang H, Shi X, Wang L, Li X, Zheng C, Gao B, et al. Intramembranous ossification and endochondral ossification are impaired differently between glucocorticoid-induced osteoporosis and estrogen deficiency-induced osteoporosis. *Sci Rep.* (2018) 8:1–13. doi: 10.1038/s41598-018-22095-1
119. Tu J, Henneicke H, Zhang Y, Stoner S, Cheng TL, Schindeler A, et al. Disruption of glucocorticoid signaling in chondrocytes delays metaphyseal fracture healing but does not affect normal cartilage and bone development. *Bone.* (2014) 69:12–22. doi: 10.1016/j.bone.2014.08.016
120. Sandberg OH, Aspenberg P. Glucocorticoids inhibit shaft fracture healing but not metaphyseal bone regeneration under stable mechanical conditions. *Bone Joint Res.* (2015) 4:170–5. doi: 10.1302/2046-3758.410.2000414
121. Cheng Y, Hootman J, Murphy L. Morbidity and mortality weekly report. prevalence of doctor-diagnosed arthritis and arthritis-attributable activity limitation: United States, 2007-2009. *MMWR Morb Mortal Wkly Rep.* (2010) 59:2007–9.
122. Loeser RF, Goldring SR, Scanzello CR, Goldring MB. Osteoarthritis: a disease of the joint as an organ. *Arthritis Rheumat.* (2012) 64:1697–707. doi: 10.1002/art.34453
123. Blagojevic M, Jinks C, Jeffery A, Jordan KP. Risk factors for onset of osteoarthritis of the knee in older adults: a systematic review and meta-analysis. *Osteoarthritis Cartil.* (2010) 18:24–33. doi: 10.1016/j.joca.2009.08.010
124. Goldring MB, Marcu KB. Cartilage homeostasis in health and rheumatic diseases. *Arthritis Res Ther.* (2009) 11:224. doi: 10.1186/ar2592
125. Tu J, Zhang P, Ji Z, Henneicke H, Li J, Kim S, et al. Disruption of glucocorticoid signalling in osteoblasts attenuates age-related surgically induced osteoarthritis. *Osteoarthr Cartil.* (2019) 27:1518–25. doi: 10.1016/j.joca.2019.04.019
126. Savvidou O, Milonaki M, Goumenos S, Flevas D, Papagelopoulos P, Moutsatsou P. Glucocorticoid signaling and osteoarthritis. *Mol Cell Endocrinol.* (2019) 480:153–66. doi: 10.1016/j.mce.2018.11.001
127. Revell PA, Mayston V, Lalor P, Mapp P. The synovial membrane in osteoarthritis: a histological study including the characterisation of the cellular infiltrate present in inflammatory osteoarthritis using monoclonal antibodies. *Ann Rheum Dis.* (1988) 47:300–7. doi: 10.1136/ard.47.4.300
128. Wu C-L, McNeill J, Goon K, Little D, Kimmerling K, Huebner J, et al. Conditional macrophage depletion increases inflammation and does not inhibit the development of osteoarthritis in obese macrophage fas-induced apoptosis-transgenic mice: conditional macrophage depletion in mafia-transgenic mice. *Arthritis Rheumatol.* (2017) 69:1772–83. doi: 10.1002/art.40161
129. Smink JJ, Buchholz IM, Hamers N, van Tilburg CM, Christis C, Sakkers RJB, et al. Short-term glucocorticoid treatment of piglets causes changes in growth plate morphology and angiogenesis. *Osteoarthritis Cartil.* (2003) 11:864–71. doi: 10.1016/S1063-4584(03)00187-0
130. Schett G, Landewé R, van der Heijde D. Tumour necrosis factor blockers and structural remodelling in ankylosing spondylitis: what is reality and what is fiction? *Ann Rheum Dis.* (2007) 66:709–11. doi: 10.1136/ard.2007.071159
131. Thambyah A, Broom N. On new bone formation in the pre-osteoarthritic joint. *Osteoarthr Cartil.* (2009) 17:456–63. doi: 10.1016/j.joca.2008.09.005
132. Dieppe PA, Lohmander LS. Pathogenesis and management of pain in osteoarthritis. *Lancet.* (2005) 365:965–73. doi: 10.1016/S0140-6736(05)71086-2
133. Sandell LJ, Aigner T. Articular cartilage and changes in arthritis: cell biology of osteoarthritis. *Arthritis Res Ther.* (2001) 3:107. doi: 10.1186/ar148
134. Dodds RA, Merry K, Littlewood A, Gowen M. Expression of mRNA for IL1 beta, IL6 and TGF beta 1 in developing human bone and cartilage. *J Histochem Cytochem.* (1994) 42:733–44. doi: 10.1177/42.6.8189035
135. van der Kraan PM, van den Berg WB. Osteophytes: relevance and biology. *Osteoarthritis Cartil.* (2007) 15:237–44. doi: 10.1016/j.joca.2006.11.006
136. Mahjoub M, Berenbaum F, Houard X. Why subchondral bone in osteoarthritis? The importance of the cartilage bone interface in osteoarthritis. *Osteoporos Int.* (2012) 23:841–6. doi: 10.1007/s00198-012-2161-0
137. Xiao Z-F, Su G-Y, Hou Y, Chen S-D, Lin D-K. Cartilage degradation in osteoarthritis: a process of osteochondral remodeling resembles the endochondral ossification in growth plate? *Med Hypotheses.* (2018) 121:183–7. doi: 10.1016/j.mehy.2018.08.023
138. Bajpayee AG, De la Vega RE, Scheu M, Varady NH, Yannatos IA, Brown LA, et al. Sustained intra-cartilage delivery of low dose dexamethasone using a cationic carrier for treatment of post traumatic osteoarthritis. *Eur Cell Mater.* (2017) 34:341–64. doi: 10.22203/eCM.v034a21
139. Geannette C, Sahr M, Mayman D, Miller TT. Ultrasound diagnosis of osteophytic impingement of the popliteus tendon after total knee replacement. *J Ultrasound Med.* (2018) 37:2279–83. doi: 10.1002/jum.14563
140. Pelletier JP, Martel-Pelletier J. Protective effects of corticosteroids on cartilage lesions and osteophyte formation in the Pond-Nuki dog model of osteoarthritis. *Arthritis Rheum.* (1989) 32:181–93. doi: 10.1002/anr.1780320211

141. Lui JC, Baron J. Effects of glucocorticoids on the growth plate. In: Ghizzoni L, Cappa M, Chrousos GP, Loche S, Maghnie MS, Karger AG, editors. *Endocrine Development*. Basel: Karger (2010). p. 187–93.
142. Blom AB, van Lent PLEM, Holthuysen AEM, van der Kraan PM, Roth J, van Rooijen N, et al. Synovial lining macrophages mediate osteophyte formation during experimental osteoarthritis. *Osteoarthr Cartil.* (2004) 12:627–35. doi: 10.1016/j.joca.2004.03.003
143. Ganova P, Gyurkovska V, Belenska-Todorova L, Ivanovska N. Functional complement activity is decisive for the development of chronic synovitis, osteophyte formation and processes of cell senescence in zymosan-induced arthritis. *Immunol Lett.* (2017) 190:213–20. doi: 10.1016/j.imlet.2017.08.023
144. van Lent PLEM, Blom AB, van der Kraan P, Holthuysen AEM, Vitters E, van Rooijen N, et al. Crucial role of synovial lining macrophages in the promotion of transforming growth factor beta-mediated osteophyte formation. *Arthritis Rheum.* (2004) 50:103–11. doi: 10.1002/art.11422
145. van den Bosch MH, Blom AB, Schelbergen RFP, Vogl T, Roth JP, Slöetjes AW, et al. Induction of canonical Wnt signaling by the alarmins S100A8/A9 in murine knee joints: implications for osteoarthritis. *Arthritis Rheumatol.* (2016) 68:152–63. doi: 10.1002/art.39420
146. Schett G, Stolina M, Dwyer D, Zack D, Uderhardt S, Krönke G, et al. Tumor necrosis factor α and RANKL blockade cannot halt bony spur formation in experimental inflammatory arthritis. *Arthritis Rheumat.* (2009) 60:2644–54. doi: 10.1002/art.24767
147. Finzel S, Kraus S, Schmidt S, Hueber A, Rech J, Engelke K, et al. Bone anabolic changes progress in psoriatic arthritis patients despite treatment with methotrexate or tumour necrosis factor inhibitors. *Ann Rheum Dis.* (2013) 72:1176–81. doi: 10.1136/annrheumdis-2012-201580
148. Huebner KD, Shrive NG, Frank CB. Dexamethasone inhibits inflammation and cartilage damage in a new model of post-traumatic osteoarthritis. *J Orthop Res.* (2014) 32:566–72. doi: 10.1002/jor.22568
149. Baschant U, Lane NE, Tuckermann J. The multiple facets of glucocorticoid action in rheumatoid arthritis. *Nat Rev Rheumatol.* (2012) 8:645–55. doi: 10.1038/nrrheum.2012.166
150. Botter SM, Glasson SS, Hopkins B, Clockaerts S, Weinans H, van Leeuwen JPTM, et al. ADAMTS5–/– mice have less subchondral bone changes after induction of osteoarthritis through surgical instability: implications for a link between cartilage and subchondral bone changes. *Osteoarthritis Cartil.* (2009) 17:636–45. doi: 10.1016/j.joca.2008.09.018
151. Kamekura S, Kawasaki Y, Hoshi K, Shimoaka T, Chikuda H, Maruyama Z, et al. Contribution of runt-related transcription factor 2 to the pathogenesis of osteoarthritis in mice after induction of knee joint instability. *Arthritis Rheumat.* (2006) 54:2462–70. doi: 10.1002/art.22041
152. van Beuningen HM, van der Kraan PM, Arntz OJ, van den Berg WB. Transforming growth factor-beta 1 stimulates articular chondrocyte proteoglycan synthesis and induces osteophyte formation in the murine knee joint. *Lab Invest.* (1994) 71:279–90.
153. Scharstuhl A, Vitters EL, van der Kraan PM, van den Berg WB. Reduction of osteophyte formation and synovial thickening by adenoviral overexpression of transforming growth factor beta/bone morphogenetic protein inhibitors during experimental osteoarthritis. *Arthritis Rheum.* (2003) 48:3442–51. doi: 10.1002/art.11328
154. Hofkens W, Schelbergen R, Storm G, van den Berg WB, van Lent PL. Liposomal targeting of prednisolone phosphate to synovial lining macrophages during experimental arthritis inhibits M1 activation but does not favor M2 differentiation. *PLoS ONE.* (2013) 8:e54016. doi: 10.1371/journal.pone.0054016
155. Hayashi K, Yamaguchi T, Yano S, Kanazawa I, Yamauchi M, Yamamoto M, et al. BMP/Wnt antagonists are upregulated by dexamethasone in osteoblasts and reversed by alendronate and PTH: potential therapeutic targets for glucocorticoid-induced osteoporosis. *Biochem Biophys Res Commun.* (2009) 379:261–6. doi: 10.1016/j.bbrc.2008.12.035
156. Luppen CA, Smith E, Spevak L, Boskey AL, Frenkel B. Bone morphogenetic protein-2 restores mineralization in glucocorticoid-inhibited MC3T3-E1 osteoblast cultures. *J Bone Miner Res.* (2003) 18:1186–97. doi: 10.1359/jbmr.2003.18.7.1186
157. Ruiz-Heiland G, Horn A, Zerr P, Hofstetter W, Baum W, Stock M, et al. Blockade of the hedgehog pathway inhibits osteophyte formation in arthritis. *Ann Rheum Dis.* (2012) 71:400–7. doi: 10.1136/ard.2010.148262
158. Siebelt M, Korthagen N, Wei W, Groen H, Bastiaansen-Jenniskens Y, Müller C, et al. Triamcinolone acetonide activates an anti-inflammatory and folate receptor-positive macrophage that prevents osteophytosis *in vivo*. *Arthritis Res Ther.* (2015) 17:352. doi: 10.1186/s13075-015-0865-1
159. Ohnaka K, Taniguchi H, Kawate H, Nawata H, Takayanagi R. Glucocorticoid enhances the expression of dickkopf-1 in human osteoblasts: novel mechanism of glucocorticoid-induced osteoporosis. *Biochem Biophys Res Commun.* (2004) 318:259–64. doi: 10.1016/j.bbrc.2004.04.025
160. Diarra D, Stolina M, Polzer K, Zwerina J, Ominsky MS, Dwyer D, et al. Dickkopf-1 is a master regulator of joint remodeling. *Nat Med.* (2007) 13:156–63. doi: 10.1038/nm1538
161. Fassio A, Idolazzi L, Viapiana O, Benini C, Vantaggiato E, Bertoldo F, et al. In psoriatic arthritis Dkk-1 and PTH are lower than in rheumatoid arthritis and healthy controls. *Clin Rheumatol.* (2017) 36:2377–81. doi: 10.1007/s10067-017-3734-2
162. Ma Y, Zhang X, Wang M, Xia Q, Yang J, Wu M, et al. The serum level of Dickkopf-1 in patients with rheumatoid arthritis: a systematic review and meta-analysis. *Int Immunopharmacol.* (2018) 59:227–32. doi: 10.1016/j.intimp.2018.04.019
163. Brunetti G, Faienza MF, Piacente L, Ventura A, Oranger A, Carbone C, et al. High dickkopf-1 levels in sera and leukocytes from children with 21-hydroxylase deficiency on chronic glucocorticoid treatment. *Am J Physiol Endocrinol Metab.* (2013) 304:E546–54. doi: 10.1152/ajpendo.00535.2012
164. Wang F-S, Ko J-Y, Yeh D-W, Ke H-C, Wu H-L. Modulation of Dickkopf-1 attenuates glucocorticoid induction of osteoblast apoptosis, adipocytic differentiation, and bone mass loss. *Endocrinology.* (2008) 149:1793–801. doi: 10.1210/en.2007-0910
165. Funck-Brentano T, Bouaziz W, Marty C, Geoffroy V, Hay E, Cohen-Solal M. Dkk-1-mediated inhibition of Wnt signaling in bone ameliorates osteoarthritis in mice. *Arthritis Rheumatol.* (2014) 66:3028–39. doi: 10.1002/art.38799
166. Tobón GJ, Youinou P, Saraux A. Autoimmunity reviews the environment, geo-epidemiology, and autoimmune disease : rheumatoid arthritis. *Autoimmun Rev.* (2009) 9:A288–92. doi: 10.1016/j.autrev.2009.11.019
167. Alamanos Y, Drosos AA. Epidemiology of adult rheumatoid arthritis. *Autoimmun Rev.* (2005) 4:130–6. doi: 10.1016/j.autrev.2004.09.002
168. McInnes IB, Schett G. The pathogenesis of rheumatoid arthritis. *N Engl J Med.* (2011) 365:2205–19. doi: 10.1056/NEJMra1004965
169. McInnes IB, Schett G. Pathogenetic insights from the treatment of rheumatoid arthritis. *Lancet.* (2017) 389:2328–37. doi: 10.1016/S0140-6736(17)31472-1
170. Sokolove J, Zhao X, Chandra PE, Robinson WH. Immune complexes containing citrullinated fibrinogen costimulate macrophages via toll-like receptor 4 and Fcγ receptor. *Arthritis Rheumat.* (2011) 63:53–62. doi: 10.1002/art.30081
171. Seibl R, Birchler T, Loeliger S, Hossle JP, Gay RE, Saurenmann T, et al. Expression and regulation of Toll-like receptor 2 in rheumatoid arthritis synovium. *Am J Pathol.* (2003) 162:1221–7. doi: 10.1016/S0002-9440(10)63918-1
172. Coutinho AE, Gray M, Brownstein DG, Salter DM, Sawatzky DA, Clay S, et al. 11B-Hydroxysteroid dehydrogenase type 1, but not type 2, deficiency worsens acute inflammation and experimental arthritis in mice. *Endocrinology.* (2012) 153:234–40. doi: 10.1210/en.2011-1398
173. Hardy RS, Fenton C, Croft AP, Naylor AJ, Begum R, Desanti G, et al. 11 Beta-hydroxysteroid dehydrogenase type 1 regulates synovitis, joint destruction, and systemic bone loss in chronic polyarthritis. *J Autoimmun.* (2018) 92:104–13. doi: 10.1016/j.jaut.2018.05.010
174. Baschant U, Frappart L, Rauchhaus U, Bruns L, Reichardt HM, Kamradt T, et al. Glucocorticoid therapy of antigen-induced arthritis depends on the dimerized glucocorticoid receptor in T cells. *Proc Natl Acad Sci USA.* (2011) 108:19317–22. doi: 10.1073/pnas.1105857108
175. Koenen M, Culemann S, Vettorazzi S, Caratti G, Frappart L, Baum W, et al. Glucocorticoid receptor in stromal cells is essential for glucocorticoid-mediated suppression of inflammation in arthritis. *Ann Rheum Dis.* (2018) 77:1610–18. doi: 10.1136/annrheumdis-2017-212762
176. Ayroldi E, Migliorati G, Bruscoli S, Marchetti C, Zollo O, Cannarile L, et al. Modulation of T-cell activation by the glucocorticoid-induced leucine zipper

factor via inhibition of nuclear factor kappaB. *Blood.* (2001) 98:743–53. doi: 10.1182/blood.V98.3.743

177. Berrebi D, Bruscoli S, Cohen N, Foussat A, Migliorati G, Bouchet-Delbos L, et al. Synthesis of glucocorticoid-induced leucine zipper. (GILZ) by macrophages: an anti-inflammatory and immunosuppressive mechanism shared by glucocorticoids and IL-10. *Blood.* (2003) 101:729–38. doi: 10.1182/blood-2002-02-0538
178. Beaulieu E, Ngo D, Santos L, Yang YH, Smith M, Jorgensen C, et al. Glucocorticoid-induced leucine zipper is an endogenous antiinflammatory mediator in arthritis. *Arthritis Rheumat.* (2010) 62:2651–61. doi: 10.1002/art.27566
179. Kassel O, Sancono A, Krätzschmar J, Kreft B, Stassen M, Cato AC. Glucocorticoids inhibit MAP kinase via increased expression and decreased degradation of MKP-1. *EMBO J.* (2001) 20:7108–16. doi: 10.1093/emboj/20.24.7108
180. Abraham SM, Lawrence T, Kleiman A, Warden P, Medghalchi M, Tuckermann J, et al. Antiinflammatory effects of dexamethasone are partly dependent on induction of dual specificity phosphatase 1. *J Exp Med.* (2006) 203:1883–9. doi: 10.1084/jem.20060336
181. Vandevyver S, Dejager L, Van Bogaert T, Kleyman A, Liu Y, Tuckermann J, et al. Glucocorticoid receptor dimerization induces MKP1 to protect against TNF-induced inflammation. *J Clin Invest.* (2012) 122:2130–40. doi: 10.1172/JCI60006
182. Vattakuzhi Y, Abraham SM, Freidin A, Clark AR, Horwood NJ. Dual-specificity phosphatase 1-null mice exhibit spontaneous osteolytic disease and enhanced inflammatory osteolysis in experimental arthritis. *Arthritis Rheum.* (2012) 64:2201–10. doi: 10.1002/art.34403
183. Perretti M, D'Acquisto F. Annexin A1 and glucocorticoids as effectors of the resolution of inflammation. *Nat Rev Immunol.* (2009) 9:62–70. doi: 10.1038/nri2470
184. Patel HB, Kornerup KN, Sampaio AL, D'Acquisto F, Seed MP, Girol AP, et al. The impact of endogenous annexin A1 on glucocorticoid control of inflammatory arthritis. *Ann Rheum Dis.* (2012) 71:1872–80. doi: 10.1136/annrheumdis-2011-201180
185. Tuckermann JP, Kleiman A, Moriggl R, Spanbroek R, Neumann A, Illing A, et al. Macrophages and neutrophils are the targets for immune suppression by glucocorticoids in contact allergy. *J Clin Invest.* (2007) 117:1381–90. doi: 10.1172/JCI28034
186. Misharin AV, Cuda CM, Saber R, Turner JD, Gierut AK, Haines GK, et al. Nonclassical Ly6C^{-} monocytes drive the development of inflammatory arthritis in mice. *Cell Rep.* (2014) 9:591–604. doi: 10.1016/j.celrep.2014.09.032
187. Buttgereit F, Zhou H, Kalak R, Gaber T, Spies CM, Huscher D, et al. Transgenic disruption of glucocorticoid signaling in mature osteoblasts and osteocytes attenuates K/BxN mouse serum-induced arthritis *in vivo*. *Arthritis Rheum.* (2009) 60:1998–2007. doi: 10.1002/art.24619
188. Tu J, Stoner S, Fromm PD, Wang T, Chen D, Tuckermann J, et al. Endogenous glucocorticoid signaling in chondrocytes attenuates joint inflammation and damage. *FASEB J.* (2018) 32:478–87. doi: 10.1096/fj.201700659R

7

Physical Activity and Bone Health: What is the Role of Immune System? A Narrative Review of the Third Way

Giovanni Lombardi[1,2*], *Ewa Ziemann*[2] **and** *Giuseppe Banfi*[1,3]

[1] *Laboratory of Experimental Biochemistry & Molecular Biology, IRCCS Istituto Ortopedico Galeazzi, Milan, Italy,*
[2] *Department of Physiology and Pharmacology, Faculty of Rehabilitation and Kinesiology, Gdansk University of Physical Education and Sport, Gdansk, Poland,* [3] *Vita-Salute San Raffaele University, Milan, Italy*

***Correspondence:**
Giovanni Lombardi
giovanni.lombardi@grupposandonato.it

Bone tissue can be seen as a physiological hub of several stimuli of different origin (e.g., dietary, endocrine, nervous, immune, skeletal muscle traction, biomechanical load). Their integration, at the bone level, results in: (i) changes in mineral and protein composition and microarchitecture and, consequently, in shape and strength; (ii) modulation of calcium and phosphorous release into the bloodstream, (iii) expression and release of hormones and mediators able to communicate the current bone status to the rest of the body. Different stimuli are able to act on either one or, as usual, more levels. Physical activity is the key stimulus for bone metabolism acting in two ways: through the biomechanical load which resolves into a direct stimulation of the segment(s) involved and through an indirect load mediated by muscle traction onto the bone, which is the main physiological stimulus for bone formation, and the endocrine stimulation which causes homeostatic adaptation. The third way, in which physical activity is able to modify bone functions, passes through the immune system. It is known that immune function is modulated by physical activity; however, two recent insights have shed new light on this modulation. The first relies on the discovery of inflammasomes, receptors/sensors of the innate immunity that regulate caspase-1 activation and are, hence, the tissue triggers of inflammation in response to infections and/or stressors. The second relies on the ability of certain tissues, and particularly skeletal muscle and adipose tissue, to synthesize and secrete mediators (namely, myokines and adipokines) able to affect, profoundly, the immune function. Physical activity is known to act on both these mechanisms and, hence, its effects on bone are also mediated by the immune system activation. Indeed, that immune system and bone are tightly connected and inflammation is pivotal in determining the bone metabolic status is well-known. The aim of this narrative review is to give a complete view of the exercise-dependent immune system-mediated effects on bone metabolism and function.

Keywords: exercise, training, biomechanical loading, inflammatory mediators, inflammasomes

INTRODUCTION

Exercise, particularly when energetically demanding and sustained, affects all human tissues and organs. Different kinds of exercise (e.g., endurance, high intensity, resistance) have different effects on tissues and organs homeostasis and, consequently, different kinds of training require different adaptive changes that might take place (1). Bone is importantly affected by exercise and bone cells metabolism forcefully adapts to training. This metabolic adaptation reflects, on long-term basis, in a micro-architectural, and possibly macro-architectural, redefinition of bone shape and structure. The biological meaning of this phenomena resides in the physical adaptation of bones (in terms of shape, mass, and strength) to the changed environmental conditions (applied forces) (2). However, the bony response to exercise does not only depend on the biomechanical stimulus but equally relies on other systemic mechanisms that make the bone a center for the integration of the signals generated during and following the exercise (3). A main signal is the metabolic one: bone metabolism is highly-demanding in terms of energy; parallel, during exercise the energy needs increase with the increasing duration and intensity. Being not a lifesaving function, bone metabolism is partially blocked in response to acute exercise, regardless the degree of biomechanical load. This block mainly pertains the anabolic function (osteoblastic function, i.e., bone formation) while leaves almost unaltered the catabolic side (osteoclastic function, i.e., bone resorption). The acute unbalance toward bone resorption makes the calcium, stored in the bone matrix, available to skeletal muscles (SKM) and cardiac muscle for contraction and to the brain to sustain the neuromuscular function (4). On the other hand, the chronically established bone metabolic response to training is driven by the degree of load: weight-bearing/high impact activities (e.g., plyometric) shift the balance toward bone formation and on average increase bone mass and bone mineral density (BMD). Equally demanding activities featured by a low/absent biomechanical load (e.g., swimming, cycling) shift the balance toward resorption and causes a decrease in the average bone mass and BMD (3). Another key signal, generated during and following exercise and affecting bone metabolism, is the immune/inflammatory one. Inflammation, acute and chronic, is a main determinant for bone metabolism and the plethora of inflammatory mediators, produced under either physiologic or pathologic conditions, affects bone cells. Noteworthy, in last 15 years an interdisciplinary branch of study embracing (but not limited to) endocrinology, immunology, orthopedics, and rheumatology, namely osteoimmunology, has developed quickly thus becoming a central subject in metabolic diseases of bone (5). A key role of the osteoimmune networking has been highlighted by the clinical success and safety, over the classical anti-resorptive drugs (6, 7), of the fully human monoclonal antibody denosumab used in the treatment of primary and secondary osteoporosis, in both males and females (8), which is an inhibitor of the prototypic osteoimmunological signaling pathway, the RANK/RANKL system, as described elsewhere (9). Acute exercise represents a powerful inflammatory stimulus itself while the inflammatory response to training is a handbook example of adaptation to a continuous stimulus. Exercise, indeed, initiates a series of inflammatory events, which ultimately, if chronically continued, positively affects health. The inflammatory response to exercise, however, takes place in the immune system (IS), involving mainly the innate compartment with fallouts on the humoral immunity, as well as in tissues other than the IS, e.g., SKM, white and brown adipose tissues (WAT, BAT), brain, liver (3, 10, 11). Notably, the acute response elicited by exercise in terms of inflammatory mediators is often very similar to that observed during pathological acute and chronic inflammatory conditions (e.g., sepsis, obesity, autoimmune diseases, tumors) but what determines the net result of this response (pro- vs. anti-inflammatory) is the milieu in which this response is generated, together with its temporal length and the site of production. As an example, interleukin (IL)-6 expression is strongly induced by time, intensity and type of muscle contractions-dependently as well as in sepsis (various origin) but, in the latter case, it is driven by the previous increase in another cytokine, the tumor necrosis factor (TNF)-α (12). Based on the interdependence between bone and IS, it is implicit that the acute inflammatory response induced by exercise- and the modulation of the inflammatory status induced by chronic training both affect bone cells differentiation and function and, in turn, the bone metabolism. It should be kept in mind that, other than a target of these endocrine and inflammatory stimuli, the bone is itself a source of these mediators and, hence, it actively enters in the regulation/modulation network of the homeostasis (3).

This review aims at summarizing the experimental evidences about the exercise- and training-dependent effects on bone mediated by the IS and the other inflammatory sources in order to depict additional, and less explored, link between bone and inflammation as further mechanisms by which the physically active status is a main determinant for health.

In order to go deep into the description, it is necessary to introduce some key concepts, relative to the exercise physiology, that will help the reader in fully understand the biological meaning underlying the homeostatic response. About the types of muscle actions, one can distinguish between static (isometric) and dynamic (isotonic) actions. During the static (isometric) action, muscles generate force without changing length due to an external resistance (weight of an object) greater than the force produced by the muscle; despite the energy expenditure, no work is done due to lack of movement. The isotonic action, instead, can be either (i) concentric, when muscles produce enough force to overcome the external resistance and the muscle contraction results in a work, or (ii) eccentric, when the muscles lengthens while generate a force due to the opposite movement of the external resistance and the sarcomere shortening (13). Another series of concepts regard the terms physical activity (PA), exercise, and training. PA is defined as any bodily movement produced by SKM resulting in an energy consumption. Everyone performs PA in order to sustain life but the amount is subject to personal. The term "exercise," instead, although often erroneously used interchangeably with PA, is defined as a PA featured by planning, structure, and repetitiveness, which is aimed at maintaining or improving the

TABLE 1 | Common and distinctive features of physical activity and exercise.

Physical Activity	Exercise
Body movement generated by skeletal muscles	Body movement generated by skeletal muscles
Variable energy expenditure	Variable energy expenditure
Positive correlation with physical fitness	Positive correlation with physical fitness
	Planned, structured, and repetitive
	Aimed at maintain/improve physical fitness

physical fitness (14). The common and distinctive features of PA and exercise are summarized in **Table 1**.

When a single bout of exercise (acute exercise) is continued over the time, in the same fashion, it is defined training (exercise training). Finally, the different types of exercise and training can be categorized as follows: (i) endurance, mainly based on the aerobic metabolism (e.g., distance running, road cycling, swimming, triathlon), (ii) resistance (also known as strength), mainly based on the anaerobic metabolism (e.g., weight lifting, discus, hammer, and javelin throw) (15).

HOW DO EXERCISE AND TRAINING AFFECT BONE METABOLISM?

The responsiveness of bone to mechanical stimulation was first theorized by Frost who postulated, with the "mechanostat" hypothesis, bone mass and structure remain constant around a certain threshold of mechanical strains. Bone formation takes place when the strain increases above this threshold, and it results in an increased bone stiffness. When the strain experienced by the bone segment is lower than this threshold bone loss can take place (16). Later, it was shown that the threshold itself is modifiable by several factors, mainly endocrine [parathyroid hormone (PTH), sex hormones, etc.] (17). However, despite its importance, the mechanical strains induced by strenuous PA is very small degree attesting to up to 0.3% (3,000 microstrain) (18). Based on that, it is likely that bone cells are exposed to and integrate different PA-generated mechanical stimuli that altogether imply an amplification of the environmental stimulation. A further level of complexity is due to the fact that different types of bone cells are anatomically exposed to different combinations of stimuli. Bone marrow and endosteal osteoblasts experience the pressure forces generated within the marrow cavity. Osteocytes buried into the matrix with their interconnecting long cellular processes running within the fluid-filled canalicular network experience dynamic fluid flow pressure, shear stress forces, and dynamic electric fields (due to the transit of charged ions in the interstitial fluid). Mature osteoclasts and their precursors, residing in the bone marrow, may be exposed to mechanical stimulation due to dynamic pressure (19). Bone mechanosensitivity is mediated by several cellular components (e.g., membrane, membrane proteins, cytoskeleton, cilia, ion channels). Shear stress and pressure deform the plasma membrane and, consequently, to the cytoskeleton and, in turn, through integrins to the protein machinery mediating the cell-to-matrix adhesion and to the nucleus where it induces the expression of downstream genes (20). In osteoblast, the deformation of the plasma membrane is associated with the activation of ion channels (21), as in osteocytes, whose cilia, protruding out of the dendritic extensions, sense fluid flow and activate channel-mediated ion fluxes that modulate the Wnt signaling pathway (22).

The different nature of the mechanical stimuli together with the number of cell structures involved in mechanosensitivity imply the integration of the different signals generated (19). Indeed, the physical stimulus is translated into several chemical signals including calcium, mitogen-activated protein kinase (MAPK), Wnt, and RhoA/ROCK pathways. For instance, the Frizzled-LRP5/6-mediated activation of Wnt induces the expression of osteoblastic factors, as RUNX2 that promotes the commitment of mesenchymal stem cells (MSCs) toward the osteoblast lineage, induces proliferation and differentiation of pre-osteoblast, and stimulates mineralization. Hence, exercise shifts the adipogenic-to-osteogenic equilibrium, governing the MSC fate, toward the osteoblastic commitment (23, 24). By modulating the OPG and RANKL expression in osteoblasts, Wnt signaling also downregulates osteoclastogenesis and osteoclast activity (25). A key mechanism regulating the Wnt activity that underlies the exercise-associated effects on bone is mediated by sclerostin (Sost) (26). Osteocytes constitutively produce Sost that inhibits the Wnt pathway, thereby osteoblastogenesis and bone formation. Loading activates a molecular response that inhibits Sost expression and, then, allow the activation of Wnt signaling. Noteworthy, also prostaglandin E2 (PGE2), which is induced by strain sensing, by activating its receptors EP2 and EP4, facilitates the nuclear translocation of β-catenin and its transcriptional action (27). Finally, the intracellular signaling generated following mechanical stimulation can be propagated to neighbor cells as calcium (e.g., between osteoblasts and osteocytes) or adenosine triphosphate (ATP; e.g., osteoblast-to-osteoclast) transients through the gap junction network (28, 29).

Another way by which exercise and recovery beneficially affects bone metabolism, mineral content, and structure is by increasing the blood flow to the bone and the consequent improved supply of nutrients supporting its metabolic needs (30, 31). Indeed, also from this point of view, bone is a really active tissue as demonstrated by the fact that blood flow to the bone and glucose uptake within the bone tissue are increased in response to exercise (32). However, as exercise load increases blood flow offs due to the sympathetic response that shifts the flow to the active SKM. Moreover, perfusion in bone, which ranges over a window wider than that expected during exercise, is mainly ruled by chemoreceptors, and hence nutrients, rather than by hypoxia (33). The exercise-induced enhanced bone perfusion also causes an increased efflux of stem cells from bone marrow (e.g., endothelial precursors) (34), consequently to the endothelial production of nitric oxide (35) and sympathetic nervous system activation (36). Finally, exercise-induced muscular-derived adenosine could solve another key role in bone blood flow determination (37).

The Effect of Acute Exercise

Despite the key role of loading, the bone tissue response of the to a single bout of exercise is mainly driven by the exercise-dependent metabolic requests of noble organs and of those organs that are directly involved in the activity. In other terms, during PA, and mostly dependent upon its intensity and duration, the metabolic needs of non-life saving organs (e.g., the bone, skin, gut) are somehow "sacrificed" in order to have all the fuels available for being used by brain, SKM, and liver (3). After the conclusion of the PA, during recovery, and with the chronic and/or long-term repetition of the act, the loading/impact-induced anabolic response takes place. This means that during PA the bone metabolism is mostly unbalanced toward resorption. This is also a consequence of the key role of bone in calcium homeostasis: PA implies the usage of calcium in terms of functioning of the contractile machinery of the SKM, release, and recycling of neurotransmitters and hormones. Being resorbed, bone make the calcium promptly available. Indeed, two activities both characterized by high energy expenditures but differentiated by kind of biomechanical loading, one featured by high load and impact (mountain ultra-trail) while the other non-impact/loading (cycling), both display an anti-anabolic/pro-catabolic acute response of the bone to the activity (38, 39).

By considering the biomechanical aspects, only dynamic stimuli can generate an osteogenic response that, instead, is not induced by static loading (40) and strain amplitude, number of cycles and interval between the cycles are important, as well (41, 42). Indeed, the anabolic response can be desensitized by long-lasting activities while interval rest between the load cycles may have an osteogenic effect (43, 44). On the contrary, inter-cycles resting activates some mechanotransduction-sensitizing mechanisms that sustain the osteogenic response (28).However, too high magnitudes or number of cycles of load may fatigue the bone tissue and consequently can cause microdamage that, in turns, result in a series of catabolic events including local bone resorption (45).

The Effect of Chronic Exercise and Training

Life-long PA is associated with a better bone quality, thus potentially resulting in a stronger bone, e.g., improved cross-sectional area, BMD, and moments of inertia. These features, for example, and have been observed in gymnasts vs. non-gymnasts (46, 47), and dominant vs. non-dominant limbs of racquet sports players (48) or triple jumpers (49). By applying the same external force, the deformation experienced by "weak bones" is greater than that of "strong bones" and, consequently, it elicits in larger tissue strains. This results in a greater anabolic response in the weaker bone that attempts to become stronger (50). In experimental models, loads causing high strains induce bone formation in loaded areas, while areas with lower peak strains featured by reduced bone formation or even increased bone catabolism (51). Site-specific adaptation to loads takes also place in human: in women, after skeletal maturity, the adaptation to load is related to the energy equivalent strain, which means that regions undergone to high-level strain experience bone apposition than regions undergone to low-level strain (50).

However, the bone adaptation to chronic PA and training mainly depends upon the kind of activity. This was clearly demonstrated by Nikander et al. (52), who evaluate the bone quality of the narrowest section of the femoral neck [areal BMD (aBMD), hip structure analysis (HSA), cross-sectional area (CSA), subperiosteal width (W), and section modulus of strength (Z)] in 225 premenopausal women performing different sports. Women performing high-impact (volleyball, hurdling) and odd-impact (squash, soccer, speed skating, step-aerobic) loading sports displayed the highest aBMD (+23 and +29% vs. non-athletic women), CSA (+22 and +27%), and Z (+22 and +26%) even following adjustment for age-, weight-, and height. Contrarily, low-impact (orienteering, cross-country skiing) and non-impact (cycling, swimming) repetitive loading activities were associated with no gains in bone quality, compared with the inactive controls (52). A Cochrane review evaluating the preventive and therapeutic effects of training on postmenopausal osteoporosis established that exercise has a small (about 3%) but significant effect on bone mass and BMD. According to the meta-analysis, femoral bone mass mostly benefits from high-force non- weight-bearing exercises (e.g., resistance strength training of the lower limbs). Vertebral bone mass, instead, mostly benefits from the combination of exercises featured by different types of dynamic loading. Consequently, the risk of fracture across all exercise groups was not significantly different compared to the control groups (53). Exercise-based, either preventing or therapeutic, strategies aimed at affecting bone health might account for this finding. Indeed, based on our recent overview of systematic reviews and meta-analyses, lifelong age-specific exercise is effective in sustaining bone health in women. School-based short bouts of high-impact plyometric exercises positively affect peak bone mass in young girls, while combined-impact exercises represent the best exercise modality to preserve/improve BMD in both pre- and post-menopausal women (54).

Beside the quite well-depicted effects of chronic exercising on the physical feature of the bone, the effects on blood flow or metabolism of human bone are scarce (33). Although neglected, these studies are of key importance since they highlight a role for bone in regulating the whole-body metabolism (55–57) and also because the bone is central in the release of vascular precursor and immune cells. Thus, it emerges that by influencing bone status, exercise training could potentially affect vascular impairments in pathological conditions such as diabetes (33) and it may regulate the release of immune cells into the circulation and, hence, to directly control the inflammatory status.

As important as loading, or even more important, is detraining. Constant load (use of the skeleton) is essential for osteocyte survival and in case of bone immobilization osteocyte apoptosis occurs (58). Parallel, detraining causes bone loss and, hence, training might be continued to maintain bone mass (59) since unloading and disuse increase bone resorption rate. This situation is encountered, for instance, in astronauts under weightlessness conditions, spinal cord injured patients, and elderly people forced to either partial or total immobilization (19). Unloading affects both the cortical and trabecular portions of the bone: spinal cord injured subjects experience a 20–40% decrease in cortical thickness (60) and an average 14% (range 2–80%) in trabecular density (61); for astronauts the mean BMD loss of the trabecular compartment was 4% at the lumbar spine and 12% at the proximal femur (62).

HOW DO EXERCISE AND TRAINING AFFECT THE INFLAMMATORY RESPONSE AND THE IMMUNE FUNCTION?

Exercise profoundly affects the normal functioning of the IS with immune responses to single bouts being transient while an immune adaptation is likely to take place with training. Exercise dose is important in determining the entity of the immune response: prolonged intense training can have depressive effects (e.g., increased infection risk), while regular moderate-intensity exercise has more balanced effects that mainly results in the improvement of the baseline immune reactivity (63). Several evidences support this effect, chronic exercise has been demonstrated to improve immune, and hence health and behavioral outcomes, in several conditions of deregulated immune response, such as aging, obesity, cancer, and chronic viral infections (e.g., HIV) as well as in preventing their onset (63–66). Interestingly, acute exercise is effective in improving vaccines response (63). These effects are mediated, from one hand, by the cells of the IS belonging to both the innate and adaptive branches and, from the other hand, by all the cells of the body that are induced to express either a pro-inflammatory or anti-inflammatory phenotype. Exercise activates inflammatory cascades involving cells belonging to both the innate and adaptive immunity branches, cytokines, and mediators with active roles in inflammation (myokines, adipokines) that are in turn responsible for the generation of an environment in which recovery, regeneration, and adaptation take place. Exercise duration, mode, and intensity are the determinants for the exercise-induced inflammatory response. At the same time, training exerts anti-inflammatory actions through several distinct mechanisms involving metabolic, endocrine, and immune mediators of various tissues and organs (67). However, exercise exerts its anti-inflammatory effect only after the activation of pro-inflammatory cascades (67).

A special mention might be spent about cortisol. Although this adrenal hormone has anti-inflammatory immunosuppressant actions, and its occasionally increased circulating concentration (e.g., following PA) are beneficial in reducing inflammation, its chronically high levels (i.e., hypercortisolism) and deregulated rhythms are associated with aging and age-associated low-grade inflammation (68). Cortisol and the other endogenous glucocorticoids (GCs) are the final products of the neuroendocrine hypothalamus-pituitary-adrenal cortex (HPA) axis that is responsible for the regulation of both the energy balance and stress response. The physiological circadian fluctuations of GC levels allow the correct functioning of the intermediate metabolism and the development and the maintenance of the homeostasis of a wide all the body tissues, including the bone. Indeed, GCs are essential for bone modeling and remodeling as they promote osteoblastogenesis to maintain the bone architecture (69). Excessive energy intake (unbalanced energy intake-to-energy expenditure ratio) and adiposity are associated with chronic inflammation and stress which are in turn responsible for a deregulated of the HPA axis. Moreover, hypercortisolism is associated with a deregulated energy metabolism that in turn is responsible for the maintenance of the chronic inflammatory state (70). PA, by acting as a chronoenhancer, also impacting on the HPA axis, is able to improve the GC response in healthy subjects as well as to restore the circadian rhythm in age-associated low-grade inflammation dependent hypercortisolism and, hence, to improve the related comorbidities (68).

Effects of Exercise and Training on Inflammation

Effect of Acute Exercise

A single exercise bout starts a series of timely-defined inflammatory events, which mainly depend upon mode, intensity, duration, and training status (i.e., familiarity with the exercise). This cascade starts with a pro-inflammatory phase (1.5–24 h post-exercise) which is then followed by an anti-inflammatory phase that sustains SKM regeneration (24–72 h post-exercise). The exercise-induced inflammatory response is evidenced by the rise of the circulating levels of myokines (i.e., IL-6) and anti-inflammatory mediators (IL-10, IL-1ra). Moreover, exercise downregulates the expression, on the surface of antigen-presenting cells (APCs, e.g., monocytes) of those receptors involved in the recognition of danger signals, i.e., toll-like receptors (TLRs) (67). TLRs are highly evolutionarily conserved transmembrane proteins involved in the recognition of classes of molecules non-specifically associated with pathogens (pathogen-associated molecular patterns, PAMPs) and "danger signals" non-specifically induced/released following tissue damage due to physical, chemical, or biological agents (danger-associated molecular patterns, DAMPs) (71). TLRs activation leads to the expression of inflammatory cytokines. Acute exercise affects the expression of TLRs on monocytes and, hence, by desensitizing these cells to pro-inflammatory stimulation, this results in a push toward the anti-inflammatory phenotype. 2.5 h of cycling at 60% of VO_2max induces a significant decrease in the expression of TLRs on CD14+ monocytes, compared to rest, immediately (TLR2, about −25%) and 1 h post-exercise (TLR1, −60%, TLR2 and TLR4, −50%, TLR3, −30%) (72).

Effect of Chronic Exercise and Training

There are several potential tissue-specific anti-inflammatory mechanisms associated with regular PA and these include reductions in body fat (particularly, visceral fat), enhanced expression and release of contracting muscle-derived anti-inflammatory mediators, downregulated expression of TLRs in monocytes and macrophages, increased expression of anti-oxidant species counteracting the exercise-associated rise in reactive oxygen species (ROS) generation (73).

Exercise causes transient elevations in IL-6 coming from exercising SKM (74). Contrarily, during inflammation, and especially chronic low-grade inflammation, IL-6 is produced in a slightly chronically elevated manner and, in this case, the source is represented by immune cells and hepatocytes (3). Muscle-derived IL-6 has anti-inflammatory effects by inducing other anti-inflammatory cytokines (e.g., IL-1ra and IL-10) that antagonize the pro-inflammatory IL-1β and TNF-α (12). IL-6, but also the exercise-related increased energy needs, stimulate the release of cortisol that has an immunosuppressant activity (74). The logic around the IL-6 release by the contracting muscle resides in its activity aimed at increasing the usage and delivery of energetic substrates to the myocytes, in concert with the stress hormones (e.g., cortisol, epinephrine). By acting in autocrine and paracrine fashions, indeed, IL-6 stimulates the cellular uptake and the oxidation of glucose and fatty acids by the SKM itself; contemporary, by acting in an endocrine fashion, it induces lipolysis at the AT level and glycogenolysis and gluconeogenesis. The insulin-mimetic effect of IL-6 on glucose uptake is of particular interest. The binding of IL-6 with the IL-6Rα/gp130Rβ receptor complex leads to the activation of AMPK that triggers the plasma membrane translocation of intracellular vesicles bearing the insulin-dependent glucose transporter (GLUT4) allowing glucose uptake regardless the insulin status. This accounts for the beneficial effects of PA on the metabolic function also in impaired glucose tolerance and insulin resistance (75). Moreover, other than stimulating the release of IL-6, exercise training generates an appropriate environment making the IL-6 effect distinctly anti-inflammatory: for instance, aerobic training reduces the expression of TNF-α and IL-1α by mononuclear cells and induces IL-4, IL-10, and TGF-β1 in subjects at high-risks of heart disease (76).

Training exerts its effects by also reducing the activation potential of the innate immune response activation in terms of TLRs in an age-independent manner. Young (18–35 years of age) and elderly (65–80 years of age) active subjects have a one third reduced expression of TLR4 on CD14+ monocytes' surface, compared to their inactive counterparts. Moreover, 12-week of either endurance or resistance training halved TLR4 expression in monocytes from these inactive (old and young) subjects to a level comparable to those found in active age-matched controls, while the intervention was ineffective in the already active subjects (72).

The anti-inflammatory effect of training might is also the result of the modulation of nitric oxide (NO) and ROS production and the consequent activation of their downstream pathways. Exercise induces the synthesis of NO and ROS which are important in inducing anti-inflammatory defensive mechanisms especially by targeting muscle gene expression (77). In the case of ROS, with training, the cyclic exercise-induced spiked production (contrarily to what happens in chronic inflammation) causes the activation of an adaptive response that, in turn, protects SKM from exposure to the exercise-dependent increase of ROS itself. This phenomenon accounts also for the decreased expression of TNFα that may further inflammation (77).

The AT is determinant in defining the inflammatory status. The association of physical inactivity and high caloric intake results in adipocyte and AT hypertrophy. As adipocytes grow, the oxygen supply becomes limiting and the consequent hypoxic stress leads to cell death and necrosis. Necrosis recalls macrophages and potently induces an inflammatory response (78). Notably, this process seems to involve mainly the visceral AT that has a higher inflammatory potential than the subcutaneous one. Exercise-induced caloric imbalance causes lipolysis, aimed at mobilizing fats to be used as fuel by the exercising muscle, with a reduction of the adipocytes' size and, thereby, hypoxic stress and inflammation (79).

Effects of Exercise and Training on Immune Functions

Exercise profoundly affects the IS functioning. An exercise bout causes an important redistribution of leukocytes as a consequence of the hemodynamic response and the increased blood levels of catecholamine and glucocorticoids, but the effects depend upon exercise intensity and duration. Prolonged periods of intensive training can impair immune functions, and particularly those of T-cells, natural killer (NK)-cells, and neutrophils; in elite athletes, during periods of heavy training and competition, mucosal immunity is also affected determining an increased risk of infections of the upper respiratory tract. Contrarily, regular moderate-intensity activities are beneficial having immune-enhancing effects and, as stated above, throughout the reductions of inflammation, increased immune cells turnover, enhanced immune surveillance, and improvement of psychological stress status (63).

Effect of Acute Exercise

An exercise bout increases both the absolute and relative leukocyte counts. Transient leucocytosis takes place already after brief (minutes) dynamic exercise and is more sustained in the case of prolonged endurance exercise (80) and returns to pre-exercise levels within 6–24 h (63). Neutrophils and lymphocytes are mainly involved in this response while a smaller contribute is given by monocytes. The response, however, differs for these cells: during the early phase of recovery (30–60 min after exercise), the neutrophilia is associated with lymphocytopenia that can be particularly pronounced until clinically relevant low levels ($<1.0 \cdot 10^9$/L, which means −30 to −50% compared to pre-exercise values) and can last up to 6 h (80). Other features also characterize this response. Exercise tends to mobilize cytotoxic cells (e.g., NK-cells, and CD8+ and γδ T-cells) (81) and non-lymphocyte effector cells (e.g., CD16+ monocytes and CD16- neutrophils) (82, 83). The exercise-dependent mobilization mainly involves those cells with a higher migration potential, e.g., leukocytes expressing high levels of integrins and intracellular adhesion molecules (84) and a wide range of chemokine receptors (85). Finally, in these leukocytes the expression of adrenoreceptors (β2-ARs) and glucocorticoid receptors is upregulated, and are therefore they are highly responsive to catecholamines and cortisol (81, 86, 87), this indicates that leukocyte trafficking between the blood and tissues is strongly influenced by both the sympathetic branch of the nervous system and the HPA axis activation.

Other than being dislodged from liver, lung, and spleen endothelia due to the exercise-induced increased blood pressure- and cardiac output-mediated shear stress (80), leucocytes come from lymph nodes, intestines, bone marrow, thymus, and SKM that contain large numbers of white cells. The contribution of primary (i.e., bone marrow, thymus) and some secondary (i.e., lymph nodes), lymphoid organs to the initial exercise-induced leucocytosis is limited, since their content in mature/differentiated cells. The bone marrow likely sustains neutrophilia during recovery from prolonged exercise, while lymph nodes and thymus mainly sustain the restoration of the blood lymphocyte count following the transient lymphocytopenia (63).

About innate immunity, submaximal exercises enhance neutrophil chemotaxis (88), phagocytosis (89), and spontaneous degranulation (90). Also the neutrophil oxidative burst is affected by the exercise although in an intensity-and duration-dependent fashion: cycling at 50 and 80% of VO_2max have enhancing and impairing effects, respectively; moreover, during recovery from moderate-intensity exercise the oxidative burst is enhanced while it is impaired following exhaustive and prolonged activities (91, 92). Also NK-cell cytotoxicity is quickly induced by exercise but this response is followed by a delayed suppression during recovery but this likely mirroring changes in their number (93).

Adaptive immunity appears to be both augmented and inhibited depending on intensity, duration, and modality of exercise (63). In trained triathletes, following a half-Ironman race, an intradermal inoculation containing several recall antigens caused a reduced 48 h-delayed-type compared to both resting triathletes and moderately trained healthy men (94).

Effect of Chronic Exercise and Training

In general, high-intensity and high-volume training is thought to cause short- or long-term immune depressive states that can increase infection risk. Repeated bouts of strenuous exercise, performed without adequate recovery, result in a chronic state of impaired immunity (80). The decline in the count of circulating immune cells is associated with the increased susceptibility to infections: although athletes and healthy age-matched controls have comparable absolute and relative leukocyte counts, endurance athletes may experience reduced resting lymphocyte (runners) and NK-cell (swimmers, cyclists) counts (95–97). Functional declines in adaptive immunity associated with prolonged intensive training are related to unbalanced expression of pro- and anti-inflammatory cytokines and increased plasma levels of stress hormone (e.g., cortisol) (98).

Contrary to the strenuous, exhaustive exercise typically practiced by athletes, moderate-intensity training has beneficial effects on immune function (99). Moreover, exercise mode (i.e., aerobic, resistance, or combined) as well as the condition on which the intervention is addressed are main determinants of the immune effects. Indeed, moderate-intensity exercise training associates with a life-long improvement/maintenance of several aspects of the immune function (99, 100), such as increased response to vaccine (101, 102), viral infections (103, 104), and tumors (105–107), enhanced neutrophil phagocytic activity (108), T-cell proliferation (93, 109), NK-cell cytotoxic activity (93, 110), basal level of cytokines (111) and IL-2 production (112) and decreased number of senescent T-cells (113) and inflammatory response to bacterial challenge (114).

The enhanced adaptive immune response is also sustained by the improvement in systemic low-grade inflammation, driven by the improved inflammatory status of the AT, and hence in the associated adipokine profile (described above). Indeed, the downregulation of TLRs on the surface of monocytes (115) together with the direct exercise-induced M1 (pro-inflammatory)-to-M2 (anti-inflammatory) shift in macrophage phenotype, reduces the infiltration of the AT and, hence, its inflammatory status (116). The stress-related hormones released during exercise that have anti-inflammatory properties are responsible of a further stimulus: cortisol acting as an immunomodulatory and immunosuppressant compound and adrenaline that downregulates the expression of the inflammatory mediators IL-1β and TNF (73, 117). Exercise also decreases the content of cholesterol of the cell membranes that may improve T-cell receptor signaling and the translocation of MHC molecules for antigen presentation (118).

IMMUNO-MEDIATED EFFECTS OF EXERCISE AND TRAINING ON BONE

Inflammasome Activation and Bone Metabolism

The innate immune function depends upon the recognition, by germline-encoded pattern-recognition receptors (PRRs), of PAMPs, derived from invading pathogens, and DAMPs, induced by endogenous stresses. PAMPs-/DAMPs-dependent activation of PRRs triggers the downstream signaling cascades and induces the expression of type I interferons (IFN-α, IFN-β) and pro-inflammatory cytokines (119). Inflammasomes are multimeric protein complexes assembling within the cytosol after sensing PAMPs or DAMPs (120, 121). They serve as scaffolds to recruit the inactive zymogen pro-caspase-1 that oligomerizes allowing the auto-proteolytic cleavage into active caspase-1. Active caspase-1 cleaves the precursor cytokines pro-IL-1β and pro-IL-18 generating the biologically active forms (122–124). Furthermore, when activated, caspase-1 can activate a series of intracellular events that lead to a form of cell-death mediated by inflammation which is known with the term of pyroptosis (125, 126). Several PRRs families are involved in inflammasomes activation, in both mice and humans, including the nucleotide-binding domain, leucine-rich repeat containing proteins (NLRs, NOD-like receptors), and absent in melanoma 2-like receptors (ALRs, AIM2-like receptors) (127). Following stimulation, the relevant NLR or ALR oligomerizes and becomes a caspase-1-activating scaffold. Inflammasomes have been linked to several auto-inflammatory and autoimmune diseases, neurodegenerative diseases (e.g., multiple sclerosis, Alzheimer's disease, Parkinson's disease), and metabolic disorders [atherosclerosis, type-2 diabetes (T2DM), obesity] (126). Inflammasomes play either causative or contributing roles in inflammatory diseases onset, and also increase the severity of the condition in response to host-derived factors (119). Many PRRs can sense metabolic signals, such as free fatty acids (FFAs) and ceramides (CERs), whose blood concentrations increase during aging. These signals activate critical inflammatory signaling cascade pathways, such as IκBα kinase/nuclear factor-κB (IKK/NF-κB), endoplasmic reticulum (ER) stress-induced unfolded protein response (UPR), and NLRP3 inflammasome. Notably, other than in immune cells, PRRs are expressed in several metabolically active tissues (liver, SKM, AT) where they prime the inflammatory cascades (128).

Besides the established role of inflammation (and age-associated low-grade inflammation) in the pathogenesis of osteoporosis (129–131), very recent findings have linked it to inflammasomes activation. PA counteracts all the molecular mechanisms involved in inflammatory signaling cascades and inflammasome complexes activation (128). In post-menopausal osteoporosis, IL-18 blood levels are increased while those of its antagonist, IL-18BP, are decreased. According to Mansoori et al., IL-18BP enhanced murine osteoblast differentiation and inhibits the activation of NLRP3 inflammasome and caspase-1, *in vitro*, and improved the metabolic and bone statuses in ovariectomized rats (a rodent model of post-menopausal OP) (132). Further evidences derived from the association of NLRP3 mutations with arthropathy and OP (133) and the SIRT1-dependent inhibition of osteogenic differentiation and enhancement adipogenic differentiation, in mesenchymal stem cells (MSC), following lipopolysaccharide (LPS)-induced NLRP3 inflammasome activation (134). It is known that bone matrix organic and inorganic components, released during high-rate bone turnover (e.g., chronic low-grade inflammation, estrogen deficiency, primary hyperparathyroidism), promote osteoclastogenesis. This process, however, was importantly reduced in Nlrp3$^{-/-}$ cells and mice and pharmacologic inhibition of bone resorption (with bisphosphonates, e.g., zoledronic acid) attenuated inflammasome activation *in vivo*. These evidences suggest that the DAMPs-NLRP3 inflammasome axis may represent a novel mechanism supporting bone resorption (135).

PA effectively counteracts all the molecular mechanisms involved in the inflammatory signaling cascades (e.g., IKK/NF-κB, ER-UPR, inflammasomes) although the evidences about the effects of exercise on inflammasome are currently limited to NLRP3 activation and only in mouse models and in obesity. According to Ringseis, in obese mice both endurance (treadmill, 80% VO_2max, 10 weeks) and resistance exercise (intermittent vertical holding, 10 weeks) decrease NLRP3 mRNA in AT and IL-18 in plasma (128). A number of human studies demonstrated that PA reduces plasma IL-18 levels providing the evidence for the exercise-dependent NLRP3 pathway inhibition: 12-week aerobic interval training in males and females with metabolic syndrome; 6-month aerobic training (50–85% VO_2max) in overweight T2DM individuals; 8-week high-intensity training on a rowing ergometer ($\geq$70% VO_2max) in obese. In diet-induced obese rats, exercise strongly reverses TLR4 signaling and IKKβ phosphorylation in AT, SKM, and liver, suggesting a priming role for the exercise-induced inhibition of NLRP3 inflammasome. Key primers of NLRP3 activation are saturated FFA and CERs, whose circulating levels are increased in aging and metabolic dysfunctions while are decreased in response to exercise in obese animals and humans. Exercise may also reduce ER stress that primes NLRP3 activation via ROS production and NF-κB activation (128).

Extra-Immune Systemic Inflammation and Bone Metabolism

Beside the above described prototypic adipo-myokine IL-6 with its anti-inflammatory actions (induction of IL-10 and IL-1ra and inhibition of IL-1β and TNFα), SKM and AT secrete a plethora of active molecules that act in autocrine, paracrine, and hormone-like fashion the blood concentrations of many of which have been associated with several metabolic, immune-related, and age-related pathological conditions (3). It is well-known that the post-exercise rise of circulating IL-6 is supported by SKM (136) but contrarily, chronically slightly elevated blood IL-6 are found in metabolic conditions such as metabolic syndrome and insulin resistance, obesity, and T2DM (137–139). In these cases, the main source of IL-6 is represented by the visceral AT, the liver, and the activated immune cells upon NF-κB signaling (140). Indeed, in both overweight and lean males the contribution of the AT to the circulating amount of IL-6 is mainly in the post-exercise phase (141).

In bone, IL-6 stimulates bone resorption by enhancing osteoclastogenesis/osteoclast differentiation throughout the induction of RANKL expression (142, 143) and by inducing prostaglandin E2 (PGE2) expression in osteoblasts (144–146). Bones from IL-6 transgenic mice developed osteoporosis in association with an increased number of osteoclasts and decreased osteoblasts while, on the contrary, IL-6 knock out (KO) improved the arthritis phenotype, associated with a reduced osteoclast recruitment at the erosion sites, in a murine model of arthritis (147, 148). Ovariectomy in rats, model of postmenopausal osteoporosis, decreased trabecular bone volume (TBV) and impaired hormone and inflammatory profile (decreased estradiol and calcitonin and increased bone-derived IL-1β, IL-6, and cyclooxygenase-2). Contrarily, the treadmill-exercised counterparts displayed an overall improved phenotype (149). Parallel, postmenopausal women have BMD and muscle strength correlated with soluble IL-6 (150).

Low-impact high-intensity interval training (HIIT) acutely increased bone alkaline phosphatase activity (BAP) and the expression of OPG, RANKL, and pro-inflammatory cytokines (IL-1α, IL-1β, IL-6, TNFα) while decreased bone resorption [N-terminal cross-linked telopeptide of type I collagen (NTx)] (151). In obese subjects (n= 173), the degree of obesity and BMD were related to IL-6 levels (in males), osteocalcin (in females), C-reactive protein (CRP), and leptin indicating that adiposity and systemic inflammation are associated with low BMD (152). In obese, a 32-week combined loading training improved muscle strength and BMD at various sites along with an improved metabolic/inflammatory status (decreased CRP, interferon (IFN)-γ, IL-6) (153).

The leukemia inhibitory factor (LIF), a myokine belonging to the IL-6 superfamily, stimulates the proliferation of satellite cell which is essential in post-injury muscle regeneration (e.g., exercise-induced muscle damage, EIMD) and SKM hypertrophy (154). It was induced, at least in term of mRNA, by acute aerobic and resistance exercises (155). In bone, LIF stimulates bone turnover, osteoblast proliferation and bone matrix deposition, and prostaglandin-induced bone resorption depending on the differentiation stage of the target cells: enhancement of differentiation in progenitors, inhibition of function (e.g., mineralization) in mature osteoblasts (156). Exercise-induced LIF acts on periosteal osteoblast in order to modulate their activity (157).

IL-7 is essential for T-cell and B-cell development (136) but it is also expressed by the contracting muscles where it acts paracrinally to induce migration in satellite cells (158). As such, IL-7 mediates the oestrogens deficiency-induced bone loss: it induces RANKL and TNFα expression in T-cells (159) and, hence, it activates mature osteoclast and stimulates the progenitors differentiation (160) as also observed *in vivo* in mice following systemic administration (161). It also promotes survival and differentiation of dendritic cells, B220+ subset, into osteoclasts (162). However, despite their beneficial effects on bone, exercise and training seem to increase the SKM expression of IL-7. Indeed, plasma IL-7 has been found to be induced, in elite female soccer players, after a 90-min soccer games (163), 30-min post resistance exercise but not after 12 weeks of resistance training (164), while the mRNA expression level was induced in SKM by 11-week long strength training (158). Therefore, as IL-6, the biological significance of SKM- and IS-derived IL-7 resides into basal-to-peak ratio (3).

In addition, IL-15 is considered an exercise-related myokine although the effect of exercise on its expression and secretion by the SKM are not well-understood. Current evidences account for a role of IL-15 in the first phase of adaptation to exercise since it has been found upregulated (in muscle and in blood) in inactive/normally active subjects following an acute bout of exercise but not following the completion of a training program (165). Indeed, IL-15 mRNA expression in SKM was not affected by a 3-h treadmill run in trained subjects (marathon runners) (166) as well as in healthy physically active men after 3-h cycling (167). However, despite no changes in plasma levels after 12-week endurance training, the protein content in SKM was increased (167). Increased blood IL-15 was found after a 30-min run on a treadmill at 70% of maximum heart rate in untrained healthy young men (168), acute resistance exercise in young healthy inactive subjects but not after 10-week chronic training (169) as well as SKM mRNA, in healthy normally active men, after an heavy bout resistance exercise (170). IL-15 is a powerful inducer of TNF-α expression, and hence of RANKL, in osteoblasts and stromal cells, resulting in enhanced osteoclastogenesis. Furthermore, in rat bone marrow cultures, it stimulates pre-osteoclasts differentiation independently from TNF-α (171). IL-15 acts synergistically with RANKL in osteoclastogenesis by activating ERK (172). These data suggest that IL-15 positively regulate osteoclastogenesis (173).

Myostatin, is a member of the transforming growth factor beta (TGF-β) superfamily [also known as growth-differentiation factor (GDF)-8], negatively regulates SKM hypertrophy and hyperplasia (174) and it may cause SKM mass loss during aging (sarcopenia) and with metabolic and inflammatory conditions (175, 176). As such it is negatively regulated by PA (acute endurance (177), acute resistance (178–180), chronic (6-month) aerobic training in overweight and obese men (181). The recovery strategy seems to have in determining the net effect of exercise (182). Different factors act as antagonist of myostatin and among them follistatin (FST) (183), follistatin-like 1 (FSTL1) (184), and decorin (185). Acute resistance exercise did not affect follistatin mRNA expression in SKM from lean young and old men (180) while it had enhancing effects in postmenopausal women (179). Decorin mRNA expression in SKM was induced by chronic combined strength and endurance training (186) but also by acute endurance exercise (187) and, in terms of plasma levels, by acute resistance exercise (186). FSTL1 plasma levels were increased in young healthy men after acute endurance exercise (188) while chronic strength training induced mRNA expression in SKM (189). Myostatin has direct effects on osteoclastogenesis (190). Indeed, osteoclasts number on trabecular bone surfaces is increased in unloading conditions in both wild-type and myostatin KO mice (191), however myostatin deficiency suppresses subperiosteal resorption with unloading, suggesting that at least a part of the effects myostatin on osteoclasts are localized to the muscle-bone interface (192). Wnt-independent bone resorption consequent to strong endurance effort (e.g., ultramarathon) has been associated to increased myostatin and decreased FST (193). FST and its related factors (FSTL1, FSTL3, decorin) are induced by exercise and their importance in bone and muscle development is evidenced in the severe phenotypes consequent to their mutation. Fstl3$^{-/-}$ mice experienced frequent fractures together with the loss of mechanosensitivity which led to the loss of bone gain and Sost response to exercise. Importantly, a decreased FSTL3 expression is associated with aging (176). FST is induced by hyper-gravity and inhibited by microgravity (194).

Although its indisputable role as a myokine (195), brain-derived neurotrophic factor (BDNF) is mostly expressed in the brain, as is its receptor (196, 197), indeed 70–80% of the circulating protein origins from brain (9). BDNF plasma levels are raised by acute endurance and high-intensity, but not low-intensity, exercise in both males and females (195, 198–200) and also in response to chronic endurance training in young adult males (201). On the other hand, 10-week chronic resistance exercise did not affect BDNF serum levels compared to physically inactive (202). Interestingly, BDNF plasma concentrations were found to be lower in young compared to middle-aged women. After high-intensity resistance exercise BDNF follows a biphasic response featured by a decrease 1 h and an increase 24 h post exercise (203). On the contrary, 12-week moderate aerobic training (nordic walking) increased circulating BDNF in middle-aged women in association with improvement in cognitive functions (204). The BDNF receptor, TrkB, is expressed by active trabecular osteoblasts, growth plate hypertrophic chondrocytes during intramembranous ossification, and in osteoblasts and endothelial cells in fracture healing site (205, 206). Mice BDNF conditional KO in brain, beside the metabolic phenotype (hyperphagia, increased abdominal AT, obesity, leptin resistance), displayed increased femur length, high BMD and BMC (207).

The chemokine MCP-1 (also known as CCL2) is the primary ligand for the CCR2 receptor, which is normally expressed on monocyte/macrophages. As such it is a key regulator of osteoclastogenesis and has a pivotal role in inflammation and tumor-induced osteolysis (208). It is also an adipo-myokine acting as chemoattractant for monocytes and T lymphocytes (209). MCP-1 expression in SKM is strongly induced by acute and chronic resistance exercise, in terms of both mRNA and protein (164, 210), in healthy young and elderly (211). Also acute endurance activities (70% VO_2max for 40 min, high-intensity treadmill running) increase mRNA expression in SKM in lean, obese, and T2DM (164), and circulating protein in well-trained male runners subjects (212). Therefore, expression of MCP-1 seems to be influenced by the intensity of the exercise rather than the kind of activity. Moreover, MCP-1 is affected by acute exercise while its response is not affected by training in both young and elderly healthy subjects, males and females, regardless the type of activity (211, 213).

The pro-inflammatory TNFα, the prototypic early mediator of local inflammation and initiator of the acute phase response, is expressed, other than from the immune cells, also by AT and SKM. In the AT, its expression is related to the fat mass (140) while in the SKM, the mRNA expression is inhibited following training (endurance and resistance) (214, 215). The muscle expression is neither affected by the metabolic status, being comparable between lean, overweight, and T2DM, nor by acute exercise (141, 216, 217). Circulating TNFα concentrations, however, are inversely related with the amount of PA (218) but, contrarily to moderate-intensity exercise, high-intensive training causes a temporary rise in systemic inflammation (e.g., TNFα) during recovery in response to muscle damage (10) as a propaedeutic step needed for the following regeneration (219). TNF-α is a powerful stimulus for bone resorption and is strikingly implicated in inflammatory bone diseases (220). By activating NF-κB signaling, it induces osteoclast differentiation form progenitors in the presence of M-CSF and in the absence of RANKL (221) and it also enhance RANKL sensitivity in osteoclast progenitors by inducing the expression of RANK (222). TNF-α can accelerate RANKL-dependent osteoclastogenesis by activating NF-κB and AP-1 throughout TRAF2/5 and MAPKs cascades (223) and RANKL enhances TNFα-induced osteoclastogenesis via TRAF6-independent signaling (224). TNF-α stimulates osteoclastogenesis also indirectly by inducing the expression of M-CSF and RANKL stromal cells, osteoblasts, and activated T cells (161, 225).

Visfatin/NAMP (alternatively known as pre-B cell colony-enhancing factor, PEBF) (226) is synthesized as both an intracellular form, acting as nicotinamide phosphoribosyltransferase (eNAMPT) in NAD biosynthesis, and extracellular one, visfatin, mainly secreted by the visceral AT, acting as an insulin-mimetic, pro-inflammatory/immuno-modulating adipokine (227). Its circulating levels are associated with obesity/fat mass, insulin resistance (228), and the energy-bone crosstalk (57). NAMPT expression was two-fold higher in SKM of athletes compared to that found in SKM from sedentary obese, non-obese, and T2DM subjects (229). However, in obese (>30 kg/m^2) men no difference circulating visfatin concentrations were found between subjects with high and low cardiorespiratory fitness (230). NAMPT mRNA expression and protein content in the SKM of the exercising leg was doubled compared to the non-exercising limb, of non-obese sedentary individuals after 3 weeks of one-legged endurance exercise training endurance training (231). Acute exercise, instead, affects eNAMPT/visfatin in an intensity-dependent manner: 3-h cycling at 60% VO_2max had no effect (232) while an acute bout of high-intensity running-based anaerobic sprint exercise had an inductive effect (233). *In vitro* visfatin stimulates osteoblast proliferation through the activation of insulin-receptor (234), induces osteoblastic differentiation in association with inhibition of OC expression (235), inhibits osteoclastogenesis throughout the suppression of RANK and NF-AT pathways (236), stimulates adipogenesis in mesenchymal stem cells (MSC) throughout the induction of PPAR-γ (237). Plasma visfatin did not differ between less than moderately trained subjects and experienced ultramarathon runners but, in this latter group it was two-fold induced after a mountain ultramarathon (39). Similarly, despite the worse metabolic profile, sedentary subjects had comparable serum visfatin concentration than professional rowers (238). Patients with metabolic syndrome had higher plasma visfatin than their age-matched counterparts which was correlated with lumbar spine BMD in men (239).Furthermore, in different women population (Chinese, Iranian) visfatin independently predicted BMD (240, 241) although it was not correlated with either BMD or BMC in a cohort of adolescent female athletes, participating in different sports (242).

Adiponectin is a prototypic adipokines that increases fatty acid oxidation and glucose uptake in SKM while inhibiting hepatic gluconeogenesis (243) and its circulating levels are inversely related to BMI and adiposity (244). It has anti-inflammatory effects since it inhibits expression and secretion of TNFα in macrophages and induces the expression of IL-10 (245, 246). Although it is considered a classical adipokine, adiponectin is also expressed by the SKM (247, 248). Plasma adiponectin levels are decreased in obesity and insulin resistance but the SKM expression of its receptors (AdipoR1 and R2) is increased (249). Acute exercise has no clear effects on circulating adiponectin with researches depicting inductive (250, 251), depressing (141) or no effects (252–256), regardless the metabolic state of the subjects. Contrarily, in healthy lean and overweight and obese subjects with impaired glucose tolerance, endurance training increased plasma adiponectin levels and induced the expression of AdipoR1/R2 in SKM (257). In highly-trained professional cyclists, plasma adiponectin was increased during a 3-week stage race (38). Fatouros and co-workers, instead, reported that high-intensity, but not moderate-intensity, either acute or chronic resistance exercise increased plasma adiponectin levels (258, 259), suggest that exercise intensity is a key determinant of the regulation of adiponectin release in blood. Among the adipokines, adiponectin is the most closely associated with BMD (negative) and fracture risk (positively) regardless gender and menopausal status (260). Hence, it exerts negative effects on bone mass although it is inversely associated with fat mass, promotes insulin sensitivity, and fat oxidation. However, bone osteocalcin induces adiponectin expression in adipocytes that, in turn, improves glucose tolerance (261, 262). AdipoRs and adiponectin are expressed by osteoblasts and osteoclasts (263, 264). Current evidences suggest that adiponectin acts autocrinally/paracrinally to simulate osteoblast function, while systemic adiponectin has inhibitory effects on osteoblasts activity while enhances osteoclastogenesis (265, 266).

Leptin is another adipokine involved in the regulation of energy homeostasis (267) it is an adiposity signal that suppresses appetite. As for adiponectin, also leptin is expressed in SKM (268) but the relative contribution of AT and SKM to circulating leptin has been not fully understood (165). Leptin and leptin receptor KO mice (ob$^{-/-}$ and db$^{-/-}$) which are obese have also higher bone mass and intracerebroventricular infusions improved the metabolic status and reverted the high bone mass phenotype (269). Leptin effects on bone formation are mediated by the sympathetic nervous system (SNS), independently from AT, indeed by high bone mass phenotype obtained following the inhibition adrenergic signaling cannot corrected by intracerebroventricular infusion of leptin (270, 271). In strenuous exercise-induced hypogonadal women, leptin induced oestrogens that partially improved the bone phenotype (272). Circulating leptin was decreased in highly trained professional cyclists during a 3-week stage race (38) and in experienced ultramarathon runners after a mountain ultramarathon (39). However, in these runners resting levels of leptin were significantly lower than their less than moderately trained counterparts (39). Interestingly, in competing professional cyclists the decrease in leptin was associated with increased bone resorption and GluOC-to-GlaOC ratio (38). Similarly, 8-week aerobic training decreased fat mass and leptin, improved insulin sensitivity, and increased both total OC and GluOC in obese young males experienced (273). On the contrary, in competing ultramarathon runners, a comparable trend in leptin was associated with a reduced GluOC-to-GlaOC ratio (39). Finally, soluble leptin, insulin, and OC were increased by bed rest independently from resistive vibration exercises (274). These data indicate that load may regulate leptin release. Leptin mRNA expression in AT after acute endurance exercise were found either unaffected (275) or decreased in lean and overweight subjects (141). Several studies have shown a delayed (24–48 h post exercise) reduction of circulating leptin levels in healthy active men (276–279). Taken together, the current evidences suggest that exercise training decreases plasma leptin levels, while is ineffective on mRNA expression in AT (165). Weight loss in elderly obese accelerated bone turnover but PA can attenuates BMD decrease and stimulated a greater decrease in circulating leptin (280). The detrimental bony effects of leptin also depends upon its pro-inflammatory action: stimulation of neutrophil chemotaxis and phagocytic function, induction of pro-inflammatory cytokines in monocytes, and induction of T helper (Th)-1 cytokines (246). These data suggest that the exercise-dependent beneficial effects on bone may be also mediated by the exercise-dependent reduction in circulating leptin (3).

Resistin, an inflammatory marker, is positively associated with fat mass, waist circumference, and obesity-related diseases, and it causes oxidative stress and nitric oxide production downregulating, thus, determining endothelial dysfunction (281, 282). Both circulating levels and AT mRNA expression are not affected by acute endurance training in overweight and lean males (141, 253). However, the baseline training status of the subjects seems to affect the resistance exercise-dependent response to exercise with regularly training subjects experiencing a decrease over 6 months (281). Also osteoclasts, osteoblasts, and bone marrow-derived MSC express resistin, and *in vitro* it may stimulate both osteoclastogenesis and osteoblastogenesis (234, 235). Similarly to visfatin, resistin induces PPAR-γ expression in MSC and, thus, the adipogenic differentiation (237). It has been negatively associated with BMD (240, 283), although not definitively (284–286), and in postmenopause its circulating levels are doubled compared to premenopause (287). Resistin correlated positively with previous osteoporotic fractures and much more in the presence of diabetes (288).

Irisin is a newly discovered myokine released into the circulation following the cleavage, mediated by unknown proteases, of the transmembrane glycoprotein fibronectin type III domain containing 5 (FNDC5). In target cells, mainly white adipocytes, it induces the expression of the mitochondrial uncoupling protein 1 (Ucp1) that uncouples the respiratory chain from the oxidative phosphorylation: the energy derived from the oxidation of energy substrates (e.g., carbohydrates, fatty acids), and generated by the passage along electrochemical gradient of the electrons, is released as heat. This process normally occurs in the thermogenic BAT rather than in fat-storing WAT. Irisin induces a metabolic shift in the white adipocytes, namely browning, making them expressing an intermediate beige phenotype (289). Irisin is induced by exercise and its circulating levels are higher in trained, males and young subjects than in sedentary, females, and elderly, as a function of the muscle mass and the muscle activation level (290). Along with animal studies (291), researches in human have highlighted that high-intensity acute exercise (292), endurance training (293, 294), cold exposure (295), lifestyle changes as in obese children (296) and pregnant women (297) all increase blood irisin in association with an improved metabolic status. However, these results have not been always replicated and there are still doubts about its physiology (182, 291). Such discrepancies could be, at least partially, imputed to the methodological issues emerged about some commercially available immunoassays when compared to the gold standard mass spectrometry-based method (298). Irisin is also expressed by the AT and respond to PA as for its muscle counterpart (299, 300). Other than being directly induced by exercise, irisin expression is regulated by several exercise-modulated factors such as BDNF, myostatin, follistatin, TGFβ, FFAs, cytokines, betatrophin (291). Irisin could be a link between exercise and BDNF expression (289). Indeed, 30-day voluntary free running-wheel induced FNDC5 expression in mice hippocampus, which in turn into and increased expression of BDNF (301). This correlation might support the neuroprotective effects of exercise. Still, data directly evaluating the impact of exercise (especially in human), its time duration and intensity on irisin, BDNF, and cognitive function are unclear. By affecting adiposity, irisin can improve the inflammatory status and, recently, a direct relationship between irisin concentrations and inflammatory markers in metabolic syndrome has been described (302). Irisin is involved in the SKM-bone endocrine connection and it its involvement in bone mass gain in muscle disease-associated osteopenia has been proposed (303). Irisin levels have been, indeed, associated with osteoporotic fractures in postmenopausal women (304) with an inverse correlation with fat mass and PA status (305). *In vitro*, irisin promotes osteoblast differentiation while *in vivo* it induces osteoblast proliferation and differentiation, inhibits osteoclast activity, increases cortical BMD (306), and prevents muscle atrophy-induced bone loss (307).

Adaptive Immunity Activation and Bone Metabolism

Besides the role of innate immunity, several examples exist about the interplay between bone and IS. First of all, as already stated, osteoclasts are monocytic/macrophagic origin and M-CSF, a key cytokine for this lineage is also important in osteoclast differentiation (308) and antigen-presenting cells, such as dendritic cells, retain the capability to transdifferentiate into bone-resorbing osteoclasts (309, 310). Moreover, several soluble mediators regulate osteoblasts and osteoclasts differentiation and activity (311). Interestingly, a subset of osteogenic cells, called N-cadherin-positive spindle-shaped osteoblasts are an integral part of the hematopoietic stem cell (HSC) niche and solve a key role in the maintenance of the HSC pool that gives rise to all blood and immune cells (312).

When activate, under inflammatory conditions (e.g., autoimmune diseases, inflammatory bowel diseases, periodontal infections), T- and B-lymphocytes secrete RANKL and TNFα that stimulate osteoclast differentiation and function and, therefore, bone resorption (313). However, under physiological conditions, B-cells represent an important source of the osteoclast inhibitor OPG. For instance, human tonsil B-cells secrete OPG and the activation of the CD40 costimulatory pathway on these cells, *in vitro*, further induced OPG expression (314); parallel, bone marrow B-cells contribute up to 64% of the total OPG, in mice (315). Consequently, B-cells KO mice experienced increased bone resorption rate, reduced BMD and bone mass, in association with low circulating OPG; the restoration of the B-cells pool into young B-cell prevented the bone phenotype. The ligand of CD40, CD40L, is mainly expressed by activated T-cells and the deletion of either CD40 or CD40L on T-cells caused a powerful inhibition of OPG expression in B-cells and bone loss (315). It is, thus, suggested that under physiological conditions B-cells, regulated by the T-cells co-stimulatory action, protect the skeleton by secreting OPG, while under inflammatory conditions B- and T-cells negatively affect bone metabolism by secreting RANKL and inflammatory cytokines (316).

Postmenopause-related estrogen deficiency gives an explicative example. Indeed, oestrogens mediate powerful anti-inflammatory effects and loss of estrogen causes significant proliferation of T- and B-lymphocytes (129, 317). This was demonstrated by the fact that while ovariectomized wild-type rats experienced bone loss, T-cell-deficient null mice were protected by osteoclastic bone resorption (318). RANKL is secreted by activated T but not in conditions of estrogen deficiency, in mice. Contrary, in this condition, circulating and tissue TNFα is raised (318, 319) and TNFα and TNFRI (p55) KO in mice prevented ovariectomy-induced bone loss (318). In agreement to this model, estrogen loss causes the expansion of TNFα-secreting T-cells and TNFα sustains and amplifies the RANKL-induced osteoclast-mediated bone resorption (320). IL-7 expression in several tissues anticipates T-cells expansion (321); this cytokine increases the sensitivity of T-cells to otherwise tolerogenic antigens and, hence, decreases the antigen-dependent T-cell activation threshold (320). Consequently, the differentiation of T-cells into the different T helper subsets (i.e., Th1) leads to TNFα secretion along with IFNγ, that upregulates the expression of CIITA in macrophage, a transcription factor that in turn upregulates MHCII expression and, hence, antigen presentation to T-cells, further amplifying T-cells activation (317). Also the Th17 subset is induced in this process; these cells secrete IL-17A a pro-osteoclastogenic cytokine that induces expression RANKL in osteoblasts. IL-17 expression is raised by ovariectomy (322): treatment with anti-IL-17 antibodies (323) or the IL-17 gene deletion (324) improves bone loss in ovariectomized mice. The downregulation of TGFβ is another step in this process. TGFβ is expressed in response to oestrogens and has immunosuppressive effects by inducing regulatory T-cells (Tregs) that down-regulate T-cells activation (316).

Importantly, T-cell activation-dependent ovariectomy-induced bone loss depends upon antigen stimulation. Indeed, ovariectomy in mice with silenced antigen presentation due to a mutated T-cell receptor, only responsive to chicken ovalbumin: when no antigen is presented, mice were fully protected from ovariectomy-induced bone loss while, after exogenous administration of ovalbumin (i.e., the antigen) the bone response was retained (317). Evidence suggests that, in human, these antigens are derived from the gut microbiota (325, 326) since the gut permeability is regulated by oestrogens (326).

T-cells are critical in the mechanisms of action of parathyroid Hormone (PTH) in bone (327). Chronic elevated production of PTH (hyperparathyroidism, HPT) causes skeletal and extra-skeletal diseases: primary HPT (PHPT) is associated with increased bone turnover and osteopenia (328), while secondary HPT (SHPT) is involved in the pathogenesis of age-associated osteoporosis (329). Continuous PTH infusion mimics PHPT and SHPT, while intermittent administration has pro-anabolic effects on bone (330). T-cells express PTH-1R, the functional G protein coupled PTH receptor and they may contribute to the catabolic effect of PTH, *in vivo* (327, 331). Continuous PTH treatment at doses that mimic HPT failed to induce osteoclast formation, bone resorption, and cortical bone depletion in mice deficient for T-cells (331). On the contrary, intermittent PTH stimulates Wnt10b expression in bone marrow CD8+ T-cells and activate the canonical Wnt signaling in pre-osteoblasts (332).

Currently, there are no available study depicting the effects of the exercise on the relationship between adaptive IS and bone cell function. Hence, in order to improve the use of PA as a therapy for bone loss it is necessary to increase the knowledge in this field.

PRACTICAL IMPLICATIONS, CONCLUSIONS, AND PERSPECTIVES

The complex net of physiological connections linking bone metabolism and IS branches in relationship with physical exercise is, now, only a little depicted. The great majority of the current knowledge concern the inflammation-mediated effects of PA while, only a few is known about the adaptive immunity-mediated effects.

Chronic PA is a powerful stimulus for bone and lifelong exercising is the most effective strategy to improve bone mass (in childhood and adolescence) and to keep bone health (in adulthood and older ages). However, there is no consensus on the best kind of PA to be prescribed at this purpose. There are evidences that sustain the effectiveness of load and impact and this is further improved when the activity is carried on in an intermittent way (54). Therefore, the role of loading is central in this discussion but, importantly, the direct effect of the applied forces onto the skeleton on the immune function are not known and this point must be developed in the next years.

AUTHOR CONTRIBUTIONS

GL conception, drafting, and reviewing the article. EZ drafting and reviewing the article. GB drafting and reviewing.

FUNDING

This work has been funded by an unrestricted grant from the Italian Ministry of Health and grant from the National Science Centre (Poland) No. 2018/29/B/NZ7/02094.

REFERENCES

1. McLaughlin M, Jacobs I. Exercise is medicine, but does it interfere with medicine? *Exerc Sport Sci Rev.* (2017) 45:127–35. doi: 10.1249/JES.0000000000000111
2. Banfi G, Lombardi G, Colombini A, Lippi G. Bone metabolism markers in sports medicine. *Sports Med.* (2010) 40:697–714. doi: 10.2165/11533090-000000000-00000
3. Lombardi G, Sanchis-Gomar F, Perego S, Sansoni V, Banfi G. Implications of exercise-induced adipo-myokines in bone metabolism. *Endocrine* (2016) 54:284–305. doi: 10.1007/s12020-015-0834-0
4. Daly RM, Duckham RL, Gianoudis J. Evidence for an interaction between exercise and nutrition for improving bone and muscle health. *Curr Osteoporos Rep.* (2014) 12:219–26. doi: 10.1007/s11914-014-0207-2
5. Terashima A, Takayanagi H. Overview of osteoimmunology. *Calcif Tissue Int.* (2018) 102:503–11. doi: 10.1007/s00223-018-0417-1
6. Miller PD, Bolognese MA, Lewiecki EM, McClung MR, Ding B, Austin M, et al. Effect of denosumab on bone density and turnover in postmenopausal women with low bone mass after long-term continued, discontinued, and restarting of therapy: a randomized blinded phase 2 clinical trial. *Bone* (2008) 43:222–9. doi: 10.1016/j.bone.2008.04.007
7. McClung MR, Lewiecki EM, Geller ML, Bolognese MA, Peacock M, Weinstein RL, et al. Effect of denosumab on bone mineral density and biochemical markers of bone turnover: 8-year results of a phase 2 clinical trial. *Osteoporos Int.* (2013) 24:227–35. doi: 10.1007/s00198-012-2052-4
8. Cosman F, de Beur SJ, LeBoff MS, Lewiecki EM, Tanner B, Randall S, et al. Clinician's guide to prevention and treatment of osteoporosis. *Osteoporos Int.* (2014) 25:2359–81. doi: 10.1007/s00198-014-2794-2
9. Bekker PJ, Holloway DL, Rasmussen AS, Murphy R, Martin SW, Leese PT, et al. A single-dose placebo-controlled study of AMG 162, a fully human monoclonal antibody to RANKL, in postmenopausal women. *J Bone Miner Res.* (2004) 19:1059–66. doi: 10.1359/JBMR.040305
10. Pedersen BK, Akerstrom TC, Nielsen AR, Fischer CP. Role of myokines in exercise and metabolism. *J Appl Physiol.* (2007) 103:1093–8. doi: 10.1152/japplphysiol.00080.2007
11. Weigert C, Hoene M, Plomgaard P. Hepatokines-a novel group of exercise factors. *Pflugers Arch.* (2018). doi: 10.1007/s00424-018-2216-y. [Epub Ahead of Print].
12. Petersen AM, Pedersen BK. The anti-inflammatory effect of exercise. *J Appl Physiol.* (2005) 98:1154–62. doi: 10.1152/japplphysiol.00164.2004
13. Rivera-Brown AM, Frontera WR. Principles of exercise physiology: responses to acute exercise and long-term adaptations to training. *PM R* (2012) 4:797–804. doi: 10.1016/j.pmrj.2012.10.007
14. Caspersen CJ, Powell KE, Christenson GM. Physical activity, exercise, and physical fitness: definitions and distinctions for health-related research. *Public Health Rep.* (1985) 100:126–31.
15. Hawley JA. Molecular responses to strength and endurance training: are they incompatible? *Appl Physiol Nutr Metab.* (2009) 34:355–61. doi: 10.1139/H09-023
16. Frost HM. Bone's mechanostat: a 2003 update. *Anat Rec A Discov Mol Cell Evol Biol.* (2003) 275:1081–101. doi: 10.1002/ar.a.10119
17. Price JS, Sugiyama T, Galea GL, Meakin LB, Sunters A, Lanyon LE. Role of endocrine and paracrine factors in the adaptation of bone to mechanical loading. *Curr Osteoporos Rep.* (2011) 9:76–82. doi: 10.1007/s11914-011-0050-7
18. Rubin CT. Skeletal strain and the functional significance of bone architecture. *Calcif Tissue Int.* (1984) 36(Suppl. 1):S11–8. doi: 10.1007/BF02406128
19. Kjaer M, Jorgensen NR, Heinemeier K, Magnusson SP. Exercise and regulation of bone and collagen tissue biology. *Prog Mol Biol Transl Sci.* (2015) 135:259–91. doi: 10.1016/bs.pmbts.2015.07.008
20. Katsumi A, Orr AW, Tzima E, Schwartz MA. Integrins in mechanotransduction. *J Biol Chem.* (2004) 279:12001–4. doi: 10.1074/jbc.R300038200
21. Duncan RL, Hruska KA, Misler S. Parathyroid hormone activation of stretch-activated cation channels in osteosarcoma cells (UMR-106.01). *FEBS Lett.* (1992) 307:219–23. doi: 10.1016/0014-5793(92)80771-8
22. Coughlin TR, Voisin M, Schaffler MB, Niebur GL, McNamara LM. Primary cilia exist in a small fraction of cells in trabecular bone and marrow. *Calcif Tissue Int.* (2015) 96:65–72. doi: 10.1007/s00223-014-9928-6
23. Zayzafoon M, Gathings WE, McDonald JM. Modeled microgravity inhibits osteogenic differentiation of human mesenchymal stem cells and increases adipogenesis. *Endocrinology* (2004) 145:2421–32. doi: 10.1210/en.2003-1156
24. David V, Martin A, Lafage-Proust MH, Malaval L, Peyroche S, Jones DB, et al. Mechanical loading down-regulates peroxisome proliferator-activated receptor gamma in bone marrow stromal cells and favors osteoblastogenesis at the expense of adipogenesis. *Endocrinology* (2007) 148:2553–62. doi: 10.1210/en.2006-1704
25. Xiong J, Onal M, Jilka RL, Weinstein RS, Manolagas SC, O'Brien CA. Matrix-embedded cells control osteoclast formation. *Nat Med.* (2011) 17:1235–41. doi: 10.1038/nm.2448
26. Lombardi G, Lanteri P, Colombini A, Mariotti M, Banfi G. Sclerostin concentrations in athletes: role of load and gender. *J Biol Regul Homeost Agents* (2012) 26:157–63.
27. Qin YX, Hu M. Mechanotransduction in musculoskeletal tissue regeneration: effects of fluid flow, loading, and cellular-molecular pathways. *Biomed Res Int.* (2014) 2014:863421. doi: 10.1155/2014/863421
28. Jorgensen NR, Henriksen Z, Brot C, Eriksen EF, Sorensen OH, Civitelli R, et al. Human osteoblastic cells propagate intercellular calcium signals by two different mechanisms. *J Bone Miner Res.* (2000) 15:1024–32. doi: 10.1359/jbmr.2000.15.6.1024

29. Jorgensen NR, Henriksen Z, Sorensen OH, Eriksen EF, Civitelli R, Steinberg TH. Intercellular calcium signaling occurs between human osteoblasts and osteoclasts and requires activation of osteoclast P2X7 receptors. *J Biol Chem.* (2002) 277:7574–80. doi: 10.1074/jbc.M104608200
30. McCarthy I. The physiology of bone blood flow: a review. *J Bone Joint Surg Am.* (2006) 88(Suppl. 3):4–9. doi: 10.2106/00004623-200611001-00002
31. Feng X, McDonald JM. Disorders of bone remodeling. *Annu Rev Pathol.* (2011) 6:121–45. doi: 10.1146/annurev-pathol-011110-130203
32. Heinonen I, Kemppainen J, Kaskinoro K, Langberg H, Knuuti J, Boushel R, et al. Bone blood flow and metabolism in humans: effect of muscular exercise and other physiological perturbations. *J Bone Miner Res.* (2013) 28:1068–74. doi: 10.1002/jbmr.1833
33. Heinonen I, Kalliokoski KK, Hannukainen JC, Duncker DJ, Nuutila P, Knuuti J. Organ-specific physiological responses to acute physical exercise and long-term training in humans. *Physiology (Bethesda)* (2014) 29:421–36. doi: 10.1152/physiol.00067.2013
34. Schuler G, Adams V, Goto Y. Role of exercise in the prevention of cardiovascular disease: results, mechanisms, and new perspectives. *Eur Heart J.* (2013) 34:1790–9. doi: 10.1093/eurheartj/eht111
35. Laufs U, Werner N, Link A, Endres M, Wassmann S, Jurgens K, et al. Physical training increases endothelial progenitor cells, inhibits neointima formation, and enhances angiogenesis. *Circulation* (2004) 109:220–6. doi: 10.1161/01.CIR.0000109141.48980.37
36. Katayama Y, Battista M, Kao WM, Hidalgo A, Peired AJ, Thomas SA, et al. Signals from the sympathetic nervous system regulate hematopoietic stem cell egress from bone marrow. *Cell* (2006) 124:407–21. doi: 10.1016/j.cell.2005.10.041
37. Ham J, Evans BA. An emerging role for adenosine and its receptors in bone homeostasis. *Front Endocrinol.* (2012) 3:113. doi: 10.3389/fendo.2012.00113
38. Lombardi G, Lanteri P, Graziani G, Colombini A, Banfi G, Corsetti R. Bone and energy metabolism parameters in professional cyclists during the Giro d'Italia 3-weeks stage race. *PLoS ONE* (2012) 7:e42077. doi: 10.1371/journal.pone.0042077
39. Sansoni V, Vernillo G, Perego S, Barbuti A, Merati G, Schena F, et al. Bone turnover response is linked to both acute and established metabolic changes in ultra-marathon runners. *Endocrine* (2017) 56:196–204. doi: 10.1007/s12020-016-1012-8
40. Burr DB, Robling AG, Turner CH. Effects of biomechanical stress on bones in animals. *Bone* (2002) 30:781–6. doi: 10.1016/S8756-3282(02)00707-X
41. Rubin CT, Lanyon LE. Regulation of bone formation by applied dynamic loads. *J Bone Joint Surg Am.* (1984) 66:397–402. doi: 10.2106/00004623-198466030-00012
42. Rubin CT, Lanyon LE. Regulation of bone mass by mechanical strain magnitude. *Calcif Tissue Int.* (1985) 37:411–7. doi: 10.1007/BF02553711
43. Robling AG, Burr DB, Turner CH. Partitioning a daily mechanical stimulus into discrete loading bouts improves the osteogenic response to loading. *J Bone Miner Res.* (2000) 15:1596–602. doi: 10.1359/jbmr.2000.15.8.1596
44. Srinivasan S, Weimer DA, Agans SC, Bain SD, Gross TS. Low-magnitude mechanical loading becomes osteogenic when rest is inserted between each load cycle. *J Bone Miner Res.* (2002) 17:1613–20. doi: 10.1359/jbmr.2002.17.9.1613
45. Kennedy OD, Laudier DM, Majeska RJ, Sun HB, Schaffler MB. Osteocyte apoptosis is required for production of osteoclastogenic signals following bone fatigue *in vivo*. *Bone* (2014) 64:132–7. doi: 10.1016/j.bone.2014.03.049
46. Bareither ML, Troy KL, Grabiner MD. Bone mineral density of the proximal femur is not related to dynamic joint loading during locomotion in young women. *Bone* (2006) 38:125–9. doi: 10.1016/j.bone.2005.07.003
47. Dowthwaite JN, Rosenbaum PF, Scerpella TA. Mechanical loading during growth is associated with plane-specific differences in vertebral geometry: a cross-sectional analysis comparing artistic gymnasts vs. non-gymnasts. *Bone* (2011) 49:1046–54. doi: 10.1016/j.bone.2011.07.033
48. Kontulainen S, Sievanen H, Kannus P, Pasanen M, Vuori I. Effect of long-term impact-loading on mass, size, and estimated strength of humerus and radius of female racquet-sports players: a peripheral quantitative computed tomography study between young and old starters and controls. *J Bone Miner Res.* (2003) 18:352–9. doi: 10.1359/jbmr.2003.18.2.352
49. Heinonen A, Sievanen H, Kyrolainen H, Perttunen J, Kannus P. Mineral mass, size, and estimated mechanical strength of triple jumpers' lower limb. *Bone* (2001) 29:279–85. doi: 10.1016/S8756-3282(01)00574-9
50. Bhatia VA, Edwards WB, Johnson JE, Troy KL. Short-term bone formation is greatest within high strain regions of the human distal radius: a prospective pilot study. *J Biomech Eng.* (2015) 137. doi: 10.1115/1.4028847
51. Lambers FM, Schulte FA, Kuhn G, Webster DJ, Muller R. Mouse tail vertebrae adapt to cyclic mechanical loading by increasing bone formation rate and decreasing bone resorption rate as shown by time-lapsed in vivo imaging of dynamic bone morphometry. *Bone* (2011) 49:1340–50. doi: 10.1016/j.bone.2011.08.035
52. Nikander R, Sievanen H, Heinonen A, Kannus P. Femoral neck structure in adult female athletes subjected to different loading modalities. *J Bone Miner Res.* (2005) 20:520–8. doi: 10.1359/JBMR.041119
53. Howe TE, Shea B, Dawson LJ, Downie F, Murray A, Ross C, et al. Exercise for preventing and treating osteoporosis in postmenopausal women. *Cochrane Database Syst Rev.* (2011) CD000333. doi: 10.1002/14651858.CD000333.pub2
54. Xu J, Lombardi G, Jiao W, Banfi G. Effects of exercise on bone status in female subjects, from young girls to postmenopausal women: an overview of systematic reviews and meta-analyses. *Sports Med.* (2016) 46:1165–82. doi: 10.1007/s40279-016-0494-0
55. Motyl KJ, McCabe LR, Schwartz AV. Bone and glucose metabolism: a two-way street. *Arch Biochem Biophys.* (2010) 503:2–10. doi: 10.1016/j.abb.2010.07.030
56. Karsenty G, Ferron M. The contribution of bone to whole-organism physiology. *Nature* (2012) 481:314–20. doi: 10.1038/nature10763
57. Lombardi G, Perego S, Luzi L, Banfi G. A four-season molecule: osteocalcin. Updates in its physiological roles. *Endocrine* (2015) 48:394–404. doi: 10.1007/s12020-014-0401-0
58. Basso N, Heersche JN. Effects of hind limb unloading and reloading on nitric oxide synthase expression and apoptosis of osteocytes and chondrocytes. *Bone* (2006) 39:807–14. doi: 10.1016/j.bone.2006.04.014
59. Dalsky GP. The role of exercise in the prevention of osteoporosis. *Compr Ther.* (1989) 15:30–7.
60. Lee TQ, Shapiro TA, Bell DM. Biomechanical properties of human tibias in long-term spinal cord injury. *J Rehabil Res Dev.* (1997) 34:295–302.
61. Frey-Rindova P, de Bruin ED, Stussi E, Dambacher MA, Dietz V. Bone mineral density in upper and lower extremities during 12 months after spinal cord injury measured by peripheral quantitative computed tomography. *Spinal Cord* (2000) 38:26–32. doi: 10.1038/sj.sc.3100905
62. Lang T, LeBlanc A, Evans H, Lu Y, Genant H, Yu A. Cortical and trabecular bone mineral loss from the spine and hip in long-duration spaceflight. *J Bone Miner Res.* (2004) 19:1006–12. doi: 10.1359/JBMR.040307
63. Simpson RJ, Kunz H, Agha N, Graff R. Exercise and the regulation of immune functions. *Prog Mol Biol Transl Sci.* (2015) 135:355–80. doi: 10.1016/bs.pmbts.2015.08.001
64. Handschin C, Spiegelman BM. The role of exercise and PGC1alpha in inflammation and chronic disease. *Nature* (2008) 454:463–9. doi: 10.1038/nature07206
65. Beavers KM, Brinkley TE, Nicklas BJ. Effect of exercise training on chronic inflammation. *Clin Chim Acta* (2010) 411:785–93. doi: 10.1016/j.cca.2010.02.069
66. Lemanne D, Cassileth B, Gubili J. The role of physical activity in cancer prevention, treatment, recovery, and survivorship. *Oncology (Williston Park)* (2013) 27:580–5.
67. Allen J, Sun Y, Woods JA. Exercise and the regulation of inflammatory responses. *Prog Mol Biol Transl Sci.* (2015) 135:337–54. doi: 10.1016/bs.pmbts.2015.07.003
68. Vitale JA, Lombardi G, Weydahl A, Banfi G. Biological rhythms, chronodisruption and chrono-enhancement: the role of physical activity as synchronizer in correcting steroids circadian rhythm in metabolic dysfunctions and cancer. *Chronobiol Int.* (2018) 35:1185–97. doi: 10.1080/07420528.2018.1475395
69. Suarez-Bregua P, Guerreiro PM, Rotllant J. Stress, glucocorticoids and bone: a review from mammals and fish. *Front Endocrinol.* (2018) 9:526. doi: 10.3389/fendo.2018.00526

70. Paredes S, Ribeiro L. Cortisol: the villain in metabolic syndrome? *Rev Assoc Med Bras.* (2014) 60:84–92. doi: 10.1590/1806-9282.60.01.017
71. Mifsud EJ, Tan AC, Jackson DC. TLR agonists as modulators of the innate immune response and their potential as agents against infectious disease. *Front Immunol.* (2014) 5:79. doi: 10.3389/fimmu.2014.00079
72. Gleeson M, McFarlin B, Flynn M. Exercise and Toll-like receptors. *Exerc Immunol Rev.* (2006) 12:34–53.
73. Gleeson M, Bishop NC, Stensel DJ, Lindley MR, Mastana SS, Nimmo MA. The anti-inflammatory effects of exercise: mechanisms and implications for the prevention and treatment of disease. *Nat Rev Immunol.* (2011) 11:607–15. doi: 10.1038/nri3041
74. Steensberg A, Fischer CP, Keller C, Moller K, Pedersen BK. IL-6 enhances plasma IL-1ra, IL-10, and cortisol in humans. *Am J Physiol Endocrinol Metab.* (2003) 285:E433–7. doi: 10.1152/ajpendo.00074.2003
75. Pedersen BK. The diseasome of physical inactivity–and the role of myokines in muscle–fat cross talk. *J Physiol.* (2009) 587(Pt 23):5559–68. doi: 10.1113/jphysiol.2009.179515
76. Smith JK, Dykes R, Douglas JE, Krishnaswamy G, Berk S. Long-term exercise and atherogenic activity of blood mononuclear cells in persons at risk of developing ischemic heart disease. *JAMA* (1999) 281:1722–7. doi: 10.1001/jama.281.18.1722
77. Scheele C, Nielsen S, Pedersen BK. ROS and myokines promote muscle adaptation to exercise. *Trends Endocrinol Metab.* (2009) 20:95–9. doi: 10.1016/j.tem.2008.12.002
78. Trayhurn P. Hypoxia and adipose tissue function and dysfunction in obesity. *Physiol Rev.* (2013) 93:1–21. doi: 10.1152/physrev.00017.2012
79. Vieira VJ, Valentine RJ, Wilund KR, Antao N, Baynard T, Woods JA. Effects of exercise and low-fat diet on adipose tissue inflammation and metabolic complications in obese mice. *Am J Physiol Endocrinol Metab.* (2009) 296:E1164–71. doi: 10.1152/ajpendo.00054.2009
80. Walsh NP, Gleeson M, Shephard RJ, Gleeson M, Woods JA, Bishop NC, et al. Position statement. Part one: Immune function and exercise. *Exerc Immunol Rev.* (2011) 17:6–63.
81. Anane LH, Edwards KM, Burns VE, Drayson MT, Riddell NE, van Zanten JJ, et al. Mobilization of gammadelta T lymphocytes in response to psychological stress, exercise, and beta-agonist infusion. *Brain Behav Immun.* (2009) 23:823–9. doi: 10.1016/j.bbi.2009.03.003
82. Steppich B, Dayyani F, Gruber R, Lorenz R, Mack M, Ziegler-Heitbrock HW. Selective mobilization of CD14(+)CD16(+) monocytes by exercise. *Am J Physiol Cell Physiol.* (2000) 279:C578–86. doi: 10.1152/ajpcell.2000.279.3.C578
83. Peake J, Wilson G, Hordern M, Suzuki K, Yamaya K, Nosaka K, et al. Changes in neutrophil surface receptor expression, degranulation, and respiratory burst activity after moderate- and high-intensity exercise. *J Appl Physiol.* (2004) 97:612–8. doi: 10.1152/japplphysiol.01331.2003
84. Simpson RJ, Florida-James GD, Whyte GP, Guy K. The effects of intensive, moderate and downhill treadmill running on human blood lymphocytes expressing the adhesion/activation molecules CD54 (ICAM-1), CD18 (beta2 integrin) and CD53. *Eur J Appl Physiol.* (2006) 97:109–21. doi: 10.1007/s00421-006-0146-4
85. Bosch JA, Berntson GG, Cacioppo JT, Dhabhar FS, Marucha PT. Acute stress evokes selective mobilization of T cells that differ in chemokine receptor expression: a potential pathway linking immunologic reactivity to cardiovascular disease. *Brain Behav Immun.* (2003) 17:251–9. doi: 10.1016/S0889-1591(03)00054-0
86. Schedlowski M, Hosch W, Oberbeck R, Benschop RJ, Jacobs R, Raab HR, et al. Catecholamines modulate human NK cell circulation and function via spleen-independent beta 2-adrenergic mechanisms. *J Immunol.* (1996) 156:93–9.
87. Dimitrov S, Lange T, Born J. Selective mobilization of cytotoxic leukocytes by epinephrine. *J Immunol.* (2010) 184:503–11. doi: 10.4049/jimmunol.0902189
88. Ortega E. Neuroendocrine mediators in the modulation of phagocytosis by exercise: physiological implications. *Exerc Immunol Rev.* (2003) 9:70–93.
89. Nieman DC, Nehlsen-Cannarella SL, Fagoaga OR, Henson DA, Utter A, Davis JM, et al. Effects of mode and carbohydrate on the granulocyte and monocyte response to intensive, prolonged exercise. *J Appl Physiol.* (1998) 84:1252–9. doi: 10.1152/jappl.1998.84.4.1252
90. Bishop NC, Gleeson M, Nicholas CW, Ali A. Influence of carbohydrate supplementation on plasma cytokine and neutrophil degranulation responses to high intensity intermittent exercise. *Int J Sport Nutr Exerc Metab.* (2002) 12:145–56. doi: 10.1123/ijsnem.12.2.145
91. Pyne DB. Regulation of neutrophil function during exercise. *Sports Med.* (1994) 17:245–58. doi: 10.2165/00007256-199417040-00005
92. Suzuki K, Nakaji S, Yamada M, Liu Q, Kurakake S, Okamura N, et al. Impact of a competitive marathon race on systemic cytokine and neutrophil responses. *Med Sci Sports Exerc.* (2003) 35:348–55. doi: 10.1249/01.MSS.0000048861.57899.04
93. Nieman DC, Miller AR, Henson DA, Warren BJ, Gusewitch G, Johnson RL, et al. Effects of high- vs. moderate-intensity exercise on natural killer cell activity. *Med Sci Sports Exerc.* (1993) 25:1126–34. doi: 10.1249/00005768-199310000-00008
94. Bruunsgaard H, Hartkopp A, Mohr T, Konradsen H, Heron I, Mordhorst CH, et al. *In vivo* cell-mediated immunity and vaccination response following prolonged, intense exercise. *Med Sci Sports Exerc.* (1997) 29:1176–81. doi: 10.1097/00005768-199709000-00009
95. Baj Z, Kantorski J, Majewska E, Zeman K, Pokoca L, Fornalczyk E, et al. Immunological status of competitive cyclists before and after the training season. *Int J Sports Med.* (1994) 15:319–24. doi: 10.1055/s-2007-1021067
96. Gleeson M, McDonald WA, Pyne DB, Clancy RL, Cripps AW, Francis JL, et al. Immune status and respiratory illness for elite swimmers during a 12-week training cycle. *Int J Sports Med.* (2000) 21:302–7. doi: 10.1055/s-2000-313
97. Horn PL, Pyne DB, Hopkins WG, Barnes CJ. Lower white blood cell counts in elite athletes training for highly aerobic sports. *Eur J Appl Physiol.* (2010) 110:925–32. doi: 10.1007/s00421-010-1573-9
98. Hough J, Corney R, Kouris A, Gleeson M. Salivary cortisol and testosterone responses to high-intensity cycling before and after an 11-day intensified training period. *J Sports Sci.* (2013) 31:1614–23. doi: 10.1080/02640414.2013.792952
99. Simpson RJ, Lowder TW, Spielmann G, Bigley AB, LaVoy EC, Kunz H. Exercise and the aging immune system. *Ageing Res Rev.* (2012) 11:404–20. doi: 10.1016/j.arr.2012.03.003
100. Simpson RJ, Bosch JA. Special issue on exercise immunology: current perspectives on aging, health and extreme performance. *Brain Behav Immun.* (2014) 39:1–7. doi: 10.1016/j.bbi.2014.03.006
101. Kohut ML, Arntson BA, Lee W, Rozeboom K, Yoon KJ, Cunnick JE, et al. Moderate exercise improves antibody response to influenza immunization in older adults. *Vaccine* (2004) 22:2298–306. doi: 10.1016/j.vaccine.2003.11.023
102. Woods JA, Keylock KT, Lowder T, Vieira VJ, Zelkovich W, Dumich S, et al. Cardiovascular exercise training extends influenza vaccine seroprotection in sedentary older adults: the immune function intervention trial. *J Am Geriatr Soc.* (2009) 57:2183–91. doi: 10.1111/j.1532-5415.2009.02563.x
103. Perna FM, LaPerriere A, Klimas N, Ironson G, Perry A, Pavone J, et al. Cardiopulmonary and CD4 cell changes in response to exercise training in early symptomatic HIV infection. *Med Sci Sports Exerc.* (1999) 31:973–9. doi: 10.1097/00005768-199907000-00009
104. Lowder T, Padgett DA, Woods JA. Moderate exercise protects mice from death due to influenza virus. *Brain Behav Immun.* (2005) 19:377–80. doi: 10.1016/j.bbi.2005.04.002
105. Fairey AS, Courneya KS, Field CJ, Bell GJ, Jones LW, Mackey JR. Randomized controlled trial of exercise and blood immune function in postmenopausal breast cancer survivors. *J Appl Physiol.* (2005) 98:1534–40. doi: 10.1152/japplphysiol.00566.2004
106. Hojman P, Dethlefsen C, Brandt C, Hansen J, Pedersen L, Pedersen BK. Exercise-induced muscle-derived cytokines inhibit mammary cancer cell growth. *Am J Physiol Endocrinol Metab.* (2011) 301:E504–10. doi: 10.1152/ajpendo.00520.2010
107. Khandekar MJ, Cohen P, Spiegelman BM. Molecular mechanisms of cancer development in obesity. *Nat Rev Cancer* (2011) 11:886–95. doi: 10.1038/nrc3174
108. Yan H, Kuroiwa A, Tanaka H, Shindo M, Kiyonaga A, Nagayama A. Effect of moderate exercise on immune senescence in men. *Eur J Appl Physiol.* (2001) 86:105–11. doi: 10.1007/s004210100521

109. Shinkai S, Kohno H, Kimura K, Komura T, Asai H, Inai R, et al. Physical activity and immune senescence in men. *Med Sci Sports Exerc.* (1995) 27:1516–26. doi: 10.1249/00005768-199511000-00008
110. Woods JA, Ceddia MA, Wolters BW, Evans JK, Lu Q, McAuley E. Effects of 6 months of moderate aerobic exercise training on immune function in the elderly. *Mech Ageing Dev.* (1999) 109:1–19. doi: 10.1016/S0047-6374(99)00014-7
111. Pedersen BK, Bruunsgaard H. Possible beneficial role of exercise in modulating low-grade inflammation in the elderly. *Scand J Med Sci Sports* (2003) 13:56–62. doi: 10.1034/j.1600-0838.2003.20218.x
112. Drela N, Kozdron E, Szczypiorski P. Moderate exercise may attenuate some aspects of immunosenescence. *BMC Geriatr.* (2004) 4:8. doi: 10.1186/1471-2318-4-8
113. Spielmann G, McFarlin BK, O'Connor DP, Smith PJ, Pircher H, Simpson RJ. Aerobic fitness is associated with lower proportions of senescent blood T-cells in man. *Brain Behav Immun.* (2011) 25:1521–9. doi: 10.1016/j.bbi.2011.07.226
114. Phillips MD, Flynn MG, McFarlin BK, Stewart LK, Timmerman KL. Resistance training at eight-repetition maximum reduces the inflammatory milieu in elderly women. *Med Sci Sports Exerc.* (2010) 42:314–25. doi: 10.1249/MSS.0b013e3181b11ab7
115. McFarlin BK, Flynn MG, Phillips MD, Stewart LK, Timmerman KL. Chronic resistance exercise training improves natural killer cell activity in older women. *J Gerontol A Biol Sci Med Sci.* (2005) 60:1315–8. doi: 10.1093/gerona/60.10.1315
116. Kawanishi N, Yano H, Yokogawa Y, Suzuki K. Exercise training inhibits inflammation in adipose tissue via both suppression of macrophage infiltration and acceleration of phenotypic switching from M1 to M2 macrophages in high-fat-diet-induced obese mice. *Exerc Immunol Rev.* (2010) 16:105–18.
117. Mastorakos G, Pavlatou M, Diamanti-Kandarakis E, Chrousos GP. Exercise and the stress system. *Hormones (Athens)* (2005) 4:73–89.
118. Shaikh SR, Edidin M. Polyunsaturated fatty acids, membrane organization, T cells, and antigen presentation. *Am J Clin Nutr.* (2006) 84:1277–89. doi: 10.1093/ajcn/84.6.1277
119. Guo H, Callaway JB, Ting JP. Inflammasomes: mechanism of action, role in disease, and therapeutics. *Nat Med.* (2015) 21:677–87. doi: 10.1038/nm.3893
120. Martinon F, Burns K, Tschopp J. The inflammasome: a molecular platform triggering activation of inflammatory caspases and processing of proIL-beta. *Mol Cell* (2002) 10:417–26. doi: 10.1016/S1097-2765(02)00599-3
121. Lamkanfi M, Dixit VM. Mechanisms and functions of inflammasomes. *Cell* (2014) 157:1013–22. doi: 10.1016/j.cell.2014.04.007
122. Howard AD, Kostura MJ, Thornberry N, Ding GJ, Limjuco G, Weidner J, et al. IL-1-converting enzyme requires aspartic acid residues for processing of the IL-1 beta precursor at two distinct sites and does not cleave 31-kDa IL-1 alpha. *J Immunol.* (1991) 147:2964–9.
123. Ghayur T, Banerjee S, Hugunin M, Butler D, Herzog L, Carter A, et al. Caspase-1 processes IFN-gamma-inducing factor and regulates LPS-induced IFN-gamma production. *Nature* (1997) 386:619–23. doi: 10.1038/386619a0
124. Gu Y, Kuida K, Tsutsui H, Ku G, Hsiao K, Fleming MA, et al. Activation of interferon-gamma inducing factor mediated by interleukin-1beta converting enzyme. *Science* (1997) 275:206–9. doi: 10.1126/science.275.5297.206
125. Lamkanfi M, Dixit VM. Inflammasomes and their roles in health and disease. *Annu Rev Cell Dev Biol.* (2012) 28:137–61. doi: 10.1146/annurev-cellbio-101011-155745
126. Strowig T, Henao-Mejia J, Elinav E, Flavell R. Inflammasomes in health and disease. *Nature* (2012) 481:278–86. doi: 10.1038/nature10759
127. Takeuchi O, Akira S. Pattern recognition receptors and inflammation. *Cell* (2010) 140:805–20. doi: 10.1016/j.cell.2010.01.022
128. Ringseis R, Eder K, Mooren FC, Kruger K. Metabolic signals and innate immune activation in obesity and exercise. *Exerc Immunol Rev.* (2015) 21:58–68.
129. Miyaura C, Onoe Y, Inada M, Maki K, Ikuta K, Ito M, et al. Increased B-lymphopoiesis by interleukin 7 induces bone loss in mice with intact ovarian function: similarity to estrogen deficiency. *Proc Natl Acad Sci USA.* (1997) 94:9360–5. doi: 10.1073/pnas.94.17.9360
130. Pietschmann P, Mechtcheriakova D, Meshcheryakova A, Foger-Samwald U, Ellinger I. Immunology of osteoporosis: a mini-review. *Gerontology* (2016) 62:128–37. doi: 10.1159/000431091
131. Fougere B, Boulanger E, Nourhashemi F, Guyonnet S, Cesari M. Chronic inflammation: accelerator of biological aging. *J Gerontol A Biol Sci Med Sci.* (2017) 72:1218–25. doi: 10.1093/gerona/glw240
132. Mansoori MN, Shukla P, Kakaji M, Tyagi AM, Srivastava K, Shukla M, et al. IL-18BP is decreased in osteoporotic women: prevents Inflammasome mediated IL-18 activation and reduces Th17 differentiation. *Sci Rep.* (2016) 6:33680. doi: 10.1038/srep33680
133. Snouwaert JN, Nguyen M, Repenning PW, Dye R, Livingston EW, Kovarova M, et al. An NLRP3 mutation causes arthropathy and osteoporosis in humanized mice. *Cell Rep.* (2016) 17:3077–88. doi: 10.1016/j.celrep.2016.11.052
134. Wang L, Chen K, Wan X, Wang F, Guo Z, Mo Z. NLRP3 inflammasome activation in mesenchymal stem cells inhibits osteogenic differentiation and enhances adipogenic differentiation. *Biochem Biophys Res Commun.* (2017) 484:871–7. doi: 10.1016/j.bbrc.2017.02.007
135. Alippe Y, Wang C, Ricci B, Xiao J, Qu C, Zou W, et al. Bone matrix components activate the NLRP3 inflammasome and promote osteoclast differentiation. *Sci Rep.* (2017) 7:6630. doi: 10.1038/s41598-017-07014-0
136. Pedersen BK, Febbraio MA. Muscles, exercise and obesity: skeletal muscle as a secretory organ. *Nat Rev Endocrinol.* (2012) 8:457–65. doi: 10.1038/nrendo.2012.49
137. Kern PA, Ranganathan S, Li C, Wood L, Ranganathan G. Adipose tissue tumor necrosis factor and interleukin-6 expression in human obesity and insulin resistance. *Am J Physiol Endocrinol Metab.* (2001) 280:E745–51. doi: 10.1152/ajpendo.2001.280.5.E745
138. Duncan BB, Schmidt MI, Pankow JS, Ballantyne CM, Couper D, Vigo A, et al. Low-grade systemic inflammation and the development of type 2 diabetes: the atherosclerosis risk in communities study. *Diabetes* (2003) 52:1799–805. doi: 10.2337/diabetes.52.7.1799
139. Dandona P, Aljada A, Bandyopadhyay A. Inflammation: the link between insulin resistance, obesity and diabetes. *Trends Immunol.* (2004) 25:4–7. doi: 10.1016/j.it.2003.10.013
140. Eckardt K, Gorgens SW, Raschke S, Eckel J. Myokines in insulin resistance and type 2 diabetes. *Diabetologia* (2014) 57:1087–99. doi: 10.1007/s00125-014-3224-x
141. Hojbjerre L, Rosenzweig M, Dela F, Bruun JM, Stallknecht B. Acute exercise increases adipose tissue interstitial adiponectin concentration in healthy overweight and lean subjects. *Eur J Endocrinol.* (2007) 157:613–23. doi: 10.1530/EJE-07-0213
142. Jilka RL, Hangoc G, Girasole G, Passeri G, Williams DC, Abrams JS, et al. Increased osteoclast development after estrogen loss: mediation by interleukin-6. *Science* (1992) 257:88–91. doi: 10.1126/science.1621100
143. Le Goff B, Blanchard F, Berthelot JM, Heymann D, Maugars Y. Role for interleukin-6 in structural joint damage and systemic bone loss in rheumatoid arthritis. *Joint Bone Spine* (2010) 77:201–5. doi: 10.1016/j.jbspin.2010.03.002
144. Palmqvist P, Persson E, Conaway HH, Lerner UH. IL-6, leukemia inhibitory factor, and oncostatin M stimulate bone resorption and regulate the expression of receptor activator of NF-kappa B ligand, osteoprotegerin, and receptor activator of NF-kappa B in mouse calvariae. *J Immunol.* (2002) 169:3353–62. doi: 10.4049/jimmunol.169.6.3353
145. Saidenberg-Kermanac'h N, Cohen-Solal M, Bessis N, De Vernejoul MC, Boissier MC. Role for osteoprotegerin in rheumatoid inflammation. *Joint Bone Spine* (2004) 71:9–13. doi: 10.1016/S1297-319X(03)00131-3
146. Axmann R, Bohm C, Kronke G, Zwerina J, Smolen J, Schett G. Inhibition of interleukin-6 receptor directly blocks osteoclast formation *in vitro* and *in vivo*. *Arthritis Rheum.* (2009) 60:2747–56. doi: 10.1002/art.24781
147. De Benedetti F, Pignatti P, Vivarelli M, Meazza C, Ciliberto G, Savino R, et al. *In vivo* neutralization of human IL-6 (hIL-6) achieved by immunization of hIL-6-transgenic mice with a hIL-6 receptor antagonist. *J Immunol.* (2001) 166:4334–40. doi: 10.4049/jimmunol.166.7.4334
148. Wong PK, Quinn JM, Sims NA, van Nieuwenhuijze A, Campbell IK, Wicks IP. Interleukin-6 modulates production of T lymphocyte-derived

cytokines in antigen-induced arthritis and drives inflammation-induced osteoclastogenesis. *Arthritis Rheum.* (2006) 54:158–68. doi: 10.1002/art.21537

149. Li L, Chen X, Lv S, Dong M, Zhang L, Tu J, et al. Influence of exercise on bone remodeling-related hormones and cytokines in ovariectomized rats: a model of postmenopausal osteoporosis. *PLoS ONE* (2014) 9:e112845. doi: 10.1371/journal.pone.0112845
150. Park JH, Park KH, Cho S, Choi YS, Seo SK, Lee BS, et al. Concomitant increase in muscle strength and bone mineral density with decreasing IL-6 levels after combination therapy with alendronate and calcitriol in postmenopausal women. *Menopause* (2013) 20:747–53. doi: 10.1097/GME.0b013e31827cabca
151. Mezil YA, Allison D, Kish K, Ditor D, Ward WE, Tsiani E, et al. Response of bone turnover markers and cytokines to high-intensity low-impact exercise. *Med Sci Sports Exerc.* (2015) 47:1495–502. doi: 10.1249/MSS.0000000000000555
152. Aguirre L, Napoli N, Waters D, Qualls C, Villareal DT, Armamento-Villareal R. Increasing adiposity is associated with higher adipokine levels and lower bone mineral density in obese older adults. *J Clin Endocrinol Metab.* (2014) 99:3290–7. doi: 10.1210/jc.2013-3200
153. Marques EA, Mota J, Viana JL, Tuna D, Figueiredo P, Guimaraes JT, et al. Response of bone mineral density, inflammatory cytokines, and biochemical bone markers to a 32-week combined loading exercise programme in older men and women. *Arch Gerontol Geriatr.* (2013) 57:226–33. doi: 10.1016/j.archger.2013.03.014
154. Broholm C, Laye MJ, Brandt C, Vadalasetty R, Pilegaard H, Pedersen BK, et al. LIF is a contraction-induced myokine stimulating human myocyte proliferation. *J Appl Physiol.* (2011) 111:251–9. doi: 10.1152/japplphysiol.01399.2010
155. Broholm C, Mortensen OH, Nielsen S, Akerstrom T, Zankari A, Dahl B, et al. Exercise induces expression of leukaemia inhibitory factor in human skeletal muscle. *J Physiol.* (2008) 586:2195–201. doi: 10.1113/jphysiol.2007.149781
156. Malaval L, Aubin JE. Biphasic effects of leukemia inhibitory factor on osteoblastic differentiation. *J Cell Biochem Suppl.* (2001) 36:63–70. doi: 10.1002/jcb.1086
157. Sims NA, Johnson RW. Leukemia inhibitory factor: a paracrine mediator of bone metabolism. *Growth Factors* (2012) 30:76–87. doi: 10.3109/08977194.2012.656760
158. Haugen F, Norheim F, Lian H, Wensaas AJ, Dueland S, Berg O, et al. IL-7 is expressed and secreted by human skeletal muscle cells. *Am J Physiol Cell Physiol.* (2010) 298:C807–16. doi: 10.1152/ajpcell.00094.2009
159. Zhao R. Immune regulation of osteoclast function in postmenopausal osteoporosis: a critical interdisciplinary perspective. *Int J Med Sci.* (2012) 9:825–32. doi: 10.7150/ijms.5180
160. Lee SK, Surh CD. Role of interleukin-7 in bone and T-cell homeostasis. *Immunol Rev.* (2005) 208:169–80. doi: 10.1111/j.0105-2896.2005.00339.x
161. Weitzmann MN, Cenci S, Rifas L, Brown C, Pacifici R. Interleukin-7 stimulates osteoclast formation by up-regulating the T-cell production of soluble osteoclastogenic cytokines. *Blood* (2000) 96:1873–8.
162. Toraldo G, Roggia C, Qian WP, Pacifici R, Weitzmann MN. IL-7 induces bone loss *in vivo* by induction of receptor activator of nuclear factor kappa B ligand and tumor necrosis factor alpha from T cells. *Proc Natl Acad Sci USA.* (2003) 100:125–30. doi: 10.1073/pnas.0136772100
163. Andersson H, Bohn SK, Raastad T, Paulsen G, Blomhoff R, Kadi F. Differences in the inflammatory plasma cytokine response following two elite female soccer games separated by a 72-h recovery. *Scand J Med Sci Sports* (2010) 20:740–7. doi: 10.1111/j.1600-0838.2009.00989.x
164. Kraemer WJ, Hatfield DL, Comstock BA, Fragala MS, Davitt PM, Cortis C, et al. Influence of HMB supplementation and resistance training on cytokine responses to resistance exercise. *J Am Coll Nutr.* (2014) 33:247–55. doi: 10.1080/07315724.2014.911669
165. Gorgens SW, Eckardt K, Jensen J, Drevon CA, Eckel J. Exercise and regulation of adipokine and myokine production. *Prog Mol Biol Transl Sci.* (2015) 135:313–36. doi: 10.1016/bs.pmbts.2015.07.002
166. Nieman DC, Davis JM, Henson DA, Walberg-Rankin J, Shute M, Dumke CL, et al. Carbohydrate ingestion influences skeletal muscle cytokine mRNA and plasma cytokine levels after a 3-h run. *J Appl Physiol.* (2003) 94:1917–25. doi: 10.1152/japplphysiol.01130.2002
167. Rinnov A, Yfanti C, Nielsen S, Akerstrom TC, Peijs L, Zankari A, et al. Endurance training enhances skeletal muscle interleukin-15 in human male subjects. *Endocrine* (2014) 45:271–8. doi: 10.1007/s12020-013-9969-z
168. Tamura Y, Watanabe K, Kantani T, Hayashi J, Ishida N, Kaneki M. Upregulation of circulating IL-15 by treadmill running in healthy individuals: is IL-15 an endocrine mediator of the beneficial effects of endurance exercise? *Endocr J.* (2011) 58:211–5. doi: 10.1507/endocrj.K10E-400
169. Riechman SE, Balasekaran G, Roth SM, Ferrell RE. Association of interleukin-15 protein and interleukin-15 receptor genetic variation with resistance exercise training responses. *J Appl Physiol.* (2004) 97:2214–9. doi: 10.1152/japplphysiol.00491.2004
170. Nielsen AR, Mounier R, Plomgaard P, Mortensen OH, Penkowa M, Speerschneider T, et al. Expression of interleukin-15 in human skeletal muscle effect of exercise and muscle fibre type composition. *J Physiol.* (2007) 584(Pt 1):305–12. doi: 10.1113/jphysiol.2007.139618
171. Ogata Y, Kukita A, Kukita T, Komine M, Miyahara A, Miyazaki S, et al. A novel role of IL-15 in the development of osteoclasts: inability to replace its activity with IL-2. *J Immunol.* (1999) 162:2754–60.
172. Okabe I, Kikuchi T, Mogi M, Takeda H, Aino M, Kamiya Y, et al. IL-15 and RANKL play a synergistically important role in osteoclastogenesis. *J Cell Biochem.* (2017) 118:739–47. doi: 10.1002/jcb.25726
173. Amarasekara DS, Yun H, Kim S, Lee N, Kim H, Rho J. Regulation of osteoclast differentiation by cytokine networks. *Immune Netw.* (2018) 18:e8. doi: 10.4110/in.2018.18.e8
174. McPherron AC, Lawler AM, Lee SJ. Regulation of skeletal muscle mass in mice by a new TGF-beta superfamily member. *Nature* (1997) 387:83–90. doi: 10.1038/387083a0
175. Hamrick MW. A role for myokines in muscle-bone interactions. *Exerc Sport Sci Rev.* (2011) 39:43–7. doi: 10.1097/JES.0b013e318201f601
176. Nam J, Perera P, Gordon R, Jeong YH, Blazek AD, Kim DG, et al. Follistatin-like 3 is a mediator of exercise-driven bone formation and strengthening. *Bone* (2015) 78:62–70. doi: 10.1016/j.bone.2015.04.038
177. Harber MP, Crane JD, Dickinson JM, Jemiolo B, Raue U, Trappe TA, et al. Protein synthesis and the expression of growth-related genes are altered by running in human vastus lateralis and soleus muscles. *Am J Physiol Regul Integr Comp Physiol.* (2009) 296:R708–14. doi: 10.1152/ajpregu.90906.2008
178. Kim JS, Cross JM, Bamman MM. Impact of resistance loading on myostatin expression and cell cycle regulation in young and older men and women. *Am J Physiol Endocrinol Metab.* (2005) 288:E1110–9. doi: 10.1152/ajpendo.00464.2004
179. Dalbo VJ, Roberts MD, Sunderland KL, Poole CN, Stout JR, Beck TW, et al. Acute loading and aging effects on myostatin pathway biomarkers in human skeletal muscle after three sequential bouts of resistance exercise. *J Gerontol A Biol Sci Med Sci.* (2011) 66:855–65. doi: 10.1093/gerona/glr091
180. Dieli-Conwright CM, Spektor TM, Rice JC, Sattler FR, Schroeder ET. Hormone therapy and maximal eccentric exercise alters myostatin-related gene expression in postmenopausal women. *J Strength Cond Res.* (2012) 26:1374–82. doi: 10.1519/JSC.0b013e318251083f
181. Hittel DS, Axelson M, Sarna N, Shearer J, Huffman KM, Kraus WE. Myostatin decreases with aerobic exercise and associates with insulin resistance. *Med Sci Sports Exerc.* (2010) 42:2023–9. doi: 10.1249/MSS.0b013e3181e0b9a8
182. Jaworska J, Micielska K, Kozłowska M, Wnorowski K, Skrobecki J, Radzimin L, et al. A 2-week specific volleyball training supported by the whole body cryostimulation protocol induced an increase of growth factors and counteracted deterioration of physical performance. *Front Physiol.* (2018) 9:1711. doi: 10.3389/fphys.2018.01711
183. Amthor H, Nicholas G, McKinnell I, Kemp CF, Sharma M, Kambadur R, et al. Follistatin complexes Myostatin and antagonises Myostatin-mediated inhibition of myogenesis. *Dev Biol.* (2004) 270:19–30. doi: 10.1016/j.ydbio.2004.01.046
184. Shi Y, Massague J. Mechanisms of TGF-beta signaling from cell membrane to the nucleus. *Cell* (2003) 113:685–700. doi: 10.1016/S0092-8674(03)00432-X
185. Miura T, Kishioka Y, Wakamatsu J, Hattori A, Hennebry A, Berry CJ, et al. Decorin binds myostatin and modulates its activity to muscle cells. *Biochem Biophys Res Commun.* (2006) 340:675–80. doi: 10.1016/j.bbrc.2005.12.060

186. Kanzleiter T, Rath M, Gorgens SW, Jensen J, Tangen DS, Kolnes AJ, et al. The myokine decorin is regulated by contraction and involved in muscle hypertrophy. *Biochem Biophys Res Commun.* (2014) 450:1089–94. doi: 10.1016/j.bbrc.2014.06.123
187. Heinemeier KM, Bjerrum SS, Schjerling P, Kjaer M. Expression of extracellular matrix components and related growth factors in human tendon and muscle after acute exercise. *Scand J Med Sci Sports* (2013) 23:e150–61. doi: 10.1111/j.1600-0838.2011.01414.x
188. Gorgens SW, Raschke S, Holven KB, Jensen J, Eckardt K, Eckel J. Regulation of follistatin-like protein 1 expression and secretion in primary human skeletal muscle cells. *Arch Physiol Biochem.* (2013) 119:75–80. doi: 10.3109/13813455.2013.768270
189. Norheim F, Raastad T, Thiede B, Rustan AC, Drevon CA, Haugen F. Proteomic identification of secreted proteins from human skeletal muscle cells and expression in response to strength training. *Am J Physiol Endocrinol Metab.* (2011) 301:E1013–21. doi: 10.1152/ajpendo.00326.2011
190. Dankbar B, Fennen M, Brunert D, Hayer S, Frank S, Wehmeyer C, et al. Myostatin is a direct regulator of osteoclast differentiation and its inhibition reduces inflammatory joint destruction in mice. *Nat Med.* (2015) 21:1085–90. doi: 10.1038/nm.3917
191. Hamrick MW, Shi X, Zhang W, Pennington C, Thakore H, Haque M, et al. Loss of myostatin (GDF8) function increases osteogenic differentiation of bone marrow-derived mesenchymal stem cells but the osteogenic effect is ablated with unloading. *Bone* (2007) 40:1544–53. doi: 10.1016/j.bone.2007.02.012
192. Bettis T, Kim BJ, Hamrick MW. Impact of muscle atrophy on bone metabolism and bone strength: implications for muscle-bone crosstalk with aging and disuse. *Osteoporos Int.* (2018) 29:1713–20. doi: 10.1007/s00198-018-4570-1
193. Kerschan-Schindl K, Thalmann MM, Weiss E, Tsironi M, Foger-Samwald U, Meinhart J, et al. Changes in serum levels of myokines and wnt-antagonists after an ultramarathon race. *PLoS ONE* (2015) 10:e0132478. doi: 10.1371/journal.pone.0132478
194. Kawao N, Morita H, Obata K, Tatsumi K, Kaji H. Role of follistatin in muscle and bone alterations induced by gravity change in mice. *J Cell Physiol.* (2018) 233:1191–201. doi: 10.1002/jcp.25986
195. Matthews VB, Astrom MB, Chan MH, Bruce CR, Krabbe KS, Prelovsek O, et al. Brain-derived neurotrophic factor is produced by skeletal muscle cells in response to contraction and enhances fat oxidation via activation of AMP-activated protein kinase. *Diabetologia* (2009) 52:1409–18. doi: 10.1007/s00125-009-1364-1
196. Huang EJ, Reichardt LF. Neurotrophins: roles in neuronal development and function. *Annu Rev Neurosci.* (2001) 24:677–736. doi: 10.1146/annurev.neuro.24.1.677
197. Rasmussen P, Brassard P, Adser H, Pedersen MV, Leick L, Hart E, et al. Evidence for a release of brain-derived neurotrophic factor from the brain during exercise. *Exp Physiol.* (2009) 94:1062–9. doi: 10.1113/expphysiol.2009.048512
198. Gold SM, Schulz KH, Hartmann S, Mladek M, Lang UE, Hellweg R, et al. Basal serum levels and reactivity of nerve growth factor and brain-derived neurotrophic factor to standardized acute exercise in multiple sclerosis and controls. *J Neuroimmunol.* (2003) 138:99–105. doi: 10.1016/S0165-5728(03)00121-8
199. Ferris LT, Williams JS, Shen CL. The effect of acute exercise on serum brain-derived neurotrophic factor levels and cognitive function. *Med Sci Sports Exerc.* (2007) 39:728–34. doi: 10.1249/mss.0b013e31802f04c7
200. Schmidt-Kassow M, Schadle S, Otterbein S, Thiel C, Doehring A, Lotsch J, et al. Kinetics of serum brain-derived neurotrophic factor following low-intensity versus high-intensity exercise in men and women. *Neuroreport* (2012) 23:889–93. doi: 10.1097/WNR.0b013e32835946ca
201. Griffin EW, Mullally S, Foley C, Warmington SA, O'Mara SM, Kelly AM. Aerobic exercise improves hippocampal function and increases BDNF in the serum of young adult males. *Physiol Behav.* (2011) 104:934–41. doi: 10.1016/j.physbeh.2011.06.005
202. Goekint M, De Pauw K, Roelands B, Njemini R, Bautmans I, Mets T, et al. Strength training does not influence serum brain-derived neurotrophic factor. *Eur J Appl Physiol.* (2010) 110:285–93. doi: 10.1007/s00421-010-1461-3
203. Gmiat A, Micielska K, Kozlowska M, Flis DJ, Smaruj M, Kujach S, et al. The impact of a single bout of high intensity circuit training on myokines' concentrations and cognitive functions in women of different age. *Physiol Behav.* (2017) 179:290–7. doi: 10.1016/j.physbeh.2017.07.004
204. Gmiat A, Jaworska J, Micielska K, Kortas J, Prusik K, Prusik K, et al. Improvement of cognitive functions in response to a regular Nordic walking training in elderly women - A change dependent on the training experience. *Exp Gerontol.* (2018) 104:105–12. doi: 10.1016/j.exger.2018.02.006
205. Yamashiro T, Fukunaga T, Yamashita K, Kobashi N, Takano-Yamamoto T. Gene and protein expression of brain-derived neurotrophic factor and TrkB in bone and cartilage. *Bone* (2001) 28:404–9. doi: 10.1016/S8756-3282(01)00405-7
206. Kilian O, Hartmann S, Dongowski N, Karnati S, Baumgart-Vogt E, Hartel FV, et al. BDNF and its TrkB receptor in human fracture healing. *Ann Anat.* (2014) 196:286–95. doi: 10.1016/j.aanat.2014.06.001
207. Camerino C, Zayzafoon M, Rymaszewski M, Heiny J, Rios M, Hauschka PV. Central depletion of brain-derived neurotrophic factor in mice results in high bone mass and metabolic phenotype. *Endocrinology* (2012) 153:5394–405. doi: 10.1210/en.2012-1378
208. Coniglio SJ. Role of tumor-derived chemokines in osteolytic bone metastasis. *Front Endocrinol.* (2018) 9:313. doi: 10.3389/fendo.2018.00313
209. Qin S, LaRosa G, Campbell JJ, Smith-Heath H, Kassam N, Shi X, et al. Expression of monocyte chemoattractant protein-1 and interleukin-8 receptors on subsets of T cells: correlation with transendothelial chemotactic potential. *Eur J Immunol.* (1996) 26:640–7. doi: 10.1002/eji.1830260320
210. Vella L, Caldow MK, Larsen AE, Tassoni D, Della Gatta PA, Gran P, et al. Resistance exercise increases NF-kappaB activity in human skeletal muscle. *Am J Physiol Regul Integr Comp Physiol.* (2012) 302:R667–73. doi: 10.1152/ajpregu.00336.2011
211. Della Gatta PA, Garnham AP, Peake JM, Cameron-Smith D. Effect of exercise training on skeletal muscle cytokine expression in the elderly. *Brain Behav Immun.* (2014) 39:80–6. doi: 10.1016/j.bbi.2014.01.006
212. Peake JM, Suzuki K, Hordern M, Wilson G, Nosaka K, Coombes JS. Plasma cytokine changes in relation to exercise intensity and muscle damage. *Eur J Appl Physiol.* (2005) 95:514–21. doi: 10.1007/s00421-005-0035-2
213. Ogawa K, Sanada K, Machida S, Okutsu M, Suzuki K. Resistance exercise training-induced muscle hypertrophy was associated with reduction of inflammatory markers in elderly women. *Mediators Inflamm.* (2010) 2010:171023. doi: 10.1155/2010/171023
214. Greiwe JS, Cheng B, Rubin DC, Yarasheski KE, Semenkovich CF. Resistance exercise decreases skeletal muscle tumor necrosis factor alpha in frail elderly humans. *FASEB J.* (2001) 15:475–82. doi: 10.1096/fj.00-0274com
215. Gielen S, Adams V, Mobius-Winkler S, Linke A, Erbs S, Yu J, et al. Anti-inflammatory effects of exercise training in the skeletal muscle of patients with chronic heart failure. *J Am Coll Cardiol.* (2003) 42:861–8. doi: 10.1016/S0735-1097(03)00848-9
216. Febbraio MA, Steensberg A, Starkie RL, McConell GK, Kingwell BA. Skeletal muscle interleukin-6 and tumor necrosis factor-alpha release in healthy subjects and patients with type 2 diabetes at rest and during exercise. *Metabolism* (2003) 52:939–44. doi: 10.1016/S0026-0495(03)00105-7
217. Plomgaard P, Nielsen AR, Fischer CP, Mortensen OH, Broholm C, Penkowa M, et al. Associations between insulin resistance and TNF-alpha in plasma, skeletal muscle and adipose tissue in humans with and without type 2 diabetes. *Diabetologia* (2007) 50:2562–71. doi: 10.1007/s00125-007-0834-6
218. Golbidi S, Laher I. Exercise induced adipokine changes and the metabolic syndrome. *J Diabetes Res.* (2014) 2014:726861. doi: 10.1155/2014/726861
219. Paulsen G, Mikkelsen UR, Raastad T, Peake JM. Leucocytes, cytokines and satellite cells: what role do they play in muscle damage and regeneration following eccentric exercise? *Exerc Immunol Rev.* (2012) 18:42–97.
220. Walsh MC, Kim N, Kadono Y, Rho J, Lee SY, Lorenzo J, et al. Osteoimmunology: interplay between the immune system and bone metabolism. *Annu Rev Immunol.* (2006) 24:33–63. doi: 10.1146/annurev.immunol.24.021605.090646
221. Azuma Y, Kaji K, Katogi R, Takeshita S, Kudo A. Tumor necrosis factor-alpha induces differentiation of and bone resorption by osteoclasts. *J Biol Chem.* (2000) 275:4858–64. doi: 10.1074/jbc.275.7.4858
222. Komine M, Kukita A, Kukita T, Ogata Y, Hotokebuchi T, Kohashi O. Tumor necrosis factor-alpha cooperates with receptor activator of

nuclear factor kappaB ligand in generation of osteoclasts in stromal cell-depleted rat bone marrow cell culture. *Bone* (2001) 28:474–83. doi: 10.1016/S8756-3282(01)00420-3

223. Park ES, Choi S, Shin B, Yu J, Yu J, Hwang JM, et al. Tumor necrosis factor (TNF) receptor-associated factor (TRAF)-interacting protein (TRIP) negatively regulates the TRAF2 ubiquitin-dependent pathway by suppressing the TRAF2-sphingosine 1-phosphate (S1P) interaction. *J Biol Chem.* (2015) 290:9660–73. doi: 10.1074/jbc.M114.609685
224. Yao Z, Lei W, Duan R, Li Y, Luo L, Boyce BF. RANKL cytokine enhances TNF-induced osteoclastogenesis independently of TNF receptor associated factor (TRAF) 6 by degrading TRAF3 in osteoclast precursors. *J Biol Chem.* (2017) 292:10169–79. doi: 10.1074/jbc.M116.771816
225. Kitaura H, Kimura K, Ishida M, Kohara H, Yoshimatsu M, Takano-Yamamoto T. Immunological reaction in TNF-alpha-mediated osteoclast formation and bone resorption *in vitro* and *in vivo*. *Clin Dev Immunol.* (2013) 2013:181849. doi: 10.1155/2013/181849
226. Fukuhara A, Matsuda M, Nishizawa M, Segawa K, Tanaka M, Kishimoto K, et al. Visfatin: a protein secreted by visceral fat that mimics the effects of insulin. *Science* (2005) 307:426–30. doi: 10.1126/science.1097243
227. Lombardi G, Banfi G. Effects of sample matrix and storage conditions on full-length visfatin measurement in blood. *Clin Chim Acta* (2015) 440:140–2. doi: 10.1016/j.cca.2014.11.006
228. Sommer G, Garten A, Petzold S, Beck-Sickinger AG, Bluher M, Stumvoll M, et al. Visfatin/PBEF/Nampt: structure, regulation and potential function of a novel adipokine. *Clin Sci.* (2008) 115:13–23. doi: 10.1042/CS20070226
229. Costford SR, Bajpeyi S, Pasarica M, Albarado DC, Thomas SC, Xie H, et al. Skeletal muscle NAMPT is induced by exercise in humans. *Am J Physiol Endocrinol Metab.* (2010) 298:E117–26. doi: 10.1152/ajpendo.00318.2009
230. Ziemann E, Olek RA, Grzywacz T, Antosiewicz J, Kujach S, Luszczyk M, et al. Whole-body cryostimulation as an effective method of reducing low-grade inflammation in obese men. *J Physiol Sci.* (2013) 63:333–43. doi: 10.1007/s12576-013-0269-4
231. Brandauer J, Vienberg SG, Andersen MA, Ringholm S, Risis S, Larsen PS, et al. AMP-activated protein kinase regulates nicotinamide phosphoribosyl transferase expression in skeletal muscle. *J Physiol.* (2013) 591:5207–20. doi: 10.1113/jphysiol.2013.259515
232. Frydelund-Larsen L, Akerstrom T, Nielsen S, Keller P, Keller C, Pedersen BK. Visfatin mRNA expression in human subcutaneous adipose tissue is regulated by exercise. *Am J Physiol Endocrinol Metab.* (2007) 292:E24–31. doi: 10.1152/ajpendo.00113.2006
233. Ghanbari-Niaki A, Saghebjoo M, Soltani R, Kirwan JP. Plasma visfatin is increased after high-intensity exercise. *Ann Nutr Metab.* (2010) 57:3–8. doi: 10.1159/000313936
234. Thommesen L, Stunes AK, Monjo M, Grosvik K, Tamburstuen MV, Kjobli E, et al. Expression and regulation of resistin in osteoblasts and osteoclasts indicate a role in bone metabolism. *J Cell Biochem.* (2006) 99:824–34. doi: 10.1002/jcb.20915
235. Xie H, Tang SY, Luo XH, Huang J, Cui RR, Yuan LQ, et al. Insulin-like effects of visfatin on human osteoblasts. *Calcif Tissue Int.* (2007) 80:201–10. doi: 10.1007/s00223-006-0155-7
236. Moschen AR, Geiger S, Gerner R, Tilg H. Pre-B cell colony enhancing factor/NAMPT/visfatin and its role in inflammation-related bone disease. *Mutat Res.* (2010) 690:95–101. doi: 10.1016/j.mrfmmm.2009.06.012
237. Li Y, He X, Li Y, He J, Anderstam B, Andersson G, et al. Nicotinamide phosphoribosyltransferase (Nampt) affects the lineage fate determination of mesenchymal stem cells: a possible cause for reduced osteogenesis and increased adipogenesis in older individuals. *J Bone Miner Res.* (2011) 26:2656–64. doi: 10.1002/jbmr.480
238. Sliwicka E, Nowak A, Zep W, Leszczynski P, Pilaczynska-Szczesniak L. Bone mass and bone metabolic indices in male master rowers. *J Bone Miner Metab.* (2015) 33:540–6. doi: 10.1007/s00774-014-0619-1
239. Iacobellis G, Iorio M, Napoli N, Cotesta D, Zinnamosca L, Marinelli C, et al. Relation of adiponectin, visfatin and bone mineral density in patients with metabolic syndrome. *J Endocrinol Invest.* (2011) 34:e12–5. doi: 10.1007/BF03346703
240. Zhang H, Xie H, Zhao Q, Xie GQ, Wu XP, Liao EY, et al. Relationships between serum adiponectin, apelin, leptin, resistin, visfatin levels and bone mineral density, and bone biochemical markers in post-menopausal Chinese women. *J Endocrinol Invest.* (2010) 33:707–11. doi: 10.1007/BF03346674
241. Tohidi M, Akbarzadeh S, Larijani B, Kalantarhormozi M, Ostovar A, Assadi M, et al. Omentin-1, visfatin and adiponectin levels in relation to bone mineral density in Iranian postmenopausal women. *Bone* (2012) 51:876–81. doi: 10.1016/j.bone.2012.08.117
242. Gruodyte R, Jurimae J, Cicchella A, Stefanelli C, Passariello C, Jurimae T. Adipocytokines and bone mineral density in adolescent female athletes. *Acta Paediatr.* (2010) 99:1879–84. doi: 10.1111/j.1651-2227.2010.01905.x
243. Yamauchi T, Iwabu M, Okada-Iwabu M, Kadowaki T. Adiponectin receptors: a review of their structure, function and how they work. *Best Pract Res Clin Endocrinol Metab.* (2014) 28:15–23. doi: 10.1016/j.beem.2013.09.003
244. Han SH, Quon MJ, Kim JA, Koh KK. Adiponectin and cardiovascular disease: response to therapeutic interventions. *J Am Coll Cardiol.* (2007) 49:531–8. doi: 10.1016/j.jacc.2006.08.061
245. Moschen AR, Kaser A, Enrich B, Mosheimer B, Theurl M, Niederegger H, et al. Visfatin, an adipocytokine with proinflammatory and immunomodulating properties. *J Immunol.* (2007) 178:1748–58. doi: 10.4049/jimmunol.178.3.1748
246. Santos MJ, Fonseca JE. Metabolic syndrome, inflammation and atherosclerosis - the role of adipokines in health and in systemic inflammatory rheumatic diseases. *Acta Reumatol Port.* (2009) 34:590–8.
247. Delaigle AM, Jonas JC, Bauche IB, Cornu O, Brichard SM. Induction of adiponectin in skeletal muscle by inflammatory cytokines: *in vivo* and *in vitro* studies. *Endocrinology* (2004) 145:5589–97. doi: 10.1210/en.2004-0503
248. Van Berendoncks AM, Garnier A, Beckers P, Hoymans VY, Possemiers N, Fortin D, et al. Functional adiponectin resistance at the level of the skeletal muscle in mild to moderate chronic heart failure. *Circ Heart Fail.* (2010) 3:185–94. doi: 10.1161/CIRCHEARTFAILURE.109.885525
249. Bluher M, Bullen JW Jr, Lee JH, Kralisch S, Fasshauer M, Kloting N, et al. Circulating adiponectin and expression of adiponectin receptors in human skeletal muscle: associations with metabolic parameters and insulin resistance and regulation by physical training. *J Clin Endocrinol Metab.* (2006) 91:2310–6. doi: 10.1210/jc.2005-2556
250. Saunders TJ, Palombella A, McGuire KA, Janiszewski PM, Despres JP, Ross R. Acute exercise increases adiponectin levels in abdominally obese men. *J Nutr Metab.* (2012) 2012:148729. doi: 10.1155/2012/148729
251. Christiansen T, Bruun JM, Paulsen SK, Olholm J, Overgaard K, Pedersen SB, et al. Acute exercise increases circulating inflammatory markers in overweight and obese compared with lean subjects. *Eur J Appl Physiol.* (2013) 113:1635–42. doi: 10.1007/s00421-013-2592-0
252. Ferguson MA, White LJ, McCoy S, Kim HW, Petty T, Wilsey J. Plasma adiponectin response to acute exercise in healthy subjects. *Eur J Appl Physiol.* (2004) 91:324–9. doi: 10.1007/s00421-003-0985-1
253. Jamurtas AZ, Theocharis V, Koukoulis G, Stakias N, Fatouros IG, Kouretas D, et al. The effects of acute exercise on serum adiponectin and resistin levels and their relation to insulin sensitivity in overweight males. *Eur J Appl Physiol.* (2006) 97:122–6. doi: 10.1007/s00421-006-0169-x
254. Bobbert T, Wegewitz U, Brechtel L, Freudenberg M, Mai K, Mohlig M, et al. Adiponectin oligomers in human serum during acute and chronic exercise: relation to lipid metabolism and insulin sensitivity. *Int J Sports Med.* (2007) 28:1–8. doi: 10.1055/s-2006-924028
255. Bouassida A, Lakhdar N, Benaissa N, Mejri S, Zaouali M, Zbidi A, et al. Adiponectin responses to acute moderate and heavy exercises in overweight middle aged subjects. *J Sports Med. Phys Fitness* (2010) 50:330–5.
256. Numao S, Katayama Y, Hayashi Y, Matsuo T, Tanaka K. Influence of acute aerobic exercise on adiponectin oligomer concentrations in middle-aged abdominally obese men. *Metabolism* (2011) 60:186–94. doi: 10.1016/j.metabol.2009.12.011
257. Bruun JM, Helge JW, Richelsen B, Stallknecht B. Diet and exercise reduce low-grade inflammation and macrophage infiltration in adipose tissue but not in skeletal muscle in severely obese subjects. *Am J Physiol Endocrinol Metab.* (2006) 290:E961–7. doi: 10.1152/ajpendo.00506.2005
258. Fatouros IG, Tournis S, Leontsini D, Jamurtas AZ, Sxina M, Thomakos P, et al. Leptin and adiponectin responses in overweight inactive elderly following resistance training and detraining are intensity related. *J Clin Endocrinol Metab.* (2005) 90:5970–7. doi: 10.1210/jc.2005-0261

259. Fatouros IG, Chatzinikolaou A, Tournis S, Nikolaidis MG, Jamurtas AZ, Douroudos II, et al. Intensity of resistance exercise determines adipokine and resting energy expenditure responses in overweight elderly individuals. *Diabetes Care* (2009) 32:2161–7. doi: 10.2337/dc08-1994
260. Biver E, Salliot C, Combescure C, Gossec L, Hardouin P, Legroux-Gerot I, et al. Influence of adipokines and ghrelin on bone mineral density and fracture risk: a systematic review and meta-analysis. *J Clin Endocrinol Metab.* (2011) 96:2703–13. doi: 10.1210/jc.2011-0047
261. Sucunza N, Barahona MJ, Resmini E, Fernandez-Real JM, Ricart W, Farrerons J, et al. A link between bone mineral density and serum adiponectin and visfatin levels in acromegaly. *J Clin Endocrinol Metab.* (2009) 94:3889–96. doi: 10.1210/jc.2009-0474
262. Ruscica M, Steffani L, Magni P. Adiponectin interactions in bone and cartilage biology and disease. *Vitam Horm.* (2012) 90:321–39. doi: 10.1016/B978-0-12-398313-8.00012-9
263. Berner HS, Lyngstadaas SP, Spahr A, Monjo M, Thommesen L, Drevon CA, et al. Adiponectin and its receptors are expressed in bone-forming cells. *Bone* (2004) 35:842–9. doi: 10.1016/j.bone.2004.06.008
264. Shinoda Y, Yamaguchi M, Ogata N, Akune T, Kubota N, Yamauchi T, et al. Regulation of bone formation by adiponectin through autocrine/paracrine and endocrine pathways. *J Cell Biochem.* (2006) 99:196–208. doi: 10.1002/jcb.20890
265. Zhang Y, Zhou P, Kimondo JW. Adiponectin and osteocalcin: relation to insulin sensitivity. *Biochem Cell Biol.* (2012) 90:613–20. doi: 10.1139/o2012-022
266. Sadie-Van Gijsen H, Crowther NJ, Hough FS, Ferris WF. The interrelationship between bone and fat: from cellular see-saw to endocrine reciprocity. *Cell Mol Life Sci.* (2013) 70:2331–49. doi: 10.1007/s00018-012-1211-2
267. Munzberg H, Morrison CD. Structure, production and signaling of leptin. *Metabolism* (2015) 64:13–23. doi: 10.1016/j.metabol.2014.09.010
268. Wang J, Liu R, Hawkins M, Barzilai N, Rossetti L. A nutrient-sensing pathway regulates leptin gene expression in muscle and fat. *Nature* (1998) 393:684–8. doi: 10.1038/31474
269. Upadhyay J, Farr OM, Mantzoros CS. The role of leptin in regulating bone metabolism. *Metabolism* (2015) 64:105–13. doi: 10.1016/j.metabol.2014.10.021
270. Takeda S, Elefteriou F, Levasseur R, Liu X, Zhao L, Parker KL, et al. Leptin regulates bone formation via the sympathetic nervous system. *Cell* (2002) 111:305–17. doi: 10.1016/S0092-8674(02)01049-8
271. Zaidi M, Buettner C, Sun L, Iqbal J. Minireview: the link between fat and bone: does mass beget mass? *Endocrinology* (2012) 153:2070–5. doi: 10.1210/en.2012-1022
272. Sienkiewicz E, Magkos F, Aronis KN, Brinkoetter M, Chamberland JP, Chou S, et al. Long-term metreleptin treatment increases bone mineral density and content at the lumbar spine of lean hypoleptinemic women. *Metabolism* (2011) 60:1211–21. doi: 10.1016/j.metabol.2011.05.016
273. Kim YS, Nam JS, Yeo DW, Kim KR, Suh SH, Ahn CW. The effects of aerobic exercise training on serum osteocalcin, adipocytokines and insulin resistance on obese young males. *Clin Endocrinol.* (2015) 82:686–94. doi: 10.1111/cen.12601
274. Yang C, Chen J, Wu F, Li J, Liang P, Zhang H, et al. Effects of 60-day head-down bed rest on osteocalcin, glycolipid metabolism and their association with or without resistance training. *Clin Endocrinol.* (2014) 81:671–8. doi: 10.1111/cen.12535
275. Keller P, Keller C, Steensberg A, Robinson LE, Pedersen BK. Leptin gene expression and systemic levels in healthy men: effect of exercise, carbohydrate, interleukin-6, and epinephrine. *J Appl Physiol.* (2005) 98:1805–12. doi: 10.1152/japplphysiol.00592.2004
276. Essig DA, Alderson NL, Ferguson MA, Bartoli WP, Durstine JL. Delayed effects of exercise on the plasma leptin concentration. *Metabolism* (2000) 49:395–9. doi: 10.1016/S0026-0495(00)90396-2
277. Olive JL, Miller GD. Differential effects of maximal- and moderate-intensity runs on plasma leptin in healthy trained subjects. *Nutrition* (2001) 17:365–9. doi: 10.1016/S0899-9007(01)00522-6
278. Phillips MD, Patrizi RM, Cheek DJ, Wooten JS, Barbee JJ, Mitchell JB. Resistance training reduces subclinical inflammation in obese, postmenopausal women. *Med Sci Sports Exerc.* (2012) 44:2099–110. doi: 10.1249/MSS.0b013e3182644984
279. Yang CB, Chuang CC, Kuo CS, Hsu CH, Tsao TH. Effects of an acute bout of exercise on serum soluble leptin receptor (sOB-R) levels. *J Sports Sci.* (2014) 32:446–51. doi: 10.1080/02640414.2013.828848
280. Shah K, Armamento-Villareal R, Parimi N, Chode S, Sinacore DR, Hilton TN, et al. Exercise training in obese older adults prevents increase in bone turnover and attenuates decrease in hip bone mineral density induced by weight loss despite decline in bone-active hormones. *J Bone Miner Res.* (2011) 26:2851–9. doi: 10.1002/jbmr.475
281. Varady KA, Bhutani S, Church EC, Phillips SA. Adipokine responses to acute resistance exercise in trained and untrained men. *Med Sci Sports Exerc.* (2010) 42:456–62. doi: 10.1249/MSS.0b013e3181ba6dd3
282. Codoner-Franch P, Alonso-Iglesias E. Resistin: insulin resistance to malignancy. *Clin Chim Acta* (2015) 438:46–54. doi: 10.1016/j.cca.2014.07.043
283. Oh KW, Lee WY, Rhee EJ, Baek KH, Yoon KH, Kang MI, et al. The relationship between serum resistin, leptin, adiponectin, ghrelin levels and bone mineral density in middle-aged men. *Clin Endocrinol.* (2005) 63:131–8. doi: 10.1111/j.1365-2265.2005.02312.x
284. Peng XD, Xie H, Zhao Q, Wu XP, Sun ZQ, Liao EY. Relationships between serum adiponectin, leptin, resistin, visfatin levels and bone mineral density, and bone biochemical markers in Chinese men. *Clin Chim Acta* (2008) 387:31–5. doi: 10.1016/j.cca.2007.08.012
285. Pluskiewicz W, Adamczyk P, Marek B, Czekajlo A, Drozdzowska B, Kajdaniuk D, et al. Adiponectin and resistin in relationship with skeletal status in women from the RAC-OST-POL study. *Endokrynol Pol.* (2012) 63:427–31.
286. Mohiti-Ardekani J, Soleymani-Salehabadi H, Owlia MB, Mohiti A. Relationships between serum adipocyte hormones (adiponectin, leptin, resistin), bone mineral density and bone metabolic markers in osteoporosis patients. *J Bone Miner Metab.* (2014) 32:400–4. doi: 10.1007/s00774-013-0511-4
287. Sowers MR, Wildman RP, Mancuso P, Eyvazzadeh AD, Karvonen-Gutierrez CA, Rillamas-Sun E, et al. Change in adipocytokines and ghrelin with menopause. *Maturitas* (2008) 59:149–57. doi: 10.1016/j.maturitas.2007.12.006
288. Fisher A, Southcott E, Li R, Srikusalanukul W, Davis M, Smith P. Serum resistin in older patients with hip fracture: relationship with comorbidity and biochemical determinants of bone metabolism. *Cytokine* (2011) 56:157–66. doi: 10.1016/j.cyto.2011.06.023
289. Bostrom P, Wu J, Jedrychowski MP, Korde A, Ye L, Lo JC, et al. A PGC1-alpha-dependent myokine that drives brown-fat-like development of white fat and thermogenesis. *Nature* (2012) 481:463–8. doi: 10.1038/nature10777
290. Jedrychowski MP, Wrann CD, Paulo JA, Gerber KK, Szpyt J, Robinson MM, et al. Detection and quantitation of circulating human irisin by tandem mass spectrometry. *Cell Metab.* (2015) 22:734–40. doi: 10.1016/j.cmet.2015.08.001
291. Mahgoub MO, D'Souza C, Al Darmaki R, Baniyas M, Adeghate E. An update on the role of irisin in the regulation of endocrine and metabolic functions. *Peptides* (2018) 104:15–23. doi: 10.1016/j.peptides.2018.03.018
292. Tsuchiya Y, Ando D, Goto K, Kiuchi M, Yamakita M, Koyama K. High-intensity exercise causes greater irisin response compared with low-intensity exercise under similar energy consumption. *Tohoku J Exp Med.* (2014) 233:135–40. doi: 10.1620/tjem.233.135
293. Miyamoto-Mikami E, Sato K, Kurihara T, Hasegawa N, Fujie S, Fujita S, et al. Endurance training-induced increase in circulating irisin levels is associated with reduction of abdominal visceral fat in middle-aged and older adults. *PLoS ONE* (2015) 10:e0120354. doi: 10.1371/journal.pone.0120354
294. Gmiat A, Mieszkowski J, Prusik K, Prusik K, Kortas J, Kochanowicz A, et al. Changes in pro-inflammatory markers and leucine concentrations in response to Nordic Walking training combined with vitamin D supplementation in elderly women. *Biogerontology* (2017) 18:535–48. doi: 10.1007/s10522-017-9694-8
295. Dulian K, Laskowski R, Grzywacz T, Kujach S, Flis DJ, Smaruj M, et al. The whole body cryostimulation modifies irisin concentration and reduces inflammation in middle aged, obese men. *Cryobiology* (2015) 71:398–404. doi: 10.1016/j.cryobiol.2015.10.143

296. Bluher S, Panagiotou G, Petroff D, Markert J, Wagner A, Klemm T, et al. Effects of a 1-year exercise and lifestyle intervention on irisin, adipokines, and inflammatory markers in obese children. *Obesity* (2014) 22:1701–8. doi: 10.1002/oby.20739
297. Szumilewicz A, Worska A, Piernicka M, Kuchta A, Kortas J, Jastrzebski Z, et al. The exercise-induced irisin is associated with improved levels of glucose homeostasis markers in pregnant women participating in 8-week prenatal group fitness program: a pilot study. *Biomed Res Int.* (2017) 2017:9414525. doi: 10.1155/2017/9414525
298. Sanchis-Gomar F, Alis R, Lippi G. Circulating irisin detection: does it really work? *Trends Endocrinol Metab.* (2015) 26:335–6. doi: 10.1016/j.tem.2015.05.004
299. Moreno-Navarrete JM, Ortega F, Serrano M, Guerra E, Pardo G, Tinahones F, et al. Irisin is expressed and produced by human muscle and adipose tissue in association with obesity and insulin resistance. *J Clin Endocrinol Metab.* (2013) 98:E769–78. doi: 10.1210/jc.2012-2749
300. Roca-Rivada A, Castelao C, Senin LL, Landrove MO, Baltar J, Belen Crujeiras A, et al. FNDC5/irisin is not only a myokine but also an adipokine. *PLoS ONE* (2013) 8:e60563. doi: 10.1371/journal.pone.0060563
301. Wrann CD, White JP, Salogiannnis J, Laznik-Bogoslavski D, Wu J, Ma D, et al. Exercise induces hippocampal BDNF through a PGC-1alpha/FNDC5 pathway. *Cell Metab.* (2013) 18:649–59. doi: 10.1016/j.cmet.2013.09.008
302. Tabak O, Simsek G, Erdenen F, Sozer V, Hasoglu T, Gelisgen R, et al. The relationship between circulating irisin, retinol binding protein-4, adiponectin and inflammatory mediators in patients with metabolic syndrome. *Arch Endocrinol Metab.* (2017) 61:515–23. doi: 10.1590/2359-3997000000289
303. Colaianni G, Cuscito C, Mongelli T, Oranger A, Mori G, Brunetti G, et al. Irisin enhances osteoblast differentiation *in vitro*. *Int J Endocrinol.* (2014) 2014:902186. doi: 10.1155/2014/902186
304. Anastasilakis AD, Polyzos SA, Makras P, Gkiomisi A, Bisbinas I, Katsarou A, et al. Circulating irisin is associated with osteoporotic fractures in postmenopausal women with low bone mass but is not affected by either teriparatide or denosumab treatment for 3 months. *Osteoporos Int.* (2014) 25:1633–42. doi: 10.1007/s00198-014-2673-x
305. Palermo A, Strollo R, Maddaloni E, Tuccinardi D, D'Onofrio L, Briganti SI, et al. Irisin is associated with osteoporotic fractures independently of bone mineral density, body composition or daily physical activity. *Clin Endocrinol.* (2015) 82:615–9. doi: 10.1111/cen.12672
306. Colaianni G, Cuscito C, Mongelli T, Pignataro P, Buccoliero C, Liu P, et al. The myokine irisin increases cortical bone mass. *Proc Natl Acad Sci USA.* (2015) 112:12157–62. doi: 10.1073/pnas.1516622112
307. Colaianni G, Mongelli T, Cuscito C, Pignataro P, Lippo L, Spiro G, et al. Irisin prevents and restores bone loss and muscle atrophy in hind-limb suspended mice. *Sci Rep.* (2017) 7:2811. doi: 10.1038/s41598-017-02557-8
308. Takayanagi H. New immune connections in osteoclast formation. *Ann NY Acad Sci.* (2010) 1192:117–23. doi: 10.1111/j.1749-6632.2009.05303.x
309. Alnaeeli M, Penninger JM, Teng YT. Immune interactions with CD4+ T cells promote the development of functional osteoclasts from murine CD11c+ dendritic cells. *J Immunol.* (2006) 177:3314–26. doi: 10.4049/jimmunol.177.5.3314
310. Lorenzo J, Horowitz M, Choi Y. Osteoimmunology: interactions of the bone and immune system. *Endocr Rev.* (2008) 29:403–40. doi: 10.1210/er.2007-0038
311. Lee SH, Kim TS, Choi Y, Lorenzo J. Osteoimmunology: cytokines and the skeletal system. *BMB Rep.* (2008) 41:495–510. doi: 10.5483/BMBRep.2008.41.7.495
312. Garrett RW, Emerson SG. Bone and blood vessels: the hard and the soft of hematopoietic stem cell niches. *Cell Stem Cell* (2009) 4:503–6. doi: 10.1016/j.stem.2009.05.011
313. Weitzmann MN, Ofotokun I. Physiological and pathophysiological bone turnover - role of the immune system. *Nat Rev Endocrinol.* (2016) 12:518–32. doi: 10.1038/nrendo.2016.91
314. Yun TJ, Chaudhary PM, Shu GL, Frazer JK, Ewings MK, Schwartz SM, et al. OPG/FDCR-1, a TNF receptor family member, is expressed in lymphoid cells and is up-regulated by ligating CD40. *J Immunol.* (1998) 161:6113–21.
315. Li Y, Toraldo G, Li A, Yang X, Zhang H, Qian WP, et al. B cells and T cells are critical for the preservation of bone homeostasis and attainment of peak bone mass *in vivo*. *Blood* (2007) 109:3839–48. doi: 10.1182/blood-2006-07-037994
316. Weitzmann MN. Bone and the immune system. *Toxicol Pathol.* (2017) 45:911–24. doi: 10.1177/0192623317735316
317. Cenci S, Toraldo G, Weitzmann MN, Roggia C, Gao Y, Qian WP, et al. Estrogen deficiency induces bone loss by increasing T cell proliferation and lifespan through IFN-gamma-induced class II transactivator. *Proc Natl Acad Sci USA.* (2003) 100:10405–10. doi: 10.1073/pnas.1533207100
318. Cenci S, Weitzmann MN, Roggia C, Namba N, Novack D, Woodring J, et al. Estrogen deficiency induces bone loss by enhancing T-cell production of TNF-alpha. *J Clin Invest.* (2000) 106:1229–37. doi: 10.1172/JCI11066
319. Pacifici R, Brown C, Puscheck E, Friedrich E, Slatopolsky E, Maggio D, et al. Effect of surgical menopause and estrogen replacement on cytokine release from human blood mononuclear cells. *Proc Natl Acad Sci USA.* (1991) 88:5134–8. doi: 10.1073/pnas.88.12.5134
320. Weitzmann MN, Pacifici R. Estrogen deficiency and bone loss: an inflammatory tale. *J Clin Invest.* (2006) 116:1186–94. doi: 10.1172/JCI28550
321. Ryan MR, Shepherd R, Leavey JK, Gao Y, Grassi F, Schnell FJ, et al. An IL-7-dependent rebound in thymic T cell output contributes to the bone loss induced by estrogen deficiency. *Proc Natl Acad Sci USA.* (2005) 102:16735–40. doi: 10.1073/pnas.0505168102
322. Tyagi AM, Srivastava K, Mansoori MN, Trivedi R, Chattopadhyay N, Singh D. Estrogen deficiency induces the differentiation of IL-17 secreting Th17 cells: a new candidate in the pathogenesis of osteoporosis. *PLoS ONE* (2012) 7:e44552. doi: 10.1371/journal.pone.0044552
323. Tyagi AM, Mansoori MN, Srivastava K, Khan MP, Kureel J, Dixit M, et al. Enhanced immunoprotective effects by anti-IL-17 antibody translates to improved skeletal parameters under estrogen deficiency compared with anti-RANKL and anti-TNF-alpha antibodies. *J Bone Miner Res.* (2014) 29:1981–92. doi: 10.1002/jbmr.2228
324. DeSelm CJ, Takahata Y, Warren J, Chappel JC, Khan T, Li X, et al. IL-17 mediates estrogen-deficient osteoporosis in an Act1-dependent manner. *J Cell Biochem.* (2012) 113:2895–902. doi: 10.1002/jcb.24165
325. Sjogren K, Engdahl C, Henning P, Lerner UH, Tremaroli V, Lagerquist MK, et al. The gut microbiota regulates bone mass in mice. *J Bone Miner Res.* (2012) 27:1357–67. doi: 10.1002/jbmr.1588
326. Li JY, Chassaing B, Tyagi AM, Vaccaro C, Luo T, Adams J, et al. Sex steroid deficiency-associated bone loss is microbiota dependent and prevented by probiotics. *J Clin Invest.* (2016) 126:2049–63. doi: 10.1172/JCI86062
327. Pacifici R. T cells: critical bone regulators in health and disease. *Bone* (2010) 47:461–71. doi: 10.1016/j.bone.2010.04.611
328. Verdelli C, Corbetta S. MECHANISMS IN ENDOCRINOLOGY: kidney involvement in patients with primary hyperparathyroidism: an update on clinical and molecular aspects. *Eur J Endocrinol.* (2017) 176:R39–52. doi: 10.1530/EJE-16-0430
329. Riggs BL, Melton LJ III. Involutional osteoporosis. *N Engl J Med.* (1986) 314:1676–86. doi: 10.1056/NEJM198606263142605
330. Canalis E, Giustina A, Bilezikian JP. Mechanisms of anabolic therapies for osteoporosis. *N Engl J Med.* (2007) 357:905–16. doi: 10.1056/NEJMra067395
331. Gao Y, Wu X, Terauchi M, Li JY, Grassi F, Galley S, et al. T cells potentiate PTH-induced cortical bone loss through CD40L signaling. *Cell Metab.* (2008) 8:132–45. doi: 10.1016/j.cmet.2008.07.001
332. Terauchi M, Li JY, Bedi B, Baek KH, Tawfeek H, Galley S, et al. T lymphocytes amplify the anabolic activity of parathyroid hormone through Wnt10b signaling. *Cell Metab.* (2009) 10:229–40. doi: 10.1016/j.cmet.2009.07.010

8

New Insights for RANKL as a Proinflammatory Modulator in Modeled Inflammatory Arthritis

Maria Papadaki[1,2], *Vagelis Rinotas*[1,2], *Foteini Violitzi*[1,2], *Trias Thireou*[1], *George Panayotou*[3], *Martina Samiotaki*[3] *and Eleni Douni*[1,2*]

[1] Laboratory of Genetics, Department of Biotechnology, Agricultural University of Athens, Athens, Greece, [2] Division of Immunology, Biomedical Sciences Research Center "Alexander Fleming", Athens, Greece, [3] Division of Molecular Oncology, Biomedical Sciences Research Center "Alexander Fleming", Athens, Greece

***Correspondence:**
Eleni Douni
douni@aua.gr

Receptor activator of nuclear factor-κB ligand (RANKL), a member of the Tumor Necrosis Factor (TNF) superfamily, constitutes the master regulator of osteoclast formation and bone resorption, whereas its involvement in inflammatory diseases remains unclear. Here, we used the human TNF transgenic mouse model of erosive inflammatory arthritis to determine if the progression of inflammation is affected by either genetic inactivation or overexpression of RANKL in transgenic mouse models. TNF-mediated inflammatory arthritis was significantly attenuated in the absence of functional RANKL. Notably, TNF overexpression could not compensate for RANKL-mediated osteopetrosis, but promoted osteoclastogenesis between the pannus and bone interface, suggesting RANKL-independent mechanisms of osteoclastogenesis in inflamed joints. On the other hand, simultaneous overexpression of RANKL and TNF in double transgenic mice accelerated disease onset and led to severe arthritis characterized by significantly elevated clinical and histological scores as shown by aggressive pannus formation, extended bone resorption, and massive accumulation of inflammatory cells, mainly of myeloid origin. RANKL and TNF cooperated not only in local bone loss identified in the inflamed calcaneous bone, but also systemically in distal femurs as shown by microCT analysis. Proteomic analysis in inflamed ankles from double transgenic mice overexpressing human TNF and RANKL showed an abundance of proteins involved in osteoclastogenesis, pro-inflammatory processes, gene expression regulation, and cell proliferation, while proteins participating in basic metabolic processes were downregulated compared to TNF and RANKL single transgenic mice. Collectively, these results suggest that RANKL modulates modeled inflammatory arthritis not only as a mediator of osteoclastogenesis and bone resorption but also as a disease modifier affecting inflammation and immune activation.

Keywords: RANKL, TNF, inflammation, arthritis, transgenic models, proteomics

INTRODUCTION

Receptor Activator of Nuclear Factor κB Ligand (RANKL), a Tumor necrosis factor (TNF) superfamily member, is the master regulator of osteoclast-induced bone resorption (1), that is necessary for the lifelong process of bone remodeling where mature bone tissue is removed from the skeleton and new bone tissue is formed by osteoblasts. RANKL binds as a trimer to its receptor RANK to promote osteoclast differentiation, activity and survival, which subsequently leads to bone resorption (2, 3). Osteoclasts derive from the myeloid lineage and have the unique ability to resorb bone through the decalcification and degradation of the bone matrix by hydrochloric acid and proteolysis, respectively (4). Genetic ablation of either RANKL or RANK results in severe osteopetrosis, a disease caused by osteoclast deficit, demonstrating that the RANKL/RANK system is indispensable for osteoclastogenesis (5–7). The function of RANKL is physiologically inhibited by the action of the decoy receptor osteoprotegerin (OPG) that binds to RANKL and prevents the process of osteoclastogenesis (8). An imbalance at the RANKL:OPG ratio caused by abundant RANKL levels is believed to be a major determinant in the development of bone loss diseases, including postmenopausal osteoporosis, a metabolic bone disease characterized by decreased bone density and increased fracture risk (9). The critical role of RANKL in osteoporosis is now well-established by the efficacy of denosumab, a human monoclonal anti-RANKL antibody, that specifically inhibits the interaction between RANKL and RANK, in postmenopausal osteoporosis (10). Although RANKL is best known for its function in osteoclastogenesis, it also plays multiple roles in the immune system (11), as it has been shown to enhance dendritic cell survival and regulates lymph node organogenesis. In addition, RANKL controls the development of autoimmune regulator $(AIRE)^+$ medullary thymic epithelial cells suggesting a key role of RANKL/RANK signals in the regulation of central tolerance. RANKL expression could also be detected in synovial fibroblasts and inflammatory cells isolated from the synovial fluid of Rheumatoid Arthritis (RA) patients, facilitating osteoclast maturation even in the absence of osteoblasts. Although the inhibition of RANKL effectively arrests progression of arthritic osteolysis, there are no evidence so far to support proinflammatory properties of RANKL (12). Thus, the role of RANKL in the progression of inflammation in RA remains unclear.

RA is a complex inflammatory disease characterized by synovial hyperplasia, cartilage damage, and bone erosions, leading to progressive disability. Inflammatory synovium, mainly including macrophage-like and fibroblast-like synoviocytes, leads to pannus formation that destroys the local articular structures through proteolytic digestion of the extracellular matrix (13). The destructive processes in RA involve a complex interplay between synovial fibroblasts, lymphocytes, macrophages, proinflammatory cytokines, and chemokines, inducing osteoclast-mediated bone resorption. TNF is a key proinflammatory cytokine in RA (14), as experimentally shown by the spontaneous development of chronic inflammatory polyarthritis upon TNF overexpression in transgenic mice (15, 16) and clinically by the efficacy of anti-TNF therapies in RA patients (17). Apart from its proinflammatory role, TNF also promotes bone resorption at sites of chronic inflammation, through the induction of osteoclastogenesis (18). Even though the RANK/RANKL signaling is also involved in local osteolysis induced by chronic inflammation, it remains unclear whether it is the absolute pathway. Previous studies have shown that proinflammatory cytokines such as TNF can compensate for RANKL during osteoclastogenesis *in vitro* (19–21), whereas it is unclear whether TNF can lead to osteoclastogenesis independently of RANKL, *in vivo*.

In the present study, we investigated the role of RANKL as a disease modifier in TNF-driven inflammatory arthritis employing two proprietary genetic models of RANKL-mediated pathologies; an osteopetrosis model caused by osteoclast absence due to a functional mutation in the *RANKL* gene (22) ($Rankl^{tles/tles}$ mice) and osteoporosis transgenic models that overexpress human RANKL (TgRANKL mice) displaying increased osteoclast activity and bone resorption (23). Our results showed that the onset and the progression of TNF-mediated arthritis is dramatically affected by deregulated RANKL expression, supporting an underestimated role of RANKL in inflammatory osteolytic diseases.

MATERIALS AND METHODS

Mouse Husbandry

Osteopetrotic $Rankl^{tles/tles}$ mice (22), osteoporotic Tg5516 and Tg5519 mice (23), and arthritic Tg197 mice (15) were maintained and bred under specific pathogen free conditions in the animal facility of Biomedical Sciences Research Center "Alexander Fleming." All animal procedures were approved and carried out in strict accordance with the guidelines of the Institutional Animal Care and Use Committee and the Region of Attica Veterinarian Office.

Arthritic Clinical Score

Arthritis was evaluated macroscopically weekly in ankle joints in a blinded manner using the following semi-quantitative arthritis score (24); 0: no arthritis (normal appearance and grip strength); (1) mild arthritis (joint swelling); (2) moderate arthritis (severe joint swelling and digit deformation, no grip strength); and (3) severe arthritis (ankylosis detected on flexion and severely impaired movement). Grip strength was evaluated as regards the ability of the mouse to grasp the cage grid cover.

Histological Processing and Scoring of Joints

Ankle joints and femurs were fixed in 10% formalin overnight at 4°C, decalcified in 13% EDTA for 14 days, and embedded in paraffin. Sections of 5 μm thickness were stained with hematoxylin and eosin, and the histopathologic score was evaluated microscopically, in a blinded manner using a modified scoring system (24) as follows; 0: no detectable pathology; 1: hyperplasia of the synovial membrane and presence of polymorphonuclear infiltrates; 2: pannus and fibrous tissue formation and focal subchondral bone erosion; 3: articular cartilage destruction and bone erosion; 4: extensive articular cartilage destruction and bone erosion, and 5: massive destruction of ankle joint with undefined structure. Osteoclasts were stained for TRAP (Tartrate Resistant Acid Phosphatase) activity using the leukocyte acid phosphatase kit 386A (Sigma-Aldrich), whereas cartilage was stained with Toluidine Blue (Sigma-Aldrich). TRAP staining was quantified as an osteoclast surface fraction (percentage of osteoclast surface in total bone surface, Oc.S/BS, %) focusing either in the bone marrow compartment area or the pannus-bone interface area using the open source software for bone histomorphometry "TrapHisto" (25).

MicroCT Analysis

Bone samples (ankles and femurs) were fixed in 10% formalin overnight at 4°C and then washed and stored in PBS. Microarchitecture of the ankle joints and the distal femurs from 6 weeks old mice was evaluated using a high-resolution SkyScan1172 microtomographic (microCT) imaging system (Bruker). Images were acquired at 50 KeV, 100 μA with a 0.5 mm aluminum filter. Three-dimensional reconstructions (8.8 mm cubic resolution) were generated using NRecon software (Bruker) as previously described (26). For the trabecular area of the calcaneous bone, we assessed the bone volume fraction (BV/TV, %), and trabecular number (Tb.N, mm^{-1}). Calcaneous trabecular geometry was assessed using 75 continuous CT slides (300 μm) located at trabecular area underneath the growth plate of the calcaneous bone. For the trabecular area of the distal femur bone we assessed the bone volume fraction (BV/TV, %), and the trabecular number (Tb.N, mm^{-1}). Femoral trabecular geometry was assessed using 300 continuous CT slides (1,800 μm) located at the trabecular area underneath the growth plate. Femural cortical geometry was assessed using 100 continuous CT slides (600 μm) located at the femoral midshaft, where the bone volume fraction (BV/TV, %) and the bone volume (Ct.BV, mm^3) were measured.

Flow Cytometry

Mice were sacrificed, ankle joints were removed and cells were extracted from the synovium based on a modified protocol (27). In brief, synovial tissue from ankle joints was minced in RPMI medium containing 5% FBS, glutamine and freshly made Collagenase type II isolated from *Clostridium histolyticum* (Worthington) and incubated in a shaking waterbath for 90 min at 37°C. Single cell suspensions were generated through pushing the tissue on a size-40 metallic mesh disc (Sigma-Aldrich). Cells were filtered through a 100-μm sheet, centrifuged, resuspended in FACS buffer (1% FBS in PBS) and counted using a hematocytometer. 10^6 cells were plated in a 96 V-bottom well plate (Costar) and stained with antibodies against CD45-Alexa 700, CD11b-PE, Gr1-FITC, TCRα-APC/Cy7, and B220-PerCP (Biolegend). Cells were incubated for 30 min at 4°C, and then were washed and transferred to tubes for analysis. BD FACS Canto II Flow Cytometer (BD Biosciences) was used for processing the samples and results were analyzed with FlowJo v7.6 software.

Quantitative Expression Analysis

Total RNA was extracted from ankle joints using a monophasic solution of guanidine isothiocyanate and phenol according to the manufacturer's instructions (TRI Reagent, MRC). After removal of DNA remnants with DNase I treatment (Sigma-Aldrich), first strand cDNA was synthesized using 2 μg of total RNA and MMLV reverse transcriptase (Sigma-Aldrich). Templates were amplified with SsoFast EvaGreen Master Mix (Bio-Rad Laboratories) on the CFX96 real time PCR instrument (Bio-Rad Laboratories). Quantitative Real Time PCR (qPCR) was performed at 55°C for all genes (except: IL6 at 58°C) for 40 cycles. Specific primer pairs (Eurofins Genomics) were used for the quantitative expression as follows (sequences 5′ to 3′, sense and antisense): *human RANKL:* ACGCGTATT TACAGCCAGTG and CCCGTAATTGCTCCAATCTG; *mouse RANKL:* TGTACTTTCGAGCGCAGATG and AGGCTTGTT TCATCCTCCTG; *human TNF:* GAGGCCAAGCCCTGGTATG and CGGGCCGATTGATCTCAGC; *mouse TNF:* CAGGCG GTGCCTATGTCTC and CGATCACCCCGAAGTTCAGTAG; *mouse IL-1β:* ATCTTTTGGGGTCCGTCAACT and CCCTCA CACTCAGATCATCTTCT; and *mouse IL-6*: TAGTCCTTC CTACCCCAATTTCC and TTGGTCCTTAGCCACTCCTTC. The samples were normalized to GAPDH expression (TTA GCACCCCTGGCCAAGG and CTTACTCCTTGGAGGCCA TG). Relative expression was calculated as the fold difference compared with control values using BioRad CFX96™. For each experiment at least three biological and two technical replicates were used.

Proteomics

For the proteomic analysis, ankle joints were isolated from 6-week-old WT, Tg5519, Tg197 and Tg197/Tg5519 mice (6–8 mice per genotype).

Protein Extraction and Lysis

Ankle joints from the four different genotypes (WT, Tg5519, Tg197, and Tg197/Tg5519) were ground to powder in liquid nitrogen using a pestle and mortar and solubilized in 150 μl lysis buffer containing 100 mM Tris-HCl, pH 7.6, 4% SDS and freshly made 100 mM DTT. Samples were incubated for 3 min at 95°C, followed by 20 min incubation in a sonication water bath in order to shear the DNA. Finally, the samples were centrifuged at 17,000 × g for 30 min at 4°C and the supernatants were transferred to new tubes.

Protein Digestion

The protein extracts were processed according to the Filter Aided Sample Preparation (FASP) protocol using spin filter devices with 10 kDa cutoff (Sartorius, VN01H02). 40 μl lysate were diluted in 8 M Urea/100 mM Tris-HCl pH 8.5, the filters were extensively washed with the urea solution, covered with 10 mg/ml iodoacetamide in the urea solution and incubated for 30 min in the dark for the alkylation of cysteines. The proteins on the top of the filters were washed three times with 50 mM ammonium bicarbonate and finally the proteins were digested adding 1 μg trypsin/LysC mix in 80 μl 50 mM ammonium bicarbonate solution (Mass spec grade, Promega) and incubated overnight at 37°C. The peptides were eluted by centrifugation, followed by speed-vac-assisted solvent removal, reconstitution in 0.1% formic acid, 2% acetonitrile in water, and transferring to LC-MS glass sample vials. Peptide concentration was determined by nanodrop absorbance measurement at 280 nm.

Ultra High Pressure NanoLC

2.5 μg peptides were injected and pre-concentrated with a flow of 3 μl/ min for 10 min using a C18 trap column (Acclaim PepMap100, 100 μm × 2 cm, Thermo Scientific) and then loaded onto a 50 cm C18 column (75 μm ID, particle size 2 μm, 100 Å, Acclaim PepMap RSLC, Thermo Scientific). The binary pumps of the HPLC (RSLCnano, Thermo Scientific) consisted of solution A

(2% v/v ACN in 0.1% v/v formic acid) and solution B (80% ACN in 0.1% formic acid). The peptides were separated using a linear gradient of 4–40% B in 450 min at a flow rate of 300 nl/min. The column was placed in an oven operating at 35°C.

MS/MS

The purified peptides were ionized through nanoESI and analyzed by an LTQ Orbitrap XL Mass spectrometer (Thermo Fisher Scientific). Full scan MS spectra were acquired in the orbitrap (m/z 300–1,600) using profile mode with a data-dependent acquisition method were the resolution was set to 60,000 at m/z 400 and the automatic gain control target at 10^6 ions. The six most intense ions were sequentially isolated for collision-induced MS/MS fragmentation and their detection in the linear ion trap. Dynamic exclusion was set to 1 min and activated for 90 sec. Ions with single charge states were excluded. Lockmass of m/z 445.120025 was used for internal calibration. Xcalibur (Thermo Scientific) was used to control the system and acquire the raw files.

Data Analysis

The raw files were analyzed using MaxQuant (version 1.6.0.16), the complete Uniprot *Mus musculus (228 311 entries / Oct-2016)* and a common contaminants database by the Andromeda search engine. The search parameters used were strict trypsin specificity, allowing up to two missed cleavages. Oxidation of methionines, deamidation of asparagine and glutamine residues and N-terminal acetylation were set as variable modifications. Cysteine carbamidomethylation was set as a fixed modification. "Second peptide" option was enabled. The protein and peptide false discovery rate (FDR) was set to 0.01 for both proteins and peptides with a minimum length of seven amino acids that was determined by searching a reverse database. Protein abundance was calculated on the basis of the normalized spectral protein intensity as label free quantitation (LFQ intensity) enabling the "match between runs" option (set at 0.7 min). LFQ was performed with a minimum ratio count of 2.

Proteomics Statistical Analysis

The statistical analysis was performed using Perseus (version 1.6.1.3) (28). Proteins identified as contaminants, "reverse" and "only identified by site" were filtered out. The LFQ intensities were transformed to logarithmic values (log2(x)). The biological replicas were grouped together. The protein groups were filtered to obtain at least 4 valid values in at least one group. A total of 2,009 label free quantified proteins were subjected to statistical analysis with ANOVA test (permutation based FDR with 0.05 cutoff) for the comparison of all groups. The 1,019 statistically significant proteins were then Z-scored, visualized by Euclidean hierarchical clustering and grouped into three main clusters (I, II and III) consisting of 403, 179, and 437 proteins, respectively. Tukey's honestly significant difference (THSD) was performed on the ANOVA significant hits to determine in exactly which pairwise group comparisons, a given protein was differentially expressed. Enrichment analysis was performed with ClueGO (29) (version 3.6.1), a Cytoscape plug-in, using KEGG (30) pathways database. Only pathways that had p-value <0.05 (hypergeometric test with Benjamini–Hochberg correction) were considered and "is Specific" was set to 60%. Default values were used for the other parameters.

Statistical Analysis

All results are expressed as mean ± standard error mean (SEM). Statistical significance was calculated for two groups using Student's t-tests or the Mann-Whitney test for non-parametric distribution. The log-rank test was used for survival curve comparison. One-Way analysis of variance (ANOVA) and Tukey *post-hoc* test was performed to compare means of multiple groups. P-values <0.05 were considered significant; $^{*}p < 0.05$, $^{**}p < 0.01$, $^{***}p < 0.001$ when not otherwise specified.

RESULTS

Significant Attenuation of TNF-Mediated Inflammatory Arthritis in the Absence of Functional RANKL

To elucidate the role of RANKL in the progression of TNF-mediated inflammatory arthritis *in vivo*, we generated Tg197/Rankl$^{tles/tles}$ mice by crossing Tg197 arthritic mice overexpressing human TNF with Rankl$^{tles/tles}$ osteopetrotic mice carrying a functional mutation in the *RANKL* gene (22). The Tg197 transgenic mouse model spontaneously develops inflammatory arthritis characterized by swelling of the ankles, infiltration of inflammatory cells, synovial hyperplasia, articular cartilage destruction and bone erosion, closely resembling the human pathology of rheumatoid arthritis. Rankl$^{tles/tles}$ mice, expressing an inactive form of RANKL incapable of forming trimers, are osteopetrotic due to osteoclast absence (22). Tg197/Rankl$^{tles/tles}$ mice also displayed an osteopetrotic phenotype as shown by failure of tooth eruption, and growth retardation similarly to Rankl$^{tles/tles}$ mice, whereas an improvement was observed in their survival percentage compared to Rankl$^{tles/tles}$ mice even though not significant (**Figures 1A,B**). Macroscopically, arthritis appeared in Tg197 mice at 3 weeks of age as detected by mild swelling of the ankle joint, which progressed with severe joint swelling and distortion accompanied by movement deterioration by the 10th week of age, the end point of the study (**Figure 1C**). However, arthritis signs were not detected in Tg197/Rankl$^{tles/tles}$ mice throughout the study period (**Figure 1C**). Histological analysis at 10 weeks of age, when Tg197 control mice reached the peak of disease, demonstrated a dramatic attenuation of inflammatory arthritis in Tg197/Rankl$^{tles/tles}$ mice, as shown by moderate synovial hyperplasia (**Figures 1D,E**). These results indicate that RANKL loss significantly attenuates inflammatory arthritis onset and progression.

RANKL-Independent Formation of Osteoclasts in TNF-Driven Inflammatory Arthritis

So far, it has been shown that RANKL is necessary for the physiological process of bone remodeling. However, it is unclear whether osteoclasts can be formed in a TNF-driven inflammatory

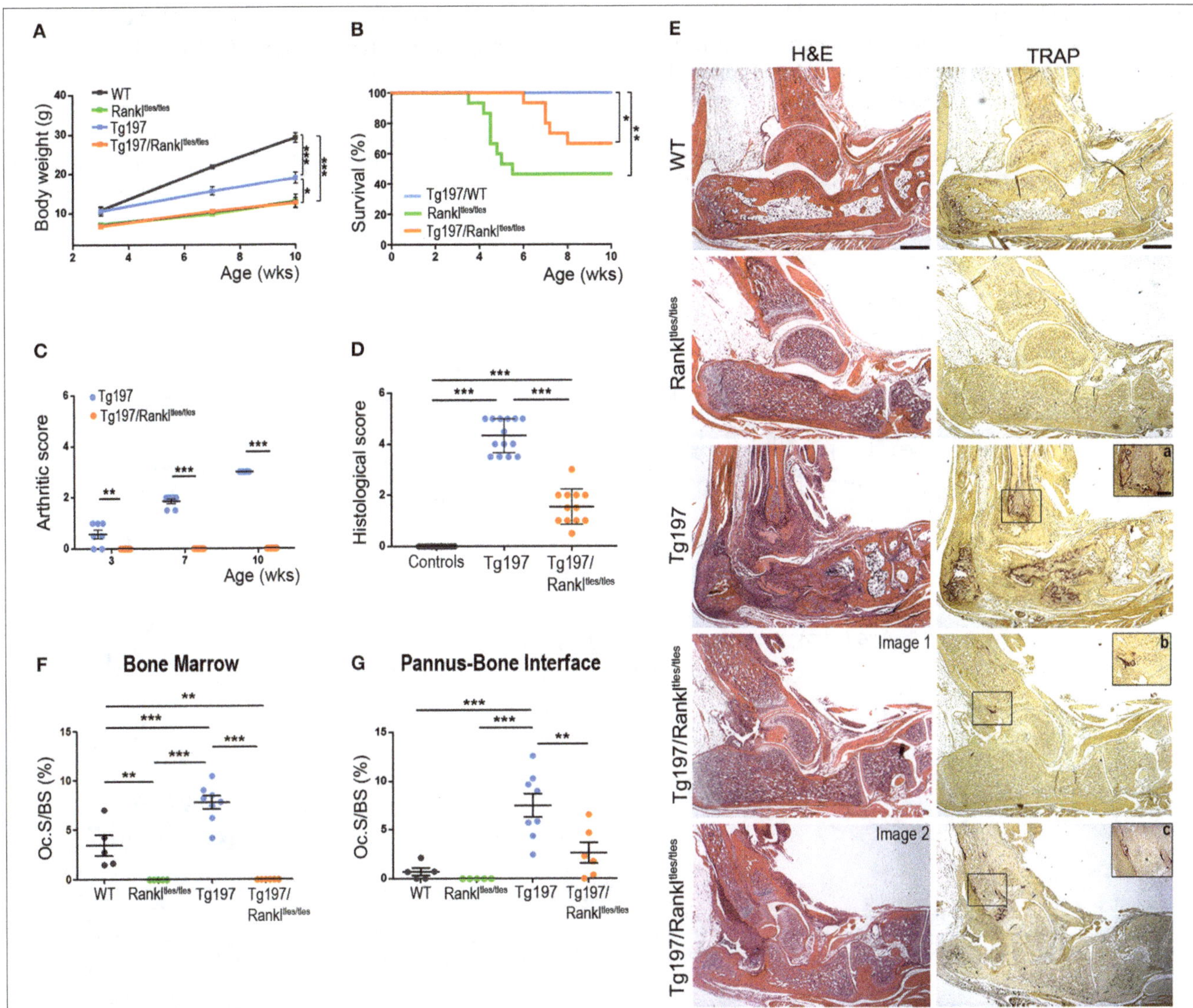

FIGURE 1 | Dramatic attenuation of TNF-driven arthritis upon RANKL genetic inactivation. Tg197/Rankl$^{tles/tles}$ mice and sex-matched control littermates WT (Rankl$^{tles/+}$), Tg197 (Tg197/Rankl$^{tles/+}$), and Rankl$^{tles/tles}$ were assessed until the 10th week of age for **(A)** body weight gain ($n = 6$–7 per genotype), **(B)** percent survival ($n = 15$ per genotype), **(C)** clinical arthritic score (from 0 to 3) in both ankles for each mouse ($n = 7$ per genotype), and **(D)** histological arthritic score (from 0 to 5) in both ankles for each mouse at 10 weeks of age ($n = 12$–14 per genotype). Control group includes Rankl$^{tles/+}$ and Rankl$^{tles/tles}$ mice. **(E)** Representative histological images of hematoxylin/eosin (H&E) and Tartrate-resistant acid phosphatase (TRAP) stained ankle joint sections from two Tg197/Rankl$^{tles/tles}$ mice, displaying either mild (Image 1), or moderate inflammatory arthritis (Image 2), and their littermate controls at 10 weeks of age. Boxed areas at TRAP staining show a higher magnification of regions harboring TRAP+ cells in Tg197 **(a)** and Tg197/Rankl$^{tles/tles}$ mice **(b,c)**. Scale bars: 300 μm at H&E and TRAP, 80 μm at boxed areas in TRAP. TRAP staining was measured as osteoclast surface fraction (Oc.S/BS, %) quantification in **(F)** the bone marrow compartment area, and **(G)** the pannus-bone interface ($n = 5$–8 per genotype). Data represent mean values ± SEM. One-Way ANOVA and Tukey *post-hoc* test was performed for statistical analysis of more than two groups and Mann-Whitney test was performed for statistical analysis between two groups. The log-rank test was used for survival curve comparison. Asterisks mark statistically significant difference ($^{*}p < 0.05$, $^{**}p < 0.01$, $^{***}p < 0.001$).

environment even without RANKL signaling *in vivo*. To investigate this possibility, we analyzed the hematoxylin/eosin stained sections for osteopetrosis and in parallel we stained serial sections from all experimental groups with Tartrate-resistant acid phosphatase (TRAP), which is an osteoclastic marker. As expected, Rankl$^{tles/tles}$ mice failed to develop TRAP+ osteoclasts and developed osteopetrosis, whereas enhanced osteoclastogenesis and bone resorption was identified in arthritic Tg197 mice at sites of pannus invasion into bone (**Figures 1E–G**). However, TNF overexpression failed to reverse the RANKL-mediated osteopetrotic phenotype in Tg197/Rankl$^{tles/tles}$ mice, which was further confirmed by the absence of osteoclastogenesis in the bone marrow compartment (**Figures 1E,F**). Instead, TRAP+ osteoclasts were identified in the inflamed synovium of Tg197/Rankl$^{tles/tles}$ mice (**Figures 1E,G**), indicating RANKL-independent mechanisms of osteoclastogenesis at sites of

TNF-induced inflammation *in vivo*. Notably, the extent of osteoclastogenesis, either limited or moderate, depended on arthritis severity in Tg197/Rankl$^{tles/tles}$ ankles (**Figures 1E,G**). Collectively, our results suggest that TNF overexpression can induce RANKL-independent osteoclastogenesis at sites of inflammatory invasion into the ankle joints but cannot compensate for RANKL in bone remodeling *in vivo* as the osteopetrotic phenotype is not affected.

RANKL Overexpression Exacerbates TNF-Driven Inflammatory Arthritis

We next investigated whether the progression of inflammatory arthritis in the TNF transgenic model was affected by human RANKL (huRANKL) overexpression. This was achieved by crossing Tg197 mice with the TgRANKL transgenic lines Tg5516 and Tg5519 that express huRANKL at a physiological relevant tissue-specific pattern. Tg5516 mice expressing huRANKL at

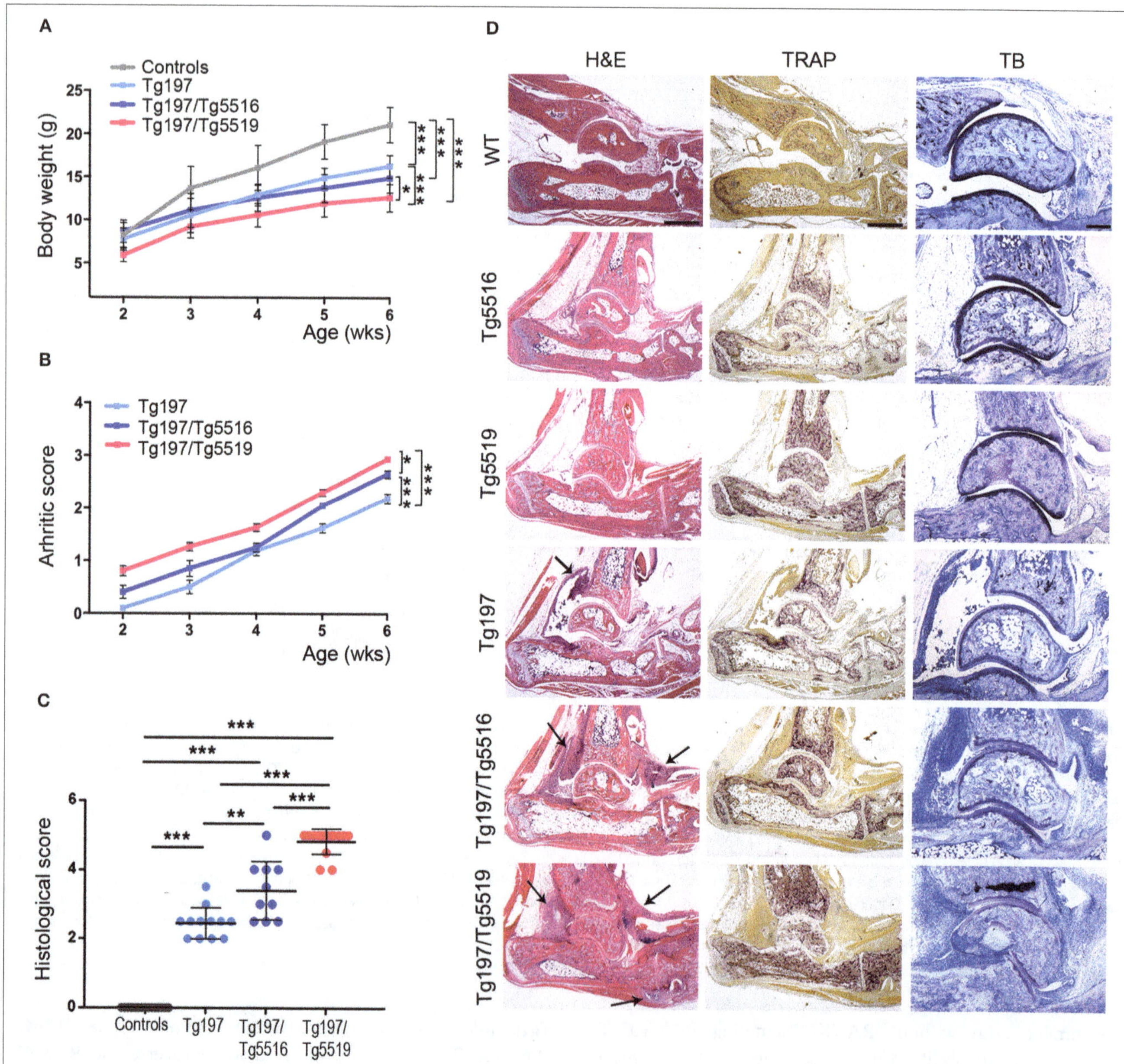

FIGURE 2 | RANKL overexpression exacerbates TNF-driven arthritis. Assessment of arthritis progression was conducted in Tg197/TgRANKL mice (Tg197/Tg5516, Tg197/Tg5519), Tg197 and sex-matched control littermates (WT, Tg5516, and Tg5519) till the 6th week of age. **(A)** Body weight curves ($n = 10$ per genotype), **(B)** clinical arthritic scores ($n = 10$–15 per genotype), **(C)** histological arthritic score ($n = 10$–15 per genotype), and **(D)** representative ankle joint sections from each genotype ($n = 10$–15) at the 6th week of age stained with hematoxylin/eosin (H&E), TRAP for osteoclasts and Toluidine Blue (TB) for articular cartilage destruction. Arrows at H&E indicate focal pannus invasion into subchondral bone regions. Scale bars: 300 μm at H&E and TRAP; 150 μm at TB. Data represent mean values ± SEM. One-Way ANOVA and Tukey *post-hoc* test was performed. Asterisks mark statistically significant difference (* $p < 0.05$, ** $p < 0.01$, *** $p < 0.001$).

low levels develop mild trabecular bone loss, while a more severe osteoporotic phenotype is identified in the Tg5519 line overexpressing huRANKL with features of severe trabecular bone loss and cortical porosity (23). Simultaneous overexpression of RANKL and TNF in Tg197/TgRANKL mice resulted in an aggressive arthritic phenotype, characterized by earlier arthritis onset and exacerbated clinical symptoms, such as reduced body weight gain and increased arthritis scores compared to Tg197 arthritic control mice (**Figures 2A,B**). Histopathological analysis at 6 weeks of age, when arthritic manifestations in Tg197 mice were restricted on synovial hyperplasia and focal pannus formation, showed significantly increased arthritis progression in Tg197/Tg5519 mice characterized by aggravated inflammatory pannus formation, increased osteoclastogenesis, massive bone destruction and surface cartilage degradation as indicated by staining with hematoxylin/eosin, TRAP and Toluidine blue (**Figures 2C,D**). Similarly, Tg197/Tg5516 mice displayed an exacerbation of inflammatory arthritis compared to Tg197 mice but to a lesser extent as regards Tg197/Tg5519 mice, indicating a RANKL dose effect on arthritis progression (**Figures 2C,D**).

A hallmark of RA is the accumulation of inflammatory cells such as monocytes, neutrophils and lymphocytes in the proliferating synovium that penetrates the cartilage and the bone in the form of pannus causing aberrant joint destruction. So far, the role of RANKL in inflammation remains enigmatic. To examine whether the exacerbated arthritis phenotype developed in Tg197/TgRANKL mice correlates with an increased inflammatory profile, we analyzed the synovial tissue for inflammatory cells through flow cytometry (**Figure 3**). Our analysis showed a significant increase in the number of infiltrated cells extracted from Tg197/Tg5519 inflamed ankles compared to Tg197 mice (Tg197/Tg5519: $13.15 \pm 2.72 \times 10^6$ cells vs. Tg197: $4.39 \pm 0.16 \times 10^6$ cells), supporting arthritis exacerbation. More specifically, $CD45^+$ hematopoietic-derived cell infiltrates were increased 4 times in the synovium of Tg197/Tg5519 mice compared to Tg197 mice (Tg197/Tg5519: $9.59 \pm 2.2 \times 10^6$ cells vs. Tg197: $2.51 \pm 0.09 \times 10^6$ cells), while no statistical changes were identified between Tg5519 and WT mice (**Figure 3A**). The synovium of Tg197/Tg5519 mice was infiltrated by 2-fold more $CD11b^+Gr1^-$ monocytes/macrophages (Tg197/Tg5519: $2.91 \pm 0.28 \times 10^6$ cells vs. Tg197: $1.36 \pm 0.11 \times 10^6$ cells), and 5-fold more $CD11b^+Gr1^+$ granulocytes (Tg197/Tg5519: $2.4 \pm 0.73 \times 10^6$ cells vs. Tg197: $0.44 \pm 0.04 \times 10^6$ cells) than Tg197 mice, where monocytes and synovial macrophages are the dominant inflammatory cells (**Figure 3B**). The absolute numbers of B220+ B lymphocytes (Tg197/Tg5519: $0.98 \pm 0.11 \times 10^6$ cells vs. Tg197: $0.51 \pm 0.06 \times 10^6$ cells) and TCRα+ T lymphocytes (Tg197/Tg5519: $1.27 \pm 0.27 \times 10^6$ cells vs. Tg197: $0.5 \pm 0.05 \times 10^6$ cells) were also significantly increased in comparison to Tg197 mice, however to a lesser extent than myeloid cells (**Figure 3B**).

As regards the percentage of inflammatory cells in the arthritic synovium, flow cytometry revealed a statistical increase of the percentage of $CD45^+$ hematopoietic cells in Tg197/Tg5519 mice compared to Tg197, supporting exacerbation of inflammation (**Figure 3C**). Even though the percentages of B and T lymphocytes were rather low in the inflamed synovium of double transgenic mice (Tg197/Tg5519) and arthritic mice (Tg197), $CD11b^+/Gr1^-$ macrophages/monocytes were prevalent in Tg197, while $CD11b^+/Gr1^+$ granulocytes in Tg197/Tg5519 mice (**Figure 3D**), indicating probable differences in pathogenic mechanisms. Similarly, inflamed synovium from Tg197/Tg5516 mice also contained increased numbers and percentages of $CD45^+$ hematopoietic cells (Tg197/Tg5516: $72.4 \pm 1.2\%$ cells vs. Tg197: $59.02 \pm 0.37\%$) and $CD11b^+/Gr1^+$ granulocytes (Tg197/Tg5516: $15.63 \pm 0.62\%$ vs. Tg197: $10.9 \pm 1\%$) compared to Tg197. Collectively, the aberrant co-expression of TNF and RANKL, modifies the inflammatory profile in the inflamed ankles toward a massive accumulation of inflammatory cells mainly of myeloid origin.

Furthermore, the cytokine profile of the inflamed ankle joints was investigated through qPCR. Expression analysis for endogenous RANKL showed a progressive increase in Tg197 and Tg197/Tg5519 mice compared to control groups WT and Tg5519, indicating a positive correlation with arthritis severity (**Figure 3E**). Similarly, the expression levels of the huRANKL transgene were significantly increased in Tg197/Tg5519 mice compared to Tg5519 mice (**Figure 3F**), supporting an impact of the arthritic milieu in the regulation of the transgene's expression since it carries regulatory regions. In contrast, the expression levels of the endogenous TNF and those of the human TNF transgene were similar between Tg197 and Tg197/Tg5519 mice (**Figures 3E,F**), excluding their possible involvement in arthritis aggravation upon RANKL overexpression. We also investigated the expression of two proinflammatory cytokines, IL-6 and IL-1b in inflamed ankles (**Figures 3G–I**). Both cytokines were significantly upregulated in Tg197 mice compared to WT mice. The expression level of IL-6, a proinflammatory cytokine of the acute phase response that promotes neutrophil production, was further 1.5-fold increased in Tg197/Tg5519 mice compared to Tg197 (**Figure 3G**), in line with the granulocytic arthritic phenotype developed in such mice (**Figures 3B,D**). Instead, IL-1b, a proinflammatory cytokine expressed by activated macrophages, was 2-fold decreased in Tg197/Tg5519 compared to Tg197 mice (**Figure 3I**), which could be explained by the proportional decrease of macrophages in the inflamed synovium of Tg197/Tg5519 mice (**Figure 3D**).

Cooperative Effect of RANKL and TNF in Local and Systemic Bone Resorption

We further investigated whether the exacerbated arthritis phenotype identified in Tg197/TgRANKL mice affected bone erosion locally. Histological examination of the inflamed ankles from Tg197/TgRANKL mice showed pronounced inflammatory bone destruction. To quantify bone loss locally, we performed microcomputed tomography (microCT) at the trabecular region of the calcaneous bone, which is proximal to the inflamed synovium and contains an organized trabecular structure. Both TgRANKL osteoporotic mice and Tg197 arthritic mice showed trabecular bone loss in the calcaneous bone at 6 weeks of age (**Figure 4**), while the calcaneous bone loss was further exacerbated in Tg197/RANKL mice compared

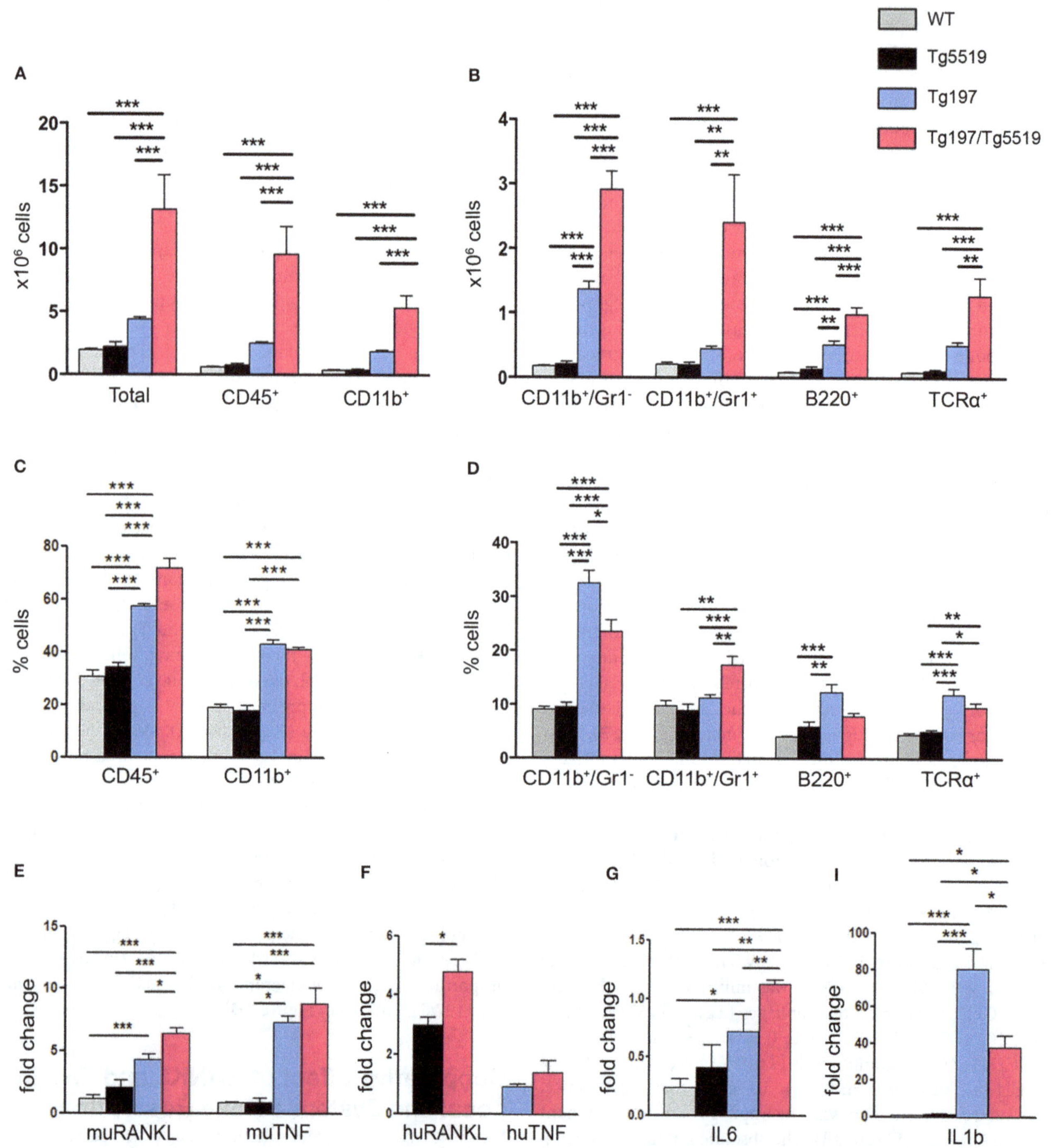

FIGURE 3 | Increased inflammatory cell infiltration in the synovium of Tg197/TgRANKL mice. **(A,B)** Absolute cell counts and **(C,D)** percentage of synovial subpopulations from 6 week-old Tg197/Tg5519 mice and sex-matched littermates (WT, Tg5519, Tg197) as determined by flow cytometry using antibodies against CD45 (hematopoietic cells), CD11b (myeloid cells), Gr1 (granulocytes), B220 (B lymphocytes) and TCRα (T lymphocytes) ($n = 4$–5 per genotype). qPCR analysis in inflamed ankles from 6 week-old Tg197/Tg5519 mice and littermate controls ($n = 3$–4) for **(E)** mouse RANKL and mouse TNF, **(F)** human RANKL and human TNF, **(G)** IL6 and **(I)** IL1b cytokine. Data represent mean values ± SEM. One-Way ANOVA and Tukey *post-hoc* test was performed for more than two groups and Student's *t*-test for two groups. Asterisks mark statistically significant difference ($^{*}p < 0.05$, $^{**}p < 0.01$, $^{***}p < 0.001$).

to the control littermate groups (WT, TgRANKL, Tg197). In the severe osteoporotic model Tg5519 the presence of the huTNF transgene promoted bone loss in an additive manner. Assessment of the trabecular bone volume fraction (BV/TV, %) demonstrated a 28% reduction in Tg5519, 46% in Tg197 and 73% in Tg197/Tg5519 compared to WT

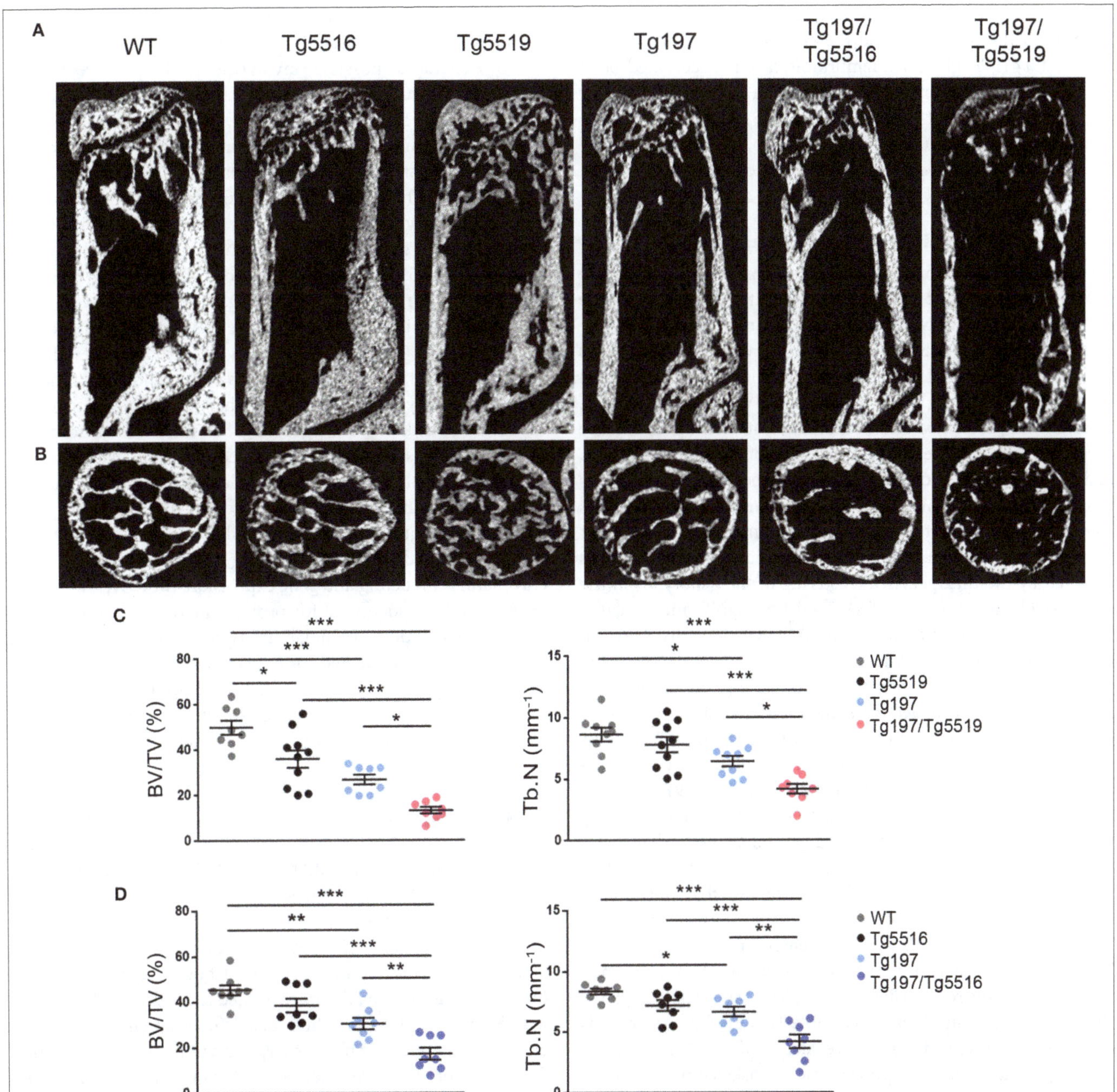

FIGURE 4 | Synergistic effect of RANKL and TNF in inflamed bone loss. MicroCT analysis in the trabecular region of the calcaneous bone from mice of each group at 6 weeks of age as shown by **(A)** representative longitudinal sections and **(B)** cross-sectional sections. Quantitative measurements with microCT in the trabecular area of the calcaneous bone for BV/TV (Bone Volume/Total Volume, %), and Tb.N (Trabecular Number per mm) in **(C)** Tg197/Tg5519 and littermates ($n = 8$–10, equal number of sexes per genotype), and **(D)** Tg197/Tg5516 and littermates ($n = 8$, equal number of sexes per genotype). Data represent mean values ± SEM. One-Way ANOVA and Tukey *post-hoc* test was performed for more than two groups. Asterisks mark statistically significant difference (*$p < 0.05$, **$p < 0.01$, ***$p < 0.001$).

group (**Figures 4A–C**). Furthermore, a synergistic effect was identified when huTNF was introduced in the mild osteoporosis model Tg5516, as Tg197/Tg5516 mice displayed a 62% reduction in BV/TV, while Tg5516 and Tg197 together reached a 48% reduction compared to WT (**Figure 4D**). These results indicate that the exacerbated arthritis developed in Tg197/TgRANKL mice coincides with a cooperative local bone loss.

To investigate whether simultaneous overexpression of RANKL and TNF also affected other skeletal sites outside of the inflamed ankles, we analyzed both metaphyseal and diaphyseal regions in distal femurs from Tg197, TgRANKL, and

Tg197/TgRANKL mice (**Figure 5**). Similarly to the calcaneous bone, both the trabecular and the cortical regions of the non-inflamed Tg197/TgRANKL femurs displayed exacerbated bone loss. The severe osteoporotic phenotype in Tg5519 was further aggravated, while mild osteoporosis in Tg5516 mice converted to severe osteoporosis upon huTNF expression, indicating that TNF and RANKL also cooperate in systemic bone loss.

Proteomic Analysis of Inflamed Joints

To identify altered biological processes and changes in the proteome at osteolytic inflammatory arthritis aggravated by the overexpression of RANKL, we utilized a comparative proteomic approach using LC-MS/MS and label free quantitation in ankles from 6 week-old Tg197/Tg5519 transgenic mice and control groups, including Tg197, Tg5519, and WT littermate mice. Analysis was performed on whole ankle joints in order to capture deregulated protein networks at the time of isolation while also maintaining all the populations and the potential interactions in inflamed ankles. For each ankle we quantified 2,009 proteins using label-free quantitation (LFQ) determined by the MaxQuant software (31, 32). We achieved high biological reproducibility as reflected by the unsupervised clustering of the genotypes in the composed heatmap (**Figure 6A**). To define significant regulated proteins, we performed one-way ANOVA analysis between the four genotypes and identified 1,019 significantly regulated proteins (**Figure 6A**). Hierarchical clustering of significantly regulated proteins revealed three major groups. Cluster I consists of 403 proteins, Cluster II of 179 and Cluster III of 437 proteins (**Figure 6A**). Bioinformatic "annotation enrichment analysis" in these clusters using ClueGO/CluePedia software (29) identified the main biological pathways (KEGG database) regulated by these proteins. Cluster I contained proteins involved in basic metabolic processes such as citrate cycle (TCA), oxidative phosphorylation or glycolysis/gluconeogenesis that were found specifically downregulated in arthritic groups Tg197 and Tg197Tg5519 (**Figure 6B** and **Supplementary Table 1**). Cluster II is composed mostly of ribosomal proteins which are enriched in huRANKL overexpressing mice Tg5519 and Tg197/Tg5519 (**Figure 6C** and **Supplementary Table 2**). Enrichment analysis in Cluster III revealed a high prevalence of proteins involved in phagosome, lysosome, proteasome, cytoskeleton regulation, leukocyte transendothelial migration and Fcγ-receptor-mediated phagocytosis in arthritic Tg197 and Tg197/Tg5519 mice compared to control groups Tg5519 and WT (**Figure 6D** and **Supplementary Table 3**), suggesting activation of immune responses.

To elucidate the most prominent proteins involved in RA aggravation by RANKL, Tukey's honestly significant difference was performed on the ANOVA significant hits. A total of 231 proteins, 120 downregulated and 111 upregulated, were found statistically altered in Tg197/Tg5519 compared to Tg197 mice. Enrichment analysis in downregulated proteins based on KEGG pathway database revealed classification to processes related with metabolism, and muscle contraction (**Figure 7A** and **Supplementary Table 4**). In contrast, the upregulated proteins were grouped to processes associated with RA, protein processing and amino acid metabolism (**Figure 7B** and **Supplementary Table 5**).

To exclude a possible involvement of the osteoporotic background in the deregulated proteins identified in Tg197/Tg5519 compared to Tg197, we examined which of the above mentioned 231 differentially expressed proteins were also statistically significant between Tg197/Tg5519 and Tg5519 mice. This analysis revealed 65 proteins downregulated (**Supplementary Table 6**) and 36 upregulated (**Figure 7C, Table 1**) in Tg197/Tg5519 compared to control groups Tg197 and Tg5519. Subcategorization of the 65 significantly downregulated proteins in Tg197/Tg5519 mice based on their biological function, showed that the majority of the proteins participated in metabolic processes of carbohydrates, lipids, amino acids and nucleotides as well as in mitochondrial function (**Supplementary Table 6**). On the other hand, the proteome of the inflamed ankles from Tg197/Tg5519 mice was enriched for proteins expressed in activated osteoclasts and vacuolar-type H+ ATPase subunits either osteoclast-specific or ubiquitous (**Figure 7C, Table 1**), indicating extended bone resorption. Similarly, upregulation was observed for proteins involved in DNA, RNA and protein processing, suggesting activation of chromatin remodeling and gene expression. Moreover, increased levels have been identified for proteins involved in intracellular signal transduction, vacuolar transport and cell migration. Many of the upregulated proteins have been implicated in inflammatory responses, and cell proliferation regulation that fully correlate with the aggressive inflammatory phenotype developed in the ankles of Tg197/Tg5519 mice.

DISCUSSION

The importance of the RANKL/RANK/OPG system in the development of bone destruction in RA has been recently established, since RANKL is highly expressed in the synovial tissue of RA patients (33–35) and inhibition of RANKL with denosumab results in amelioration of bone destruction in RA (36, 37). Paradoxically, there are limited clinical trials that inhibit RANKL in RA, and from the available ones an effectiveness has been demonstrated for bone resorption but not for inflammation during a short-term treatment period from 6 to 12 months (36–39). Thus, the role of RANKL in the progression of inflammation in RA remains unclear. Here, we investigated if the progression of TNF-mediated erosive inflammatory arthritis is affected either by genetic inactivation (22) or overexpression of RANKL in transgenic mouse models (23). Our previous studies have shown that the G278R substitution identified in Rankl$^{tles/tles}$ mice allows normal RANKL gene expression and protein production but abrogates RANKL trimer formation and subsequently receptor binding. Therefore, mutant RANKL lacks biological activity as it fails to induce osteoclastogenesis both *ex vivo* and *in vivo* leading to an osteopetrotic phenotype (22). Our results demonstrated that modeled arthritis was significantly attenuated in the absence of functional RANKL, as shown by the absence of clinical arthritis signs and significant decrease in synovial hyperplasia. The unexpected improvement of survival in Tg197/Rankl$^{tles/tles}$

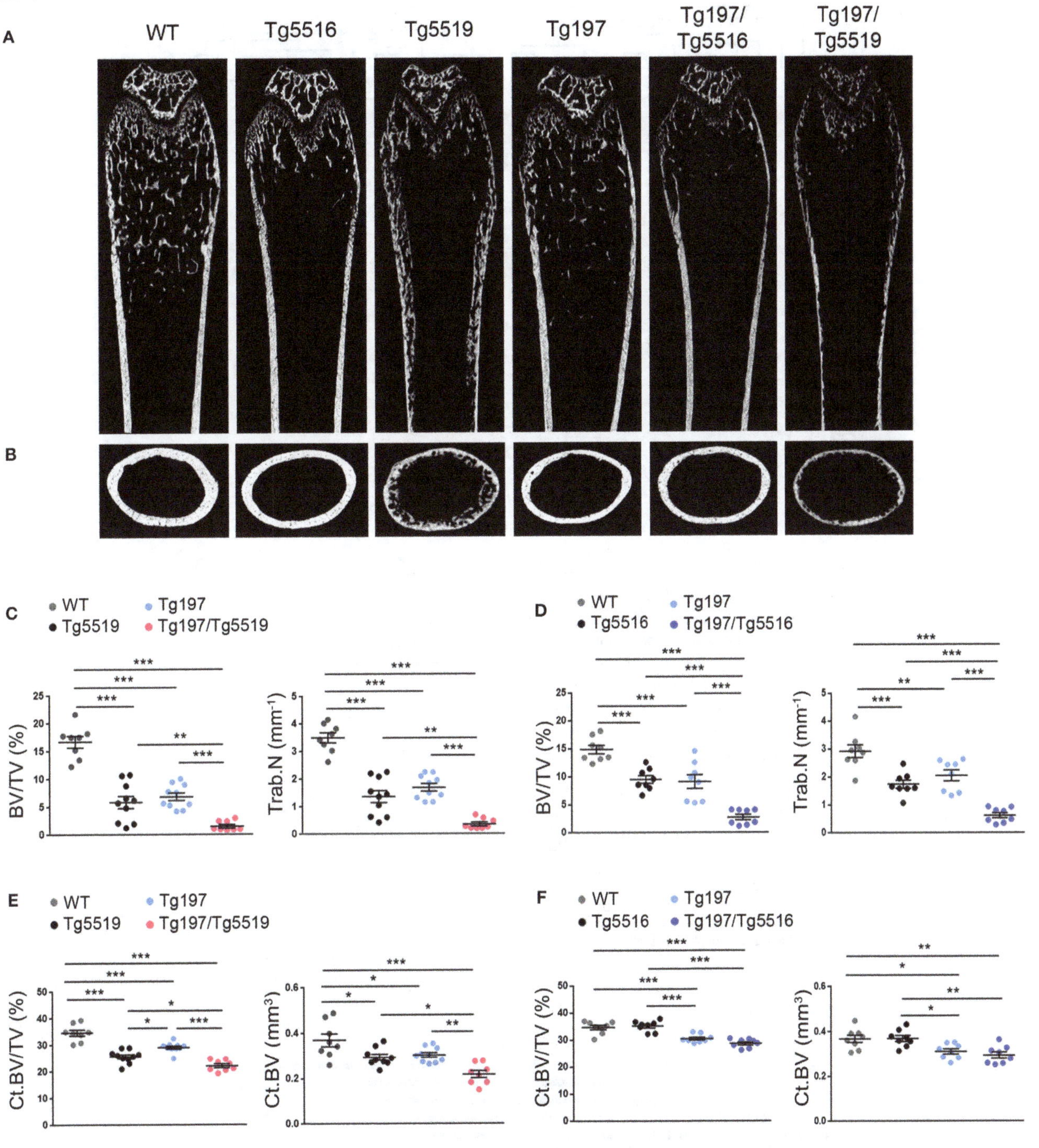

FIGURE 5 | Cooperative effect of RANKL and TNF in systemic bone loss. MicroCT analysis in the distal femur from mice of each genotype at 6 weeks of age as shown by **(A)** representative longitudinal sections and **(B)** cross-sectional sections at mid-diaphysis. Quantitative analysis with microCT of trabecular bone in the metaphyseal region of the distal femur of **(C)** Tg197/Tg5519 mice and their littermate controls ($n = 8$–10, equal number of sexes per genotype) and **(D)** Tg197/Tg5516 mice and their littermate controls ($n = 8$, equal number of sexes per genotype) for BV/TV (Bone Volume/Total Volume, %), and Tb.N (Trabecular Number per mm). Quantitative analysis with microCT of cortical bone in the mid-diaphyseal region of the femur of **(E)** Tg197/Tg5519 mice compared to their littermate controls ($n = 8$–10, equal number of sexes per genotype), and **(F)** Tg197/Tg5516 and their littermates ($n = 8$, equal number of sexes per genotype) for Ct.BV/TV (Cortical Bone Volume/Total Volume, %), and Ct. BV (Cortical Bone Volume, mm^3). Data represent mean values ± SEM. One-Way ANOVA and Tukey *post-hoc* test was performed for more than two groups. Asterisks mark statistically significant difference ($^*p < 0.05$, $^{**}p < 0.01$, $^{***}p < 0.001$).

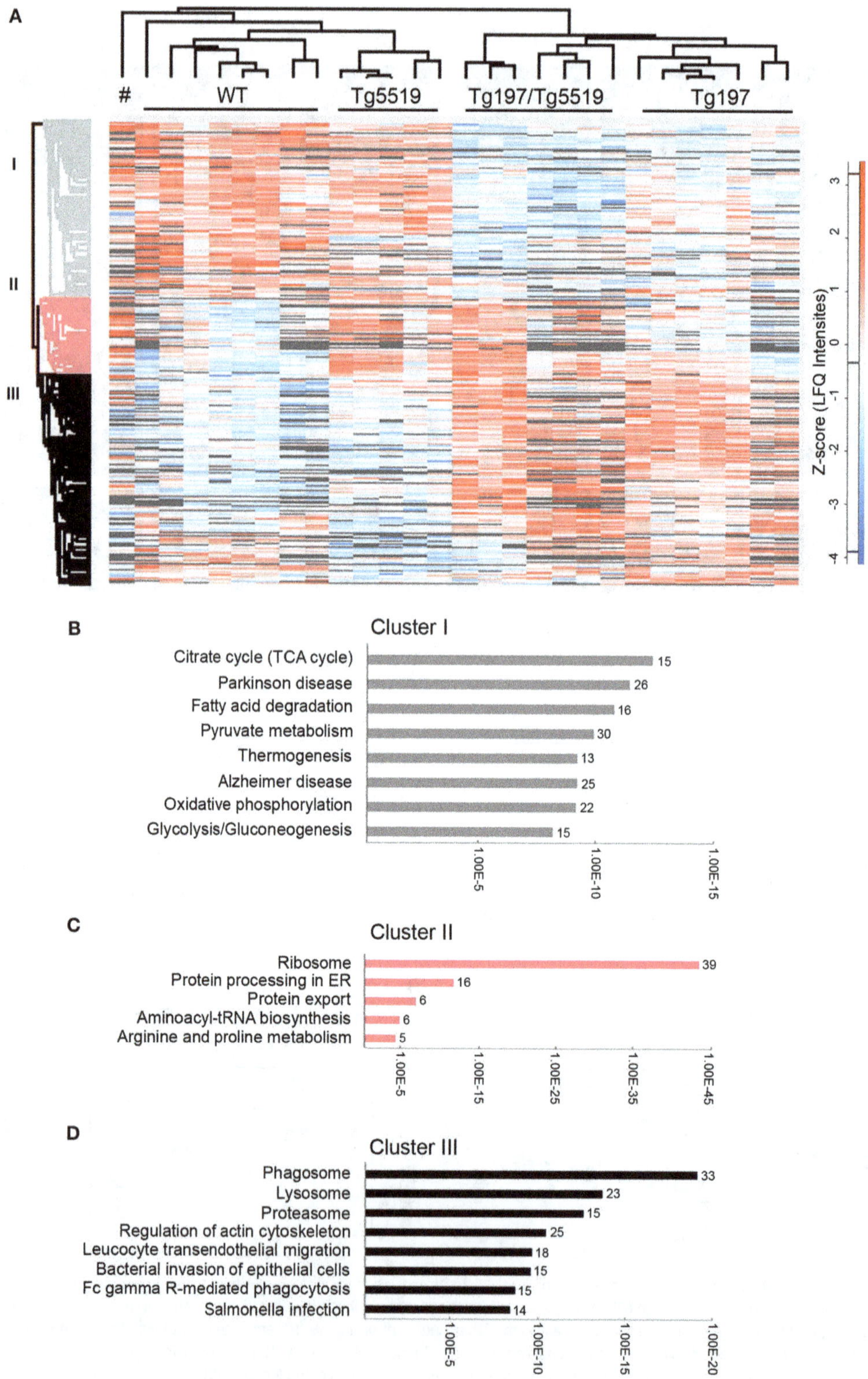

FIGURE 6 | Proteomic analysis in inflamed ankle joints of Tg197/TgRANKL mice. Comparative proteomic analysis using LC-MS/MS and label free quantitation in ankles from 6 week-old Tg197/Tg5519 mice and control groups including Tg197, Tg5519, and WT littermate mice ($n = 6$–8 biological replicas). **(A)** Heat map of statistical significant proteins (one-way ANOVA analysis). Columns represent each individual sample, labeled on top, and each row represents single proteins with an assigned color from blue (low expression) to red (high expression). Not detectable proteins are colored gray. Hierarchical Euclidean clustering created 3 protein clusters (gray, pink, and black). # indicates one Tg5519 mouse. Annotation enrichment analysis was performed using KEGG pathways database for **(B)** cluster I, **(C)** cluster II, and **(D)** cluster III.

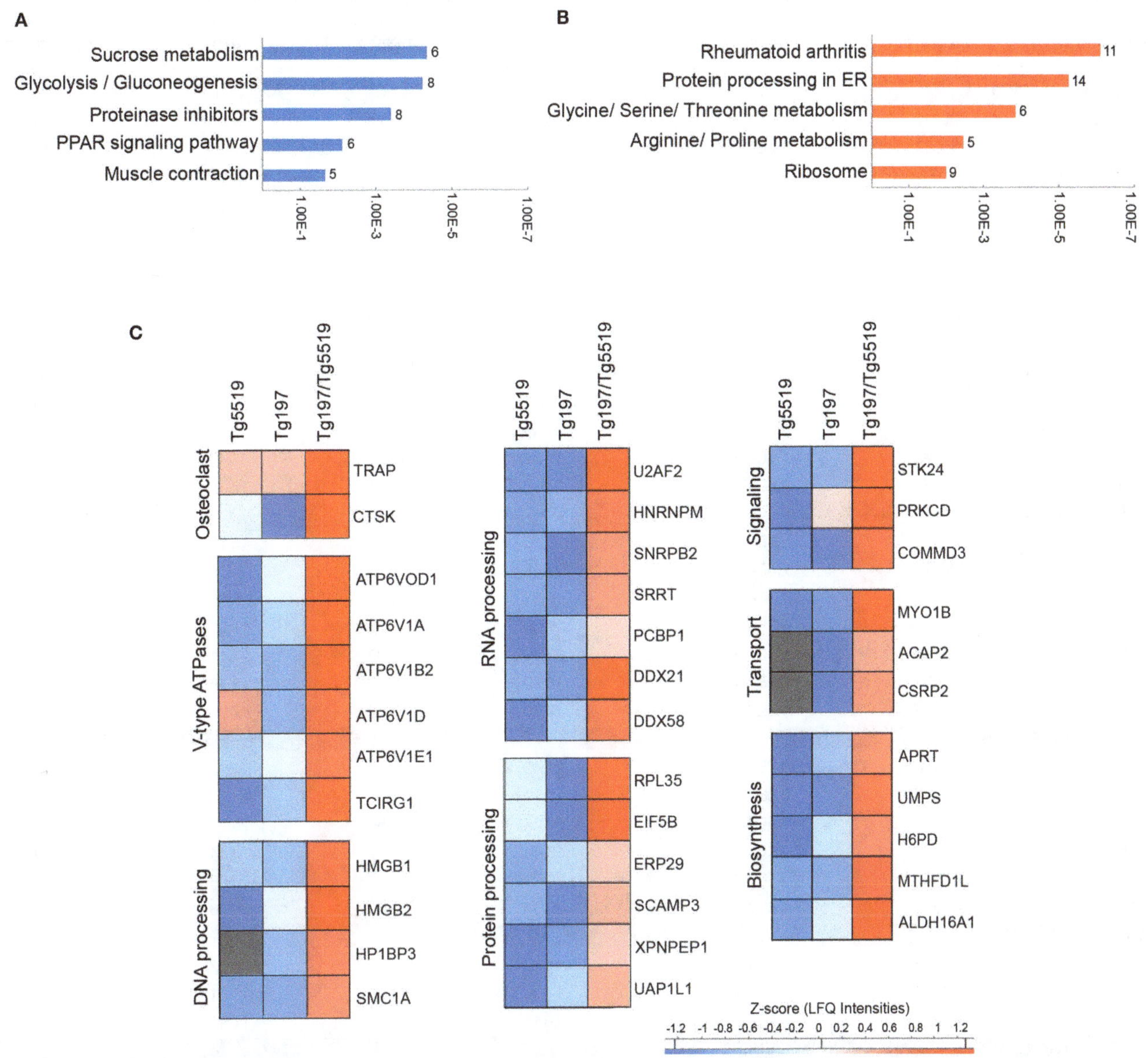

FIGURE 7 | Identification of upregulated proteins in the inflamed ankles of Tg197/TgRANKL mice. Enrichment annotation analysis based on KEGG database for **(A)** downregulated and **(B)** upregulated proteins in Tg197/Tg5519 compared to Tg197 mice. Bars represent the –Log(*p*-value) of pathways and the associated number of genes is presented at the end of the bar. **(C)** Abundance heat maps for proteins upregulated in Tg197/Tg5519 mice compared to Tg197 and Tg5519 control mice (Tukey's analysis). The average abundance of biological replicas ($n = 6$–8) is represented in each cell of the heat map.

mice compared to control Rankl$^{tles/tles}$ mice, could indicate a compensatory role for TNF in a RANKL-null background and needs further investigation. It is possible that the observed amelioration of arthritis is caused by the osteopetrotic phenotype rather than RANKL inactivation *per se*. In contrast, previous reports using c-fos deficient osteopetrotic mice crossed with TNF arthritic mice demonstrated that osteopetrosis is dispensable for TNF-mediated arthritis as synovial inflammation was not affected whereas bone resorption was blocked (40), supporting RANKL involvement in arthritis as shown in Tg197/Rankl$^{tles/tles}$ mice. Moreover, it is also possible that the attenuation of arthritis identified in Tg197/Rankl$^{tles/tles}$ mice is caused by the failure of RANKL deficient mice to develop a functional immune system (5, 6, 22).

Although several studies have revealed that TNF mediates osteoclastogenesis using *in vitro* cell culture systems (19, 20), there is still a central controversy of whether TNF can compensate for RANKL during osteoclastogenesis *in vivo*. Even though administration of high doses of exogenous TNF leads to the formation of osteoclast-like cells in RANK knockout mice at the site of calvarial injection (41), introduction of the Tg3647 TNF-expressing transgenic model displaying late

TABLE 1 | Proteins identified significantly overexpressed in the ankles from Tg197/Tg5519 mice compared to those isolated from their littermates Tg197, and Tg5519.

Gene Name	Protein ID	ANOVA *p*-value	WT	Tg5519	Tg197	Tg197/Tg5519
OSTEOCLAST ACTIVITY						
Acp5 (Trap)	Q05117	5.1E-08	18.46	21.24	21.24	22.73
Ctsk	P55097	2.2E-04	0.00	19.14	17.94	20.61
V-TYPE ATPASES						
Atp6v0d1	P51863	8.8E-07	18.26	19.14	19.52	20.05
Atp6v1a	P50516	7.0E-10	21.83	22.60	22.74	23.37
Atp6v1b2	P62814	1.2E-10	21.20	22.03	22.01	22.73
Atp6v1d	P57746	1.9E-08	17.95	19.33	18.78	19.47
Atp6v1e1	P50518	1.5E-08	20.34	21.33	21.50	21.85
Tcirg1	Q9JHF5	2.2E-08	18.13	19.23	19.59	20.57
DNA PROCESSING						
Hmgb1	P63158	9.5E-03	21.69	21.06	20.96	22.48
Hmgb2	P30681	8.3E-05	20.44	19.78	20.59	21.66
Hp1bp3	Q3TEA8	1.2E-03	17.51	0.00	17.47	18.22
Smc1a	Q9CU62	2.6E-02	17.38	17.11	17.13	17.75
RNA PROCESSING						
U2af2	P26369	2.7E-04	19.10	18.86	18.83	19.91
Hnrnpm	Q9D0E1	2.5E-03	21.95	22.03	22.06	22.46
Snrpd2	Q9CQI7	1.3E-02	19.58	19.11	18.96	19.68
Srrt	Q99MR6	5.3E-03	17.36	17.31	17.25	18.03
Pcbp1	P60335	1.3E-03	22.19	21.93	22.11	22.39
Ddx21	Q9JIK5	9.7E-04	18.70	18.82	18.76	19.64
Ddx58	Q6Q899	1.5E-03	17.00	17.40	17.77	18.56
PROTEIN PROCESSING						
Rpl35	Q6ZWV7	3.7E-03	20.45	21.16	20.43	22.08
Eif5b	Q05D44	9.0E-06	17.17	17.64	17.03	18.64
Erp29	P57759	7.5E-05	20.24	20.59	20.77	21.09
Scamp3	O35609	1.7E-03	18.44	18.62	18.54	18.95
Xpnpep1	Q6P1B1	9.1E-03	20.79	20.63	20.68	20.98
Uap1l1	Q3TW96	1.4E-05	20.54	20.69	20.96	21.34
SIGNAL TRANSDUCTION						
Stk24	Q99KH8	5.9E-04	17.66	17.96	18.02	19.43
Prkcd	P28867	7.6E-06	17.96	18.36	19.31	19.83
Commd3	Q63829	1.8E-02	0.00	17.98	17.91	18.70
VACUOLAR TRANSPORT, ENDOCYTOSIS, INVASIVENESS						
Myo1b	P46735	2.2E-03	17.84	18.23	18.27	19.08
Acap2	Q6ZQK5	7.8E-03	17.72	0.00	17.82	18.36
Csrp2	P97314	5.1E-05	18.22	0.00	18.37	19.36
BIOSYNTHETIC PROCESS						
Aprt	P08030	9.7E-06	19.19	19.41	19.72	20.38
Umps	P13439	2.3E-02	0.00	17.31	17.35	18.34
H6pd	Q8CFX1	6.2E-07	18.94	19.07	19.31	19.58
Mthfd1l	Q3V3R1	4.0E-04	19.55	19.73	19.75	20.25
Aldh6a1	Q9EQ20	7.2E-03	22.27	22.04	21.68	21.53

Logarithmic LFQ mean values are provided for each genotype.

onset arthritis in a RANK knockout background, showed that upon TNF overexpression osteoclastogenesis does not occur in the absence of RANKL/RANK signaling (42). Our results demonstrated that TNF overexpression could not compensate for RANKL-mediated osteopetrosis in Tg197/Rankl$^{tles/tles}$ mice, supported by the absence of osteoclasts in the bone marrow compartment. The fact that osteoclasts were identified between the pannus and bone interface in Tg197/Rankl$^{tles/tles}$ mice, indicates that this effect is driven by TNF-induced inflammation *in vivo*. However, the involvement of a subtle RANKL signaling in TNF-driven osteoclastogenesis cannot be excluded and needs further investigation. Similarly, previous reports have shown that induction of K/BxN serum transfer arthritis in RANK-deleted mice, resulted in osteoclastogenesis in the inflamed synovium but not in the bone marrow, supporting RANKL-indepedent mechanisms for osteoclast formation *in vivo* in a sufficiently inflamed environment (43).

Following a similar approach, the effect of RANKL overexpression in arthritis progression was studied in Tg197/TgRANKL double transgenic mice that simultaneously overexpress TNF and RANKL. Our results demonstrated that abundance of RANKL accelerated TNF-driven arthritis onset and disease severity characterized by massive osteoclastogenesis and bone resorption, aggressive pannus expansion and immense infiltration of inflammatory cells mainly of myeloid origin. Even though in the inflamed ankles of Tg197 mice the dominant inflammatory cells were $CD11b^{+}Gr1^{-}$ monocytes and synovial macrophages, the synovium of Tg197/Tg5519 mice had a 5-fold increase in $CD11b^{+}Gr1^{+}$ granulocytes and 2-fold in $CD11b^{+}Gr1^{-}$ monocytes/macrophages. The percent composition of various infiltrated populations showed a clear prevalence of granulocytes in TNF-driven arthritis upon RANKL overexpression. Neutrophils, the most abundant type of granulocytes, are short-lived and highly motile cells that constitute an essential component in innate immune system, as they are among the first cells that arrive in inflamed tissues (44). They are involved in various chronic inflammatory diseases such as RA, where are found in synovial fluid and rheumatoid pannus. It has been previously demonstrated that the membrane-associated form of RANKL is expressed in healthy blood neutrophils as well as in SF neutrophils (45), suggesting a role for inflammatory neutrophils infiltrated at the hypertrophied synovium, in osteoclastogenesis and bone resorption. Apart from that, RANKL was recently demonstrated to potently activate human neutrophil degranulation (46) and treatment with anti-RANKL improved cardiac infarct size and function by potentially impacting on neutrophil-mediated injury and repair (47). Thus, the dramatic increase in the population of granulocytes in inflamed ankles from Tg197/Tg5519 mice could promote bone destruction.

Proteomics, the largescale study of the proteome, has emerged as a powerful technique to identify biomarkers for diagnosis, prognosis, disease monitoring and discovery of novel disease targets in RA (48). To identify proteome alterations in osteolytic inflammatory arthritis aggravated by the overexpression of RANKL, we utilized a comparative proteomic approach in inflamed ankles from Tg197/Tg5519 and control mice. Our analysis revealed 65 significantly downregulated proteins in Tg197/Tg5519 mice compared to Tg197 and Tg5519 mice, while their classification based on biological function, showed that the majority of the proteins participated in metabolic processes of carbohydrates, lipids, amino acids and nucleotides as well as in mitochondrial function. These results indicate that severe inflammation developed in the ankles of Tg197/Tg5519 mice is related to altered metabolic profile and probably mitochondria dysfunction as many mitochondrial proteins were downregulated (**Supplementary Table 6**). In RA the inflamed joint is profoundly hypoxic as a result of dysregulated angiogenesis, impaired mitochondrial function and inflammation, which leads to a bioenergetic crisis. Under these conditions synovial cells display adaptive survival responses, which in conjunction with altered metabolism, activate key transcriptional signaling pathways that further exacerbate inflammation (49). Notably, there is also downregulation of proteins functioning as protease inhibitors, such as Alpha-1-antitrypsin encoded by the *SERPINA1* gene, that protect tissues from enzymes of inflammatory cells, especially neutrophil elastase (50), suggesting extensive tissue damage in Tg197/Tg5519 mice. Moreover, downregulation of proteins involved in muscle contraction in Tg197/Tg5519 mice is indicative of muscle degeneration caused by movement impairment due to severe arthritis progression.

In contrast, the proteome of the inflamed ankles from Tg197/Tg5519 mice was enriched for proteins expressed in activated osteoclasts, including TRAP and cathepsin K (CTSK), and vacuolar-type H+ ATPase subunits. TRAP prompts the dephosphorylation of bone matrix phosphoproteins and allows osteoclast migration, and further resorption to occur (51), while Cathepsin K, a member of cysteine proteases, is involved in the degradation of bone matrix proteins, especially type I collagen (52). Apart from bone resorption, Cathepsin K plays an important role in the immune system as shown by suppression of experimental arthritis through its pharmacological inhibition (53). The vacuolar type H+ ATPases (V-ATPase) are ATP-driven proton pumps that establish and maintain the acidic environment of intracellular organelles, including secretory granules, endosomes, and lysosomes, as well as extracellular compartments by specialized cells (54). Within intracellular membranes, V-ATPases function in a variety of processes, including antigen processing in dendritic cells and lysosomal degradation, while their presence in the plasma membrane mediates extracellular acidification (55). The mammalian V-ATPase proton pump is a macromolecular complex composed of at least 14 subunits that are expressed and function in a tissue-specific manner. Genetic studies implicate a critical role for subunits ATP6V1B2, ATP6V1C1, ATPV0D2, and ATP6V0A3 (TCIRG1) in osteoclast activity as relevant mutations lead to osteopetrosis (56). Osteoclasts employ plasma membrane V-ATPases to release hydrogen ions (H+) into the resorption lacunae in order to dissolve the mineral component of bone and concomitantly to enhance the activity of enzymes that digest the organic matrix (56). The fact that Tg197/Tg5519 inflamed ankles overexpress various V-ATPase subunits either osteoclast specific such as ATP6V1B2, and TCIRG1 or ubiquitous ATP6V1A, ATP6V1E1, and ATPV0D1 indicates an overwhelming osteoclastic activity that causes massive joint destruction, which is also confirmed by the histological analysis. Upregulated V-ATPase subunits could also have an impact on inflammatory responses such as phagocytosis, cytokine secretion and exocytosis of neutrophil granules (57, 58). Notably, recent studies have shown that in inflammatory conditions, osteoclasts can differentiate from dendritic cells in the presence of RANKL and behave as antigen-presenting cells (59). Therefore, increased osteoclastogenesis identified in Tg197/TgRANKL mice could not only contribute to bone destruction, but may also participate in perpetuating the inflammatory response.

In inflamed ankles from Tg197/Tg5519 mice there is also upregulated expression of proteins involved in DNA, RNA and protein processing, suggesting activation of chromatin remodeling and gene expression. Of special importance are DNA binding proteins, HMGB1 and HMGB2, members of the High-mobility group box (HMGB) family displaying two functions. In the nucleus, HMGB proteins bind to DNA in a DNA structure-dependent but nucleotide sequence-independent manner to function in chromatin remodeling. Extracellularly, HMGB proteins function as alarmins or damage-associated molecular pattern (DAMP) molecules, which are endogenous molecules released upon tissue damage to activate the immune system and drive inflammatory responses (60). Circulating HMGB1, the prototype member, has a crucial role in sterile inflammation caused by tissue injury or mitochondria damage, while its levels are increased in many human inflammatory diseases such as rheumatoid arthritis and their associated experimental models (61–63). Secreted HMGB1 binds to several immune receptors, principally toll-like receptors (TLRs) and through activation of NF-κB signaling (64) triggers inflammation by inducing cytokine release and recruitment of leucocytes. Thus, upregulation of HMGB1 and HMGB2 in inflamed ankles suggests extensive tissue damage and sustained inflammatory responses.

Moreover, proteomic analysis in Tg197/Tg5519 inflamed ankles identified high expression of RNA-binding proteins involved in mRNA splicing, and miRNA biogenesis. Among these proteins, U2AF2 (U2 Small Nuclear RNA Auxiliary Factor 2) is a central splicing complex member involved in pre-mRNA splicing and 3′-end processing (65) with an impact in the regulation of transcriptome in activated CD4 T lymphocytes (66). Moreover, HNRNPM (Heterogeneous nuclear ribonucleoprotein M), a component of the spliceosome machinery, promotes alternative spicing, cell proliferation and progression of breast cancer (67), while SRRT (Serrate, RNA Effector Molecule) participates to mRNA splicing and primary miRNA processing (68), it is involved in cell cycle progression at S phase, and its genetic deletion resulted in defective hematopoiesis in bone marrow and thymus (69). DDX21 and DDX58, as RNA helicases unwind their RNA substrates, and are involved in multiple biological processes related to RNA metabolism, including viral dsRNA sensing by innate cells, initiation of host antiviral responses and production of proinflammatory cytokines (70). Emerging evidence indicate that HMGBs bind to immunogenic nucleic acids (promiscuous sensing), which is required for subsequent recognition by specific pattern recognition receptors (discriminative sensing) such as DDXs to activate the innate immune responses. Such helicases also interact with endogenous RNAs regulating ribosome biogenesis (71) or translation of specific targets such as NF-κB1 (72). This category of nuclear RNA-binding proteins suggests increased transcription, RNA biogenesis and processing, while it remains unclear whether there is a specific correlation with regulation of inflammatory genes.

As regards intracellular signal transduction, there is abundance of protein kinases such as Serine/threonine kinase (STK24), and Protein kinase Cδ (PKCδ) in Tg197/T5519 ankles. STK24 plays an important role in controlling interleukin 17 (IL-17)-triggered inflammation and autoimmune diseases, since STK24 deficiency or knockdown markedly inhibited IL-17-induced phosphorylation of NF-κB and impaired IL-17-induced chemokines and cytokines expression (73). PKCδ, a signaling kinase with multiple downstream target proteins, is an essential regulator of peripheral B-cell development with a critical role in immune homeostasis. Among its main roles, PKCδ is responsible for the regulation of survival, proliferation, and apoptosis in a variety of cells including lymphocytes, while deficiency in PKCδ leads to systemic autoimmunity (74). Moreover, COMM domain-containing protein 3 (COMMD3) is an uncharacterised member of the COMMD family of proteins that interact with NF-κB and modulate its response (75).

Another group of proteins found upregulated in Tg197/Tg5519 ankles are involved in intracellular vesicular transport, endocytosis and invasiveness in extracellular matrix. MYO1B (Myosin IB) along with actin have been implicated in the control of secretory granule biogenesis and invagination of the plasma membrane during endocytosis (76). ACAP2 (ArfGAP With Coiled-Coil, Ankyrin Repeat And PH Domains 2), is a GTPase-activating protein that plays central role in endocytosis and FcγR-mediated phagocytosis (77), while CRP2 (Cysteine Rich Protein 2) is a new cytoskeletal component of invadopodia promoting breast cancer cell invasiveness and metastasis (78).

To our knowledge, this is the first study showing a proinflammatory role of RANKL in modeled arthritis apart from its well-established bone resorbing properties. A similar effect of RANKL has been identified in experimental periodontitis as RANKL antagonists inhibit both tissue inflammation and bone loss (79). Given that RA is a heterogeneous disease and so far the effect of denosumab in RA has been addressed only for a 12-month period, further studies are needed to investigate the inflammatory properties of RANKL in RA patients. Our results support that RANKL synergizes with TNF not only in local and systemic bone resorption but also in the inflammatory phenotype developed in modeled arthritis. Abundance of RANKL in TNF-driven arthritis worsens arthritis severity as shown by an increase in bone resorption, inflammatory cells and protein biomarkers indicative of extented osteoclastogenesis, tissue damage and activation of the immune system. Moreover, RANKL is essential for physiological and inflammation-induced bone remodeling, while TNF induces osteoclastogenesis *in vivo* at contact sites between synovium and bone. Therefore, RANKL provides an interesting candidate for resolution of inflammatory resorption in RA, whereas a dual inhibition of RANKL and TNF seems a promising therapeutic approach for severe inflammatory osteolytic arthritis.

AUTHOR CONTRIBUTIONS

ED conceived and designed the study, supervised experiments, and wrote the manuscript. MP performed and analyzed the majority of experiments and prepared the manuscript. VR performed microCT analysis and edited the manuscript. FV and MS conducted proteomic analysis and edited the manuscript. TT performed statistic analysis in proteomics data. GP provided scientific insight and edited the manuscript.

FUNDING

This work was supported by the Seventh Framework Programme Marie Curie Initial Training Network Osteoimmune Grant FP7-PEOPLE-2011-ITN-289150 (to ED).

ACKNOWLEDGMENTS

We thank Professor George Kollias (Biomedical Sciences Research Center Alexander Fleming) for kindly providing Tg197 human TNF transgenic mice.

REFERENCES

1. Fuller K, Wong B, Fox S, Choi Y, Chambers TJ. TRANCE is necessary and sufficient for osteoblast-mediated activation of bone resorption in osteoclasts. *J Exp Med.* (1998) 188:997–1001. doi: 10.1084/jem.188.5.997
2. Lacey DL, Timms E, Tan HL, Kelley MJ, Dunstan CR, Burgess T, et al. Osteoprotegerin ligand is a cytokine that regulates osteoclast differentiation and activation. *Cell* (1998) 93:165–76. doi: 10.1016/S0092-8674(00)81569-X
3. Yasuda H, Shima N, Nakagawa N, Yamaguchi K, Kinosaki M, Mochizuki S, et al. Osteoclast differentiation factor is a ligand for osteoprotegerin/osteoclastogenesis-inhibitory factor and is identical to TRANCE/RANKL. *Proc Natl Acad Sci USA.* (1998) 95:3597–602. doi: 10.1073/pnas.95.7.3597
4. Seeman E, Delmas PD. Bone quality–the material and structural basis of bone strength and fragility. *N Engl J Med.* (2006) 354:2250–61. doi: 10.1056/NEJMra053077
5. Kong YY, Yoshida H, Sarosi I, Tan HL, Timms E, Capparelli C, et al. OPGL is a key regulator of osteoclastogenesis, lymphocyte development and lymph-node organogenesis. *Nature* (1999) 397:315–23. doi: 10.1038/16852
6. Kim D, Mebius RE, MacMicking JD, Jung S, Cupedo T, Castellanos Y, Rho J, et al. Regulation of peripheral lymph node genesis by the tumor necrosis factor family member TRANCE. *J Exp Med.* (2000) 192:1467–78. doi: 10.1084/jem.192.10.1467
7. Dougall WC, Glaccum M, Charrier K, Rohrbach K, Brasel K, De Smedt T, et al. RANK is essential for osteoclast and lymph node development. *Genes Dev.* (1999) 13:2412–24. doi: 10.1101/gad.13.18.2412
8. Simonet WS, Lacey DL, Dunstan CR, Kelley M, Chang MS, Lüthy R, et al. Osteoprotegerin: a novel secreted protein involved in the regulation of bone density. *Cell* (1997) 89:309–19. doi: 10.1016/S0092-8674(00)80209-3
9. Darby AJ. Bone formation and resorption in postmenopausal osteoporosis. *Lancet* (1981) 2:536. doi: 10.1016/S0140-6736(81)90931-4
10. Cummings SR, San Martin J, McClung MR, Siris ES, Eastell R, Reid IR, et al. Denosumab for prevention of fractures in postmenopausal women with osteoporosis. *N Engl J Med.* (2009) 361:1914. doi: 10.1056/NEJMoa0809493
11. Leibbrandt A, Penninger JM. Novel functions of RANK(L) signaling in the immune system. *Adv Exp Med Biol.* (2010) 658:77–94. doi: 10.1007/978-1-4419-1050-9_9
12. Tanaka Y. Clinical immunity in bone and joints. *J Bone Miner Metab* (2018). doi: 10.1007/s00774-018-0965-5. [Epub ahead of print].
13. Firestein GS. Evolving concepts of rheumatoid arthritis. *Nature* (2003) 423:356–61. doi: 10.1038/nature01661
14. Feldmann M, Brennan FM, Foxwell BM, Maini RN. The role of TNF alpha and IL-1 in rheumatoid arthritis. *Curr Dir Autoimmun.* (2001) 3:188–99. doi: 10.1159/000060522)
15. Keffer J, Probert L, Cazlaris H, Georgopoulos S, Kaslaris E, Kioussis D, et al. Transgenic mice expressing human tumour necrosis factor: a predictive genetic model of arthritis. *EMBO J.* (1991) 10:4025–31. doi: 10.1002/J.1460-2075.1991.TB04978.X
16. Kontoyiannis D, Pasparakis M, Pizarro TT, Cominelli F, Kollias G. Impaired on/off regulation of TNF biosynthesis in mice lacking TNF AU- rich elements: implications for joint and gut-associated immunopathologies. *Immunity* (1999) 10:387–98. doi: 10.1016/S1074-7613(00)80038-2
17. Elliott MJ, Maini RN, Feldmann M, Long-Fox A, Charles P, Bijl H, et al. Repeated therapy with monoclonal antibody to tumour necrosis factor alpha (cA2) in patients with rheumatoid arthritis. *Lancet* (1994) 344:1125–7. doi: 10.1016/S0140-6736(94)90632-7
18. Boyce BF, Li P, Yao Z, Zhang Q, Badell IR, Schwarz EM, et al. TNF-alpha and pathologic bone resorption. *Keio J Med.* (2005) 54:127–31. doi: 10.2302/kjm.54.127
19. Azuma Y, Kaji K, Katogi R, Takeshita S, Kudo A. Tumor necrosis factor-alpha induces differentiation of and bone resorption by osteoclasts. *J Biol Chem.* (2000) 275:4858–64. doi: 10.1074/jbc.275.7.4858
20. Kobayashi K, Takahashi N, Jimi E, Udagawa N, Takami M, Kotake S, et al. Tumor necrosis factor stimulates osteoclast differentiation by a mechanism independent of the Odf/rankl-rank interaction. *J Exp Med.* (2000) 191:275–86. doi: 10.1084/jem.191.2.275
21. Fuller K, Murphy C, Kirstein B, Fox SW, Chambers TJ. TNFα potently activates osteoclasts, through a direct action independent of and strongly synergistic with RANKL. *Endocrinology* (2002) 143:1108–18. doi: 10.1210/en.143.3.1108
22. Douni E, Rinotas V, Makrinou E, Zwerina J, Penninger JM, Eliopoulos E, et al. A RANKL G278R mutation causing osteopetrosis identifies a functional amino acid essential for trimer assembly in RANKL and TNF. *Hum Mol Genet.* (2012) 21:784–98. doi: 10.1093/hmg/ddr510
23. Rinotas V, Niti A, Dacquin R, Bonnet N, Stolina M, Han CY, et al. Novel genetic models of osteoporosis by overexpression of human RANKL in transgenic mice. *J Bone Miner Res.* (2014) 29:1158–69. doi: 10.1002/jbmr.2112
24. Douni E, Sfikakis PP, Haralambous S, Fernandes P, Kollias G. Attenuation of inflammatory polyarthritis in TNF transgenic mice by diacerein: comparative analysis with dexamethasone, methotrexate and anti-TNF protocols. *Arthritis Res Ther.* (2004) 6:R65–72. doi: 10.1186/ar1028
25. van 't Hof RJ, Rose L, Bassonga E, Daroszewska A. Open source software for semi-automated histomorphometry of bone resorption and formation parameters. *Bone* (2017) 99:69–79. doi: 10.1016/j.bone.2017.03.051
26. Bouxsein ML, Boyd SK, Christiansen BA, Guldberg RE, Jepsen KJ, Müller R. Guidelines for assessment of bone microstructure in rodents using micro-computed tomography. *J Bone Miner Res.* (2010) 25:1468–86. doi: 10.1002/jbmr.141
27. Armaka M, Gkretsi V, Kontoyiannis D, Kollias G. A standardized protocol for the isolation and culture of normal and arthritogenic murine synovial fibroblasts. *Protoc Exch* (2009). doi: 10.1038/nprot.2009.102
28. Tyanova S, Cox J. Perseus: a bioinformatics platform for integrative analysis of proteomics data in cancer research. *Methods Mol Biol.* (2018) 1711:133–48. doi: 10.1007/978-1-4939-7493-1_7
29. Bindea G, Mlecnik B, Hackl H, Charoentong P, Tosolini M, Kirilovsky A, et al. ClueGO: a cytoscape plug-in to decipher functionally grouped gene ontology and pathway annotation networks. *Bioinformatics* (2009) 25:1091–3. doi: 10.1093/bioinformatics/btp101
30. Ogata H, Goto S, Sato K, Fujibuchi W, Bono H, Kanehisa M. KEGG: kyoto encyclopedia of genes and genomes. *Nucleic Acids Res.* (1999) 27:29–34. doi: 10.1093/nar/27.1.29
31. Cox J, Mann M. Maxquant enables high peptide identification rates, individualized p.p.b.-range mass accuracies and proteome-wide protein quantification. *Nat Biotechnol.* (2008) 26:1367–72. doi: 10.1038/nbt.1511

32. Cox J, Hein MY, Luber CA, Paron I, Nagaraj N, Mann M. Accurate proteome-wide label-free quantification by delayed normalization and maximal peptide ratio extraction, termed maxlfq. *Mol Cell Proteomics* (2014) 13:2513–26. doi: 10.1074/mcp.M113.031591
33. Gravallese EM, Manning C, Tsay A, Naito A, Pan C, Amento E, et al. Synovial tissue in rheumatoid arthritis is a source of osteoclast differentiation factor. *Arthritis Rheum.* (2000) 43:250–8. doi: 10.1002/1529-0131(200002)43:2<250::AID-ANR3>3.0.CO;2-P
34. Shigeyama Y, Pap T, Kunzler P, Simmen BR, Gay RE, Gay S. Expression of osteoclast differentiation factor in rheumatoid arthritis. *Arthritis Rheum.* (2000) 43:2523–30. doi: 10.1002/1529-0131(200011)43:11<2523::AID-ANR20>3.0.CO;2-Z
35. Takayanagi H, Iizuka H, Juji T, Nakagawa T, Yamamoto A, Miyazaki T, et al. Involvement of receptor activator of nuclear factor κB ligand/osteoclast differentiation factor in osteoclastogenesis from synoviocytes in rheumatoid arthritis. *Arthritis Rheum.* (2000) 43:259–69. doi: 10.1002/1529-0131(200002)43:2<259::AID-ANR4>3.0.CO;2-W
36. Cohen SB, Dore RK, Lane NE, Ory PA, Peterfy CG, Sharp JT, et al. Denosumab treatment effects on structural damage, bone mineral density, and bone turnover in rheumatoid arthritis: a twelve-month, multicenter, randomized, double-blind, placebo-controlled, phase II clinical trial. *Arthritis Rheum.* (2008) 58:1299–309. doi: 10.1002/art.23417
37. Takeuchi T, Tanaka Y, Ishiguro N, Yamanaka H, Yoneda T, Ohira T, et al. Effect of denosumab on Japanese patients with rheumatoid arthritis: a dose-response study of AMG 162 (Denosumab) in patients with rheumatoid arthritis on methotrexate to validate inhibitory effect on bone erosion (DRIVE) - A 12-month, multicentre, randomi. *Ann Rheum Dis.* (2016) 75:983–90. doi: 10.1136/annrheumdis-2015-208052
38. Sharp JT, Tsuji W, Ory P, Harper-Barek C, Wang H, Newmark R. Denosumab prevents metacarpal shaft cortical bone loss in patients with erosive rheumatoid arthritis. *Arthritis Care Res.* (2010) 62:537–44. doi: 10.1002/acr.20172
39. Deodhar A, Dore RK, Mandel D, Schechtman J, Shergy W, Trapp R, et al. Denosumab-mediated increase in hand bone mineral density associated with decreased progression of bone erosion in rheumatoid arthritis patients. *Arthritis Care Res.* (2010) 62:569–74. doi: 10.1002/acr.20004
40. Redlich K, Hayer S, Ricci R, David J, Tohidast-Akrad M, Kollias G, et al. Osteoclasts are essential for TNF-alpha-mediated joint destruction. *J Clin Invest.* (2002) 110:1419–27. doi: 10.1172/JCI15582
41. Li J, Sarosi I, Yan XQ, Morony S, Capparelli C, Tan HL, et al. RANK is the intrinsic hematopoietic cell surface receptor that controls osteoclastogenesis and regulation of bone mass and calcium metabolism. *Proc Natl Acad Sci USA.* (2000) 97:1566–71. doi: 10.1073/pnas.97.4.1566
42. Li P, Schwarz EM, O'Keefe RJ, Ma L, Boyce BF, Xing L. RANK signaling is not required for TNFalpha-mediated increase in CD11(hi) osteoclast precursors but is essential for mature osteoclast formation in TNFalpha-mediated inflammatory arthritis. *J Bone Miner Res.* (2004) 19:207–13. doi: 10.1359/JBMR.0301233
43. O'Brien W, Fissel BM, Maeda Y, Yan J, Ge X, Gravallese EM, et al. RANK-independent osteoclast formation and bone erosion in inflammatory arthritis. *Arthritis Rheumatol.* (2016) 68:2889–900. doi: 10.1002/art.39837
44. Lipsky PE, Davis LS, Cush JJ, Oppenheimer-Marks N. The role of cytokines in the pathogenesis of rheumatoid arthritis. *Springer Semin Immunopathol.* (1989) 11:123–62. doi: 10.1007/BF00197186
45. Poubelle PE, Chakravarti A, Fernandes MJ, Doiron K, Marceau AA. Differential expression of RANK, RANK-L, and osteoprotegerin by synovial fluid neutrophils from patients with rheumatoid arthritis and by healthy human blood neutrophils. *Arthritis Res Ther.* (2007) 9:R25. doi: 10.1186/ar2137
46. Quercioli A, Mach F, Bertolotto M, Lenglet S, Vuilleumier N, Galan K, et al. Receptor activator of NF-κB ligand (RANKL) increases the release ofneutrophil products associated with coronary vulnerability. *Thromb Haemost.* (2012) 107:124–39. doi: 10.1160/TH11-05-0324
47. Carbone F, Crowe LA, Roth A, Burger F, Lenglet S, Braunersreuther V, et al. Treatment with anti-RANKL antibody reduces infarct size and attenuates dysfunction impacting on neutrophil-mediated injury. *J Mol Cell Cardiol.* (2016) 94:82–94. doi: 10.1016/j.yjmcc.2016.03.013
48. Park Y-J, Chung MK, Hwang D, Kim W-U. Proteomics in rheumatoid arthritis research. *Immune Netw.* (2015) 15:177–85. doi: 10.4110/in.2015.15.4.177
49. Fearon U, Canavan M, Biniecka M, Veale DJ. Hypoxia, mitochondrial dysfunction and synovial invasiveness in rheumatoid arthritis. *Nat Rev Rheumatol.* (2016) 12:385–97. doi: 10.1038/nrrheum.2016.69
50. Potempa J, Korzus E, Travis J. The serpin superfamily of proteinase inhibitors: structure, function, and regulation. *J Biol Chem.* (1994) 269:15957–60. doi: 10.1021/ed056pA86.2
51. Ek-Rylander B, Flores M, Wendel M, Heinegard D, Andersson G. Dephosphorylation of osteopontin and bone sialoprotein by osteoclastic tartrate-resistant acid phosphatase. Modulation of osteoclast adhesion *in vitro*. *J Biol Chem.* (1994) 269:14853–6. doi: 10.1111/j.1095-8649.2004.00473.x
52. Bossard MJ, Tomaszek TA, Thompson SK, Amegadzie BY, Hanning CR, Jones C, et al. Proteolytic activity of human osteoclast cathepsin K: expression, purification, activation, and substrate identification. *J Biol Chem.* (1996) 271:12517–24. doi: 10.1074/jbc.271.21.12517
53. Asagiri M, Hirai T, Kunigami T, Kamano S, Gober HJ, Okamoto K, et al. Cathepsin K-dependent toll-like receptor 9 signaling revealed in experimental arthritis. *Science* (2008) 319:624–7. doi: 10.1126/science.1150110
54. Cotter K, Stransky L, McGuire C, Forgac M. Recent insights into the structure, regulation, and function of the V-ATPases. *Trends Biochem Sci.* (2015) 40:611–22. doi: 10.1016/j.tibs.2015.08.005
55. Trombetta ES, Ebersold M, Garrett W, Pypaert M, Mellman I. Activation of lysosomal function during dendritic cell maturation. *Science* (2003) 299:1400–3. doi: 10.1126/science.1080106
56. Qin A, Cheng TS, Pavlos NJ, Lin Z, Dai KR, Zheng MH. V-ATPases in osteoclasts: structure, function and potential inhibitors of bone resorption. *Int J Biochem Cell Biol.* (2012) 44:1422–35. doi: 10.1016/j.biocel.2012.05.014
57. Gilman-Sachs A, Tikoo A, Akman-Anderson L, Jaiswal M, Ntrivalas E, Beaman K. Expression and role of a2 vacuolar-ATPase (a2V) in trafficking of human neutrophil granules and exocytosis. *J Leukoc Biol.* (2015) 97:1121–31. doi: 10.1189/jlb.3A1214-620RR
58. Scherer O, Steinmetz H, Kaether C, Weinigel C, Barz D, Kleinert H, et al. Targeting V-ATPase in primary human monocytes by archazolid potently represses the classical secretion of cytokines due to accumulation at the endoplasmic reticulum. *Biochem Pharmacol.* (2014) 91:490–500. doi: 10.1016/j.bcp.2014.07.028
59. Ibáñez L, Abou-Ezzi G, Ciucci T, Amiot V, Belaïd N, Obino D, et al. Inflammatory Osteoclasts Prime TNFα-Producing CD4+T Cells and Express CX3CR1. *J Bone Miner Res.* (2016) 31:1899–908. doi: 10.1002/jbmr.2868
60. Lotze MT, Tracey KJ. High-mobility group box 1 protein (HMGB1): nuclear weapon in the immune arsenal. *Nat Rev Immunol.* (2005) 5:331–42. doi: 10.1038/nri1594
61. Yanai H, Ban T, Wang Z, Choi MK, Kawamura T, Negishi H, et al. HMGB proteins function as universal sentinels for nucleic-acid-mediated innate immune responses. *Nature* (2009) 462:99–103. doi: 10.1038/nature08512
62. Andersson U, Tracey KJ. HMGB1 is a therapeutic target for sterile inflammation and infection. *Annu Rev Immunol.* (2011) 29:139–62. doi: 10.1146/annurev-immunol-030409-101323
63. Taniguchi N, Kawakami Y, Maruyama I, Lotz M. HMGB proteins and arthritis. *Hum Cell* (2018) 31:1–9. doi: 10.1007/s13577-017-0182-x
64. Park JS, Svetkauskaite D, He Q, Kim JY, Strassheim D, Ishizaka A, et al. Involvement of toll-like receptors 2 and 4 in cellular activation by high mobility group box 1 protein. *J Biol Chem.* (2004) 279:7370–7. doi: 10.1074/jbc.M306793200
65. Millevoi S, Loulergue C, Dettwiler S, Karaa SZ, Keller W, Antoniou M, et al. An interaction between U2AF 65 and CF Imlinks the splicing and 3′ end processing machineries. *EMBO J.* (2006) 25:4854–64. doi: 10.1038/sj.emboj.7601331
66. Whisenant TC, Peralta ER, Aarreberg LD, Gao NJ, Head SR, Ordoukhanian P, et al. The activation-induced assembly of an RNA/protein interactome centered on the splicing factor U2AF2 regulates gene expression in human CD4 T cells. *PLoS ONE* (2015) 10:e0144409. doi: 10.1371/journal.pone.0144409
67. Yang W-H, Ding M-J, Cui G-Z, Yang M, Dai D-L. Heterogeneous nuclear ribonucleoprotein M promotes the progression of breast cancer by regulating the axin/β-catenin signaling pathway. *Biomed Pharmacother.* (2018) 105:848–55. doi: 10.1016/j.biopha.2018.05.014

68. Gruber JJ, Zatechka DS, Sabin LR, Yong J, Lum JJ, Kong M, et al. Ars2 Links the nuclear cap-binding complex to RNA interference and cell proliferation. *Cell* (2009) 138:328–39. doi: 10.1016/j.cell.2009.04.046
69. Elahi S, Egan SM, Holling GA, Kandefer RL, Nemeth MJ, Olejniczak SH. The RNA binding protein Ars2 supports hematopoiesis at multiple levels. *Exp Hematol.* (2018) 64:45–58.e9. doi: 10.1016/j.exphem.2018.05.001
70. Steimer L, Klostermeier D. RNA helicases in infection and disease. *RNA Biol.* (2012) 9:751–71. doi: 10.4161/rna.20090
71. Xing YH, Yao RW, Zhang Y, Guo CJ, Jiang S, Xu G, et al. SLERT regulates DDX21 rings associated with Pol I transcription. *Cell* (2017) 169:664–78.e16. doi: 10.1016/j.cell.2017.04.011
72. Zhang H-X, Liu Z-X, Sun Y-P, Zhu J, Lu S-Y, Liu X-S, et al. Rig-I regulates NF-B activity through binding to Nf- b1 3′-UTR mRNA. *Proc Natl Acad Sci USA.* (2013) 110:6459–64. doi: 10.1073/pnas.1304432110
73. Jiang Y, Tian M, Lin W, Wang X, Wang X. Protein kinase serine/threonine kinase 24 positively regulates interleukin 17-induced inflammation by promoting IKK complex activation. *Front Immunol.* (2018) 9:1–16. doi: 10.3389/fimmu.2018.00921
74. Salzer E, Santos-Valente E, Keller B, Warnatz K, Boztug K. Protein kinase C δ: a gatekeeper of immune homeostasis. *J Clin Immunol.* (2016) 36:631–40. doi: 10.1007/s10875-016-0323-0
75. Bartuzi P, Hofker MH, van de Sluis B. Tuning NF-κB activity: a touch of COMMD proteins. *Biochim Biophys Acta* (2013) 1832:2315–21. doi: 10.1016/j.bbadis.2013.09.014
76. Delestre-Delacour C, Carmon O, Laguerre F, Estay-Ahumada C, Courel M, Elias S, et al. Myosin 1b and F-actin are involved in the control of secretory granule biogenesis. *Sci Rep.* (2017) 7:5172. doi: 10.1038/s41598-017-05 617-1
77. Egami Y, Fujii M, Kawai K, Ishikawa Y, Fukuda M, Araki N. Activation-inactivation cycling of Rab35 and ARF6 is required for phagocytosis of zymosan in RAW264 macrophages. *J Immunol Res.* (2015) 2015:429439. doi: 10.1155/2015/429439
78. Hoffmann C, Mao X, Dieterle M, Moreau F, Absi A Al, Steinmetz A, et al. CRP2, a new invadopodia actin bundling factor critically promotes breast cancer cell invasion and metastasis. *Oncotarget* (2016) 7:13688–705. doi: 10.18632/oncotarget.7327
79. Yuan H, Gupte R, Zelkha S, Amar S. Receptor activator of nuclear factor kappa B ligand antagonists inhibit tissue inflammation and bone loss in experimental periodontitis. *J Clin Periodontol.* (2011) 38:1029–36. doi: 10.1111/j.1600-051X.2011.01780.x

9

Compromised Bone Healing in Aged Rats is Associated with Impaired M2 Macrophage Function

Julia Löffler[1,2], F. Andrea Sass[1,2], Sebastian Filter[1], Alexander Rose[1], Agnes Ellinghaus[1,2], Georg N. Duda[1,2†] and Anke Dienelt[1,2†]*

[1] Julius Wolff Institute and Center for Musculoskeletal Surgery, Charité-Universitätsmedizin Berlin, Corporate Member of Freie Universität Berlin, Berlin Institute of Health, Humboldt-Universität zu Berlin, Berlin, Germany, [2] Berlin Institute of Health Center for Regenerative Therapies, Charité-Universitätsmedizin Berlin, Corporate Member of Freie Universität Berlin, Berlin Institute of Health, Humboldt-Universität zu Berlin, Berlin, Germany

***Correspondence:**
Georg N. Duda
georg.duda@charite.de

† These authors have contributed equally to this work as senior authors

Fracture repair is initiated by a multitude of immune cells and induction of an inflammatory cascade. Alterations in the early healing response due to an aged adaptive immune system leads to impaired bone repair, delayed healing or even formation of non-union. However, immuno-senescence is not limited to the adaptive immunity, but is also described for macrophages, main effector cells from the innate immune system. Beside regulation of pro- and anti-inflammatory signaling, macrophages contribute to angiogenesis and granulation tissue maturation. Thus, it seems likely that an altered macrophage function due to aging may affect bone repair at various stages and contribute to age related deficiencies in bone regeneration. To prove this hypothesis, we analyzed the expression of macrophage markers and angiogenic factors in the early bone hematoma derived from young and aged osteotomized Spraque Dawley rats. We detected an overall reduced expression of the monocyte/pan-macrophage markers CD14 and CD68 in aged rats. Furthermore, the analysis revealed an impaired expression of anti-inflammatory M2 macrophage markers in hematoma from aged animals that was connected to a diminished revascularization of the bone callus. To verify that the age related disturbed bone regeneration was due to a compromised macrophage function, CD14+ macrophage precursors were transplanted locally into the osteotomy gap of aged rats. Transplantation rescued bone regeneration partially after 6 weeks, demonstrated by a significantly induced deposition of new bone tissue, reduced fibrosis and significantly improved callus vascularization.

Keywords: bone regeneration, macrophage, monocyte, CD14+ cells, aging, angiogenesis, compromised healing

HIGHLIGHTS

- Compromised bone regeneration in aged rats is connected to a reduced expression of the pan-macrophage markers CD14 and CD68.
- Anti-inflammatory M2 macrophage markers are decreased in the early callus from aged animals.
- Macrophage mediated angiogenesis is impaired in the early callus of aged animals.
- Transplantation of CD14 macrophage precursors rescues impaired bone regeneration in aged rats partially.

INTRODUCTION

Fracture repair is a highly orchestrated process that involves a distinct pro- to anti-inflammatory signaling cascade in the hematoma, angiogenesis, coordinated extracellular matrix deposition and progression toward endochondral ossification (1). Comorbidities associated with an altered immune response, such as advanced age, diabetes, or rheumatoid arthritis, have been shown to reduce the initial biological potential of the fracture hematoma and may impair regeneration (2–4). In addition, disturbances in the revascularization or unbalanced expression of angiogenic growths factors can delay bone regeneration and eventually lead to the formation of atrophic pseudarthrosis (1, 5–8). Several studies report on the interconnection of immune cells, inflammation, and angiogenic processes. Especially monocytes and macrophages, cells from the innate immune system, are reported to regulate bone homeostasis and repair, as well as tissue vascularization (9, 10). In this context, optimal fracture repair is steered by a collaboration from infiltrating and bone-resident macrophages (11). In dependence of their surroundings, activated macrophages can adopt different functions that are characterized by a pro-inflammatory M1 (classically activated), and an anti-inflammatory M2 phenotype (alternatively activated). M1 macrophages produce large amounts of pro-inflammatory cytokines, as TNFa and IL-1b, and induce Th1 responses. In contrast, the so called M2 phenotype produces IL-10, IL-1 receptor type α, and TGF-β, induces Th2 immune responses, and contribute to angiogenesis, wound healing progression and granulation tissue maturation (12–16). Particularly M2 macrophages have shown to be highly diverse in their functionality and activation patterns. Over the last years, several M2 subsets have been identified (M2a, M2b, and M2c), even repolarization toward M1 phenotypes has been observed, highlighting the great plasticity of macrophages (17, 18).

However, detailed information on the diverse functions of even the more simplified concept of M1 and M2 macrophages during bone repair are rare. While Loi et al. demonstrated that a transition from M1 toward M2 phenotypes highly promotes bone formation *in vitro*, studies analyzing the impact of the different macrophage phenotypes in biologically compromised healing situations, as advanced age, are missing (19). We hypothesized that biologically impaired bone regeneration is connected to disturbances in macrophage functionality and alterations in the M1/M2 macrophage populations. To prove this hypothesis, we investigated the impact of M1/M2 macrophages on bone healing in aged rats more in detail.

MATERIALS AND METHODS

Animal Studies

For the *in vivo* animal studies 3 and 12 month old female ex-breeder Sprague Dawley rats from Charles River WIGA Deutschland GmbH were used. These aged rats, that had a minimum of 3 L served as models for biologically impaired fracture healing that develop a non-union, when no additional treatment is applied (4, 20–22). Animal experiments were conducted in compliance with the ARRIVE guidelines and according to the policies and principles of the Animal Welfare Act, the National Institutes of Health Guide for the Care and Use of Laboratory Animals, and the National Animal Welfare Guidelines. All animal experiments were approved by the local legal representative (Institutional Animal Care and Use Committees, LaGeSo, G0120/14, G0172/15). Animals were anesthetized with 0.3 mg/kg Medetomidin DomitorH and 60 mg/kg Ketamin by intraperitoneal injection prior to surgical procedure. Additionally, 20 mg/kg Tramadol was administered as analgesia. Forty-five milligram per kilogram Clindamycin was administered by subcutaneous injection and eyes were prevented from drying out by application of eye balm. A longitudinal skin incision was made over the left femur. The bone was exposed by blunt fascia dissections. An in-house developed unilateral external fixator was mounted to stabilize the bone, made of stainless steel and titanium as published previously (20, 23). For an exact placement of the four wire holes, a drilling template was used for every procedure. After incision of the titanium wires, the external fixator bar was placed on the wires and a standardized 2 mm gap was sawn by osteotomy into the femoral bone. To ensure reproducibility of the gap size a sawing template was used at all times. Muscle fascia and skin were closed using absorbable and non-absorbable sutures, respectively. Animals received an anesthetic antagonist and were placed under red light until awakening. Post-surgical analgesia was given by addition of Tramadol (25 ml/l) to the drinking water for 3 days. Fracture healing was assessed after 3 and 7 days, as well as after 6 weeks by euthanization and femur dissection. Animal IDs, weights and group sizes can be found in **Table 1**.

Intraoperative Cell Transplantation

For the intraoperative cell transplantation of PBMCs or CD14+ cells into the osteotomy gap, 15 ml cardiac blood were drawn from 12-month-old donor rats. Subsequently, PBMCs were isolated by application of a density gradient using Histopaque-1083 (Sigma-Aldrich). The CD14+ subset was further extracted from the PBMC population using positive Magnetic Activated Cell Sorting by application of a murine CD14+ antibody (clone: biG, Abnova), combined with anti-mouse IgG microbeads from Miltenyi Biotec. Per blood clot 2×10^5 of either PBMCs (including CD14+ cells) or CD14+ cells were re-suspended in 200 μl autologous blood, that was drawn just prior to the surgical procedure (including 10 μl sodium citrate, to prevent clotting). The osteotomy procedure was performed as described above. For cell transplantation groups, blood clotting was induced right before the clot was placed into the osteotomy gap by adding 7 μl $CaCl_2$ 12%Thrombin (Baxter). The lid of a 1.5 ml Eppendorf tube served as a forming device for the artificial hematoma. The clot was designed to exactly fit into the osteotomy gap (same height as gap width), but with a slightly larger diameter, to ensure that the osteotomy gap was spanned by the clot. No differences in clot quality/nature were observed at any point. It was previously shown, that bone formation after a regular healing time of 6 weeks in animals receiving an empty autologous blood clot without additional cell supplementation is comparable to the one seen in animals that received a PBMC supplemented blood clot (24, 25) thus PBMC supplemented artificial hematoma was used as control in this study rather than the autologous blood clot alone.

μCT

Bone healing was assessed *in vitro* with micro-computed tomography on formaldehyde-fixed left femurs extracted from euthanized animals 6 weeks after surgery. A region of interest (ROI) covering the 2 mm osteotomy gap plus 1 mm proximal and distal was scanned in a Viva CT 40 microCT (Scanco Medical AG) with application of a voxel size of 10.5 μm, 55 keVp, 145 μA. Bone microstructure trabecular number, trabecular space, trabecular thickness) and the key parameters of tissue and bone mineral content were assessed using the respective software from the device supplier (Scanco Software, Scanco Medical AG). 3D μCT reconstruction were done using CTvox (version 3.2.0.r1294). All analyses were performed in a blinded manner by two different observers with automatically assignment of μCT screen-numbers, to avoid bias to the treatment.

TABLE 1 | Animal numbers, weight, and group sizes for intraoperative cell transplantations.

Animal ID	Weight (g)	Weight mean	Weight SD	Read-out	Group	Group size
362	406	357	55.31	Histomorphometry/αSMA	PBMC	$n = 5$
364	326					
365	345					
369	288					
371	420					
381	407	375.3	66.14	Histomorphometry/αSMA	CD14+	$n = 7$
382	343					
385	384					
386	294					
387	318					
388	387					
390	494					
362	406	349.6	59.62	μCT	PBMC	$n = 5$
364	326					
366	308					
369	288					
371	420					
386	294	388.4	84.70	μCT	CD14+	$n = 5$
387	318					
388	387					
389	449					
390	494					

Fracture Hematoma Extraction and Gene Expression Analysis

For gene expression analysis, femurs were excised from animals euthanized 3 and 7 days after osteotomy. Surrounding muscle tissue was dissected and tissue containing the fracture callus plus 1 mm proximal and distal to the osteotomy gap was extracted and immediately transferred to liquid nitrogen. Subsequently, tissue samples were pestled while frozen in liquid nitrogen and collected in TRIzol Reagent (LifeTechnologies) afterwards. RNA was isolated according to the manufacturer's protocol, followed by determination of RNA concentration using a Nano-Drop spectrophotometer. cDNA was transcribed from 25 ng/μl RNA with iScript reverse transcriptase as indicated by the manufacturer (Bio-Rad Laboratories GmbH) and gene expression was determined via quantitative real time PCR (iQ5 Cycler, Bio-Rad Laboratories GmbH). Primer sequences (**Table 2**) were generated using the primer 3 web based software (http://primer3.ut.ee/) and tested for specificity (ePCR, http://www.ncbi.nlm.nih.gov/tools/epcr/). Expression of each gene was calculated according to the ddCT method with adjustment for primer efficiency and normalization to TATA-box binding protein (Tbp) expression by utilizing the REST software (26). The housekeeping gene Tbp was tested against others (Gapdh,

TABLE 2 | Primer sequences.

Gene	Gene name	Forward 5′-3′	Reverse 5′-3′
CD14	Cluster of differentiation 14	aactgaagcctttctcggagc	gcataagcttcatggtcggt
CD68	Cluster of differentiation 68	tccagcaattcacctggacc	aagagaagcatggcccgaag
CD80	Cluster of differentiation 80	gctgctggttggtcttttcc	ttcttgtactcgggccacac
CCR7	C-C chemokine receptor type 7	tacatcggcgagaacaccac	caggacttggcttcgctgta
CD163	Cluster of differentiation 163	ctggagcatgaacgaggtgt	ttcctgagcatcggttgtcc
CD206	Cluster of differentiation 206	cagtttgagggcagcaagag	acactcaggagctcagcatt
Tie-2	TEK tyrosine kinase; angiopoetin receptor	tctgctctcaaggatggcaa	cacactgcagacccaaactc
Dectin	C-type lectin domain family 7 member A (CLEC7A)/Dectin	cgtcttttctggaccttgcc	acggcccttcactctgattg
PDGFα	Platelet derived growth factor alpha	ttgaacatgacccgagcaca	acacctctgtacgcgtcttg
PDGFRα	Platelet derived growth factor receptor alpha	agtgcttggtcggatcttgg	gagcatcttcacagccacct
PDGFβ	Platelet derived growth factor beta	ttgaacatgacccgagcaca	acacctctgtacgcgtcttg
PDGFRβ	Platelet derived growth factor receptor beta	cgttgcaggtggtgtttgag	acacggacagggacattgac
HIF-1α	Hypoxia-inducible factor 1, alpha subunit	tcatcagttgccacttcccc	actgggccatttctgtgtgt
VEGF	Vascular endothelial growth factor	aaagcccatgaagtggtgaa	tctgcatagtgacgttgctc
VEFGR	Vascular endothelial growth factor receptor	agaacagagctcaacgtggg	atctttgccacagtcccagg

Actb, Eif4e, B2m) and was found to be the most stable gene in all investigated samples.

Histological Analysis

Histological analyses were performed on frozen section according to the Kawamoto's film method (27). Excised femurs were fixed in a 4% PBS/PFA solution for 24 h at 4°C. For cryo-protection purposes, femurs were transferred into 10, 20, 30% sucrose solutions in ascending order for 24 h at 4°C at a time, subsequently embedded in SCEM-Medium and frozen by immersion into cold n-Hexan. Embedded and frozen samples were sectioned into 5 μm thick slices. All femurs were oriented in the same manner for the histological analyses, where the proximal part of the femur is placed on the left and the distal end of the femur on the right side of the image.

To distinguish between different calcified and soft tissues Movant Pentachrome staining was used. Prior to the staining procedure, slides were fixed with 4% PFA/PBS for 15 min. Five subsequent stainings are applied to stain mineralized bone (yellow/orange), collagen (yellow), cartilage (green/blue), osteoid (dark red), elastic fibers (orange/red), and nuclei (blue-black). After fixation samples were rehydrated for 5 min before alcian blue staining was applied for 30 min, which targets acid proteoglycans structures like chondroitin sulfate. One hour incubation in alkaline ethanol, stabilizing the blue-green pigment. Afterwards, slides were incubated in Weigert's Iron hematoxylin solution (15 min), to stain nuclei. Cell plasma was stained by brilliant crocein acid fuchsine (15 min), followed by differentiation in 0.5% acetic acid. As a last step, slides were incubated in phosphotungstic acid (20 min) and the connective tissue was stained by saffron du gatinais solution.

Vascularization analysis was performed on smooth muscle actin (αSMA) immunohistochemical staining. Slides were fixed with 4% PFA/PBS prior to the staining procedure. All subsequent staining steps were carried out in a humid chamber, at room temperature, unless stated otherwise. To block against unspecific background, samples were incubated with 2% normal horse serum before overnight application of the primary antibody (α-SMA, Dako M0851) at 4°C. Thirty minutes incubation with the secondary antibody (biotinylated anti-mouse IGG, rat-adsorbed, made in horse) and subsequent application of AB complex (ABC-AP Vectastain Kit—SP 5000) for 50 min. 2 × 5 min incubation with chromogen buffer before visualization of the vessels with AP- substrate (Red AP Substrate Kit, Vector—SK 5100). Color development was controlled under the microscope and ended by washing the slides with PBS. Nuclei were counter stained using Mayers Hämalaun for 1.5 min, unstained surrounding tissue is blued by tab water.

Pictures of the stained samples were taken with Zeiss Axioscope 40 Microscope, 10× objective (plus condenser) and the corresponding Imaging AxioVision LE Software (Carl Zeiss).

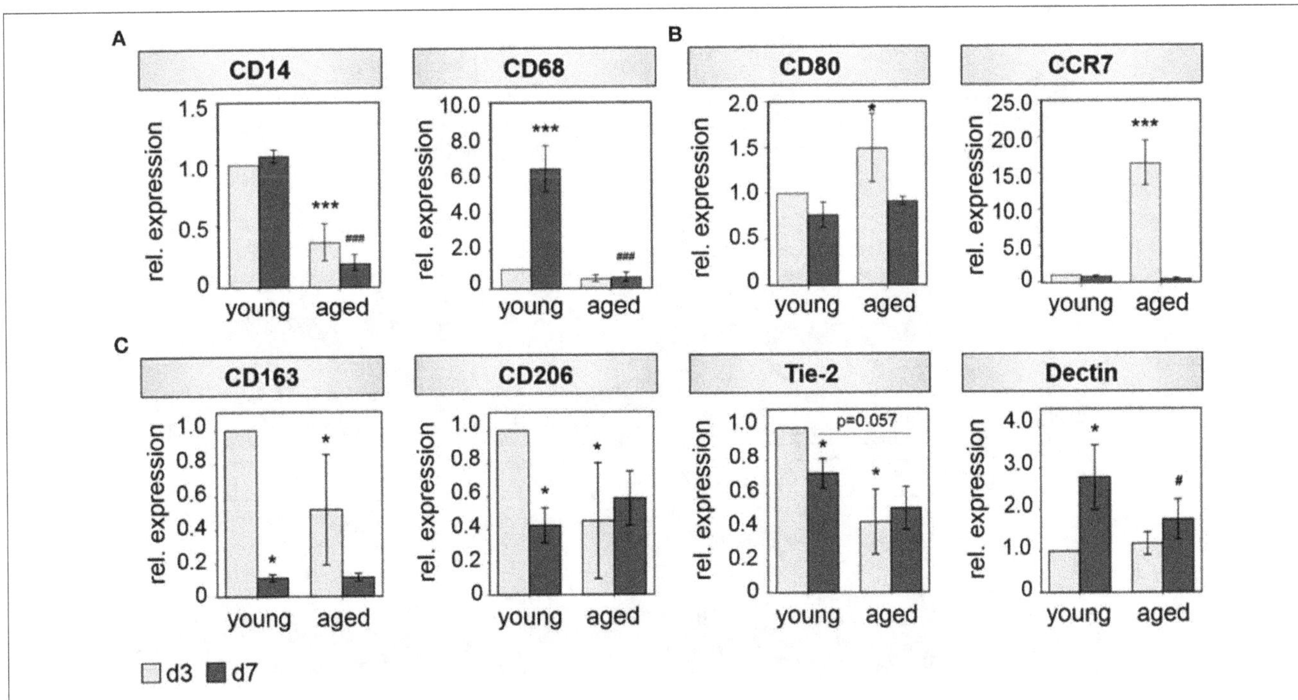

FIGURE 1 | M2 Macrophage function is impaired in bone hematoma of aged rats. **(A)** The general monocyte maker CD14 and the general mocrophage maker CD68 show a significant reduced expression 3 and 7 days after osteotomy in hematoma tissue extracted from aged animals compared to young ones. **(B)** The makers CD80 and CCR7 that are predominantly expressed by M1 macrophages show higher expression levels in fracture callus tissue from aged animals at day 3. **(C)** Marker genes that are mostly expressed by M2 macrophages (CD163, CD206, Tie-2, Dectin) show a significantly diminished expression in hematoma tissue from aged animals compared to the expression found in fracture hematoma extracted from young animals. $n = 4$–5, *significant to young d3, *$p < 0.05$;**$p < 0.001$; #significant to young d7, #$p < 0.05$; ###$p < 0.001$, ANOVA.

Tissue quantification was done with ImageJ (Version 1.44p; http://rsbweb.nih.gov/ij/) using a semi-automated method on blinded sections. Vessels were counted manually in a blinded approach. Inclusion criteria included a clear endothelial cell border, a visible lumen and non-muscle association. A region of interest (ROI) including the osteotomy gap and 1 mm proximal and distal to it was investigated.

Statistics

Determined values are depicted as bar charts showing mean ± standard deviation. For statistical analysis SigmaPlot 11.0 was used. Data were checked for normality distribution and analyzed with Student's t-test or ANOVA using a Bonferroni correction. If normality distribution could not be confirmed, data were analyzed using a non-parametric Man Whitney U Test or a multiple pairwise comparison according to Dunn's method. A $p \leq 0.05$ was considered as significant. Each analysis was performed with three technical replicates per biological samples. The applied statistical method and the amount of individual biological samples (n) that were analyzed are indicated in the respective figure legends.

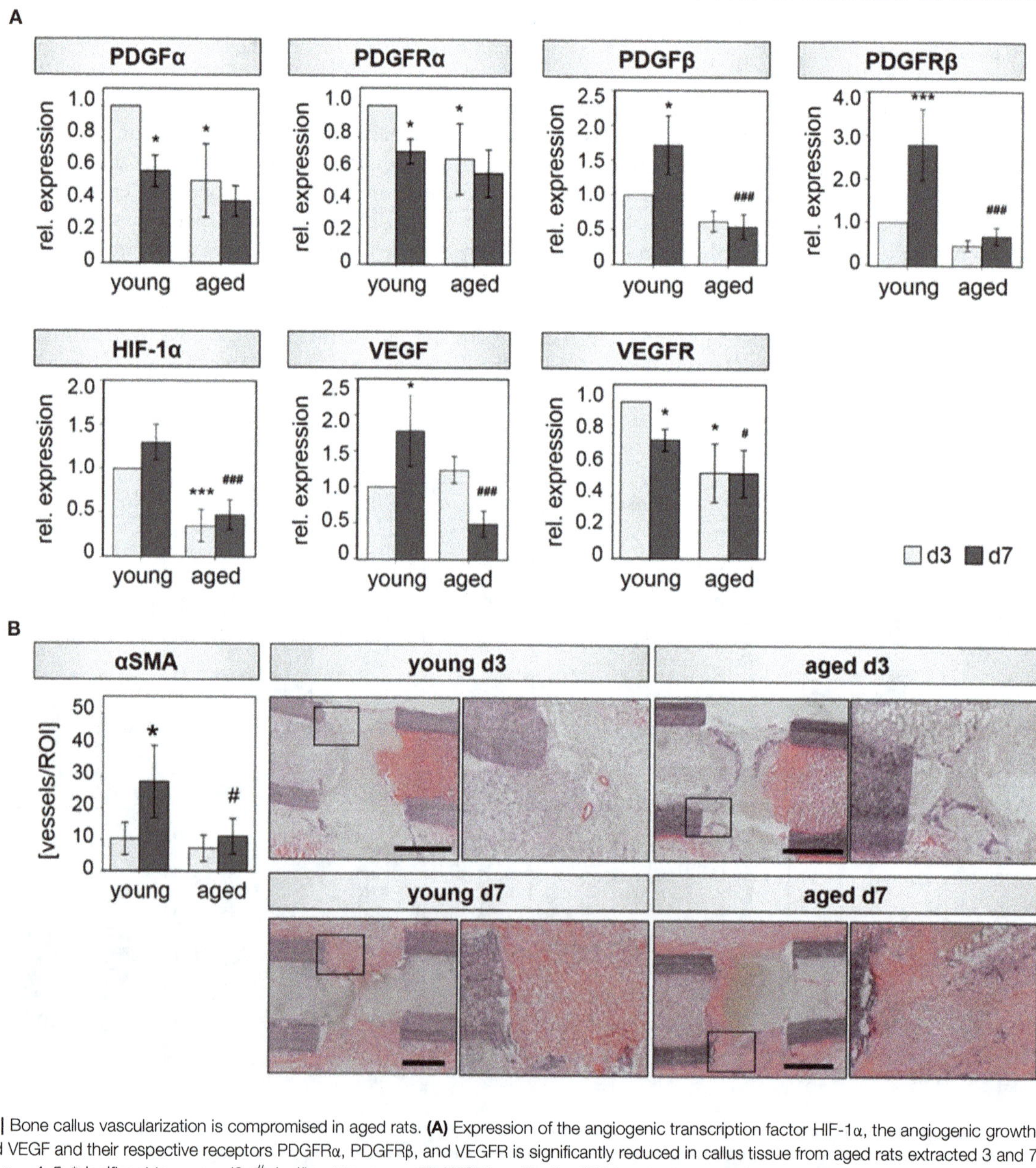

FIGURE 2 | Bone callus vascularization is compromised in aged rats. **(A)** Expression of the angiogenic transcription factor HIF-1α, the angiogenic growth factors PDGFα and VEGF and their respective receptors PDGFRα, PDGFRβ, and VEGFR is significantly reduced in callus tissue from aged rats extracted 3 and 7 days after osteotomy. $n = 4–5$, *significant to young d3; #significant to young d7, ANOVA on Ranks. **(B)** Vessel number evaluated in αSMA stained tissue sections. For each condition, the left picture shows the overview of the whole region of interest, the right picture shows the magnification of the region within the square-found in the respective overview mage. Femurs are placed in the same orientation, with the proximal side on the left and distal on the right side. y/d3, y/d7 $n = 5$, a/d3 $n = 3$, a/d7 $n = 6$, *significant to young d3, $^{*}p < 0.05$, $^{***}p < 0.001$; #significant to young d7, $^{\#}p < 0.05$, $^{\#\#\#}p < 0.001$, ANOVA.

RESULTS

Diminished Macrophage Accumulation in Bone Callus of Aged Rats

To validate our hypothesis, we analyzed the expression of commonly applied macrophage markers at early fracture healing time-points (28–32). Therefore, we extracted hematoma/callus tissue 3 and 7 days after osteotomy from young (3 months) and aged (12 months), female rats. The aged animals served hereby as a model system for impaired bone regeneration that develop a non-union without additional treatment, as we have shown previously (4, 20–22).

Interestingly, a diminished expression of monocyte/macrophage related genes was detected in bone callus tissue derived from aged animals, which develop a non-union when no additional treatment is applied. The expression of the monocyte/macrophage precursor marker CD14 and the general macrophage marker CD68 were significantly downregulated in bone callus tissue of aged animals, when compared to their expression in callus tissue derived from young animals (**Figure 1A**). Next, we investigated the expression of specific M1 and M2 macrophage polarization markers in more detail, considering the various processes, in which macrophage subsets take part during healing cascades (10, 33). The M1 markers

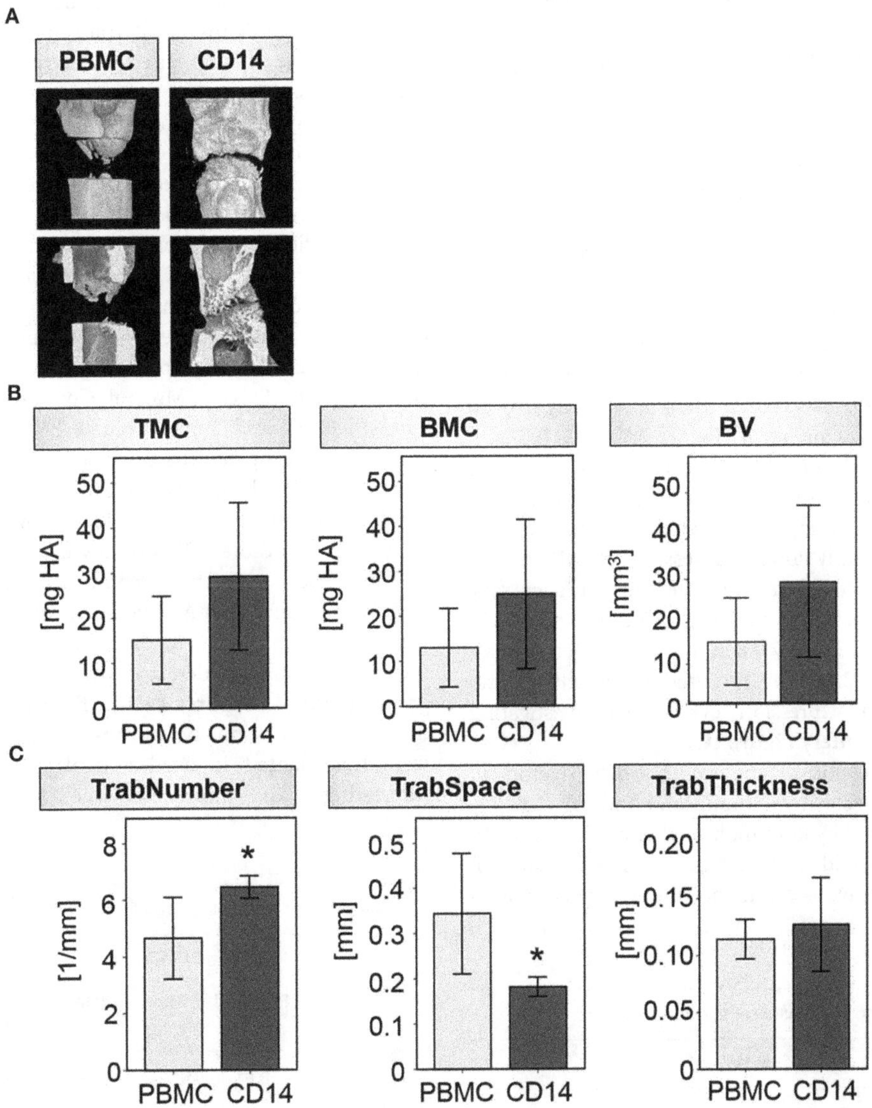

FIGURE 3 | Transplantation of CD14+ macrophage precursors partly rescues impaired bone regeneration in aged rats. **(A)** Exemplary 3D reconstructions from four individual animals receiving either PBMC or CD14+ cells locally at the osteotomy site. Bone healing was induced after CD14+ cell transplantation. **(B)** Mineral deposition was prone to be increased after CD14+ cell transplantation in the investigated ROI. **(C)** Formation of new trabeculae was significantly induced after CD14+ cell transplantation as indicated by an increased number and a reduced space between them. Thickness of the single trabeculae were unaffected by cell transplantation. $n = 5$, *significant to PBMC, $p < 0.05$, t-test.

CD80 and CCR7 showed a significant upregulation in fracture callus tissue of aged animals compared to young animals, at day 3 after osteotomy (**Figure 1B**). We further detected significant alterations, when we investigated the expression of M2 specific markers (**Figure 1C**). CD163, CD206, and Tie-2 showed lower expression levels in bone callus tissue derived from aged animals compared to younger ones (**Figure 1C**). These differences reached significance on day 3 after osteotomy. The M2 marker Dectin on the other hand, showed an upregulation from day 3 toward day 7 after osteotomy in young and aged animals. However, its expression was significantly lower in callus tissue from aged compared to young animals (**Figure 1C**). When investigating unfractured contralateral bone tissue no significant changes in marker gene expression levels could be detected (**Supplementary Figures 1A,B** and **Supplementary Table 1**).

Disturbed Callus Revascularization in Aged Rats

M2 macrophages are known to be highly involved in the regulation of angiogenic responses (34, 35). We therefore hypothesized, that the altered M2 macrophage expression profile detected in bone callus of aged animals is further accompanied with impaired revascularization of the injured bone tissue. To this end, we investigated the expression of several pro-angiogenic (growth) factors and their corresponding receptors. Indeed, we found a significantly downregulated expression of PDGFα, PDGFRα, HIF1α, and VEGFRα in fracture callus tissue of aged animals 3 days after osteotomy compared to tissue harvested from young ones (**Figure 2A**). PDGFβ and its receptor PDGFRβ did not reach statistical significance but showed the same trend of lower expression levels in fracture calli from aged animals compared to young animals at day 3 (**Figure 2A**). Significantly lower expression of HIF1α and VEGFRα was still evident 7 days after osteotomy in aged rats. In addition, expression levels of PDGFβ, PDGFRβ, and VEGF were significantly reduced at day 7 when comparing aged animals to young ones (**Figure 2A**). The analyzed genes showed no significant regulation in expression levels when investigating control tissue (**Supplementary Figure 1C**).

The decreased expression of angiogenic growth factors in aged animals is also reflected by a diminished number of newly forming vessels, identified by immunohistochemical assessment. Aged rats displayed 1.4-fold reduced numbers of alpha smooth vessel actin (αSMA) positive vessels in the callus region compared to young animals at day 3. At day 7 αSMA positive vessel numbers were reduced by a factor of 2.5 in aged animals (**Figure 2B**). Vessel diameter was also significantly reduced in hematoma tissue derived from aged animals at day 7 (**Supplementary Figure 2**).

Monocyte Transplantation Rescues Impaired Bone Healing in Aged Rats

Based on the findings discussed above, we assumed that a diminished monocyte number and possibly decreased M2 macrophage differentiation or the lack of a shift from M1 to M2 population may lead to the observed delayed healing. Enrichment of the naturally occurring monocyte/macrophage CD14+ precursor cells in the osteotomy gap region of aged animals may assist in steering a successful endogenous healing cascade. Thus, local transplantation of CD14+ cells, could improve the impaired bone regeneration observed in aged animals.

Indeed, upon local transplantation of an artificial blood clot containing CD14+ cells into the fracture gap of aged animals directly after osteotomy-induced trauma, induction of new bone formation was detected when compared to the control group (artificial blood clot containing PBMCS) (**Figure 3**). Reconstructions from μCT analysis showed a clear formation of new bone tissue within the osteotomy gap (**Figure 3A**), connected to a quantitatively increased mineral deposition in the CD14+ enriched transplantation group compared to the PBMC control group (Tissue Mineral Content-TMC, Bone Mineral Content-BMC and Bone Volume-BV) (**Table 3**; **Figure 3B**). When we investigated the microstructure of the newly formed bone more in detail, we detected a significant increase in trabecular number and a significantly diminished space between the trabeculae (**Table 3; Figures 3A,C**).

Histological evaluations confirmed the findings from the radiological analysis. A significant induction of new bone tissue mainly proximal to the bone trauma and partly within the gap region was detected in the CD14+ transplantation group (**Table 4**; **Figures 4A,B**). By trend, we also found a decreased formation of fibrous tissue, when CD14+ cells were transplanted in aged animals (**Table 4**; **Figures 4A,B**). Interestingly, the improved bone tissue regeneration after

TABLE 3 | μCT investigations 6 weeks after cell transplantation.

	PBMC	CD14
TMC [mg HA]	15.13 ± 9.70	29.19 ± 16.32
BMC [mg HA]	12.99 ± 8.71	24.84 ± 16.58
BV [mm^3]	14.95 ± 10.60	29.51 ± 18.50
Trabecular number [1/mm]	4.66 ± 1.44	6.45 ± 0.40
Trabecular space [mm]	0.34 ± 0.13	0.18 ± 0.02
Trabecular thickness [mm]	0.11 ± 0.02	0.13 ± 0.04

TABLE 4 | Histomorphometric evaluations 6 weeks after cell transplantation.

	PBMC			CD14		
	Proximal	Gap	Distal	Proximal	Gap	Distal
Mineralized tissue [% of total area]	19.27 ± 8.81	18.96 ± 10.28	11.89 ± 3.26	34.54 ± 8.65	24.13 ± 14.38	13.39 ± 5.96
Fibrotic tissue [% of total area]	n.d	20.79 ± 21.10	14.29 ± 17.60	0.91 ± 1.12	4.18 ± 4.88	2.34 ± 3.46
Cartilage [% of total area]	0.01 ± 0.03	8.95 ± 10.88	0.21 ± 0.47	0.20 ± 0.38	13.18 ± 12.55	0.75 ± 0.92
Vessel number [1/ROI]	12 ± 3	23 ± 14	14 ± 9	23 ± 15	55 ± 16	21 ± 9

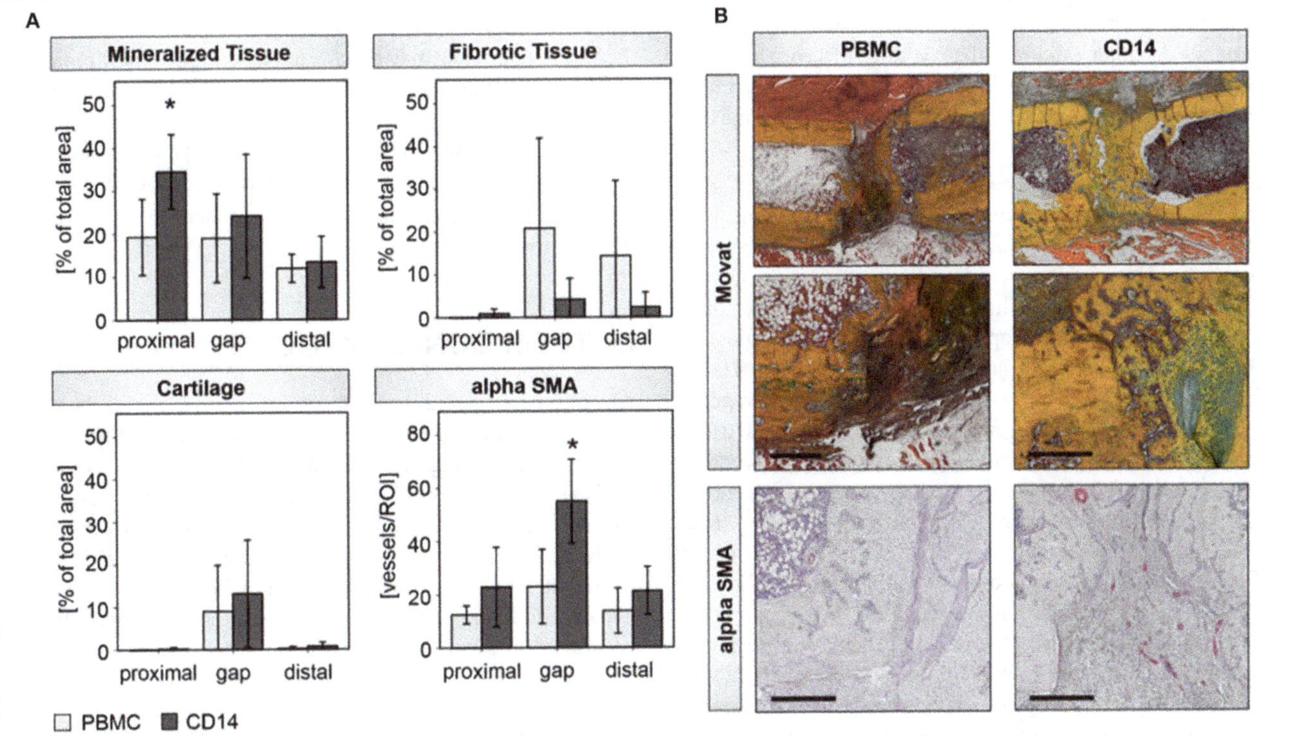

FIGURE 4 | Histological assessments verify improved bone healing after CD14+ cell transplantation aged rats. **(A)** Histomorphometric evaluations of mineralized, fibrotic, and cartilage tissue with the osteotomy gap, as well as distal and proximal to it, were done. The analysis revealed a significant induced deposition of mineralized bone matrix and by trend a diminished formation of fibrotic tissue, when aged animals received CD14+ cells locally at the osteotomy site. Number of αSMA positive vessel increased significantly in the region of interest after CD14+ cell transplantation. PBMCs $n = 5$, CD14+ $n = 7$, *significant to PBMC, $p < 0.05$. **(B)** Exemplary pictures of Movat-Pentachrom (mineralized bone, yellow/orange; collagen, yellow; cartilage, green/blue; osteoid, dark red; elastic fibers, orange/ref; nuclei, blue-black) and aSMA stained tissue sections. Femurs are placed in the same orientation, with the proximal side on the left and distal on the right side. Bar = 500 μm.

CD14+ cell transplantation was accompanied with a significant induction of new vessel formation (**Table 4**; **Figures 4A,B**).

DISCUSSION AND CONCLUSION

Macrophages are essential for bone regeneration and they participate in all stages of healing, promote collagen I deposition and matrix mineralization by osteoblasts *in vitro* and *in vivo* (9, 36, 37). Additional evidence that macrophages play important roles during bone regeneration can be obtained from studies reporting on systemic depletions of macrophages in experimental mouse models. Independent of the time point of macrophage depletion, a diminished formation of new bone matrix and an altered endochondral ossification process is visible 7–28 days after injury (36, 38).

The M1 to M2 switch plays a vital role during healing progression as reported recently by co-workers from our institute and others (19, 38). We confirm here that macrophage activity plays a significant role in bone repair and that an imbalance in the M1/M2 macrophage differentiation is associated with disturbed bone regeneration in aged rats. Furthermore, we showed that local transplantation of macrophage precursors can enhance and potentially rescue bone repair under biologically impaired conditions, presumably by an induction of M2 macrophage differentiation. Our findings highlight the potential of local cell transplantations, here monocytes/macrophages to steer bone repair, especially under compromised conditions, since we used macrophage precursors derived from circulating blood of aged matched donors for local cell transplantation, which presumably shifted the endogenous cell balance and thus promoted healing. Ongoing research further highlights a close connection between macrophages and osteogenic differentiation. A recent study, reported on the osteogenic differentiation capacity of MC3T3 pre-osteoblasts in *in vitro* co-cultures with macrophages (19). When MC3T3 cells were cultivated together with M1 macrophages that underwent an IL-4 triggered M2 switch during MC3T3 osteoblast maturation, mineralized matrix deposition was significantly induced (19). This might be due to M2 macrophage-induced BMP-2 secretion, which is a major contributor to osteogenic differentiation (39). In addition, recent studies from Gibon et al. support our hypothesis of a disturbed M1/M2 phenotype balance in aged. They could show that bone marrow macrophages isolated from aged mice have a higher pre-activated resting state and increased expression of the pro-inflammatory cytokine TNFa after activation than macrophages isolated from young animals (40). Furthermore, they described an impaired M2 polarization of bone marrow macrophages derived from aged mice (40). Recently Vi et al.

also reported that the age of macrophages is crucial for fracture repair. Parabiosis and fractionated bone marrow transplantation experiments in mice showed that young macrophages can rejuvenate healing potential of old bone marrow stromal cells, while old macrophages impair healing of young bone marrow stromal cells (41).

There is also *in vivo* evidence that M2 rather than M1 macrophages regulate bone healing. Animals that were administered with CSF-1, which is required for macrophage differentiation, have an increased abundance of M2 macrophages within the fracture site and show improved healing outcomes (36, 42). In addition, M2 macrophages are highly pro-angiogenic and secrete various growth factors, as e.g., TGF-b, TGF-a, bFGF, PDGF, and VEGF (43, 44). Thereby they might regulate revascularization and matrix maturation of the callus tissue. The angiogenic capacity of monocytes and their descendent macrophages is also proven by investigations of $Ccr2^{-/-}$ mice. Beside compromised cartilage maturation, $Ccr2^{-/-}$ mice show an impaired formation of new blood vessels within the fracture site (45). Moldovan et al. reported that the angiogenic capacity of macrophages relates to their capability to degrade extracellular matrix. Using a transgenic mouse model of ischemic cardiomyopathy, where monocytes were attracted to the myocardium by the targeted overexpression of CCL2, they showed tunnel carving by macrophages, which provide growing vessels with a path for invading capillaries (12).

However, there is still an ongoing discussion on the state of macrophage polarization and activation and its effect on bone regeneration. M1 macrophages for instance can be beneficial or deleterious for bone formation, highly depending on the study design as recently reviewed by Pajarinen et al. (9). Another possibility is that all macrophage phenotypes can promote osteogenesis, but that their effectiveness is connected to different physiological and pathophysiological states (9).

Related to these recent reports and the current study, it is still a matter of discussion whether the pro-regenerative function of M2 macrophages in bone repair is related to their angiogenic properties and/or their ability for matrix degradation and how these characteristics may be effected by compromised biological conditions. While our work gives new insights concerning the beneficial effect of local macrophage enrichment on bone healing outcome, it is limited in showing M1/M2 dynamics early after transplantation. Additional research is needed to explore the exact role of M2 macrophages and other macrophage phenotypes in the early healing cascade.

AUTHOR CONTRIBUTIONS

AD has participated in conception and design of the study, acquisition, analysis and interpretation of data, and manuscript writing and editing. JL has contributed to data acquisition, analysis and interpretation of data, and manuscript writing and editing. AE, AR, FS, and SF have participated in acquisition, analysis and interpretation of data, and manuscript editing. GD contributed to conception and design of the study, interpretation of data, and manuscript editing. All co-authors approved the final version of the submitted manuscript.

FUNDING

This work has been supported by the BCRT through funding by the German Federal Ministry of Education and Research (BMBF).

ACKNOWLEDGMENTS

We are grateful for the excellent technical assistance of Janine Mikutta, Mario Thiele, and Gabriela Korus in execution and analyses of the animal experiments.

REFERENCES

1. Schmidt-Bleek K, Petersen A, Dienelt A, Schwarz C, Duda GN. Initiation and early control of tissue regeneration-bone healing as a model system for tissue regeneration. *Expert Opin Biol Ther.* (2014) 14:247–59. doi: 10.1517/14712598.2014.857653
2. Tarantino U, Cerocchi I, Scialdoni A, Saturnino L, Feola M, Celi M, et al. Bone healing and osteoporosis. *Aging Clin Exp Res.* (2011) 23(Suppl 2):62–4. Available online at: https://www.researchgate.net/publication/51693253_Bone_healing_and_osteoporosis
3. Gorman E, Chudyk AM, Madden KM, Ashe MC. Bone health and type 2 diabetes mellitus: a systematic review. *Physiother Can.* (2011) 63:8–20. doi: 10.3138/ptc.2010-23bh
4. Strube P, Sentuerk U, Riha T, Kaspar K, Mueller M, Kasper G, et al. Influence of age and mechanical stability on bone defect healing: age reverses mechanical effects. *Bone.* (2008) 42:758–64. doi: 10.1016/j.bone.2007.12.223
5. Garcia P, Pieruschka A, Klein M, Tami A, Histing T, Holstein JH, et al. Temporal and spatial vascularization patterns of unions and nonunions: role of vascular endothelial growth factor and bone morphogenetic proteins. *J Bone Joint Surg Am.* (2012) 94:49–58. doi: 10.2106/JBJS.J.00795
6. Hankenson KD, Dishowitz M, Gray C, Schenker M. Angiogenesis in bone regeneration. *Injury.* (2011) 42:556–61. doi: 10.1016/j.injury.2011.03.035
7. Fassbender M, Strobel C, Rauhe JS, Bergmann C, Schmidmaier G, Wildemann B. Local inhibition of angiogenesis results in an atrophic non-union in a

rat osteotomy model. *Eur Cell Mater.* (2011) 22:1–11. doi: 10.22203/eCM.v022a01
8. Lienau J, Schmidt-Bleek K, Peters A, Haschke F, Duda GN, Perka C, et al. Differential regulation of blood vessel formation between standard and delayed bone healing. *J Orthop Res.* (2009) 27:1133–40. doi: 10.1002/jor.20870
9. Pajarinen J, Lin T, Gibon E, Kohno Y, Maruyama M, Nathan K, et al. Mesenchymal stem cell-macrophage crosstalk and bone healing. *Biomaterials.* (2019) 196:80–9. doi: 10.1016/j.biomaterials.2017.12.025
10. Gu QL, Yang HL, Shi Q. Macrophages and bone inflammation. *J Orthop Transl.* (2017) 10:86–93. doi: 10.1016/j.jot.2017.05.002
11. Alexander KA, Raggatt LJ, Millard S, Batoon L, Chiu-Ku Wu A, Chang MK, et al. Resting and injury-induced inflamed periosteum contain multiple macrophage subsets that are located at sites of bone growth and regeneration. *Immunol Cell Biol.* (2017) 95:7–16. doi: 10.1038/icb.2016.74
12. Moldovan NI, Goldschmidt-Clermont PJ, Parker-Thornburg J, Shapiro SD, Kolattukudy PE. Contribution of monocytes/macrophages to compensatory neovascularization: the drilling of metalloelastase-positive tunnels in ischemic myocardium. *Circ Res.* (2000) 87:378–84. doi: 10.1161/01.RES.87.5.378
13. Lucas T, Waisman A, Ranjan R, Roes J, Krieg T, Müller W, et al. Differential roles of macrophages in diverse phases of skin repair. *J Immunol.* (2010) 184:3964–77. doi: 10.4049/jimmunol.0903356
14. Okuno Y, Nakamura-Ishizu A, Kishi K, Suda T, Kubota Y. Bone marrow-derived cells serve as proangiogenic macrophages but not endothelial cells in wound healing. *Blood.* (2011) 117:5264–72. doi: 10.1182/blood-2011-01-330720
15. Capoccia BJ, Gregory AD, Link DC. Recruitment of the inflammatory subset of monocytes to sites of ischemia induces angiogenesis in a monocyte chemoattractant protein-1-dependent fashion. *J Leukoc Biol.* (2008) 84:760–8. doi: 10.1189/jlb.1107756
16. Ochoa O, Sun D, Reyes-Reyna SM, Waite LL, Michalek JE, McManus LM, et al. Delayed angiogenesis and VEGF production in CCR2$^{-/-}$ mice during impaired skeletal muscle regeneration. *Am J Physiol Regul Integr Comp Physiol.* (2007) 293:R651–61. doi: 10.1152/ajpregu.00069.2007
17. Mantovani A, Sica A, Sozzani S, Allavena P, Vecchi A, Locati M. The chemokine system in diverse forms of macrophage activation and polarization. *Trends Immunol.* (2004) 25:677–86. doi: 10.1016/j.it.2004.09.015
18. Davis MJ, Tsang TM, Qiu Y, Dayrit JK, Freij JB, Huffnagle GB, et al. Macrophage M1/M2 polarization dynamically adapts to changes in cytokine microenvironments in *Cryptococcus neoformans* infection. *mBio.* (2013) 4:e00264-13. doi: 10.1128/mBio.00264-13
19. Loi F, Córdova LA, Zhang R, Pajarinen J, Lin TH, Goodman SB, et al. The effects of immunomodulation by macrophage subsets on osteogenesis *in vitro. Stem Cell Res Ther.* (2016) 7:15. doi: 10.1186/s13287-016-0276-5
20. Preininger B, Gerigk H, Bruckner J, Perka C, Schell H, Ellinghaus A, et al. An experimental setup to evaluate innovative therapy options for the enhancement of bone healing using BMP as a benchmark–a pilot study. *Eur Cell Mater.* (2012) 23:262–71. doi: 10.22203/eCM.v023a20
21. Mehta M, Duda GN, Perka C, Strube P. Influence of gender and fixation stability on bone defect healing in middle-aged rats: a pilot study. *Clin Orthop Relat Res.* (2011) 469:3102–10. doi: 10.1007/s11999-011-1914-y
22. Strube P, Mehta M, Baerenwaldt A, Trippens J, Wilson CJ, Ode A, et al. Sex-specific compromised bone healing in female rats might be associated with a decrease in mesenchymal stem cell quantity. *Bone.* (2009) 45:1065–72. doi: 10.1016/j.bone.2009.08.005
23. Strube P, Mehta M, Putzier M, Matziolis G, Perka C, Duda GN. A new device to control mechanical environment in bone defect healing in rats. *J Biomech.* (2008) 41:2696–702. doi: 10.1016/j.jbiomech.2008.06.009
24. Sass FA, Schmidt-Bleek K, Ellinghaus A, Filter S, Rose A, Preininger B, et al. CD31+ cells from peripheral blood facilitate bone regeneration in biologically impaired conditions through combined effects on immunomodulation and angiogenesis. *J Bone Miner Res.* (2017) 32:902–12. doi: 10.1002/jbmr.3062
25. Preininger B, Duda G, Gerigk H, Bruckner J, Ellinghaus A, Sass FA, et al. CD133: enhancement of bone healing by local transplantation of peripheral blood cells in a biologically delayed rat osteotomy model. *PLoS ONE.* (2013) 8:e52650. doi: 10.1371/journal.pone.0052650
26. Pfaffl MW, Horgan GW, Dempfle L. Relative expression software tool (REST) for group-wise comparison and statistical analysis of relative expression results in real-time PCR. *Nucleic Acids Res.* (2002) 30:e36. doi: 10.1093/nar/30.9.e36
27. Kawamoto T. Use of a new adhesive film for the preparation of multi-purpose fresh-frozen sections from hard tissues, whole-animals, insects and plants. *Arch Histol Cytol.* (2003) 66:123–43. doi: 10.1679/aohc.66.123
28. Forget MA, Voorhees JL, Cole SL, Dakhlallah D, Patterson IL, Gross AC, et al. Macrophage colony-stimulating factor augments Tie2-expressing monocyte differentiation, angiogenic function, and recruitment in a mouse model of breast cancer. *PLoS ONE.* (2014) 9:e98623. doi: 10.1371/journal.pone.0098623
29. Zhou Y, Yoshida S, Kubo Y, Yoshimura T, Kobayashi Y, Nakama T, et al. Different distributions of M1 and M2 macrophages in a mouse model of laser-induced choroidal neovascularization. *Mol Med Rep.* (2017) 15:3949–56. doi: 10.3892/mmr.2017.6491
30. Sindrilaru A, Peters T, Wieschalka S, Baican C, Baican A, Peter H, et al. An unrestrained proinflammatory M1 macrophage population induced by iron impairs wound healing in humans and mice. *J Clin Invest.* (2011) 121:985–97. doi: 10.1172/JCI44490
31. Oh J, Riek AE, Weng S, Petty M, Kim D, Colonna M, et al. Endoplasmic reticulum stress controls M2 macrophage differentiation and foam cell formation. *J Biol Chem.* (2012) 287:11629–41. doi: 10.1074/jbc.M111.338673
32. Suzuki K, Meguro K, Nakagomi D, Nakajima H. Roles of alternatively activated M2 macrophages in allergic contact dermatitis. *Allergol Int.* (2017) 66:392–7. doi: 10.1016/j.alit.2017.02.015
33. Vi L, Baht GS, Whetstone H, Ng A, Wei Q, Poon R, et al. Macrophages promote osteoblastic differentiation in-vivo: implications in fracture repair and bone homeostasis. *J Bone Min Res.* (2015) 30:1090–102. doi: 10.1002/jbmr.2422
34. Jetten N, Verbruggen S, Gijbels MJ, Post MJ, De Winther MP, Donners MM. Anti-inflammatory M2, but not pro-inflammatory M1 macrophages promote angiogenesis *in vivo. Angiogenesis.* (2014) 17:109–18. doi: 10.1007/s10456-013-9381-6
35. Ferrante CJ, Leibovich SJ. Regulation of macrophage polarization and wound healing. *Adv Wound Care.* (2012) 1:10–6. doi: 10.1089/wound.2011.0307
36. Alexander KA, Chang MK, Maylin ER, Kohler T, Müller R, Wu AC, et al. Osteal macrophages promote *in vivo* intramembranous bone healing in a mouse tibial injury model. *J Bone Miner Res.* (2011) 26:1517–32. doi: 10.1002/jbmr.354
37. Chang MK, Raggatt LJ, Alexander KA, Kuliwaba JS, Fazzalari NL, Schroder K, et al. Osteal tissue macrophages are intercalated throughout human and mouse bone lining tissues and regulate osteoblast function *in vitro* and *in vivo. J Immunol.* (2008) 181:1232–44. doi: 10.4049/jimmunol.181.2.1232
38. Schlundt C, El Khassawna T, Serra A, Dienelt A, Wendler S, Schell H, et al. Macrophages in bone fracture healing: their essential role in endochondral ossification. *Bone.* (2018) 106:78–89. doi: 10.1016/j.bone.2015
39. Champagne CM, Takebe J, Offenbacher S, Cooper LF. Macrophage cell lines produce osteoinductive signals that include bone morphogenetic protein-2. *Bone.* (2002) 30:26–31. doi: 10.1016/S8756-3282(01)00638-X
40. Gibon E, Loi F, Córdova LA, Pajarinen J, Lin T, Lu L, et al. Aging affects bone marrow macrophage polarization: relevance to bone healing. *Regen Eng Transl Med.* (2016) 2:98–104. doi: 10.1007/s40883-016-0016-5
41. Vi L, Baht GS, Soderblom EJ, Whetstone H, Wei Q, Furman B, et al. Macrophage cells secrete factors including LRP1 that orchestrate the rejuvenation of bone repair in mice. *Nat Commun.* (2018) 9:5191. doi: 10.1038/s41467-018-07666-0
42. Sarahrudi K, Mousavi M, Grossschmidt K, Sela N, König F, Vécsei V, et al. The impact of colony-stimulating factor-1 on fracture healing:

an experimental study. *J Orthop Res.* (2009) 27:36–41. doi: 10.1002/jor. 20680
43. DiPietro LA, Polverini PJ. Role of the macrophage in the positive and negative regulation of wound neovascularization. *Behring Inst Mitt.* (1993) 1993:238–47.
44. Eming SA, Krieg T, Davidson JM. Inflammation in wound repair: molecular and cellular mechanisms. *J Invest Dermatol.* (2007) 127:514–25. doi: 10.1038/sj.jid.5700701
45. Xing Z, Lu C, Hu D, Yu YY, Wang X, Colnot C, et al. Multiple roles for CCR2 during fracture healing. *Dis Model Mech.* (2010) 3:451–8. doi: 10.1242/dmm.003186

10

Osteoimmunology of Oral and Maxillofacial Diseases: Translational Applications Based on Biological Mechanisms

*Carla Alvarez[1,2], Gustavo Monasterio[2], Franco Cavalla[3], Luis A. Córdova[4], Marcela Hernández[2], Dominique Heymann[5], Gustavo P. Garlet[6], Timo Sorsa[7,8], Pirjo Pärnänen[7], Hsi-Ming Lee[9], Lorne M. Golub[9], Rolando Vernal[2,10] and Alpdogan Kantarci[1]**

[1] Forsyth Institute, Cambridge, MA, United States, [2] Periodontal Biology Laboratory, Faculty of Dentistry, Universidad de Chile, Santiago, Chile, [3] Department of Conservative Dentistry, Faculty of Dentistry, Universidad de Chile, Santiago, Chile, [4] Department of Oral and Maxillofacial Surgery, Faculty of Dentistry, San Jose's Hospital and Clínica Las Condes, Universidad de Chile, Santiago, Chile, [5] INSERM, UMR 1232, LabCT, CRCINA, Institut de Cancérologie de l'Ouest, Université de Nantes, Université d'Angers, Saint-Herblain, France, [6] Department of Biological Sciences, Bauru School of Dentistry, University of São Paulo, Bauru, Brazil, [7] Department of Oral and Maxillofacial Diseases, University of Helsinki, Helsinki University Hospital, Helsinki, Finland, [8] Department of Oral Diseases, Karolinska Institutet, Stockholm, Sweden, [9] Department of Oral Biology and Pathology, School of Dental Medicine, Stony Brook University, Stony Brook, NY, United States, [10] Dentistry Unit, Faculty of Health Sciences, Universidad Autónoma de Chile, Santiago, Chile

***Correspondence:**
Alpdogan Kantarci
akantarci@forsyth.org

The maxillofacial skeleton is highly dynamic and requires a constant equilibrium between the bone resorption and bone formation. The field of osteoimmunology explores the interactions between bone metabolism and the immune response, providing a context to study the complex cellular and molecular networks involved in oro-maxillofacial osteolytic diseases. In this review, we present a framework for understanding the potential mechanisms underlying the immuno-pathobiology in etiologically-diverse diseases that affect the oral and maxillofacial region and share bone destruction as their common clinical outcome. These otherwise different pathologies share similar inflammatory pathways mediated by central cellular players, such as macrophages, T and B cells, that promote the differentiation and activation of osteoclasts, ineffective or insufficient bone apposition by osteoblasts, and the continuous production of osteoclastogenic signals by immune and local stromal cells. We also present the potential translational applications of this knowledge based on the biological mechanisms involved in the inflammation-induced bone destruction. Such applications can be the development of immune-based therapies that promote bone healing/regeneration, the identification of host-derived inflammatory/collagenolytic biomarkers as diagnostics tools, the assessment of links between oral and systemic diseases; and the characterization of genetic polymorphisms in immune or bone-related genes that will help diagnosis of susceptible individuals.

Keywords: osteoimmunology, oral, maxillofacial, periodontal disease, biomarkers

INTRODUCTION

The maxillofacial skeletal structure has a complex geometry, adapted to the high mechanical requirements of the masticatory function. In this complex system, the alveolar bone accommodates the teeth and periodontal tissues while the basal bone provides support and insertion of masticatory muscles. Also, the mandible has two bilateral vertical rami that articulate with the base of the skull to form the temporomandibular joint (TMJ). Under physiological conditions, the bone undergoes continuous remodeling in a dynamic equilibrium of bone resorption by osteoclasts and bone formation by osteoblasts, at anatomically discrete sites known as basic multicellular units (BMUs) (1). Tight control of bone remodeling at the BMUs level is necessary to conserve structural integrity as the formation component needs to replace the exact amount removed by resorption. The strict synchronization of bone resorption and formation is referred to as coupling, a term that applies to each BMUs along with the skeleton (2). Bone coupling is controlled through a complex cellular communication network regulated by the signaling between osteoblasts, their mesenchymal pre-osteoblastic precursors, osteocytes, and osteoclasts and their monocytic precursors (1). Although circulating hormones, including PTH and 1,25-dihydroxyvitamin-D3, are considered to be the critical regulators of bone remodeling, it has become clear that locally generated cytokines are the key modulators of bone-cells communication and function (2).

The field of osteoimmunology has provided insight into the mechanics of osteoclast differentiation and activation during inflammation by immune cells and their soluble products. This process is fundamentally regulated by a triad of proteins of the tumor necrosis factor/tumor necrosis factor receptor family namely the receptor activator of nuclear factor κB ligand (RANKL), its functional receptor (RANK), and its soluble decoy receptor osteoprotegerin (OPG). Both soluble and membrane-bound RANKL can induce osteoclastogenesis through RANK in osteoclast precursors. Meanwhile, OPG inhibits the interaction between RANKL and RANK, and arrests osteoclastogenesis (3, 4). Under homeostatic conditions, RANKL is produced mainly by osteocytes, which have a higher capacity to support osteoclastogenesis than osteoblasts and are essentials for bone remodeling (5, 6). Interestingly, osteoblasts also produce RANKL which acts as an acceptor for vesicular RANK produced by mature osteoclasts. The osteoblastic RANKL-RANK cross-linking triggers RANKL reverse signaling, which promotes bone formation through the increased expression of early regulators of osteoblast differentiation (7). Under inflammatory conditions, however, the sources of RANKL are increased; immune cells such as particular subtypes of T cells and B cells can also produce RANKL (8). In addition, the local secretion of pro-inflammatory cytokines, such as IL-17 can induce the production of RANKL by osteoblasts and fibroblasts with osteoclastogenic capacity (9) suggesting a highly complex network of cellular origins of RANKL activity in tissues induced by inflammation.

In addition to osteoclast differentiation, inflammation impacts bone formation. Anabolic bone apposition is generally sustained by the expression of different growth factors such as fibroblast growth factors (FGFs), platelet-derived growth factors (PDGFs), insulin-like growth factors (IGFs), tumor growth factor β (TGF-β), bone morphogenetic proteins (BMPs), and Wnt proteins, released from the bone matrix or produced locally by different cell types (10–14). In particular, the Wnt/β-catenin and Bmp/Runx2 signaling pathways are essential for bone mass maintenance by regulating the differentiation and anabolic bone-formation activity of osteoblasts and osteocytes (15, 16). However, during inflammation, the activation of the classical (or canonical) NF-κB pathway inhibits the production of bone matrix proteins by decreasing the Bmp2-stimulated Runx2 and Wnt-stimulated β-catenin binding to osteocalcin and bone sialoprotein promoters (12). Inflammation also induces the production of the Wnt/β-catenin pathway inhibitors Dickkopf factor-1 (DKK1) and sclerotin (17, 18). The decline of inflammation restores the osteoblast functions by activating the canonical Wnt/β-catenin pathway (19), which has been shown to up-regulate OPG expression and inhibit osteoclast differentiation (20). Accumulating evidence, therefore, points to the failure of endogenous inflammation-resolution pathways as an underlying factor in the initiation and progression of chronic osteolytic inflammatory diseases and their relationship with systemic diseases.

In osteolytic inflammatory diseases such as periodontal disease, apical periodontitis, maxillofacial bone sarcomas and osteoarthritis of the TMJ, inflammation results in tissue destruction by the continuous release of osteoclastogenic mediators that counteract the production of bone-coupling signals. These otherwise different diseases share similar inflammatory pathways mediated by central cellular players, such as macrophages, T and B cells, that promote the differentiation and activation of osteoclasts, ineffective or insufficient bone apposition by osteoblasts, and the continuous production of osteoclastogenic signals by immune and local stromal cells. In the present review, we focused on the immune pathways that lead to the clinical signs of bone loss in different oro-maxillofacial diseases and possible translational applications of this knowledge.

PERIODONTAL DISEASE

Definition and Pathogenesis of the Periodontal Disease

Among the osteolytic chronic inflammatory disorders of the jaws, periodontitis is the most well-defined and studied. The mechanisms underlying the pathogenesis of periodontitis are complex as periodontitis is a multifactorial disease that requires the combination of both a susceptible host and a dysbiotic polymicrobial community (21). Periodontitis is a significant public health problem due to its high prevalence, its cause of tooth loss, and its association with systemic diseases (22). Host susceptibility to periodontal diseases is the combination of genetic, epigenetic, behavioral, and environmental factors that modulate the immune response and the conditions of maintenance of the microbial community that colonizes the pathogenic biofilm (23, 24). The periodontitis-associated microbial communities not only stimulate but also exploit inflammation as a way to obtain nutrients for growth and persistence. The virulence factors of the bacteria can inhibit the antimicrobial functions and promote the pro-inflammatory and tissue-destructive properties of the host immune response to escape annihilation; consequently exacerbating and perpetuating the disease (21, 25). Thus, the interactions between the host and the microorganisms in periodontal disease are not only complex but also evolving.

Cellular and the Molecular Immune Basis of the Periodontal Disease

The immune response during periodontitis involves different elements of innate and adaptive immunity. One of the first responders during the pathogenesis of periodontitis is the complement system, first recognized in early clinical studies that associated the disease with the presence of activated complement fragments in the gingival crevicular fluid (GCF) (26, 27). The use of animal models helped to clarify the role of complement-related mechanisms during periodontitis and alveolar bone loss (26, 28). These studies have highlighted the synergistic cross-talk of the complement with TLR pathways. For example, the activation of both C5aR1 and TLR2 by specific agonists resulted in the induction of significantly higher levels of pro-inflammatory cytokines in the gingiva (28). Mice lacking C5aR1 are resistant to bone-destructive diseases such as periodontitis and arthritis (29, 30), attributed to the critical role of the anaphylatoxin receptors in initiating neutrophils and macrophages adhesion and recruitment, necessary for the induction of bone resorption (31). Also, *P. gingivalis* targets C5aR to promote its adaptive fitness by manipulating the activation of TLR2 via the C5a-C5aR axis, allowing it to escape the IL-12p70-dependent immune clearance. This C5aR1-dependent evasion mechanism is crucial for the induction of microbial dysbiosis (29, 32).

Periodontal health is particularly sensitive to neutrophil functions and dysfunctions. Both hyper- and hypo-responsiveness of neutrophils have been associated with dysregulated inflammatory response and bone loss (33). Rare diseases related to defective extravasation of circulating neutrophils (LAD-1 deficiency) or neutrophil functionality (Papillon-Lefèvre syndrome) display a severe and fast-progressive form of periodontitis (34). If neutrophils cannot reach the gingiva, there is an overproduction of IL-23, IL-17, and G-CSF in the periodontium, attributed to macrophages, which in turn induces further inflammation and osteoclastogenesis (35). *P. gingivalis* possesses virulence factors that disrupt the neutrophil responses. For example, the LPS-induced TLR2 activation and cross-talk with C5aR inhibits the Myd88 but activates the Mal-PI3K pathway; this abolishes the antimicrobial response and PI3K-mediated phagocytosis while triggering the Mal-dependent inflammation (36). *P. gingivalis* can inhibit opsonization and phagocytosis, enhance neutrophil recruitment and respiratory burst, thus incrementing the neutrophil-associated inflammation and tissue damage (37). Neutrophils may also possess a hyper-inflammatory phenotype characterized by the over-expression of reactive oxygen species and pro-inflammatory cytokines (IL-1β, IL-6, IL-8, and TNF-α), which along with their other defective functions such as phagocytosis and chemotaxis, contribute to additional tissue-damage and comorbidity with other inflammatory diseases (38, 39). In the context of osteoimmunological regulation of periodontal diseases, neutrophils display heterotypic adhesion to osteoblast and modulate their function (40) and possess a regulatory role during microbial infection by secreting the anti-inflammatory cytokine IL-10 (41). Neutrophils acquire regulatory functions by direct cell-to-cell contact with regulatory T (Treg) cells or by exogenous IL-10 stimuli. The IL-10-producing neutrophils have been found in the purulent exudate collected from periodontal pockets in patients with chronic periodontitis; their role in the resolution of periodontal inflammation still needs to be investigated (42).

Even though macrophages are in low quantities in periodontal tissues (43), they participate in the pathogenesis of periodontitis as central players by initiating or resolving inflammation, contributing to tissue repair, activating lymphocyte-mediated adaptive immunity and mediating alveolar bone resorption and apposition (44). During inflammation, tissue-resident macrophages are expanded, and circulating monocytes are recruited to be differentiated into macrophage-like cells (45). Macrophages are divided into two functionally different subtypes: M1 classically-activated macrophages, produced in response to IFN-γ, TNF-α, IL-1β, and IL-6, with pro-inflammatory, antibacterial and antiviral functions; M2 alternatively-activated macrophages, produced in response to IL-4 and IL-13, with anti-inflammatory and tissue-repair/regeneration functions that expresses high levels of IL-10 (46–48). While these classes are clearly defined in mice; in humans, macrophages represent a continuum of highly plastic effector cells, resembling a spectrum of diverse phenotype states (47). Both M1 and M2 macrophages are increased in periodontitis compared to controls, yet the M1/M2 ratio is higher in periodontitis and is associated with increased expression of M1-related molecules such as IL-1β, IL-6 and matrix metalloproteinase (MMP)-9 (48, 49). Circulating monocytes/macrophages are affected by experimental periodontitis and display an M1 phenotype by overexpressing TNF-α and IL-6 (50). The temporal analysis of inflammation to healing osteolytic periodontal lesions showed a shift in the macrophage activation from inflammatory (CD80 and TNF-α expression) to resolving (CD206 expression) phenotype, which correlated to bone loss (51).

Lymphocytes are the majority of all $CD45^+$ hematopoietic-origin cells within the normal gingival mucosa (43) and play a key role in osteoimmunology. The $CD3^+$ T cell compartment is the dominant population in both health and disease, reflecting a 10-fold increase in total inflammatory cells (43). The analysis of alveolar bone resorption during *P. gingivalis*-induced experimental periodontitis in MHC-I or MHC-II deficient mice showed the destructive role for $CD4^+$ T cells (52); yet effector-memory $CD8^+$ T cells are present in normal gingival mucosa (43) suggesting a protective role for $CD8^+$ T cells during periodontitis possibly due their ability to suppress osteoclastogenesis (53). Upon activation by the APCs, $CD4^+$ T cells are polarized into distinct effector phenotypes depending on the nature of the antigen, co-stimulatory signals, and the local cytokine milieu (22). These phenotypes are Th1, Th2, Th9, Th17, Th22, and Treg, each with a particular transcription factor, often called a master switch, that modulates the phenotypic differentiation and particular effector-functions making these phenotypes highly plastic (54). Each phenotype has different involvement in the pathogenesis of periodontitis. They can be broadly classified in two axes: (1) Th1/Th17 pro-inflammatory and osteoclastogenic and (2) Th2/Treg mechanistically implied in the arrest of the disease and progression (55). Th9 and Th22, which are relatively new-subsets, have been scantily characterized in periodontal disease. Th22 cells were increased in gingival biopsies in periodontitis, associated with the increased osteoclastic activity, and triggered upon stimulation with the periodontal pathogen *Aggregatibacter actinomycetemcomitans* (56, 57).

Th1 cells produce pro-inflammatory cytokines such as IFN-γ, IL-12, IL-1β, and TNF-α, under the control of the transcription factor T-bet (22). The Th1-type of response, mediated by the production of IFN-γ, is necessary for both the control of microbial invasion and bone loss. The induction of periodontitis with *A. actinomycetemcomitans* in IFN-γ-deficient mice resulted in a less severe bone loss but impaired host defense against the microbial challenge, followed by a disseminated bacterial infection and mice death (58). *P. gingivalis* promotes the expression of type-1 interferons by disrupting innate immunological functions through degradation of Myd88, resulting in a constitutively priming of $CD4^+$ T-cells by dendritic cells and leading to elevated IFN-γ and RANKL expression associated with increased alveolar bone loss. Blocking type-I IFN signaling prevented the destructive Th1 immune response and alveolar bone loss (59).

Th17 cells are the most osteoclastogenic type of T-cells, directly expressing and inducing RANKL expression on resident cells through IL-17 production, and necessary to sustain the host defense against the dysbiotic microbial community. Th17 cells produce IL-17A, IL-17F, and IL-22, under the control of the master switch RORγ, and the critical participation of the transcription factor STAT3 (60). In healthy individuals, Th17 cells naturally accumulate in the gingival mucosa with age and promote barrier defense. This growth depends on mechanical stimulation, such as chewing, which induces the production of IL-6 in epithelial cells, and is independent of commensal bacteria (61). The expansion of the Th17 cells during periodontitis, on the other hand, is dependent on microbial dysbiosis and requires both IL-6 and IL-23 production (62). These are predominantly resident memory Th17 cells, capable of quick responses and the primary producers of IL-17. A recent study in mice confirmed that IL-17 producing Th17 cells rather than γδT cells are involved in bone damage during periodontitis. IL-17 production is necessary for host defense against the invasion of oral bacteria (9). Also, a significant proportion of the IL-17 producing Th17 cells were exFoxp3Th17, cells that expressed high amounts of membrane-bound RANKL, suggesting that at some point, these cells might have had regulatory functions (9). Accordingly, patients with autosomal-dominant STAT3 deficiency (AD-HIES), are less susceptible to periodontitis (62).

The Th2 and Treg type of responses are implicated in the resolution of periodontitis (63). Th2 cells produce IL-4, IL-5, and IL-13, and mediate humoral immunity and mast cell activation in allergic reactions (22). Treg cells produce IL-10 and TGF-β and are crucial for the maintenance of immune homeostasis and tissue repair under the control of the master switch Foxp3 (64). Tregs inhibit osteoclast differentiation and their bone resorptive activity through the interaction of CTLA-4 with CD80/86 on osteoclasts and their precursors (29). Both Th2 and Treg cells express the chemokine receptor CCR4. The induction of periodontitis in $CCR4^{-/-}$ mice presented a significant deficiency of Treg migration, associated with increased inflammatory alveolar bone loss (63).

B cells are practically not present in normal gingival mucosa (43), but they dramatically increase as the disease progresses, making it a distinct feature of the established periodontal lesion (22). During periodontitis, stromal cells and immune cells express different cytokines and chemokines such as IL-4, IL6, IL-5, CXCL13, and APRIL that induce B cell migration and support their survival in the periodontium (65, 66). Patients with periodontitis have a significantly higher percentage of $CD19^+CD27^+CD382^-$ memory B cells and $CD138^+HLA\text{-}DR^{low}$ plasma cells while B1 cells, which have been previously described as a regulatory type of B cell ($CD20^+CD69^-CD43^+CD27^+CD11b^+$) are decreased (67, 68). B cells/plasma cells are well-known for their humoral immunity. However, periodontitis progresses despite the presence of B cells and the induction of humoral responses against periodontal bacteria. The B cell-mediated IgG-dominant immune response might contribute to the pathogenesis of periodontitis (65, 68). Most infiltrating B cells present during periodontitis produce RANKL, suggesting that they can directly induce osteoclastogenesis (8). Indeed, the induction of experimental periodontitis in B cell-deficient mice showed significantly less bone loss (65). Latest data demonstrated the existence of a regulatory B cell subtype (Bregs) that can inhibit inflammation and support Treg differentiation through their production of IL-10. Bregs cells in humans have been identified as both $CD19^+CD24^{hi}CD38^{hi}CD1d^{hi}$ and $CD19^+CD24^{hi}CD27^+$ cells (69). In mice, the functional IL-10-producing subset of Bregs, B10, have bone protective roles during periodontitis (70).

Osteoimmunological Processes in the Periodontal Disease

The periodontium offers a unique environment to understand the interactions between the immune system and bone since it combines mucosal and skeletal tissues and the interaction between the host and the oral microbiota (21). The alveolar bone is susceptible to different types of mechanical stress and is continuously remodeled by the coupled action of osteoclasts and osteoblasts within the bone surface (3, 71). As reviewed above, the immune response caused by the dysbiotic microbiota during periodontitis dramatically enhances the production of local RANKL by different immune cell types such as Th17 and B cells. However, recent studies with specific cell type-depleted animals have highlighted the impact of RANKL production by osteocytes, osteoblasts, and periodontal ligament cells on osteoclast differentiation and alveolar bone loss (72). Osteocytes respond to inflammation, specifically to IL-6 and IL-17, by producing RANKL and increasing their osteoclastogenesis (73, 74). In a *P. gingivalis* and *Fusobacterium nucleatum*-induced periodontitis model, the genetic depletion of RANKL in osteocytes decreased the alveolar bone destruction and osteoclast differentiation (75). Osteocytes react to *P. gingivalis* LPS by producing sclerostin, which reduces osteoblastic bone formation by inhibiting the Wnt/β catenin signaling pathway (76).

Osteoblasts and periodontal ligament cells also respond to IL-17, producing RANKL, and decreasing OPG production (77). The osteoblastic inflammatory-mediated RANKL production depends on the activation of the classical NF-κB pathway. The inhibition of NF-κB activation in osteoblastic lineage cells in mice reduces osteoclast numbers and RANKL expression induced by periodontal infection (72). Specific genetic depletion of RANKL production in osteoblasts and periodontal ligament cells during ligature-induced periodontitis reduces the alveolar bone resorption in an even greater extent that the RANKL depletion on CD4$^+$ cells (9). Osteocytes, osteoblasts, and periodontal ligament cells significantly contribute to osteoclastogenesis during periodontitis by translating inflammatory signals into RANKL overexpression, often paired with OPG downregulation. This process results in the disruption of the coupling of bone resorption and apposition (**Figure 1**) (77). A recent study further demonstrated that bone matrix-derived products activate the NLRP3 inflammasome and stimulate osteoclast differentiation (78). The intracellular multi-protein complex known as the inflammasome functions as a molecular platform that triggers the activation of caspase-1, necessary to proteolytically process the biologically inactive form of IL-1β and IL-18 into mature cytokines. This conversion is key since RANKL acts in concert with TNF-α or IL-1β to regulate osteoclastogenesis (79).

Translational Applications

Systematic approaches to control inflammation through immune modulation have been applied in different animal models of periodontal disease with the potential for translational applications. For instance, the blockade of the complement cascade at an earlier level, by the inhibition of C3 with AMY-101 (Cp40), is effective in a non-human primate model of periodontitis (80). This model is significantly more predictive of drug efficacy in a clinical setting since complement blockage inhibits inflammation in naturally occurring periodontitis (81). In murine models, the local delivery of CCL2 by control-delivered microparticles promoted the recruitment and differentiation of M2 macrophages, which in turn prevented alveolar bone loss (82). Similarly, the administration of CCL22-releasing microparticles prevented inflammatory bone loss by inducing the selective chemo-attraction of Treg in both murine and canine models of periodontitis (63). Rosiglitazone, a peroxisome proliferator-activated receptor (PPAR)-γ agonist, induced resolving macrophages with an M2-like phenotype that reduce bone resorption and enhance bone formation (51). The treatment with all-trans-retinoic acid or the synthetic retinoic acid receptor (RAR) agonist tamibarotene (Am80) improved the Th17/Treg balance and decreased the alveolar bone loss during periodontitis (83, 84). The treatment with RvD2 (a resolution agonist) prevented alveolar bone loss by inhibiting the systemic and gingival Th1-type of response in *P. gingivalis*-induced periodontitis (85). *In vivo* inhibition of Th17 differentiation by knocking *Stat3* or pharmaceutically inhibiting *Rorc* in CD4$^+$ T cells led to significantly reduced alveolar-bone loss (up to 70%), reflecting their critical role in the induction of bone resorption by producing IL-17 and expressing RANKL (9). The antibody-mediated neutralization of APRIL or BLyS substantially diminished the number of infiltrating B-cells and reduced bone loss during the experimental periodontitis (65). The adoptive transfer of B10 cells, previously cultured with *P. gingivalis* LPS and cytosine-phospho-guanine (CpG) oligodeoxynucleotides, into mice with *P. gingivalis* and ligature-induced periodontitis, showed a significant reduction of bone loss and gingival inflammation, associated with increased local IL-10 production (70). Also, the gingival application of an optimized combination of CD40L, IL-21, anti-Tim1, which *in vitro* induces IL-10 production on B10 cells, inhibited bone loss in ligature-induced experimental periodontitis (86). Thus, the development of immune-based therapies has been proven effective in the prevention of bone destruction during experimental periodontitis *in vivo*. Current approaches to drug delivery and local applications of these therapeutic strategies in humans are being tested.

APICAL PERIODONTITIS

Definition and Pathogenesis of the Periapical Periodontitis

The infection of periodontal tissues in the periapical area following the bacterial invasion of pulp in the root canal system leads to the inflammatory destruction of the periodontal ligament, radicular cement and alveolar bone, which are the clinical hallmarks of apical periodontitis. Interestingly, the pathogenesis underlying the clinical presentation of apical periodontitis possesses outstanding parallels with that of periodontitis (87–89). Both conditions are initiated by an infectious stimulus and share pathological mechanisms of tissue destruction (chronic and exacerbated immune response that uncouples tissue balance) as well as the susceptibility traits and the treatment approach (eradication of the infecting microorganisms) (87, 90). Indeed, epidemiological data suggest that there is a correlation between the occurrence of apical periodontitis and marginal bone loss characteristic of periodontitis (91), reinforcing the existence of a common susceptibility profile.

Cellular and Molecular Basis of the Periapical Periodontitis

Although microorganisms are essential for disease initiation, their presence is not sufficient to explain the pathologic

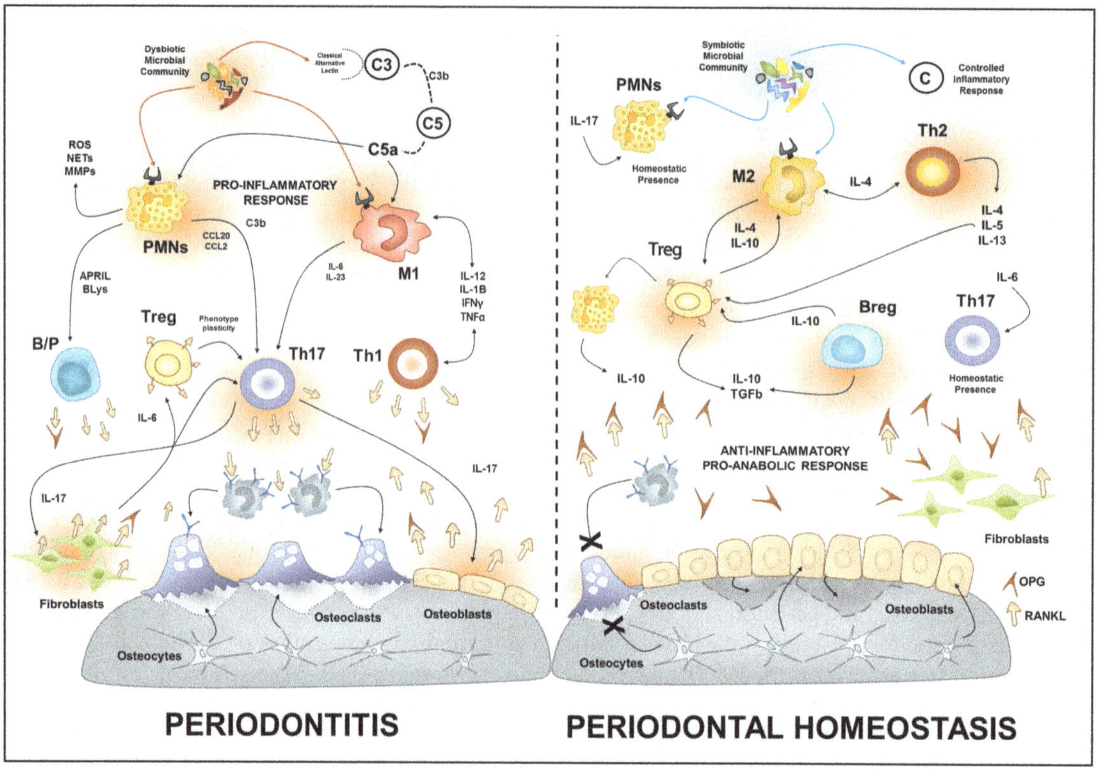

FIGURE 1 | Osteoimmunology of periodontal disease. During periodontitis, the immune response induced by the dysbiotic microbiota enhances the production of local RANKL by different immune cells types such as Th1, Th17, B cells. Additionally, the increased gingival levels of IL-17 stimulate the membrane-bound expression of RANKL in osteoblasts and periodontal ligament fibroblasts; this provokes the activation of osteoclast and bone-loss. On the contrary, in health, different immune cells such as Tregs, Bregs, M2, and Th2 cells promote an anti-inflammatory and pro-anabolic state that sustain the alveolar-bone homeostasis. PMNs, polymorph nuclear neutrophil; B/P, B and plasma cell.

phenomena that generate inflammatory destruction of the apical periodontium (92). The presence of a protected reservoir of microorganisms inside the root canal system precludes their eradication by immune defense mechanisms, generating a loop of constant activation and amplification of the immune response. Without active regulatory or suppressive signals, this amplification loop of the immune response results in a constant and exacerbated response, which causes the progressive destruction of periodontal support (87). This exacerbated immune response tampers with the normal turnover mechanisms of periodontal tissue, particularly bone, uncoupling bone formation from bone resorption leading to a net bone loss. Conversely, immunoregulatory mechanisms can provide a fine tune to immune effector mechanisms, resulting in a response that can control the spread of the infection outside the root canal system, while limiting the pathological tissue destruction. The balance shift toward deficient or excessive response can allow for infection spreading or uncontrolled periapical tissue resorption (93).

The treatment of apical periodontitis requires the disinfection of the root canal system and its obliteration with a biomaterial capable of maintaining a sterile environment and, in some refractory cases, the surgical elimination of periapical tissues (94, 95). The absence of reliable means to know in advance if the endodontic treatment will be successful or not is a critical weakness in endodontic therapy. Once the apical lesion has developed, there are no highly sensitive clinical or radiographic tools to predict if a lesion will acquire an activated phenotype -and continue to expand to the surrounding tissues- or will attain an inactive phenotype, resulting in the arrest of its progression or even remission and healing. Since not all subjects suffering from an infection of the root canal will develop apical periodontitis, it is logical to propose that a susceptibility profile is necessary for the occurrence of the disease The identification of putative genetic and molecular markers potentially responsible for the periapical immune-balance might help to discriminate susceptible or resistant subjects to improve the treatment outcome prediction (96). Additionally, periapical lesion development does not follow a linear pattern, alternating active and inactive phases, like the "bursts" progression model, described for periodontitis (97, 98). Therefore, the understanding of host response elements responsible for the switch from activity to inactivity can also contribute to elucidate the basis of susceptibility/resistance to lesions development.

From the genetic viewpoint, the overall hypothesis is that polymorphic variations in critical genes could contribute to increased risk to suffer from apical periodontitis. That possibility is investigated using a case-control approach, based on the comparison of a group of diseased subjects (i.e., cases) to an unaffected group of individuals (i.e., controls). However, in the context of periapical lesions, the use of a healthy population as control group disregards the classic case-control study definition, which states that a case-control study is designed to determine if exposure is associated with an outcome (99). The absence of the exposure (bacterial invasion of the pulp in the root canal system) disqualifies the healthy controls to be compared with susceptible individuals that develop periapical lesions upon the "exposure." The study design, therefore, should comprise groups exposed to the same causal agent required for periapical lesions development, but with distinct clinical outcomes. The inclusion of theoretically resistant individuals (i.e., presenting deep caries without periapical lesions) have been found to improve the odds of identifying genetic factors that potentially contribute to increasing the risk to periapical lesions development (100, 101). A similar approach has been used in chronic periodontitis, with the use of chronic gingivitis subjects as a theoretically resistant population (99, 102).

Despite the inherent complexity to genetic association case-control studies, another useful approach to unravel the potential influence of genetic variants in apical periodontitis pathogenesis is to perform correlation analysis between the different genotypes/alleles and host response markers. For instance, MMP1-1607 polymorphism (rs1799750) is associated with increased expression of MMP-1 mRNA. MMPs are a family of collagenolytic enzymes responsible for the degradation and remodeling of the extracellular matrix. An increase in the expression or activation of MMPs without a parallel increase in their tissue inhibitors mediate numerous pathological processes, including apical periodontitis (103). In a sample of 326 subjects, the alternative variant of MMP-1 rs1799750 was associated with increased risk to suffer from apical periodontitis. Additionally, the cytokines TNFα, IL-21, IL-17A, and IFN-γ were associated with augmented transcriptional activity of MMP-1 in apical periodontitis, favoring its development (104).

Wnt/β-catenin signaling plays an essential role in bone biology, especially in the differentiation of osteoblasts and the suppression of bone resorption (105). The Wnt family in humans consists of 19 highly conserved genes that regulate gene expression, cell behavior, cell adhesion, and cell polarity (106). The polymorphic variations on the genes WNT3 and WNT3A were associated with increased susceptibility to apical periodontitis, specifically an intronic SNP in WNT3 (rs9890413) and a promoter SNP in WNT3A (rs1745420). The WNT3 (rs9890413) SNP is in an intronic region and to this date has no known function, so its putative mechanism of action to regulate apical periodontitis susceptibility is indefinite. On the other hand, a functional assays showed that the alternate allele G in the associated WNT3A (rs1745420), located in the gene promoter, increased promoter activity by 1.5-fold in comparison to the ancestral allele C. These findings suggested that this SNP may have a regulatory role in WNT3A expression and function (data not published).

The comparison of the gene expression signatures of periapical lesions with periapical tissues known to experience bone resorption or bone formation (i.e., in pressure and tension sides of teeth submitted to orthodontic forces) may allow for the discrimination of osteolytic activity status. Using this approach, it was possible to categorize apical granulomas in "active" or "inactive" according to their molecular profile of RANKL/OPG mRNA expression (107). Once the activity of the lesion was defined, it was possible to discriminate host response patterns associated with each subset. In this context, the inflammatory signature of 110 apical granulomas (persisting apical lesion after a technically adequate endodontic treatment, requiring surgery) and 26 healthy periapical tissues as controls were characterized (108). The apical granulomas were categorized as "active" or "inactive" according to the molecular profile of RANKL/OPG mRNA expression (107). The inflammatory signature was investigated by the expression of Th1, Th2, Th9, Th17, Th22, Thf, Tr1, and Tregs cytokines/markers. The cluster analysis revealed that "active" apical lesions were characterized by increased expression of TNF-α, IFN-γ, IL-17A, and IL-21, whereas "inactive" lesions expressed increased levels of IL-4, IL-9, IL-10, IL-22, and Foxp3. Interestingly, distinct patterns of IFNγ and IL-17 expression were described in periapical lesions. Lesions presenting a high RANKL/OPG ratio (active) overexpress IFNγ and IL-17 compared with inactive lesions. Additionally, active lesions can be clustered in groups presenting distinct patterns of IFNγ and IL-17 expression, suggesting that Th1/Th17 cytokines can drive apical periodontitis development independently (108). Accordingly, different studies describe that Th1 and Th17 responses can be mutually inhibitory (109). However, the Th1/Th17 interplay seems to be way more complicated than the mutually inhibitory activity, suggesting that collaborative and inhibitory phases may coexist in different disease stages. Also, cells presenting features of both Th17 and Th1 subsets, including Tbet and IFNγ expression, have been described in inflammatory and osteolytic conditions (110).

Therefore, the activity status of apical periodontitis may be determined by the relative enrichment of different Th subsets. Indeed, leukocytes subsets such as Th2, Tregs, and MSCs mediate a natural immunoregulatory response that suppresses apical periodontitis development. IL-4 (the prototypical Th2 cytokine) was described to induce the expression of CCL22, a main chemoattractant of Tregs (63). It is noteworthy that Tregs hallmark products, such as IL-10 and TGF-β, are described to boost MSCs immunosuppressive properties (111). Therefore, while all the details regarding the potential Th2, Tregs and MSCs cooperation remain to be unraveled, the existence of a protective/regulatory cellular network in inflamed periapical tissues seems feasible (89, 108).

Impact of Osteoimmunology in the Periapical Disease

A recent study points to an unexpected potential trigger of a protective immunoregulatory response (112). While RANKL has a well-characterized role in the control of bone homeostasis, it can also play critical roles in the regulation of the immune system. Indeed, while anti-RANKL administration resulted in the arrest of periapical bone loss, it led to an unremitting pro-inflammatory response and impaired immunoregulation, restored by Tregs adoptive transfer (113). Therefore, RANKL seems to be responsible for trigger immunoregulatory feedback via Tregs induction, which in turn acts as suppressive elements (113). Notably, RANKL seems to play a fundamental role in linking the immune system with bone metabolism. Infiltrating immune cells are an important source of RANKL, but also resident bone osteoblast produce and secrete RANKL, most of the time under the regulatory influence of osteocytes following mechanical or endocrine stimulus (73, 75).

Despite the lymphocyte-centered paradigm of the most studies into apical periodontitis pathogenesis in the last decade, other leukocyte subsets (such as granulocytes) also can play significant roles in periapical lesion pathogenesis. For example, we determined that CXCL12 levels increase significantly in apical periodontitis. CXC ligand 12 (CXCL12 a.k.a. SDF-1) is a pleiotropic chemokine that regulates the influx of leukocytes to inflamed sites. In apical periodontitis, CXCL12 proved to be the primary molecular signal responsible for the recruitment of mast cells into the periapical inflammatory infiltrate during lesion development (114). This CXCL12/mast cell axis is significant as mast cells can secrete a variety of molecular signals and regulate many diseases (115, 116).

Another major cellular player during the first stages of the immune response in the pathogenesis of apical periodontitis is the neutrophil. These cells invade the apical periodontium in vast numbers and are in the front line of contention of bacterial infection. Despite being mainly associated with the direct killing of bacteria and tissue necrosis, neutrophils are also capable of releasing molecular mediators into the extracellular compartment and influencing the later stages of the response (117, 118). Accordingly, a significant increase in heat shock protein 27 (HSP27) and Serpin Family B member 1 (SERPINB1) protein levels were identified in apical periodontitis compared to healthy tissues (119). HSP27 belongs to the heat shock protein gene family and has an essential role in the inhibition of apoptosis in thermal and chemical stress, protecting the cells from injury in hostile environments (120). SERPINB1 is a potent inhibitor of neutrophil serine proteases and plays crucial roles in protecting PMN and other cells from apoptosis (121). The role of another Serpin family member (SERPINE1) has been demonstrated in the stabilization of apical lesions (122), thus pointing to a molecular pathway of Serpin family proteins regulating PMN functions and periodontal destruction in apical periodontitis. Importantly, this increased expression of HSP27 and SERPINB1 was compartmentalized to epithelial cells and infiltrating neutrophils in the inflammatory front (119). The expression of HSP27 and SERPINB1 was inversely correlated with markers of acute inflammation and markedly increased in apical lesion characterized as "stable/inactive." This evidence suggests that HSP27 and SERPINB1 could be putative markers of lesion regression and useful to follow the outcome of endodontic treatment

Ultimately, most osteoclastogenic signals are controlled by osteocytes, whether directly by secreting osteoclastogenic signals or indirectly by entering apoptosis (123–125). The inflammatory milieu characteristic of apical periodontitis creates the necessary environment to favor pro-osteoclastogenic signaling and net bone loss (72). The communication network established between osteocytes and osteoblast is capable of sensing delicate environmental changes and react to favoring the bone formation and resorption (126). The exacerbated and unrelenting immune response characteristic of apical periodontitis provides plenty of pro-resorptive signals that tilt the balance in favor of bone resorption (127, 128).

Taken together, recent findings point to a complex and multilevel regulatory network that underlies the clinical presentation of apical periodontitis (**Figure 2**). Infecting agents and immune defense mechanisms are in opposing trenches in an all-out war leading to apical lesion formation or regression. As in many other diseases characterized by inflammatory tissue destruction, the regulatory features of the immune system have a disproportionally important role in the progress and outcome of the disease. Despite extensive efforts, there is still much to be investigated and learned before we can develop a comprehensive molecular model capable of guiding changes in clinical conducts leading to improved clinical outcomes in the treatment and management of apical periodontitis.

BIOLOGICALLY-BASED DIAGNOSTICS AND THERAPEUTICS TO MANAGE ORAL AND SYSTEMIC HEALTH IN PERIODONTITIS PATIENTS

Marginal periodontitis and periapical periodontitis are the most common oral diseases involving alveolar bone loss (129). Substantial research supports the positive association between periodontitis and several systemic diseases such as cardiovascular diseases and diabetes, while growing evidence is unveiling an analog connection with periapical lesions. Recently, periodontitis has also been associated with the onset and development of oral and extraoral cancers, and their fatal outcome (130–132).

The result of periodontitis forms is a prolonged release of both host-derived inflammatory/collagenolytic mediators (e.g., arachidonic acid metabolites, cytokines, nitric oxide [NO], reactive oxygen species [ROS] and MMPs), and virulence factors generated by the dysbiotic perio-pathogens and/or endodontic pathogens in the etiologic microbial biofilm. Though this response is intended to restrain dissemination, this toxic "brew" impairs the host's immune response. The proposed mechanisms linking periodontitis and extraoral diseases involve the spread of bacteria from the oral cavity causing damage to other organs, the increase in inflammatory systemic burden, or an autoimmune response triggered by oral bacterial species (133–138).

Albeit clinical and radiographic examinations are the gold standard for the diagnosis of periodontal and periapical diseases, variations in the inflammatory profile might impact disease susceptibility and severity at both local and systemic levels (129, 139). Oral fluids (gingival crevicular fluid/GCF, mouth

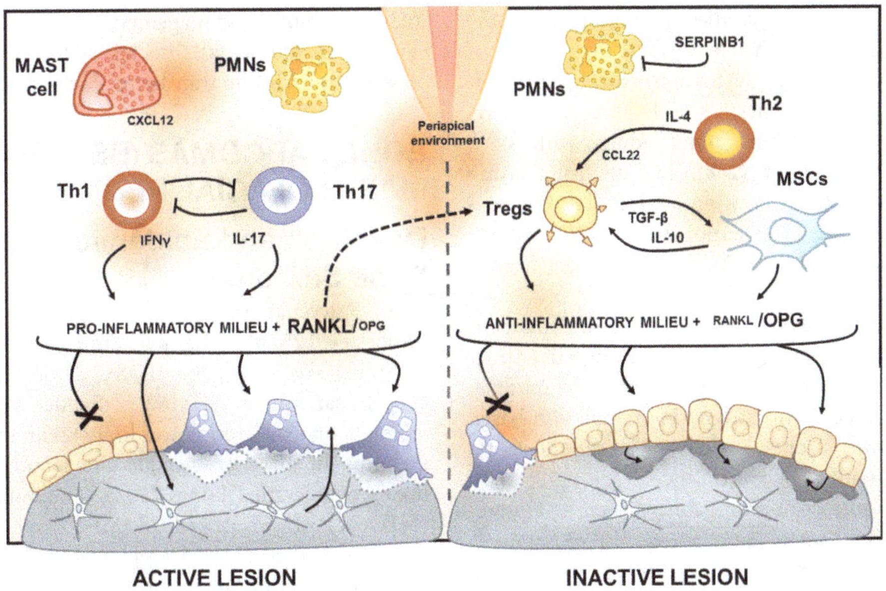

FIGURE 2 | Immunological features of active and inactive periapical lesions. In the periapical environment, the presence of endodontic pathogens and its products (such as LPS) triggers the host inflammatory immune response. The analysis of gene expression signatures of periapical lesions allows for the discrimination of osteolytic activity status in "active" or "inactive" according to RANKL/OPG expression ratio. Active periapical lesions are characterized by high RANKL/OPG ratio is an association with a pro-inflammatory milieu, which includes a high level of IFN-g and IL-17. Distinct patterns of IFNg and IL-17 expression were described in periapical lesions, suggesting that Th1 and Th17 subsets, described to be mutually inhibitory, can drive apical periodontitis development independently. The presence of PMNs and mast cells also have been associated with lesion activity. Conversely, inactive lesions are characterized by a low RANKL/OPG ratio is an association with an anti-inflammatory milieu, which is supposed to involve a cooperative immunoregulatory network composed by Th2 and Tregs subsets, as well by MSCs. The prototypical Th2 cytokine IL-4 is described to induce the expression of CCL22, a main chemoattractant of Tregs. Noteworthy, Tregs hallmark products, such as IL-10 and TGF-β, are described to boost MSCs immunosuppressive properties. Interestingly, a recent study points to RANKL as an unexpected immunoregulatory feedback trigger via Tregs induction.

rinse, and saliva samples) obtained non-invasively from the oral cavity are critical sources for factors and/or biomarkers related to the metabolic activity of periodontal tissues. Quantitative point of care (PoC)/chair-side technologies are emerging as available tools to monitor periodontal conditions, including orthodontic tooth movement, periodontitis, apical periodontitis, and peri-implantitis, whereas key inflammatory mediators can be targeted for therapeutic purposes. Complementary salivary/oral fluid MMP-8 determinations aid to identify periodontal loss and inflammation in line with clinically deepened periodontal pockets, bleeding on probing, and radiographic alveolar bone loss (140–144). MMP-8, MMP-9, TRAP-5, and MPO demonstrates very high diagnostic accuracy in GCF for discriminating periodontitis, apical periodontitis, gingivitis and/or healthy periodontium, supporting their usefulness for PoC diagnostics (129, 142). Of interest, oral fluid biomarker analysis has shown usefulness in extraoral conditions or diseases (141, 142), whereas GCF placental and inflammatory markers proved the diagnostic potential for preeclampsia (145) and gestational diabetes mellitus in pre-symptomatic women (146), revealing new emerging spectra for oral fluid applications.

Up to now, several studies have explored the associations between tooth loss, oral infections, CVD and diabetes, and it is widely accepted that low-grade systemic inflammation, as measured by CRP and other biomarkers, influences their development and progression. Currently, there is substantial evidence supporting that marginal periodontitis imparts increased risk for future atherosclerotic cardiovascular disease, in which the exacerbated inflammatory burden favors atheroma formation, maturation, and exacerbation. Periodontal treatment can reduce systemic inflammation as evidenced by a reduction in C-reactive protein (CRP), reduce the levels of oral fluid and systemic (serum) proinflammatory biomarkers of tissue destruction and improve endothelial function and subclinical atherosclerosis, but the evidence is not yet conclusive (131, 147). Periodontitis also associates with elevated risk for dysglycaemia and insulin resistance, as well as incident type 2 diabetes, whereas the latter is also an essential modifying factor for periodontitis. Evidence supports that periodontal therapy seems to improve glycemic control, although studies involving long-term follow-up are also inconclusive (133). Despite the associations between endodontic infections, CVD and diabetes have not been thoroughly explored; emerging evidence sustains an analogous link (134).

Most available mechanistic studies seeking for an association between apical periodontitis and the systemic inflammatory burden lacks adequate control for confounders. Often, a clinically heterogeneous mixture of acute and chronic forms of apical periodontitis is included, and participants are older than the main risk group, resulting in overall inconclusive evidence for hsCRP. Few recent studies accounting for these variables reported early endothelial dysfunction and up-regulation of pro-inflammatory cytokines, including IL-1, IL-2, IL-6, reactive oxygen species, as well as asymmetrical dimethylarginine in serum from young adults with CAP compared to healthy volunteers (148). Recently our group demonstrated an association between apical lesions and cardiovascular risk based on CRP serum levels concentrations (135), but the systemic effects of endodontic treatment are yet unknown (134).

Recently periodontitis was proposed as an independent risk factor for cancer development, such as digestive tract cancer, pancreatic, lung, prostate, breast, uteri, lymphoma, and hematological cancer. Moreover, in population-based studies, periodontitis was strongly linked to cancer mortality, especially in patients with pancreatic cancer (130, 149, 150). Studies demonstrate a role of microorganisms such as Human Papillomavirus (HPV), Epstein-Barr virus (EBV) and *P. gingivalis* that could be detected in inflamed periodontal tissues and might favor cancer initiation at the oral cavity or distant tissues (151–153). Recently, *Treponema denticola*, a virulent proteolytic periodontopathogen, was found to promote the onset of oro-digestive cancers (154, 155). Besides oral pathogens, the local and systemic inflammatory responses associated with periodontitis can represent an indirect mechanism that could promote cancer development (130).

Periodontitis derived-systemic low-grade inflammation can also be readily monitored in serum samples, by measuring acute-phase proteins such as C-reactive protein, to further diagnostically assess the risk. hsCRP measurement is especially recommended in subjects at intermediate cardiovascular risk to determine the need for treatment (156); hsCRP levels are also used to evaluate the success of an intervention such as the metalloproteinase inhibition with sub-antimicrobial doses of doxycycline to prevent acute coronary syndromes (MIDAS) (157, 158). In this way, biomarker's utility becomes clinically practical with the current availability of PoC chair-side biomarker analysis of oral fluids & serum, and host-modulation therapies such as non-antimicrobial doxycycline medications (Periostat®, now generic; and Oracea®) as pleiotropic MMP-inhibitors, and others such as omega-3 fatty acid derivatives (e.g., docosahexaenoic acid), i.e., the resolvins (**Figure 3**) (159–161). Thus, recently-developed strategies of personalizing the use of "host-modulation therapy," when indicated by modern PoC chair-side diagnostic tests (140, 144), may significantly enhance the beneficial outcome of both the commonly-used oral therapy (scaling & root planing, and oral hygiene instruction) and its impact on the overall medical health of the patient. Further evidence of the need for modern, biologically-based diagnostics and therapeutics to manage the oral/systemic health of the patient is continuously emerging. These findings reinforce the view that modern, biologically-based oral-systemic health management requires a "two-pronged strategy" including diagnostic monitoring in oral fluids biomarkers, and optimally therapeutic suppressing these mediators with "host-modulation therapy" combined with microbial biofilm management. Both strategies are currently available to the dental clinician as the result of long-term and substantial basic and translational research.

BONE SARCOMAS (BS) AFFECTING THE MAXILLOFACIAL REGION

Definition and Epidemiological Impact of Bone Sarcomas

Bone Sarcomas (BS) are rare primary mesenchymal bone tumors (<0.2% of malignant tumors of EUROCARE database), including osteosarcoma (OS), Ewing sarcoma (ES) and chondrosarcoma (CS) (162). BS affects more frequently the appendicular skeleton (lower limbs) than the craniomaxillofacial skeleton. In this area, maxilla and mandible are more affected bones over cranial bones (163). Thus, maxillofacial (MF) OS (MFOS), ES (MFES), and CS (MFCS) are considered malignant tumors of the maxillofacial region according to the 4th edition of the World Health Organization Classification of head and neck tumors (164). Here, we will focus specifically on MFOS, MFES, and MFCS, highlighting the role of immune response on their pathophysiology and, also, revising experimental approaches for therapy.

Maxillofacial Osteosarcoma (MFOS)

MFOS represent <10% of the total OS (165). Compared with the appendicular OS, which peaks in the 2nd and sixth decade, MFOS peaks in the 3rd decade (162, 163, 165). Typically, MFOS arise from the cancellous compartment rather than bony surfaces. MFOS affects the alveolar ridge of the mandible and posterior area of the maxilla (163, 166). MFOS can be categorized according to the predominant matrix as an osteoblastic, fibroblastic, chondroblastic, telangiectatic, or osteoclastic type (163, 165). At the X-ray imaging, MFOS appear as either as the osteolytic form with undefined margins or, the osteoblastic form, showing a sclerotic and sunburst structure caused by radiated bone spiculae (163).

Maxillofacial Ewing Sarcoma (MFES)

MFES is 1–4% of all ES which peak in both the first and second decades mainly in white Caucasian people, affecting equally both sexes (163). MFES is an aggressive, hemorrhagic, and rapidly metastatic malignant tumor affecting naso-orbital bones. MFES are characterized by an irregular lesion combining sclerosis and lucent zones compromising cortical bone. MFES also show the characteristic onion peel appearance and sunburst new bone formation, which correspond to periosteal osteogenic reaction (163).

Maxillofacial Chondrosarcoma (MFCS)

It accounts for 2% of all CS with a peak incidence during the 4th to fifth decades with a male predilection (ratio 2.4:1). It affects mostly the skull base, maxilla, and less frequent the orbit and, cartilage of the nasal septum. MFCS can be observed after malignant and benign diseases such as OS, fibrosarcoma, Paget disease, and fibrous dysplasia (163, 167).

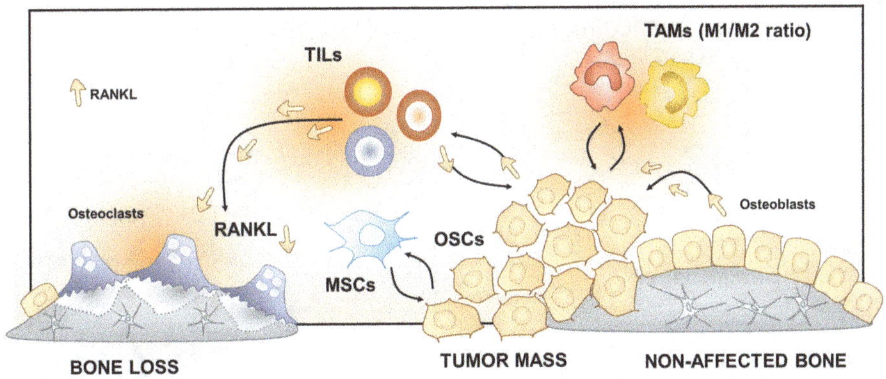

FIGURE 3 | Osteoimmunology at the osteosarcoma (OS) niche. Tumor-Associated Macrophages (TAMs), Tumor-Infiltrating Lymphocytes (TILs) and Mesenchymal Stem cells (MSCs) regulate osteosarcoma cells (OSCs) proliferation, tumor mass progression, and metastasis. The RANK/RANKL signaling leads to both OSCs progression and increased osteoclast activation and bone loss in the OS niche.

Histologically, chondrosarcoma of the craniofacial region can be divided into (a) the conventional subtype with myxoid and/or hyaline components, the most common form, is slow growing, and rarely metastatic; (b) the aggressive mesenchymal and dedifferentiated subtype, more aggressive and tends to metastasize and; the clear cell subtype, extremely rare (163). High-grade CS can induce metastasis, but local recurrence of curettage is a common feature of such tumors. Since the vast majority of literature describing the pathophysiology of BS focus on the non-maxillofacial OS, we will base our work upon these recent findings.

These three entities result from the disruption of differentiation of Mesenchymal Stem Cells (MSCs) into bone and cartilage cell lineages (168). In bone homeostasis, MSCs differentiate into stromal cells, which will contribute to both the hematopoietic and the skeletal niches (168, 169). At the skeletal niche level, stromal cells will activate transcription factors such as Runx2 to follow the osteogenic path to become functional osteoblasts or, Sox9 to follow the chondrogenic pathway to become cartilage cells (168) (**Figure 3**).

BS results from the interaction of both OS cells (OSCs), cancer stem cells, and their niche. OSCs are the malignant counterpart of osteoblasts. OSCs are mesenchymal-derived cells subjected to an initial oncogenic event altering the commitment from a mesenchymal cell toward an osteoblast by a mutation (e.g., *p53* and *Rb*) and/or aberrant Hedgehog and Notch signaling (168, 170). Within the tumor mass, cells exhibit high heterogeneous profiling that can be partly explained by the presence of cancer stem-like cells (CSCs), the clonal evolution of OSCs and the high heterogeneity of the local tumor microenvironment (168, 170). These cells are characterized by its self-renewing property, and they are proposed as responsible for tumor progression, resistance to chemotherapy, and initiate metastasis (168, 171). Based on the "seed and soil' theory of Paget, it is now well-recognized that OS, like other cancers, requires an adequate local microenvironment for its development (168, 171). This specialized microenvironment provides all metabolites and regulates the self-renewal process of CSCs (171). Interactions between OSCs, CSCs, and its niche may determine OS progression or dormancy and, potential drug resistance (171, 172).

Cellular and the Molecular Immune Basis of Bone Sarcomas

Some clinical studies correlate survival rates of OS patients with both immune markers and the immune cell (lymphocyte/macrophage) ratio (173, 174). However, the role of the immune system in OS development remains still misunderstood. The relationship among OS niche and immune response may be explained by the fact that OSCs (and also, bone cells) are surrounded by bone marrow cells occupying the same bone marrow space. Within this space, hematopoietic precursors give rise to the immune cell population, lymphoid, myeloid cells, and mast cells. These cells will regulate both innate and acquired immune responses (173). Consistently; an immune infiltrates composed by monocyte/macrophages/dendritic cells and T-lymphocytes have been identified in OS tissues (173, 174). Although B-lymphocyte and mast cells are less represented in the OS tumor mass, they are far more distributed in the interface bone-tumor. Both lymphocytes and mast cells are essential sources of RANKL, becoming key players in the activation of osteoclasts, and then contributing to the osteolytic feature of OS (173, 174).

Macrophages are essential cells participating in bone homeostasis (173, 174). Macrophages, located in the vicinity of the tumor, are known as Tumor-Associated Macrophages (TAMs) (168). TAMs control local immunity, angiogenesis, and regulate tumor cell migration and invasion (168). Also, TAMs participate in the seating of cancer cells at the metastatic site by modeling the permissiveness of the host-tissues (168). TAMs are composed by a large variety of subpopulations which have been classified initially in M1 and M2 subtypes according to their differentiation and activities. M1, the pro-inflammatory macrophage subset, are classified as anti-tumor cells and associated with excellent survival rates, and M2, the

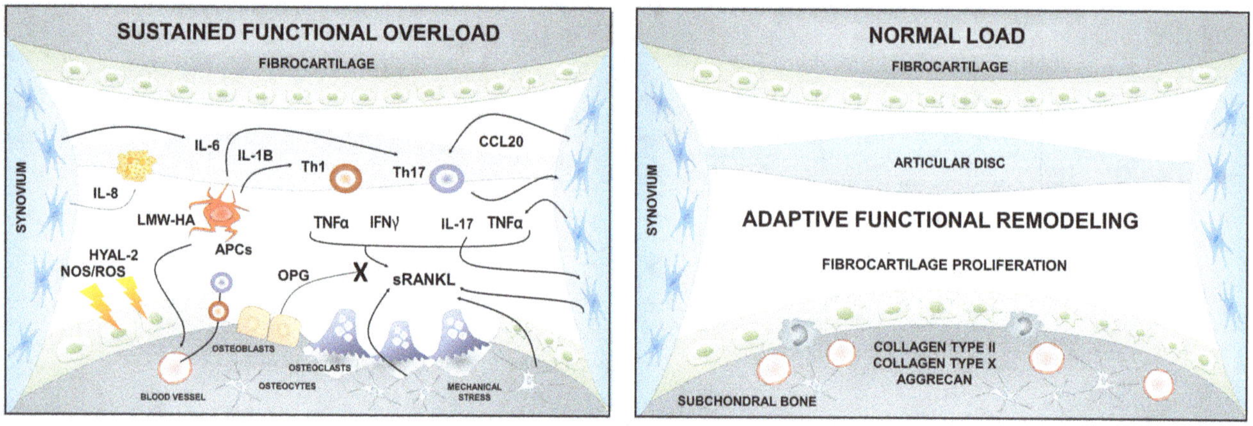

FIGURE 4 | Immune response and bone crosstalk during temporomandibular joint osteoarthritis. The sustained functional overload that exceeds the joint adaptive capacity can induce dysfunctional remodeling. This dysfunctional remodeling is characterized by increased oxidative stress, due to hypoxia/reperfusion effect, and higher levels of catabolic enzymes that degrade the fibrocartilage extracellular matrix and induce chondrocyte apoptosis. The molecular products derived from cartilage breakdown (e.g., LMW-HA or PG) can trigger the immuno-inflammatory response by interacting with APCs and finally resulting in the activation of Th17 lymphocytes and the RANK/RANKL/OPG axis, leading to subchondral bone resorption. The normal joint load of the TMJ, such as static loading during swallowing or teeth clenching, induces an adaptive functional remodeling of joint tissues and promotes fibrocartilage healing. HYAL, hyaluronidase; LMW-HA, low molecular weight hyaluronan; NOS, nitric oxide; OPG, osteoprotegerin; ROS, reactive oxygen species; sRANKL; soluble receptor activator of nuclear factor-kappa B ligand; APCs, Antigen presenting cells.

anti-inflammatory macrophage subset, as pro-tumor regulators (168, 173, 174). Thus, in OS patients, a TAM-M1 predominant ratio over TAM-M2 was associated with better survival rates and the opposite, with poor prognosis (168, 173, 174). These associations may be explained by an immunosuppressive effect on intra-tumor T-lymphocytes, and pro-angiogenic effect exerted by TAM-M2 observed both preclinical models of OS and metastatic patients (168, 173, 174).

T-infiltrating Lymphocytes (TILs) are the second more prevalent infiltrated cell type in OS tissues and OS metastasis (174). Studies showed that selected subpopulations of T-cells ($CD8^+/FOXP3^+$) exhibit high reactivity again tumor cells compared with non-infiltrating lymphocytes (175). Thus, OS patients with elevated $CD8^+/FOXP3^+$ -ratio had better survival rates confirming the immunosuppressive role of TIL in OS pathogenesis (175, 176). TILs have higher cytotoxic properties again OS cells compared with circulating T-cells; however, OSCs secrete immunosuppressive molecules preventing the activation of TILs on the tumor site (175).

Beside immune cells, Mesenchymal Stem Cells (MSCs) have been reported as an essential regulator of OS behavior (177). Indeed, both bone and the bone marrow niche are rich in MSCs that are closely located to OS cells (178). Several studies demonstrated that MSCs establish active crosstalk with OSCs controlling OS progression and/metastasis (178). MSCs and early developed pre-osteoblasts communicate with OSCs by secreted vesicles containing mRNA, proteins, and miRNA modulating OSCs proliferation and stemness (e.g., ability to form sarcospheres, expression of stem-associated genes) (179). Reciprocally, OSCs are able to educate MSCs by tumor-secreted extracellular vesicles turning MSCs into OS extracellular vesicle-educated MSCs. These cells promote tumor progression and/or metastasis via secretion of IL-6, TGF-β and IFN-γ and by inhibiting T, B and NK cell proliferation (173, 174).

Impact of Osteoimmunology in Bone Sarcomas

Bone remodeling is controlled by osteoblasts and osteoclasts, which are responsible for bone formation and resorption, respectively. Bone remodeling is regulated by the RANKL/RANK/OPG triad (180). RANKL expressed as a membranous or secreted form by stromal and osteoblastic cells which binds to RANK, a transmembranous receptor expressed by pre-osteoclast. Their interaction leads to the activation of pro-osteoclastic genes (e.g., *NFATc1*, *cathepsin K*, *TRAP*), osteoclast differentiation (osteoclastogenesis) and then, bone resorption (180, 181). OPG is secreted by stromal and osteoblastic cells acting as a soluble decoy receptor for RANKL, leading to the inhibition of osteoclastogenesis and bone loss (180, 181).

In the OS context, the fact that RANK usually is not expressed by osteoblastic cells and the recognition of $RANK^+$ OSCs have been long debated. However, human data and most of established OSC lines confirm the expression of RANK by OSC, proposing the interaction of RANK with its ligand (RANKL) as a critical contributor in OS pathogenesis (181). In this line, a preclinical genetic model of aggressive OS in a RANKL invalidated mice showed the complete blocking of OS development, confirming the critical role of RANK/RANKL signaling into OS progression (182). Moreover, human data analyzing OS tissues from patients with or without metastatic status showed that RANK is expressed in both groups, meaning that RANK expression is not related with the metastatic status, becoming a potential predisposing factor. However, the overexpression of RANKL and the lower

OPG/RANK ratio in tumors from metastatic patients lead to hypothesize that the RANKL available in the OS niche is a significant driver to tumor progression and metastasis in OS patients (181). Taken these findings together, strongly support the use of RANKL blockers as a therapeutic approach for OS progression to a metastatic status (181).

On the other hand, the RANKL/RANK/OPG triad has been associated with the pathogenesis of OS by regulating both the osteoclastic activity and, immunoregulatory effects (180, 181). However, the real contribution of osteoclasts to the pathogenesis of OS remains still controversial. Some authors propose that the RANKL-activated osteoclasts might exert a pro-tumoral function in the early stage and on the contrary, a pro-bone remodeling/anti-tumoral effect in the later stage of OS (180, 181). Moreover, osteoclasts may modulate immune response promoting an immunogenic $CD4^{+}$ T cell response upon inflammation. Taken together, osteoclasts can be considered as essential regulators of OS growth and progression through either their resorptive or their immune functions (180, 181).

Bone Sarcomas and Immune-Based Therapeutic Approaches

In contrast to CS for which the conventional therapy is based on surgery with adequate margins, current treatments of ES and OS associate chemotherapy and surgery. Chemotherapy lines combined a minimum of three cytotoxic agents among doxorubicin, cisplatin, methotrexate, and ifosfamide (168). Unfortunately, most conventional therapies used results in limited therapeutic responses, and new approaches are urgently needed explaining the high number of clinical trials with new drugs for rare cancers including immune modulators, checkpoint inhibitors and tyrosine-kinase inhibitors (168, 174, 183, 184). Among immune regulators, an activator of macrophages such as muramyl tripeptide phosphatidylethanolamine (MTPPE) showed therapeutic efficacy in the metastatic OS. Trabectedin, a cytotoxic agent, could be attractive to treat sarcomas thanks its effect on macrophage differentiation toward M1 subtypes and targeting of PD1/PDL1 may be promising therapy by disrupting the communications between cancer cells and immune protagonists (183, 184). However, future therapeutic development will require a better characterization of the critical molecular network involved in the differentiation of BS cells and their microenvironment that should lead to the identification of new therapeutic targets and will allow better stratification of the patients enrolled in clinical trials (183, 184).

OSTEOARTHRITIS OF THE TEMPOROMANDIBULAR JOINT

Definition and Pathogenesis of the Osteoarthritis of the Temporomandibular Joint

Degenerative joint disease (DJD) is characterized by the progressive breakdown of articular cartilage, variable degrees of synovial inflammation, and pathological remodeling of subchondral bone (185, 186). Osteoarthritis (OA) is considered the most common form of DJD, affecting approximately 15% of the world population, and a leading cause of pain and disability (187, 188). Although, it mainly affects load-bearing synovial joints, such as the knee, hip, spine, and finger, other joints such as the shoulder or temporomandibular joint (TMJ) could also be affected (189). The TMJ is an exceptional synovial joint that connects the jawbone to the skull and, compared to the knee joint, it is exposed only to limited load-bearing forces (189). It has different morphological, functional, biomechanical, and biological features in comparison to other synovial joints (190). In the knee joint, hyaline cartilage covers articular surfaces, while in the TMJ, the articular lining is covered by fibrocartilage, which is surrounded by an angiogenic microenvironment and is softer than hyaline cartilage (186, 191). Thus, TMJ osteoarthritis (TMJ-OA) should not be considered as a common joint disease, but rather a unique one.

Although different factors such as systemic illnesses, developmental abnormalities, disc displacement, micro-trauma, and parafunction have been associated with the etiology of TMJ-OA, functional overload has been described as its main etiologic factor (28, 189, 192, 193). Articular remodeling is an essential biological process that responds to normal functional loading and ensures the joint's homeostasis (189). However, excessive or unbalanced mechanical loading in the TMJ can induce dysfunctional articular remodeling, leading to degenerative changes (189). Two kinds of mechanical loading occur in the TMJ: Static loading, which occurs during teeth clenching, jaw bracing, and swallowing; and dynamic loading, which occurs during tooth grinding, jaw thrusting, talking, and chewing (194). For instance, the static loading applied during forced mouth opening for 1 day increases the expression of Dickkopf factor-3 (Dkkf-3), an antagonistic non-canonical member of the Wnt family, in the cartilage surface and induces the synthesis of type II and type X collagen in the inner fibrocartilage layers; thus, promoting anabolic effects over the mineralized and unmineralized condylar cartilage (195). Nevertheless, when the same force was applied for 1 week, catabolic effects and several degenerative lesions were observed in the TMJs (196, 197).

Similarly, *in vitro* experiments demonstrated that the effects of loading forces are time-dependent. After 24 h of dynamic compressive loading over condylar chondrocytes, the expression levels of aggrecan, type I and type II collagen increased, possibly as an adaptation attempt; though, after 48 h these expression levels decreased significantly, showing a catabolic effect of prolonged loading (198). Furthermore, compressive forces also promote osteoclastogenesis through the increased expression of RANKL in synovial cells (199). In brief, light forces induced with a mouth opening protocol demonstrated an anabolic effect over TMJ, while massive forces induced a catabolic effect over joint tissues (200). Dynamic overloading forces in a TMJ-OA mice model disrupted the metabolism of hyaluronan (HA), one of the central extracellular matrix (ECM) glycosaminoglycans (GAGs) of the TMJ fibrocartilage (200). In this study, the sustained loading forces significantly decreased the expression levels of hyaluronan synthase (HAS) 2 and 3 and increased the expression levels of hyaluronidase (HYAL) 2 and KIAA1199, an HA binding protein that facilitates the degradation of HA in articular cartilage (200). Interestingly, low-molecular-weight fragments of HA (LMW-HA) can act as a damage-associated molecular pattern (DAMPs), activating antigen presenting cells and initiating the immuno-inflammatory response (201, 202).

Cellular and the Molecular Immune Basis of the Osteoarthritis of the Temporomandibular Joint

Many contributing factors have been described in the progression of bone changes during TMJ-OA, including genetic factors, female hormones, catabolic enzymes, and inflammatory mediators (203). Although inflammation has considerable importance in the progression of TMJ-OA, it is classified as a "low-inflammatory arthritic condition" as opposed to rheumatoid arthritis (RA), which is considered as a "high-inflammatory condition" (204). Recent studies suggest that OA is an inflammatory disease, at least in certain patients, and that synovial inflammation is accompanied by immune cells infiltration, similarly to RA (205–207). Of these immune cells, macrophages and T lymphocytes are the most abundant cell types that infiltrate the synovia during TMJ-OA, representing approximately 65% and 22% of the total immune cells, respectively (208). Furthermore, several inflammatory cytokines and mediators are increased in the synovial fluid of TMJ-OA affected patients, such as IL-1β, IL-6, IL-17, IFN-γ, TNF-α, prostaglandin E2 (PGE2), and chemerin, suggesting a role of the immuno-inflammatory response during the pathogenesis of the TMJ-OA (209–213). In addition to metabolic or mechanical factors, chronic inflammation induces early damage of the cartilage and consequently initiates biomechanical changes in hard and soft tissues of the joint (214). Thus, the low-grade inflammation present in OA is a result of the interactions between the immune response and local factors, such as tissue breakdown and metabolic dysfunction (215).

The inflammatory response to trauma, hypoxia-reperfusion injury, or chemical-provoked wound typically occurs in the absence of microorganisms; therefore, it has been called "sterile inflammation" (216). The first step of sterile inflammation requires the presence of endogenous molecules released during tissue or cellular injury, which can act as DAMPs able to trigger the immuno-inflammatory response (216). DAMPs can be molecules derived from necrotic cell death, such as high-mobility group box 1 (HMGB1), heat shock proteins (HSPs), or purine-derived metabolites (e.g., ATP); or fragments of molecules derived from the breakdown of the ECM, such as fragments of heparan sulfate, byglican, or HA (e.g., LMW-HA) (215). At initial stages of TMJ-OA, increased local oxidative stress induces the fragmentation of HA in the synovial fluid and fibrocartilage (217–219). The oxidative stress could increase due to direct mechanical trauma, by homolytic fission, or due to hypoxia-reperfusion, and the following non-enzymatic release of reactive oxygen species (ROS) (217, 218). The molecular weight of HA decreases and LMW-HA accumulates within the joint milieu as the disease progresses leading to an increase of joint friction due to the reduction of the chondroprotective and boundary lubrication originally provided by HA (219, 220). Furthermore, LMW-HA can trigger the immune response by interacting with the toll-like receptor (TLR)-2 or TLR-4 expressed in antigen presenting cells (221). TLR activation during OA has been associated with the development of synovitis, cartilage degeneration, and disease susceptibility (222). Using an animal model of TMJ-OA, Kong et al. demonstrated that synovial inflammation changes are related to increased TLR-4 activation and enhanced IL-1β production (223). This synovial inflammatory reaction characterized by the increased levels of IL-1β induced by TLR-4 stimulation depends on the phosphorylation of p38 during the mitogen-activated protein kinase (MAPK) signaling cascade and culminates in the activation of nuclear factor-κB (NF-κB) or nuclear transcription factor activation protein-1 (AP-1) (224). Synovitis is frequently observed during the progression of TMJ-OA (225, 226). The lining layer of synovium is mainly composed of fibroblast-like cells and macrophage-like cells (227). These resident cells play a vital role in the immuno-inflammatory response and bone metabolism during OA by producing several inflammatory mediators that enhance the breakdown of joint tissues (228, 229). Synovial fibroblasts (SF) have the ability to transduce IL-17 signals by expressing different variants of the IL-17 receptor (IL-17R) (227). In response to IL-17A, SFs of the TMJ up-regulate the expression levels of the chemokines CXCL1, IL-8, and CCL20, a specific chemoattractant of Th17 lymphocytes (227). IL-17A also induces increased production of IL-6 by SFs of the TMJ (227), and IL-6 favors the Th17 cell differentiation and promotes osteoclastogenesis and bone resorption (230, 231). Thus, the increased levels of Th17-related chemokines and cytokines produced by SFs of the TMJ stimulated by IL-17A could be related to bone loss and OA progression (227).

In other synovial joints, RANKL is highly expressed on SFs (232), while in TMJ synovium, RANKL is detected in the cytoplasm of synovial lining cells, endothelial cells, and SFs (233). A recent study using Tnfsf11flox/Δ Lck-Cre mice, which lack RANKL expression in T lymphocytes, demonstrated that the absence of RANKL-producing T cells does not protect against osteoclastogenesis and bone resorption (234). On the other hand, the deletion of RANKL on SFs using Tnfsf11flox/Δ Col6a1-Cre mice was protective against osteoclastogenesis and bone loss, thus demonstrating that SFs are the primary RANKL-expressing cells, and responsible for the osteoclast formation and bone resorption during joint inflammation (234). Interestingly, TMJ chondrocytes affected by chondral degradation, may also promote osteoclastogenesis by increasing the RANKL:OPG ratio, ultimately resulting in a subchondral bone loss (235).

LMW-HA is a potent activator of APCs, in particular, dendritic cells (DCs), through the interaction with the complex TLR-4/Cluster of differentiation (CD)44/Myeloid differentiation protein (MD)-2 (236, 237). LMW-HA induces an immuno-phenotypic maturation of DCs through the up-regulation of CD44, CD83, CD80/86, intercellular adhesion molecule-1 (ICAM-1), and the major histocompatibility complex (MHC) II (238). Furthermore, DCs exposed to LMW-HA increase their capacity to stimulate alloreactive T lymphocytes to secrete IL-12, IL-1β, and TNF-α (238). Apart from that, LMW-HA could act as a co-stimulatory molecule during antigen presentation by interacting with CD44 and could also promote the activation and polarization of T lymphocytes (239). The stimulatory effects of LMW-HA over DCs are mediated by the TLR-4 complex signaling pathway, including the phosphorylation of p38 and p42/p44 MAPK and the consequent nuclear translocation of NF-κB (237). LMW-HA also increases the migratory capacity of DCs and stimulates its trafficking toward the draining lymph nodes (240). Moreover, LMW-HA can induce the polarization of DCs to conventional type 1 (cDC1) and type 2 (cDC2) subsets, by increasing the expression levels of their specific transcription factors interferon regulatory factor 4 (IRF4), neurogenic locus notch homolog protein 2 (NOTCH2), and basic leucine zipper ATF-like transcription factor 3 (BATF3) (241). Thus, cDC1 produces TNF-α and cDC2 produces IL-6 and IL-23, inducing the selective differentiation and activation of Th1 and Th17 lymphocytes (242, 243).

Peripheral Th lymphocytes are involved in the pathogenesis of OA (244). T lymphocytes from OA patients can recognize peptides presented by APCs such as the amino acid regions 16–39 and 263–282 located in the G1 domain of human cartilage proteoglycan aggrecan (PG) (245). The recognition of these PG epitopes enhances the proliferation of OA-derived T lymphocytes and increases the production of cytokines, IL-1β, IL-6, IFN-γ, and TNF-α, and CC-chemokines, CCL-2, and CCL-3 (245). Increased expression of the Th1/Th17/Th22 cytokines IL-1β, IL-17, and IL-22, chemokines CCL5, and CCL20, and chemokines receptors CCR5 and CCR7 have been detected in synovial cells of TMJ-OA affected patients (212, 246). Further, the increased levels of IL-1β, IL-17, and IL-22 significantly correlate with the enhanced RANKL expression and immunological signs of bone degeneration (246). Moreover, the synovial fluid obtained from TMJ-OA affected patients induces significantly more osteoclast maturation and activity in comparison to synovial fluid obtained from controls (246).

Although both Th1 and Th17 cells are involved in the etiology of OA, it has been reported that the IL-23/IL-17 axis is more critical than the IL-12/IFN-γ axis in the onset of the disease (247–249). Analyses of blood samples obtained from OA affected patients, and healthy donors showed a significantly higher percentage of activated CD4+ T cells and Th17 lymphocytes in the OA group, while there were no differences between the percentages of Th1 and Th2 lymphocytes among the studied groups (250). Further, increased numbers of Th17 cells have also been detected in the OA synovial membrane (251). An osteoarthritic joint milieu with low levels of TGF-β but high levels of IL-12 induces the plasticity of Th17 lymphocytes to an intermediate phenotype between Th1 and Th17 lymphocytes known as Th17/1 cells. These cells are characterized by an increased expression of the transcription factors retinoic acid-related orphan receptor C2 (RORC2), and T-box expressed in T cells (T-bet) and production of the cytokines IFN-γ and IL-17 (252). Indeed, in OA patients, both peripheral blood and synovial fluid frequencies of Th17/1 cells are significantly increased in comparison to healthy subjects or even rheumatoid arthritis patients (253). Additionally, the enrichment of Th17/1 cells in OA patients is higher in synovial fluid than serum (253). These findings suggest that Th17/1 cells could be a Th subset with a particular role during OA and; thus, need to be further evaluated in TMJ-OA.

Higher expression levels of IL-17 have been reported in either synovial membranes or synovial fluid of TMJ-OA affected patients (212, 246, 254, 255). IL-6, a key cytokine involved in Th17 polarization, is also increased in the TMJ-OA affected patients (256). *In vitro* experiments have demonstrated that IL-17A promotes synovial hyperplasia, synoviocyte invasion, cartilage breakdown, and angiogenesis (257–260). Using SFs isolated from patients with TMJ disorders, Hattori et al. determined that IL-17A upregulates the expression of IL-6, CXCL1, IL-8, and CCL20, in a dose- and time-dependent manner, promoting T lymphocyte chemoattraction toward the TMJ synovial tissues (227). However, the central role of the Th17 lymphocytes during the pathogenesis of the joint disorders is related to its RANKL-producing osteoclastogenic function (261).

Impact of Osteoimmunology in the Osteoarthritis of the Temporomandibular Joint

Different types of cells orchestrate the physiological remodeling process within the TMJ bone microenvironment. As mentioned before, osteoclasts and osteoblasts are the primary effector cells involved in the bone resorption and formation, respectively, in the articular subchondral bone. In this molecular-and-cellular-regulated process, however, the contribution of other cell types, such as osteocytes, has been considered. Osteocytes are a group of cells which differentiate from osteoblasts, that during the formation of mineralized tissues are left embedded within the bone matrix, and further contribute to the regulation of bone metabolism (262). Even though, under physiological conditions, osteoblasts are considered as the primary source of RANKL for the RANKL-induced osteoclastogenesis and consequent osteoclast-mediated subchondral bone remodeling; osteocyte-specific RANKL-deficient mice (*Tnfsf11*$^{flox/\Delta}$ *Dmp1-Cre* or *Tnfsf11*$^{flox/flox}$ *Sost-Cre* mice) present a similar osteopetrotic phenotype than RANKL-null mice; thus, demonstrating the importance of osteocytes as a primary source of RANKL (5, 263). Moreover, by using a high-purity isolation method for osteocytes and osteoblasts, Nakashima et al. evidenced that osteocytes have a stronger ability to induce and support osteoclastogenesis than osteoblasts, through higher *Tnfsf11* (encoding RANKL) mRNA expression and RANKL production (5). Apart from that, the authors demonstrated that the absence of RANKL in T cells is not critical for bone metabolism in physiological conditions (5).

Osteocytes also actively release RANKL in response to mechanical stress (5). Indeed, osteocytes contact osteoclast precursor cells and mature osteoclasts through long dendrites that reach the bone surface, which enable direct cell-cell interaction by membrane-expressed factors released in response to load forces, such as RANKL (264). A mechanical stress experiment with MLO-Y4 osteocyte-like cells revealed that *Tnfsf11* expression is remarkably induced by mechanical strength (5). In fact, during the application of orthodontic forces for bone remodeling-dependent tooth movement, osteocytes were the primary source of RANKL in response to compressive forces, thus promoting osteoclastogenesis and bone resorption (265). Conversely, increased loading forces during mastication induced by a hard diet in mice showed an increase in the osteocyte-mediated bone formation, through an increment of the levels of insulin-like growth factor (IGF)-1 and thus, promoting osteoblastogenesis (266). Therefore, the osteocyte response to mechanical load could drastically differ between the physiological context and the pathological scenario during TMJ-OA. Indeed, osteocytes adjacent to sites of bone microdamage, as occurs in subchondral bone during the advanced stage of TMJ-OA, undergo apoptosis; whereas osteocytes adjacent to this apoptotic cells upregulate the expression of osteoclastogenic and immunogenic signaling molecules, such as ATP, membrane-derived peptides, chemokines, vascular endothelial cell growth factor A (VEGFA), and RANKL (262). Besides, osteocytes exposed to extra-cellular matrix molecules derived from TMJ-OA subchondral bone osteoblasts showed decreased levels of maturation and increased levels of apoptosis due to a decrease in the integrin-β1 expression, in comparison with extra-cellular matrix molecules derived from normal subchondral bone osteoblasts (267). This suggests that the pathological behavior of osteocytes in response to the mechanical overload during the progression of TMJ-OA could be due to molecular and cellular changes occurring in the joint microenvironment.

The RANKL:OPG ratio is increased in synovial fluid obtained from TMJ-OA patients, mainly due to the increased levels of RANKL together with the decreased levels of OPG detected in the joint microenvironment (212, 268). The secretion of IL-17 by Th17 lymphocytes enhances the RANKL production by osteoblasts, osteocytes, and SFs and activates the production of other osteoclastogenic cytokines, such as TNF-α, IL-1β, and IL-6 by synovial macrophages (269). Thus, the accumulation of Th17 lymphocytes in synovial tissues may contribute to subchondral bone resorption by stimulating the RANKL-mediated osteoclast activity (270). Kikuta et al. using intravital multiphoton microscopy, have demonstrated that Th17 but not Th1 lymphocytes preferentially adhere to mature osteoclasts and that low levels of RANKL secreted by mature osteoclast-adhered Th17 lymphocytes could induce the rapid conversion from moving-non-resorptive to static-bone-resorptive osteoclast phenotype in bone (271). Besides, using a mice model of primary hyperparathyroidism, it was described that the osteocyte-mediated RANKL production induced by Th17-derived IL17A/IL17RA interaction is critical for the bone catabolic activity, revealing another potential mechanism of subchondral bone loss induction by Th17 cells during TMJ-OA (74). Altogether, these studies demonstrated a pivotal role for Th17 lymphocytes in the osteoimmunology of the TMJ-OA, through the modulation of the osteoblast/osteocyte/osteoclast activity (**Figure 4**).

Overall, the evidence presented above shows that TMJ-OA could be considered a chronic mechanically induced and immuno-inflammatory-mediated disease, mainly due to the continuous production of DAMPs during joint tissues destruction, particularly LMW-HA, the activation of a Th17-pattern of immune response and the consequent RANKL-mediated and osteoclast-induced bone resorption.

Translational Applications

For the diagnosis of the TMJ-OA, four criteria are usually used: Joint noises, chronic joint pain, joint cramping during movements of the jaw, and degenerative bone deterioration detected through imaging (111, 214, 272). However, these criteria are only observable when the disease has been established, and tissue damage has occurred; so these gold-standard criteria do not allow early symptoms detection to prevent or stop the progression of TMJ-OA. In addition, when the diagnosis has been made, the analysis of treatment success is based on exactly the same criteria and, in older adults, these criteria are unreliable, due to the subjective component of clinical symptoms and the involuntary movements that many individuals present, which diminish the sharpness of the images and in some cases making their contribution, as a complement to the diagnosis, uncertain (273).

Several research groups have proposed to incorporate competing molecular strategies that could allow the early diagnosis of TMJ-OA and the evaluation of its therapeutic success (256, 273–281). In this sense, the determination of molecular mediators associated with the inflammatory and destructive articular tissue processes characteristic of TMJ-OA is convenient; however, nowadays, there are no registered initiatives focused on the development of an alternative solution complementary to the current standards for the diagnosis of the disease.

In this sense, the validation of a diagnostic strategy based on the identification of a panel of detectable biomarkers in the synovial fluid of the TMJ and complementary to the traditional clinical-imaging methods of diagnosis of TMJ-OA is feasible. An ideal diagnostic panel should incorporate osteoimmunology markers. In this way, the identification of molecular mediators associated with the differentiation and activity of osteoblasts, osteoclasts and/or osteocytes, as well as cytokines (IL-1β, IL-6, IL-17, IL-12, and TNF-α), MMPs (MMP-8 and MMP-9), and RANKL, could be proposed as potentially sensitive and specific biomarkers to detect early degenerative changes in the TMJ.

CONCLUSIONS

The understanding of the immune-mediated bone destruction during periodontal diseases, periapical infections, maxillary bone-sarcomas, and temporomandibular joint osteoarthritis require a detailed analysis of a wide array of pathways. While each disease in the oral and maxillofacial milieu has a distinct etiological basis, recent work has demonstrated that several mechanistic aspects could share common cellular and molecular processes that are unique to the oral and maxillofacial structures. In this work, we have reviewed the cutting-edge literature in an attempt to identify the most current knowledge in the oral osteoimmunology to provide new therapeutic approaches in otherwise difficult to treat bone lesions. The characterization of the different molecules involved in immune-mediated tissue destruction has been identified to provide biomarkers that would be useful to comprehend the link between bone-destructive oral diseases, such as periodontal disease and apical periodontitis, with systemic diseases. Collectively, the work represents a unique attempt to tackle common pathways of osteoimmunology and osteoinflammation of the oral cavity, which presents a highly unique environment colonized by the highest number of bacterial species in the mammalian body and regulated by highly functional biomechanical forces created by occlusion. Thus, successful prevention and treatment of oral diseases require recognition of this complexity to design specialized therapeutic approaches and maintain the treatment outcomes.

AUTHOR CONTRIBUTIONS

CA, RV, and AK conceived the original idea and designed the manuscript. TS, PP, H-ML, LG, and MH provided the data. CA, FC, LC, GM, and MH designed the figures. GG edited the figures. All authors participated in manuscript writing and critically reviewed the manuscript. AK edited the manuscript and supervised the project.

FUNDING

This work was financially supported by grants TYH 2016251, TYH 2017251, TYH 2018229, Y1014SL017, and Y1014SL018 from the Helsinki University Hospital Research Foundation, Finland; The Finnish Dental Association Apollonia; The Karolinska Institutet, Stockholm, Sweden; NIDCR grants R01 DE012872 and R01 DE25020 NIH; and grants FONDECYT 1140904, 1160741, and 1181780 from Comisión Nacional de Investigación Científica y Tecnológica (CONICYT) from the Chilean Government. AK is supported by NIH grant AG062496.

REFERENCES

1. Furuya M, Kikuta J, Fujimori S, Seno S, Maeda H, Shirazaki M, et al. Direct cell–cell contact between mature osteoblasts and osteoclasts dynamically controls their functions *in vivo*. *Nat Commun.* (2018) 9:300. doi: 10.1038/s41467-017-02541-w
2. Sims NA, Martin TJ. Coupling the activities of bone formation and resorption: a multitude of signals within the basic multicellular unit. *BoneKEy Rep.* (2014) 3:481. doi: 10.1038/bonekey.2013.215
3. Graves DT, Li J, Cochran DL. Inflammation and uncoupling as mechanisms of periodontal bone loss. *J Dental Res.* (2011) 90:143–53. doi: 10.1177/0022034510385236
4. Takayanagi H. Inflammatory bone destruction and osteoimmunology. *J Periodontal Res.* (2005) 40:287–93. doi: 10.1111/j.1600-0765.2005.00814.x
5. Nakashima T, Hayashi M, Fukunaga T, Kurata K, Oh-Hora M, Feng JQ, et al. Evidence for osteocyte regulation of bone homeostasis through RANKL expression. *Nat Med.* (2011) 17:1231–4. doi: 10.1038/nm.2452
6. Xiong J, Onal M, Jilka RL, Weinstein RS, Manolagas SC, O'Brien CA. Matrix-embedded cells control osteoclast formation. *Nat Med.* (2011) 17:1235–41. doi: 10.1038/nm.2448
7. Ikebuchi Y, Aoki S, Honma M, Hayashi M, Sugamori Y, Khan M, et al. Coupling of bone resorption and formation by RANKL reverse signalling. *Nature.* (2018) 561:195–200. doi: 10.1038/s41586-018-0482-7
8. Kawai T, Matsuyama T, Hosokawa Y, Makihira S, Seki M, Karimbux NY, et al. B and T lymphocytes are the primary sources of RANKL in the bone resorptive lesion of periodontal disease. *Am J Pathol.* (2006) 169:987–98. doi: 10.2353/ajpath.2006.060180
9. Tsukasaki M, Komatsu N, Nagashima K, Nitta T, Pluemsakunthai W, Shukunami C, et al. Host defense against oral microbiota by bone-damaging T cells. *Nat Commun.* (2018) 9:701. doi: 10.1038/s41467-018-03147-6
10. Takei Y, Minamizaki T, Yoshiko Y. Functional diversity of fibroblast growth factors in bone formation. *Int J Endocrinol.* (2015) 2015:729352. doi: 10.1155/2015/729352
11. Davies OG, Grover LM, Lewis MP, Liu Y. PDGF is a potent initiator of bone formation in a tissue engineered model of pathological ossification. *J Tissue Eng Regenerat Med.* (2018) 12:e355-e67. doi: 10.1002/term.2320
12. Yakar S, Rosen CJ, Beamer WG, Ackert-Bicknell CL, Wu Y, Liu J-L, et al. Circulating levels of IGF-1 directly regulate bone growth and density. *J Clin Invest.* (2002) 110:771–81. doi: 10.1172/JCI0215463
13. Wu M, Chen G, Li Y-P. TGF-β and BMP signaling in osteoblast, skeletal development, and bone formation, homeostasis and disease. *Bone Res.* (2016) 4:16009. doi: 10.1038/boneres.2016.9
14. Chen Y, Alman BA. Wnt pathway, an essential role in bone regeneration. *J Cell Biochem.* (2009) 106:353–62. doi: 10.1002/jcb.22020
15. Tu X, Delgado-Calle J, Condon KW, Maycas M, Zhang H, Carlesso N, et al. Osteocytes mediate the anabolic actions of canonical Wnt/beta-catenin signaling in bone. *Proc Natl Acad Sci USA.* (2015) 112:E478-86. doi: 10.1073/pnas.1409857112
16. Phimphilai M, Zhao Z, Boules H, Roca H, Franceschi RT. BMP signaling is required for RUNX2-dependent induction of the osteoblast phenotype. *J Bone Mineral Res.* (2006) 21:637–46. doi: 10.1359/jbmr.060109
17. Ruaro B, Casabella A, Paolino S, Pizzorni C, Ghio M, Seriolo C, et al. Dickkopf-1 (Dkk-1) serum levels in systemic sclerosis and rheumatoid arthritis patients: correlation with the Trabecular Bone Score (TBS). *Clin Rheumatol.* (2018) 37:3057–62. doi: 10.1007/s10067-018-4322-9
18. Napimoga MH, Nametala C, da Silva FL, Miranda TS, Bossonaro JP, Demasi AP, et al. Involvement of the Wnt-beta-catenin signalling antagonists, sclerostin and dickkopf-related protein 1, in chronic periodontitis. *J Clin Periodontol.* (2014) 41:550–7. doi: 10.1111/jcpe.12245
19. Matzelle MM, Gallant MA, Condon KW, Walsh NC, Manning CA, Stein GS, et al. Resolution of inflammation induces osteoblast function and regulates the Wnt signaling pathway. *Arthritis Rheumat.* (2012) 64:1540–50. doi: 10.1002/art.33504
20. Glass DA II, Bialek P, Ahn JD, Starbuck M, Patel MS, Clevers H, et al. Canonical Wnt signaling in differentiated osteoblasts controls osteoclast differentiation. *Dev Cell.* (2005) 8:751-64. doi: 10.1016/j.devcel.2005.02.017
21. Hajishengallis G. Periodontitis: from microbial immune subversion to systemic inflammation. *Nat Rev Immunol.* (2015) 15:30-44. doi: 10.1038/nri3785
22. Hajishengallis G, Korostoff JM. Revisiting the Page & Schroeder model: the good, the bad and the unknowns in the periodontal host response 40 years later. *Periodontology 2000.* (2017) 75:116–51. doi: 10.1111/prd.12181
23. Papapanou PN, Sanz M, Buduneli N, Dietrich T, Feres M, Fine DH, et al. Periodontitis: Consensus report of workgroup 2 of the 2017 world workshop on the classification of periodontal and peri-implant diseases and conditions. *J Periodontol.* (2018) 45:S162–S70. doi: 10.1111/jcpe.12946
24. Kurgan S, Kantarci A. Molecular basis for immunohistochemical and inflammatory changes during progression of gingivitis to periodontitis. *Periodontology 2000.* (2018) 76:51–67. doi: 10.1111/prd.12146
25. Hajishengallis G. The inflammophilic character of the periodontitis-associated microbiota. *Mol Oral Microbiol.* (2014) 29:248-57. doi: 10.1111/omi.12065
26. Hajishengallis G. Complement and periodontitis. *Biochem Pharmacol.* (2010) 80:1992–2001. doi: 10.1016/j.bcp.2010.06.017
27. Schenkein HA, Genco RJ. Gingival fluid and serum in periodontal diseases. II. Evidence for cleavage of complement components C3, C3 proactivator

(factor B) and C4 in gingival fluid. *J Periodontol.* (1977) 48:778–84. doi: 10.1902/jop.1977.48.12.778
28. Hajishengallis G, Hajishengallis E, Kajikawa T, Wang B, Yancopoulou D, Ricklin D, et al. Complement inhibition in pre-clinical models of periodontitis and prospects for clinical application. *Semi Immunol.* (2016) 28:285–91. doi: 10.1016/j.smim.2016.03.006
29. Liang S, Krauss JL, Domon H, McIntosh ML, Hosur KB, Qu H, et al. The C5a receptor impairs IL-12-dependent clearance of Porphyromonas gingivalis and is required for induction of periodontal bone loss. *J Immunol.* (2011) 186:869–77. doi: 10.4049/jimmunol.1003252
30. Grant EP, Picarella D, Burwell T, Delaney T, Croci A, Avitahl N, et al. Essential role for the C5a receptor in regulating the effector phase of synovial infiltration and joint destruction in experimental arthritis. *J Exp Med.* (2002) 196:1461–71. doi: 10.1084/jem.20020205
31. Modinger Y, Loffler B, Huber-Lang M, Ignatius A. Complement involvement in bone homeostasis and bone disorders. *Sem Immunol.* (2018) 37:53–65. doi: 10.1016/j.smim.2018.01.001
32. Olsen I, Lambris JD, Hajishengallis G. Porphyromonas gingivalis disturbs host-commensal homeostasis by changing complement function. *J Oral Microbiol.* (2017) 9:1340085. doi: 10.1080/20002297.2017.1340085
33. Hajishengallis E, Hajishengallis G. Neutrophil homeostasis and periodontal health in children and adults. *J Dental Res.* (2014) 93:231–7. doi: 10.1177/0022034513507956
34. Hajishengallis G, Moutsopoulos NM, Hajishengallis E, Chavakis T. Immune and regulatory functions of neutrophils in inflammatory bone loss. *Semi Immunol.* (2016) 28:146–58. doi: 10.1016/j.smim.2016.02.002
35. Moutsopoulos NM, Konkel J, Sarmadi M, Eskan MA, Wild T, Dutzan N, et al. Defective neutrophil recruitment in leukocyte adhesion deficiency type I disease causes local IL-17-driven inflammatory bone loss. *Sci Transl Med.* (2014) 6:229ra40-ra40. doi: 10.1126/scitranslmed.3007696
36. Sochalska M, Potempa J. Manipulation of neutrophils by *Porphyromonas gingivalis* in the development of periodontitis. *Front Cell Infect Microbiol.* (2017) 7:197. doi: 10.3389/fcimb.2017.00197
37. Maekawa T, Krauss JL, Abe T, Jotwani R, Triantafilou M, Triantafilou K, et al. *Porphyromonas gingivalis* manipulates complement and TLR signaling to uncouple bacterial clearance from inflammation and promote dysbiosis. *Cell Host Microbe.* (2014) 15:768–78. doi: 10.1016/j.chom.2014.05.012
38. Ling MR, Chapple IL, Matthews JB. Peripheral blood neutrophil cytokine hyper-reactivity in chronic periodontitis. *Innate Immunity.* (2015) 21:714–25. doi: 10.1177/1753425915589387
39. Kantarci A, Oyaizu K, Van Dyke TE. Neutrophil-mediated tissue injury in periodontal disease pathogenesis: findings from localized aggressive periodontitis. *J Periodontol.* (2003) 74:66–75. doi: 10.1902/jop.2003.74.1.66
40. Allaeys I, Rusu D, Picard S, Pouliot M, Borgeat P, Poubelle PE. Osteoblast retraction induced by adherent neutrophils promotes osteoclast bone resorption: implication for altered bone remodeling in chronic gout. *Lab Invest.* (2011) 91:905–20. doi: 10.1038/labinvest.2011.46
41. Zhang N, Schroppel B, Lal G, Jakubzick C, Mao X, Chen D, et al. Regulatory T cells sequentially migrate from inflamed tissues to draining lymph nodes to suppress the alloimmune response. *Immunity.* (2009) 30:458–69. doi: 10.1016/j.immuni.2008.12.022
42. Lewkowicz N, Mycko MP, Przygodzka P, ćwiklińska H, Cichalewska M, Matysiak M, et al. Induction of human IL-10-producing neutrophils by LPS-stimulated Treg cells and IL-10. *Mucosal Immunol.* (2015) 9:364. doi: 10.1038/mi.2015.66
43. Dutzan N, Konkel JE, Greenwell-Wild T, Moutsopoulos NM. Characterization of the human immune cell network at the gingival barrier. *Mucosal Immunol.* (2016) 9:1163–72. doi: 10.1038/mi.2015.136
44. Hasturk H, Kantarci A, Van Dyke TE. Oral inflammatory diseases and systemic inflammation: role of the macrophage. *Front Immunol.* (2012) 3:118. doi: 10.3389/fimmu.2012.00118
45. Lavin Y, Mortha A, Rahman A, Merad M. Regulation of macrophage development and function in peripheral tissues. *Nat Rev Immunol.* (2015) 15:731–44. doi: 10.1038/nri3920
46. Murray PJ, Wynn TA. Protective and pathogenic functions of macrophage subsets. *Nat Rev Immunol.* (2011) 11:723-37. doi: 10.1038/nri3073
47. Sima C, Glogauer M. Macrophage subsets and osteoimmunology: tuning of the immunological recognition and effector systems that maintain alveolar bone. *Periodontology 2000.* (2013) 63:80–101. doi: 10.1111/prd.12032
48. Yang J, Zhu Y, Duan D, Wang P, Xin Y, Bai L, et al. Enhanced activity of macrophage M1/M2 phenotypes in periodontitis. *Arch Oral Biol.* (2018) 96:234–42. doi: 10.1016/j.archoralbio.2017.03.006
49. Yu T, Zhao L, Huang X, Ma C, Wang Y, Zhang J, et al. Enhanced activity of the macrophage M1/M2 phenotypes and phenotypic switch to M1 in periodontal infection. *J Periodontol.* (2016) 87:1092–102. doi: 10.1902/jop.2016.160081
50. Miyajima S, Naruse K, Kobayashi Y, Nakamura N, Nishikawa T, Adachi K, et al. Periodontitis-activated monocytes/macrophages cause aortic inflammation. *Sci Rep.* (2014) 4:5171. doi: 10.1038/srep05171
51. Viniegra A, Goldberg H, Cil C, Fine N, Sheikh Z, Galli M, et al. Resolving macrophages counter osteolysis by anabolic actions on bone cells. *J Dental Res.* (2018) 97:1160–9. doi: 10.1177/0022034518777973
52. Baker PJ, Dixon M, Evans RT, Dufour L, Johnson E, Roopenian DC. CD4(+) T cells and the proinflammatory cytokines gamma interferon and interleukin-6 contribute to alveolar bone loss in mice. *Infect Immunity.* (1999) 67:2804-9.
53. Cardoso EM, Arosa FA. CD8(+) T cells in chronic periodontitis: roles and rules. *Front Immunol.* (2017) 8:145. doi: 10.3389/fimmu.2017.00145
54. Bluestone JA, Mackay CR, O'Shea JJ, Stockinger B. The functional plasticity of T cell subsets. *Nat Rev Immunol.* (2009) 9:811. doi: 10.1038/nri2654
55. Garlet GP, Giannobile WV. Macrophages: the bridge between inflammation resolution and tissue repair? *J Dental Res.* (2018) 97:1079–81. doi: 10.1177/0022034518785857
56. Diaz-Zuniga J, Melgar-Rodriguez S, Rojas L, Alvarez C, Monasterio G, Carvajal P, et al. Increased levels of the T-helper 22-associated cytokine (interleukin-22) and transcription factor (aryl hydrocarbon receptor) in patients with periodontitis are associated with osteoclast resorptive activity and severity of the disease. *J Periodontal Res.* (2017) 52:893–902. doi: 10.1111/jre.12461
57. Diaz-Zuniga J, Melgar-Rodriguez S, Monasterio G, Pujol M, Rojas L, Alvarez C, et al. Differential human Th22-lymphocyte response triggered by Aggregatibacter actinomycetemcomitans serotypes. *Arch Oral Biol.* (2017) 78:26–33. doi: 10.1016/j.archoralbio.2017.02.008
58. Garlet GP, Cardoso CR, Campanelli AP, Garlet TP, Avila-Campos MJ, Cunha FQ, et al. The essential role of IFN-gamma in the control of lethal Aggregatibacter actinomycetemcomitans infection in mice. *Microb Infect.* (2008) 10:489–96. doi: 10.1016/j.micinf.2008.01.010
59. Mizraji G, Nassar M, Segev H, Sharawi H, Eli-Berchoer L, Capucha T, et al. Porphyromonas gingivalis promotes unrestrained Type I interferon production by dysregulating TAM signaling via MYD88 degradation. *Cell Rep.* (2017) 18:419–31. doi: 10.1016/j.celrep.2016.12.047
60. Yang XO, Pappu BP, Nurieva R, Akimzhanov A, Kang HS, Chung Y, et al. T helper 17 lineage differentiation is programmed by orphan nuclear receptors ROR alpha and ROR gamma. *Immunity.* (2008) 28:29–39. doi: 10.1016/j.immuni.2007.11.016
61. Dutzan N, Abusleme L, Bridgeman H, Greenwell-Wild T, Zangerle-Murray T, Fife ME, et al. On-going mechanical damage from mastication drives homeostatic Th17 cell responses at the oral barrier. *Immunity.* (2017) 46:133–47. doi: 10.1016/j.immuni.2016.12.010
62. Dutzan N, Kajikawa T, Abusleme L, Greenwell-Wild T, Zuazo CE, Ikeuchi T, et al. A dysbiotic microbiome triggers Th17 cells to mediate oral mucosal immunopathology in mice and humans. *Sci Transl Med.* (2018) 10:eaat0797. doi: 10.1126/scitranslmed.aat0797
63. Araujo-Pires AC, Vieira AE, Francisconi CF, Biguetti CC, Glowacki A, Yoshizawa S, et al. IL-4/CCL22/CCR4 axis controls regulatory T-cell migration that suppresses inflammatory bone loss in murine experimental periodontitis. *J Bone Mineral Res.* (2015) 30:412-22. doi: 10.1002/jbmr.2376
64. Alvarez C, Rojas C, Rojas L, Cafferata EA, Monasterio G, Vernal R. Regulatory T lymphocytes in periodontitis: a translational view. *Medi Inflamm.* (2018) 2018:7806912. doi: 10.1155/2018/7806912
65. Abe T, AlSarhan M, Benakanakere MR, Maekawa T, Kinane DF, Cancro MP, et al. The B cell-stimulatory cytokines BLyS and APRIL are elevated in human periodontitis and are required for B cell-dependent bone loss

in experimental murine periodontitis. *J Immunol.* (2015) 195:1427–35. doi: 10.4049/jimmunol.1500496

66. Nakajima T, Amanuma R, Ueki-Maruyama K, Oda T, Honda T, Ito H, et al. CXCL13 expression and follicular dendritic cells in relation to B-cell infiltration in periodontal disease tissues. *J Periodontal Res.* (2008) 43:635–41. doi: 10.1111/j.1600-0765.2008.01042.x
67. Demoersman J, Pochard P, Framery C, Simon Q, Boisrame S, Soueidan A, et al. B cell subset distribution is altered in patients with severe periodontitis. *PLoS ONE.* (2018) 13:e0192986. doi: 10.1371/journal.pone.0192986
68. Mahanonda R, Champaiboon C, Subbalekha K, Sa-Ard-Iam N, Rattanathammatada W, Thawanaphong S, et al. Human memory B cells in healthy gingiva, gingivitis, and periodontitis. *J Immunol.* (2016) 197:715–25. doi: 10.4049/jimmunol.1600540
69. Rosser Elizabeth C, Mauri C. Regulatory B cells: origin, phenotype, and function. *Immunity.* (2015) 42:607–12. doi: 10.1016/j.immuni.2015.04.005
70. Wang Y, Yu X, Lin J, Hu Y, Zhao Q, Kawai T, et al. B10 cells alleviate periodontal bone loss in experimental periodontitis. *Infect Immunity.* (2017) 85:e00335-17. doi: 10.1128/IAI.00335-17
71. Jonasson G, Skoglund I, Rythen M. The rise and fall of the alveolar process: dependency of teeth and metabolic aspects. *Arch Oral Biol.* (2018) 96:195–200. doi: 10.1016/j.archoralbio.2018.09.016
72. Pacios S, Xiao W, Mattos M, Lim J, Tarapore RS, Alsadun S, et al. Osteoblast lineage cells play an essential role in periodontal bone loss through activation of nuclear factor-kappa B. *Sci Rep.* (2015) 5:16694. doi: 10.1038/srep16694
73. Wu Q, Zhou X, Huang D, Ji Y, Kang F. IL-6 enhances osteocyte-mediated osteoclastogenesis by promoting JAK2 and RANKL activity *in vitro. Cell Physiol Biochem.* (2017) 41:1360–9. doi: 10.1159/000465455
74. Li J-Y, Yu M, Tyagi AM, Vaccaro C, Hsu E, Adams J, et al. IL-17 receptor signaling in osteoblasts/osteocytes mediates PTH-induced bone loss and enhances osteocytic RANKL production. *J Bone Mineral Res.* (2019) 34:349–60. doi: 10.1002/jbmr.3600
75. Graves DT, Alshabab A, Albiero ML, Mattos M, Corrêa JD, Chen S, et al. Osteocytes play an important role in experimental periodontitis in healthy and diabetic mice through expression of RANKL. *J Clin Periodontol.* (2018) 45:285–92. doi: 10.1111/jcpe.12851
76. Sakamoto E, Kido J-i, Takagi R, Inagaki Y, Naruishi K, Nagata T, et al. Advanced glycation end-product 2 and Porphyromonas gingivalis lipopolysaccharide increase sclerostin expression in mouse osteocyte-like cells. *Bone.* (2019) 122:22–30. doi: 10.1016/j.bone.2019.02.001
77. Lin D, Li L, Sun Y, Wang W, Wang X, Ye Y, et al. IL-17 regulates the expressions of RANKL and OPG in human periodontal ligament cells via TRAF6/TBK1-JNK/NF-κB pathways. *Immunology.* (2014) 144:472–85. doi: 10.1111/imm.12395
78. Alippe Y, Wang C, Ricci B, Xiao J, Qu C, Zou W, et al. Bone matrix components activate the NLRP3 inflammasome and promote osteoclast differentiation. *Sci Rep.* (2017) 7:6630. doi: 10.1038/s41598-017-07014-0
79. Wei S, Kitaura H, Zhou P, Ross FP, Teitelbaum SL. IL-1 mediates TNF-induced osteoclastogenesis. *J Clin Invest.* (2005) 115:282–90. doi: 10.1172/JCI200523394
80. Kajikawa T, Briones RA, Resuello RRG, Tuplano JV, Reis ES, Hajishengallis E, et al. Safety and efficacy of the complement inhibitor AMY-101 in a natural model of periodontitis in non-human primates. *Mol Therapy Methods Clin Dev.* (2017) 6:207–15. doi: 10.1016/j.omtm.2017.08.001
81. Maekawa T, Briones RA, Resuello RR, Tuplano JV, Hajishengallis E, Kajikawa T, et al. Inhibition of pre-existing natural periodontitis in non-human primates by a locally administered peptide inhibitor of complement C3. *J Clin Periodontol.* (2016) 43:238–49. doi: 10.1111/jcpe.12507
82. Zhuang Z, Yoshizawa-Smith S, Glowacki A, Maltos K, Pacheco C, Shehabeldin M, et al. Induction of M2 macrophages prevents bone loss in murine periodontitis models. *J Dental Res.* (2018) 98:200–8. doi: 10.1177/0022034518805984
83. Jin Y, Wang L, Liu D, Lin X. Tamibarotene modulates the local immune response in experimental periodontitis. *Int Immunopharmacol.* (2014) 23:537–45. doi: 10.1016/j.intimp.2014.10.003
84. Wang L, Wang J, Jin Y, Gao H, Lin X. Oral administration of all-trans retinoic acid suppresses experimental periodontitis by modulating the Th17/treg imbalance. *J Periodontol.* (2014) 85:740–50. doi: 10.1902/jop.2013.130132
85. Mizraji G, Heyman O, Van Dyke TE, Wilensky A. Resolvin D2 restrains Th1 immunity and prevents alveolar bone loss in murine periodontitis. *Front Immunol.* (2018) 9:785. doi: 10.3389/fimmu.2018.00785
86. Hu Y, Yu P, Yu X, Hu X, Kawai T, Han X. IL-21/anti-Tim1/CD40 ligand promotes B10 activity in vitro and alleviates bone loss in experimental periodontitis *in vivo. Biochim et Biophy Acta Mol Basis Dis.* (2017) 1863:2149–57. doi: 10.1016/j.bbadis.2017.06.001
87. Cavalla F, Araujo-Pires AC, Biguetti CC, Garlet GP. Cytokine networks regulating inflammation and immune defense in the oral cavity. *Curr Oral Health Rep.* (2014) 1:104-13. doi: 10.1007/s40496-014-0016-9
88. Cavalla F, Biguetti CC, Garlet T, Trombone A, Garlet GP. Inflammatory *Pathways of Bone Resorption in Periodontitis, in Pathogenesis of Periodontal Diseases Biological Concepts for Clinicians.* Switzerland: Springer International Publishing AG. (2018) 59-86. doi: 10.1007/978-3-319-53737-5_6
89. Francisconi CF, Vieira AE, Biguetti CC, Glowacki AJ, Trombone AP, Letra A, et al. Characterization of the protective role of regulatory T cells in experimental periapical lesion development and their chemoattraction manipulation as a therapeutic tool. *J Endodont.* (2016) 42:120–6. doi: 10.1016/j.joen.2015.09.022
90. Garlet GP. Destructive and protective roles of cytokines in periodontitis: a re-appraisal from host defense and tissue destruction viewpoints. *J Dental Res.* (2010) 89:1349-63. doi: 10.1177/0022034510376402
91. Jansson L. Relationship between apical periodontitis and marginal bone loss at individual level from a general population. *Int Dental J.* (2015) 65:71–6. doi: 10.1111/idj.12143
92. Silva N, Abusleme L, Bravo D, Dutzan N, Garcia-Sesnich J, Vernal R, et al. Host response mechanisms in periodontal diseases. *J Appl Oral Sci.* (2015) 23:329–55. doi: 10.1590/1678-775720140259
93. Repeke CE, Ferreira SB Jr, Vieira AE, Silveira EM, Avila-Campos MJ, da Silva JS, et al. Dose-response met-RANTES treatment of experimental periodontitis: a narrow edge between the disease severity attenuation and infection control. *PLoS ONE.* (2011) 6:e22526. doi: 10.1371/journal.pone.0022526
94. Tomson PL, Simon SR. Contemporary cleaning and shaping of the root canal system. *Primary Dental J.* (2016) 5:46–53. doi: 10.1308/205016816819304196
95. Darcey J, Roudsari RV, Jawad S, Taylor C, Hunter M. Modern endodontic principles. part 5: obturation. *Dental Update.* (2016) 43:114–6. doi: 10.12968/denu.2016.43.2.114
96. Menezes-Silva R, Khaliq S, Deeley K, Letra A, Vieira AR. Genetic susceptibility to periapical disease: conditional contribution of MMP2 and MMP3 genes to the development of periapical lesions and healing response. *J Endodont.* (2012) 38:604–7. doi: 10.1016/j.joen.2012.02.009
97. Hernandez M, Dutzan N, Garcia-Sesnich J, Abusleme L, Dezerega A, Silva N, et al. Host-pathogen interactions in progressive chronic periodontitis. *J Dental Res.* (2011) 90:1164–70. doi: 10.1177/0022034511401405
98. Provenzano JC, Antunes HS, Alves FR, Rocas IN, Alves WS, Silva MR, et al. Host-bacterial interactions in post-treatment apical periodontitis: a metaproteome analysis. *J Endodont.* (2016) 42:880–5. doi: 10.1016/j.joen.2016.02.013
99. Garlet GP, Trombone AP, Menezes R, Letra A, Repeke CE, Vieira AE, et al. The use of chronic gingivitis as reference status increases the power and odds of periodontitis genetic studies: a proposal based in the exposure concept and clearer resistance and susceptibility phenotypes definition. *J Clin Periodontol.* (2012) 39:323–32. doi: 10.1111/j.1600-051X.2012.01859.x
100. Dill A, Letra A, Chaves de Souza L, Yadlapati M, Biguetti CC, Garlet GP, et al. Analysis of multiple cytokine polymorphisms in individuals with untreated deep carious lesions reveals IL1B (rs1143643) as a susceptibility factor for periapical lesion development. *J Endodont.* (2015) 41:197–200. doi: 10.1016/j.joen.2014.10.016
101. Maheshwari K, Silva RM, Guajardo-Morales L, Garlet GP, Vieira AR, Letra A. Heat shock 70 protein genes and genetic susceptibility to apical periodontitis. *J Endodont.* (2016) 42:1467–71. doi: 10.1016/j.joen.2016.07.010
102. Cavalla F, Biguetti CC, Dionisio TJ, Azevedo MCS, Martins W Jr, Santos CF, et al. CCR5Delta32 (rs333) polymorphism is associated with decreased risk of chronic and aggressive periodontitis: A case-control analysis based in disease resistance and susceptibility phenotypes. *Cytokine.* (2018) 103:142–9. doi: 10.1016/j.cyto.2017.09.022

103. Cavalla F, Hernández-Ríos P, Sorsa T, Biguetti C, Hernández M. Matrix metalloproteinases as regulators of periodontal inflammation. *Int J Mol Sci.* (2017) 18:440. doi: 10.3390/ijms18 020440
104. Trombone AP, Cavalla F, Silveira EM, Andreo CB, Francisconi CF, Fonseca AC, et al. MMP1-1607 polymorphism increases the risk for periapical lesion development through the upregulation MMP-1 expression in association with pro-inflammatory milieu elements. *J Appl Oral Sci.* (2016) 24:366–75. doi: 10.1590/1678-775720160112
105. Lerner UH, Ohlsson C. The WNT system: background and its role in bone. *J Int Med.* (2015) 277:630–49. doi: 10.1111/joim.12368
106. Tan Z, Ding N, Lu H, Kessler JA, Kan L. Wnt signaling in physiological and pathological bone formation. *Histol Histopathol.* (2018) 34:18062. doi: 10.14670/HH-18-062
107. Menezes R, Garlet TP, Letra A, Bramante CM, Campanelli AP, Figueira Rde C, et al. Differential patterns of receptor activator of nuclear factor kappa B ligand/osteoprotegerin expression in human periapical granulomas: possible association with progressive or stable nature of the lesions. *J Endodont.* (2008) 34:932–8. doi: 10.1016/j.joen.2008.05.002
108. Araujo-Pires AC, Francisconi CF, Biguetti CC, Cavalla F, Aranha AM, Letra A, et al. Simultaneous analysis of T helper subsets (Th1, Th2, Th9, Th17, Th22, Tfh, Tr1 and Tregs) markers expression in periapical lesions reveals multiple cytokine clusters accountable for lesions activity and inactivity status. *J Appl Oral Sci.* (2014) 22:336–46. doi: 10.1590/1678-775720140140
109. Hu X, Ivashkiv LB. Cross-regulation of signaling pathways by interferon-gamma: implications for immune responses and autoimmune diseases. *Immunity.* (2009) 31:539–50. doi: 10.1016/j.immuni.2009.09.002
110. van Hamburg JP, Tas SW. Molecular mechanisms underpinning T helper 17 cell heterogeneity and functions in rheumatoid arthritis. *J Autoimmunity.* (2018) 87:69–81. doi: 10.1016/j.jaut.2017.12.006
111. Wang L, Zhao Y, Shi S. Interplay between mesenchymal stem cells and lymphocytes: implications for immunotherapy and tissue regeneration. *J Dental Res.* (2012) 91:1003–10. doi: 10.1177/0022034512460404
112. Francisconi CF, Vieira AE, Azevedo MCS, Tabanez AP, Fonseca AC, Trombone APF, et al. RANKL triggers treg-mediated immunoregulation in inflammatory osteolysis. *J Dental Res.* (2018) 97:917–27. doi: 10.1177/0022034518759302
113. Lin J, Yang L, Silva HM, Trzeciak A, Choi Y, Schwab SR, et al. Increased generation of Foxp3(+) regulatory T cells by manipulating antigen presentation in the thymus. *Nat Commun.* (2016) 7:10562. doi: 10.1038/ncomms10562
114. Cavalla F, Reyes M, Vernal R, Alvarez C, Paredes R, Garcia-Sesnich J, et al. High levels of CXC ligand 12/stromal cell-derived factor 1 in apical lesions of endodontic origin associated with mast cell infiltration. *J Endodont.* (2013) 39:1234–9. doi: 10.1016/j.joen.2013.06.020
115. Rivellese F, Mauro D, Nerviani A, Pagani S, Fossati-Jimack L, Messemaker T, et al. Mast cells in early rheumatoid arthritis associate with disease severity and support B cell autoantibody production. *Ann Rheumat Dis.* (2018) 77:1773–81. doi: 10.1136/annrheumdis-2018-213418
116. Cardamone C, Parente R, Feo GD, Triggiani M. Mast cells as effector cells of innate immunity and regulators of adaptive immunity. *Immunol Lett.* (2016) 178:10–4. doi: 10.1016/j.imlet.2016.07.003
117. Dallenga T, Schaible UE. Neutrophils in tuberculosis–first line of defence or booster of disease and targets for host-directed therapy? *Pathog Dis.* (2016) 74:ftw012. doi: 10.1093/femspd/ftw012
118. Pechous RD. With friends like these: the complex role of neutrophils in the progression of severe pneumonia. *Front Cell Infect Microbiol.* (2017) 7:160. doi: 10.3389/fcimb.2017.00160
119. Cavalla F, Biguetti C, Jain S, Johnson C, Letra A, Garlet GP, et al. Proteomic profiling and differential messenger RNA expression correlate HSP27 and serpin family B member 1 to apical periodontitis outcomes. *J Endodont.* (2017) 43:1486–93. doi: 10.1016/j.joen.2017.03.014
120. Singh MK, Sharma B, Tiwari PK. The small heat shock protein Hsp27: present understanding and future prospects. *J Therm Biol.* (2017) 69:149–54. doi: 10.1016/j.jtherbio.2017.06.004
121. Baumann M, Pham CT, Benarafa C. SerpinB1 is critical for neutrophil survival through cell-autonomous inhibition of cathepsin G. *Blood.* (2013) 121:3900–7. doi: 10.1182/blood-2012-09-455022
122. Garlet GP, Horwat R, Ray HL Jr, Garlet TP, Silveira EM, Campanelli AP, et al. Expression analysis of wound healing genes in human periapical granulomas of progressive and stable nature. *J Endodont.* (2012) 38:185–90. doi: 10.1016/j.joen.2011.09.011
123. Al-Dujaili SA, Lau E, Al-Dujaili H, Tsang K, Guenther A, You L. Apoptotic osteocytes regulate osteoclast precursor recruitment and differentiation *in vitro*. *J Cell Biochem.* (2011) 112:2412–23. doi: 10.1002/jcb.23164
124. Hayashida C, Ito J, Nakayachi M, Okayasu M, Ohyama Y, Hakeda Y, et al. Osteocytes produce interferon-beta as a negative regulator of osteoclastogenesis. *J Biol Chem.* (2014) 289:11545–55. doi: 10.1074/jbc.M113.523811
125. Zhao S, Zhang YK, Harris S, Ahuja SS, Bonewald LF. MLO-Y4 osteocyte-like cells support osteoclast formation and activation. *J Bone Mineral Res.* (2002) 17:2068–79. doi: 10.1359/jbmr.2002.17.11.2068
126. Buenzli PR, Sims NA. Quantifying the osteocyte network in the human skeleton. *Bone.* (2015) 75:144–50. doi: 10.1016/j.bone.2015.02.016
127. Ito N, Wijenayaka AR, Prideaux M, Kogawa M, Ormsby RT, Evdokiou A, et al. Regulation of FGF23 expression in IDG-SW3 osteocytes and human bone by pro-inflammatory stimuli. *Mol Cell Endocrinol.* (2015) 399:208–18. doi: 10.1016/j.mce.2014.10.007
128. Algate K, Haynes DR, Bartold PM, Crotti TN, Cantley MD. The effects of tumour necrosis factor-alpha on bone cells involved in periodontal alveolar bone loss; osteoclasts, osteoblasts and osteocytes. *J Periodontal Res.* (2016) 51:549–66. doi: 10.1111/jre.12339
129. Baeza M, Garrido M, Hernandez-Rios P, Dezerega A, Garcia-Sesnich J, Strauss F, et al. Diagnostic accuracy for apical and chronic periodontitis biomarkers in gingival crevicular fluid: an exploratory study. *J Clin Periodontol.* (2016) 43:34–45. doi: 10.1111/jcpe.12479
130. Corbella S, Veronesi P, Galimberti V, Weinstein R, Del Fabbro M, Francetti L. Is periodontitis a risk indicator for cancer? A meta-analysis. *PLoS ONE.* (2018) 13:e0195683. doi: 10.1371/journal.pone.0195683
131. Tonetti MS, Van Dyke TE. Periodontitis and atherosclerotic cardiovascular disease: consensus report of the Joint EFP/AAPWorkshop on Periodontitis and Systemic Diseases. *J Periodontol.* (2013) 84 (Suppl 4S):S24-s9. doi: 10.1902/jop.2013.1340019
132. Periodontal manifestations of systemic diseases and developmental and acquired conditions: Consensus report of workgroup 3 of the 2017 World Workshop on the Classification of Periodontal and Peri-Implant Diseases and Conditions. *Br Dental J.* (2018) 225:141. doi: 10.1038/sj.bdj.2018.616
133. Sanz M, Ceriello A, Buysschaert M, Chapple I, Demmer RT, Graziani F, et al. Scientific evidence on the links between periodontal diseases and diabetes: consensus report and guidelines of the joint workshop on periodontal diseases and diabetes by the International Diabetes Federation and the European Federation of Periodontology. *J Clin Periodontol.* (2018) 45:138–49. doi: 10.1111/jcpe.12808
134. Gomes MS, Blattner TC, Sant'Ana Filho M, Grecca FS, Hugo FN, Fouad AF, et al. Can apical periodontitis modify systemic levels of inflammatory markers? A systematic review and meta-analysis. *J Endodont.* (2013) 39:1205–17. doi: 10.1016/j.joen.2013.06.014
135. Garrido M, Cardenas AM, Astorga J, Quinlan F, Valdes M, Chaparro A, et al. Elevated systemic inflammatory burden and cardiovascular risk in young adults with endodontic apical lesions. *J Endodont.* (2019) 45:111–5. doi: 10.1016/j.joen.2018.11.014
136. Schenkein HA, Loos BG. Inflammatory mechanisms linking periodontal diseases to cardiovascular diseases. *J Clin Periodontol.* (2013) 40(Suppl 14):S51–69. doi: 10.1111/jcpe.12060
137. Garrido M, Dezerega A, Bordagaray MJ, Reyes M, Vernal R, Melgar-Rodriguez S, et al. C-reactive protein expression is up-regulated in apical lesions of endodontic origin in association with interleukin-6. *J Endodont.* (2015) 41:464–9. doi: 10.1016/j.joen.2014.12.021
138. Hernandez-Rios P, Pussinen PJ, Vernal R, Hernandez M. Oxidative stress in the local and systemic events of apical periodontitis. *Front Physiol.* (2017) 8:869. doi: 10.3389/fphys.2017.00869
139. Buduneli N, Kinane DF. Host-derived diagnostic markers related to soft tissue destruction and bone degradation in periodontitis. *J Clin Periodontol.* (2011) 38(Suppl 11):85–105. doi: 10.1111/j.1600-051X.2010.01670.x
140. Sorsa T, Gursoy UK, Nwhator S, Hernandez M, Tervahartiala T, Leppilahti J, et al. Analysis of matrix metalloproteinases, especially MMP-8, in gingival

creviclular fluid, mouthrinse and saliva for monitoring periodontal diseases. *Periodontology 2000.* (2016) 70:142–63. doi: 10.1111/prd.12101
141. Rathnayake N, Gieselmann DR, Heikkinen AM, Tervahartiala T, Sorsa T. Salivary Diagnostics-point-of-care diagnostics of MMP-8 in dentistry and medicine. *Diagnostics.* (2017) 7:E7 doi: 10.3390/diagnostics7010007
142. Leppilahti JM, Harjunmaa U, Jarnstedt J, Mangani C, Hernandez M, Tervahartiala T, et al. Diagnosis of newly delivered mothers for periodontitis with a novel oral-rinse aMMP-8 point-of-care test in a rural malawian population. *Diagnostics.* (2018) 8:E67. doi: 10.3390/diagnostics8030067
143. Alassiri S, Parnanen P, Rathnayake N, Johannsen G, Heikkinen AM, Lazzara R, et al. The ability of quantitative, specific, and sensitive point-of-care/chair-side oral fluid immunotests for aMMP-8 to detect periodontal and peri-implant diseases. *Dis Mark.* (2018) 2018:1306396. doi: 10.1155/2018/1306396
144. Sorsa T, Gieselmann D, Arweiler NB, Hernandez M. A quantitative point-of-care test for periodontal and dental peri-implant diseases. *Nat Rev Dis Primers.* (2017) 3:17069. doi: 10.1038/nrdp.2017.69
145. Chaparro A, Sanz A, Quintero A, Inostroza C, Ramirez V, Carrion F, et al. Increased inflammatory biomarkers in early pregnancy is associated with the development of pre-eclampsia in patients with periodontitis: a case control study. *J Periodontal Res.* (2013) 48:302–7. doi: 10.1111/jre.12008
146. Chaparro A, Zuniga E, Varas-Godoy M, Albers D, Ramirez V, Hernandez M, et al. Periodontitis and placental growth factor in oral fluids are early pregnancy predictors of gestational diabetes mellitus. *J Periodontol.* (2018) 89:1052–60. doi: 10.1002/JPER.17-0497
147. Payne JB, Golub LM, Stoner JA, Lee HM, Reinhardt RA, Sorsa T, et al. The effect of subantimicrobial-dose-doxycycline periodontal therapy on serum biomarkers of systemic inflammation: a randomized, double-masked, placebo-controlled clinical trial. *J Am Dental Assoc.* (2011) 142:262–73. doi: 10.14219/jada.archive.2011.0165
148. Cotti E, Dessi C, Piras A, Flore G, Deidda M, Madeddu C, et al. Association of endodontic infection with detection of an initial lesion to the cardiovascular system. *J Endodont.* (2011) 37:1624–9. doi: 10.1016/j.joen.2011.09.006
149. Heikkila P, But A, Sorsa T, Haukka J. Periodontitis and cancer mortality: Register-based cohort study of 68,273 adults in 10-year follow-up. *Int J Cancer.* (2018) 142:2244–53. doi: 10.1002/ijc.31254
150. Damle SG. Health consequences of poor oral health? *Contemp Clin Dent.* (2018) 9:1. doi: 10.4103/ccd.ccd_106_18
151. Hormia M, Willberg J, Ruokonen H, Syrjanen S. Marginal periodontium as a potential reservoir of human papillomavirus in oral mucosa. *J Periodontol.* (2005) 76:358–63. doi: 10.1902/jop.2005.76.3.358
152. Saygun I, Kubar A, Ozdemir A, Slots J. Periodontitis lesions are a source of salivary cytomegalovirus and Epstein-Barr virus. *J Periodontal Res.* (2005) 40:187–91. doi: 10.1111/j.1600-0765.2005.00790.x
153. Katz J, Onate MD, Pauley KM, Bhattacharyya I, Cha S. Presence of *Porphyromonas gingivalis* in gingival squamous cell carcinoma. *Int J Oral Sci.* (2011) 3:209–15. doi: 10.4248/IJOS11075
154. Nieminen MT, Listyarifah D, Hagstrom J, Haglund C, Grenier D, Nordstrom D, et al. Treponema denticola chymotrypsin-like proteinase may contribute to orodigestive carcinogenesis through immunomodulation. *Br J Cancer.* (2018) 118:428–34. doi: 10.1038/bjc.2017.409
155. Kylma AK, Jouhi L, Listyarifah D, Mohamed H, Makitie A, Remes SM, et al. Treponema denticola chymotrypsin-like protease as associated with HPV-negative oropharyngeal squamous cell carcinoma. *Br J Cancer.* (2018) 119:89–95. doi: 10.1038/s41416-018-0143-5
156. Pearson TA, Mensah GA, Alexander RW, Anderson JL, Cannon RO III, Criqui M, et al. Markers of inflammation and cardiovascular disease: application to clinical and public health practice: a statement for healthcare professionals from the Centers for Disease Control and Prevention and the American Heart Association. *Circulation.* (2003) 107:499–511. doi: 10.1161/01.CIR.0000052939.59093.45
157. Brown DL, Desai KK, Vakili BA, Nouneh C, Lee HM, Golub LM. Clinical and biochemical results of the metalloproteinase inhibition with subantimicrobial doses of doxycycline to prevent acute coronary syndromes (MIDAS) pilot trial. *Arterioscler Thromb Vasc Biol.* (2004) 24:733–8. doi: 10.1161/01.ATV.0000121571.78696.dc
158. Bench TJ, Jeremias A, Brown DL. Matrix metalloproteinase inhibition with tetracyclines for the treatment of coronary artery disease. *Pharmacol Res.* (2011) 64:561–6. doi: 10.1016/j.phrs.2011.05.002
159. Golub LM, Evans RT, McNamara TF, Lee HM, Ramamurthy NS. A non-antimicrobial tetracycline inhibits gingival matrix metalloproteinases and bone loss in Porphyromonas gingivalis-induced periodontitis in rats. *Ann NY Acad Sci.* (1994) 732:96–111. doi: 10.1111/j.1749-6632.1994.tb24728.x
160. Golub LM, Lee HM, Stoner JA, Sorsa T, Reinhardt RA, Wolff MS, et al. Subantimicrobial-dose doxycycline modulates gingival crevicular fluid biomarkers of periodontitis in postmenopausal osteopenic women. *J Periodontol.* (2008) 79:1409–18. doi: 10.1902/jop.2008.070623
161. Hamilton JA, Hasturk H, Kantarci A, Serhan CN, Van Dyke T. Atherosclerosis, periodontal disease, and treatment with resolvins. *Curr Atheroscl Rep.* (2017) 19:57. doi: 10.1007/s11883-017-0696-4
162. The EESNWG. Bone sarcomas: ESMO clinical practice guidelines for diagnosis, treatment and follow-up †. *Ann Oncol.* (2012) 23(suppl_7):vii100-vii9. doi: 10.1093/annonc/mds254
163. Razek AA. Imaging appearance of bone tumors of the maxillofacial region. *World J Radiol.* (2011) 3:125–34. doi: 10.4329/wjr.v3.i5.125
164. Wright JM, Vered M. Update from the 4th edition of the World Health Organization classification of head and neck tumours: odontogenic and maxillofacial bone tumors. *Head Neck Pathol.* (2017) 11:68–77. doi: 10.1007/s12105-017-0794-1
165. Bertin H, Guilho R, Brion R, Amiaud J, Battaglia S, Moreau A, et al. Jaw osteosarcoma models in mice: first description. *J Transl Med.* (2019) 17:56. doi: 10.1186/s12967-019-1807-5
166. Park YK, Ryu KN, Park HR, Kim DW. Low-grade osteosarcoma of the maxillary sinus. *Skeletal Radiol.* (2003) 32:161-4. doi: 10.1007/s00256-002-0577-x
167. David E, Blanchard F, Heymann MF, De Pinieux G, Gouin F, Redini F, et al. The bone niche of chondrosarcoma: a sanctuary for drug resistance, tumour growth and also a source of new therapeutic targets. *Sarcoma.* (2011) 2011:932451. doi: 10.1155/2011/932451
168. Brown HK, Schiavone K, Gouin F, Heymann MF, Heymann D. Biology of bone sarcomas and new therapeutic developments. *Calci Tiss Int.* (2018) 102:174–95. doi: 10.1007/s00223-017-0372-2
169. Chan CKF, Gulati GS, Sinha R, Tompkins JV, Lopez M, Carter AC, et al. Identification of the human skeletal stem cell. *Cell.* (2018) 175:43–56.e21. doi: 10.1016/j.cell.2018.07.029
170. Gambera S, Abarrategi A, Gonzalez-Camacho F, Morales-Molina A, Roma J, Alfranca A, et al. Clonal dynamics in osteosarcoma defined by RGB marking. *Nat Commun.* (2018) 9:3994. doi: 10.1038/s41467-018-06401-z
171. Brown HK, Tellez-Gabriel M, Heymann D. Cancer stem cells in osteosarcoma. *Cancer Lett.* (2017) 386:189–95. doi: 10.1016/j.canlet.2016.11.019
172. Vallette FM, Olivier C, Lezot F, Oliver L, Cochonneau D, Lalier L, et al. Dormant, quiescent, tolerant and persister cells: four synonyms for the same target in cancer. *Biochem Pharmacol.* (2018) 162:169–76 doi: 10.1016/j.bcp.2018.11.004
173. Dumars C, Ngyuen JM, Gaultier A, Lanel R, Corradini N, Gouin F, et al. Dysregulation of macrophage polarization is associated with the metastatic process in osteosarcoma. *Oncotarget.* (2016) 7:78343–54. doi: 10.18632/oncotarget.13055
174. Heymann MF, Lezot F, Heymann D. The contribution of immune infiltrates and the local microenvironment in the pathogenesis of osteosarcoma. *Cell Immunol.* (2017). doi: 10.1016/j.cellimm.2017.10.011
175. Koirala P, Roth ME, Gill J, Piperdi S, Chinai JM, Geller DS, et al. Immune infiltration and PD-L1 expression in the tumor microenvironment are prognostic in osteosarcoma. *Sci Rep.* (2016) 6:30093. doi: 10.1038/srep30093
176. Fritzsching B, Fellenberg J, Moskovszky L, Sapi Z, Krenacs T, Machado I, et al. CD8(+)/FOXP3(+)-ratio in osteosarcoma microenvironment separates survivors from non-survivors: a multicenter validated retrospective study. *Oncoimmunology.* (2015) 4:e990800. doi: 10.4161/2162402X.2014.990800
177. Stamatopoulos A, Stamatopoulos T, Gamie Z, Kenanidis E, Ribeiro RDC, Rankin KS, et al. Mesenchymal stromal cells for bone sarcoma treatment: Roadmap to clinical practice. *J Bone Oncol.* (2019) 16:100231. doi: 10.1016/j.jbo.2019.100231
178. Baglio SR, Lagerweij T, Perez-Lanzon M, Ho XD, Leveille N, Melo SA, et al. Blocking tumor-educated MSC paracrine activity halts

osteosarcoma progression. *Clin Cancer Res.* (2017) 23:3721–33. doi: 10.1158/1078-0432.CCR-16-2726
179. Avnet S, Di Pompo G, Chano T, Errani C, Ibrahim-Hashim A, Gillies RJ, et al. Cancer-associated mesenchymal stroma fosters the stemness of osteosarcoma cells in response to intratumoral acidosis via NF-kappaB activation. *Int J Cancer.* (2017) 140:1331–45. doi: 10.1002/ijc.30540
180. Renema N, Navet B, Heymann MF, Lezot F, Heymann D. RANK-RANKL signalling in cancer. *Biosci Rep.* (2016) 36:e00366. doi: 10.1042/BSR20160150
181. Navet B, Ando K, Vargas-Franco JW, Brion R, Amiaud J, Mori K, et al. The intrinsic and extrinsic implications of RANKL/RANK signaling in osteosarcoma: from tumor initiation to lung metastases. *Cancers.* (2018) 10:E398. doi: 10.3390/cancers10110398
182. Chen Y, Di Grappa MA, Molyneux SD, McKee TD, Waterhouse P, Penninger JM, et al. RANKL blockade prevents and treats aggressive osteosarcomas. *Sci Transl Med.* (2015) 7:317ra197. doi: 10.1126/scitranslmed.aad0295
183. Heymann MF, Brown HK, Heymann D. Drugs in early clinical development for the treatment of osteosarcoma. *Expert Opin Investigat Drugs.* (2016) 25:1265–80. doi: 10.1080/13543784.2016.1237503
184. Heymann D. Metastatic osteosarcoma challenged by regorafenib. *Lancet Oncol.* (2018) 20:12–4. doi: 10.1016/S1470-2045(18)30821-0
185. Loeser RF, Goldring SR, Scanzello CR, Goldring MB. Osteoarthritis: a disease of the joint as an organ. *Arthritis Rheum.* (2012) 64:1697–707. doi: 10.1002/art.34453
186. Vos LM, Kuijer R, Huddleston Slater JJ, Bulstra SK, Stegenga B. Inflammation is more distinct in temporomandibular joint osteoarthritis compared to the knee joint. *J Oral Maxillofac Surg.* (2014) 72:35–40. doi: 10.1016/j.joms.2013.08.022
187. Allen KD, Golightly YM. State of the evidence. *Curr Opin Rheumatol.* (2015) 27:276–83. doi: 10.1097/BOR.0000000000000161
188. Johnson VL, Hunter DJ. The epidemiology of osteoarthritis. *Best Pract Res Clin Rheumatol.* (2014) 28:5–15. doi: 10.1016/j.berh.2014.01.004
189. Tanaka E, Detamore MS, Mercuri LG. Degenerative disorders of the temporomandibular joint: etiology, diagnosis, and treatment. *J Dental Res.* (2008) 87:296–307. doi: 10.1177/154405910808700406
190. Embree MC, Kilts TM, Ono M, Inkson CA, Syed-Picard F, Karsdal MA, et al. Biglycan and fibromodulin have essential roles in regulating chondrogenesis and extracellular matrix turnover in temporomandibular joint osteoarthritis. *Am J Pathol.* (2010) 176:812–26. doi: 10.2353/ajpath.2010.090450
191. Yee G, Yu Y, Walsh WR, Lindeman R, Poole MD. The immunolocalisation of VEGF in the articular cartilage of sheep mandibular condyles. *J Craniomaxillofac Surg.* (2003) 31:244–51. doi: 10.1016/S1010-5182(03)00040-4
192. Matsumoto R, Ioi H, Goto TK, Hara A, Nakata S, Nakasima A, et al. Relationship between the unilateral TMJ osteoarthritis/osteoarthrosis, mandibular asymmetry and the EMG activity of the masticatory muscles: a retrospective study. *J Oral Rehabil.* (2010) 37:85–92. doi: 10.1111/j.1365-2842.2009.02026.x
193. Krisjane Z, Urtane I, Krumina G, Neimane L, Ragovska I. The prevalence of TMJ osteoarthritis in asymptomatic patients with dentofacial deformities: a cone-beam CT study. *Int J Oral Maxillofacial Surg.* (2012) 41:690–5. doi: 10.1016/j.ijom.2012.03.006
194. Betti BF, Everts V, Ket JCF, Tabeian H, Bakker AD, Langenbach GE, et al. Effect of mechanical loading on the metabolic activity of cells in the temporomandibular joint: a systematic review. *Clin Oral Investig.* (2018) 22:57–67. doi: 10.1007/s00784-017-2189-9
195. Utreja A, Dyment NA, Yadav S, Villa MM, Li Y, Jiang X, et al. Cell and matrix response of temporomandibular cartilage to mechanical loading. *Osteoarthr Cartilage.* (2016) 24:335-44. doi: 10.1016/j.joca.2015.08.010
196. Fujisawa T, Kuboki T, Kasai T, Sonoyama W, Kojima S, Uehara J, et al. A repetitive, steady mouth opening induced an osteoarthritis-like lesion in the rabbit temporomandibular joint. *J Dental Res.* (2003) 82:731–5. doi: 10.1177/154405910308200914
197. Sobue T, Yeh WC, Chhibber A, Utreja A, Diaz-Doran V, Adams D, et al. Murine TMJ loading causes increased proliferation and chondrocyte maturation. *J Dental Res.* (2011) 90:512–6. doi: 10.1177/0022034510390810
198. Nicodemus GD, Villanueva I, Bryant SJ. Mechanical stimulation of TMJ condylar chondrocytes encapsulated in PEG hydrogels. *J Biomed Mater Res A.* (2007) 83:323–31. doi: 10.1002/jbm.a.31251
199. Ichimiya H, Takahashi T, Ariyoshi W, Takano H, Matayoshi T, Nishihara T. Compressive mechanical stress promotes osteoclast formation through RANKL expression on synovial cells. *Oral Surg Oral Med Oral Pathol Oral Radiol Endod.* (2007) 103:334–41. doi: 10.1016/j.tripleo.2006.05.026
200. Shinohara T, Izawa T, Mino-Oka A, Mori H, Iwasa A, Inubushi T, et al. Hyaluronan metabolism in overloaded temporomandibular joint. *J Oral Rehabil.* (2016) 43:921–8. doi: 10.1111/joor.12443
201. Petrey AC, de la Motte CA. Hyaluronan, a crucial regulator of inflammation. *Front Immunol.* (2014) 5:101. doi: 10.3389/fimmu.2014.00101
202. Scheibner KA, Lutz MA, Boodoo S, Fenton MJ, Powell JD, Horton MR. Hyaluronan fragments act as an endogenous danger signal by engaging TLR2. *J Immunol.* (2006) 177:1272-81. doi: 10.4049/jimmunol.177.2.1272
203. Wang XD, Zhang JN, Gan YH, Zhou YH. Current understanding of pathogenesis and treatment of TMJ osteoarthritis. *J Dental Res.* (2015) 94:666–73. doi: 10.1177/0022034515574770
204. de Souza RF, Lovato da Silva CH, Nasser M, Fedorowicz Z, Al-Muharraqi MA. Interventions for the management of temporomandibular joint osteoarthritis. *Cochrane Database Syst Rev.* (2012) 2012:CD007261. doi: 10.1002/14651858.CD007261.pub2
205. Sakkas LI, Platsoucas CD. The role of T cells in the pathogenesis of osteoarthritis. *Arthritis Rheum.* (2007) 56:409–24. doi: 10.1002/art.22369
206. de Lange-Brokaar BJ, Ioan-Facsinay A, van Osch GJ, Zuurmond AM, Schoones J, Toes RE, et al. Synovial inflammation, immune cells and their cytokines in osteoarthritis: a review. *Osteoarthr Cartilage.* (2012) 20:1484–99. doi: 10.1016/j.joca.2012.08.027
207. Ponchel F, Burska AN, Hensor EM, Raja R, Campbell M, Emery P, et al. Changes in peripheral blood immune cell composition in osteoarthritis. *Osteoarthr Cartilage.* (2015) 23:1870-8. doi: 10.1016/j.joca.2015.06.018
208. Pessler F, Chen LX, Dai L, Gomez-Vaquero C, Diaz-Torne C, Paessler ME, et al. A histomorphometric analysis of synovial biopsies from individuals with Gulf War Veterans' Illness and joint pain compared to normal and osteoarthritis synovium. *Clin Rheumatol.* (2008) 27:1127-34. doi: 10.1007/s10067-008-0878-0
209. Kaneyama K, Segami N, Nishimura M, Suzuki T, Sato J. Importance of proinflammatory cytokines in synovial fluid from 121 joints with temporomandibular disorders. *Br J Oral Maxillofac Surg.* (2002) 40:418–23. doi: 10.1016/S0266-4356(02)00215-2
210. Kellesarian SV, Malignaggi VR, Abduljabbar T, Vohra F, Malmstrom H, Romanos GE, et al. Efficacy of scaling and root planing with and without adjunct antimicrobial photodynamic therapy on the expression of cytokines in the gingival crevicular fluid of patients with periodontitis: a systematic review. *Photodiagnosis Photodyn Ther.* (2016) 16:76–84. doi: 10.1016/j.pdpdt.2016.08.009
211. Lim WH, Toothman J, Miller JH, Tallents RH, Brouxhon SM, Olschowka ME, et al. IL-1beta inhibits TGFbeta in the temporomandibular joint. *J Dental Res.* (2009) 88:557–62. doi: 10.1177/0022034509336823
212. Vernal R, Velasquez E, Gamonal J, Garcia-Sanz JA, Silva A, Sanz M. Expression of proinflammatory cytokines in osteoarthritis of the temporomandibular joint. *Arch Oral Biol.* (2008) 53:910–5. doi: 10.1016/j.archoralbio.2008.04.004
213. Simsek Kaya G, Yapici Yavuz G, Kiziltunc A. Expression of chemerin in the synovial fluid of patients with temporomandibular joint disorders. *J Oral Rehabil.* (2018) 45:289–94 doi: 10.1111/joor.12608
214. Kalladka M, Quek S, Heir G, Eliav E, Mupparapu M, Viswanath A. Temporomandibular joint osteoarthritis: diagnosis and long-term conservative management: a topic review. *J Indian Prosthodont Soc.* (2014) 14:6–15. doi: 10.1007/s13191-013-0321-3
215. Robinson WH, Lepus CM, Wang Q, Raghu H, Mao R, Lindstrom TM, et al. Low-grade inflammation as a key mediator of the pathogenesis of osteoarthritis. *Nat Rev Rheumatol.* (2016) 12:580-92. doi: 10.1038/nrrheum.2016.136
216. Chen GY, Nunez G. Sterile inflammation: sensing and reacting to damage. *Nat Rev Immunol.* (2010) 10:826–37. doi: 10.1038/nri2873
217. Milam SB. Pathogenesis of degenerative temporomandibular joint arthritides. *Odontology.* (2005) 93:7–15. doi: 10.1007/s10266-005-0056-7
218. Milam SB, Zardeneta G, Schmitz JP. Oxidative stress and degenerative temporomandibular joint disease: a proposed hypothesis. *J Oral Maxillofac Surg.* (1998) 56:214–23. doi: 10.1016/S0278-2391(98)90872-2

219. Wei L, Xiong H, Li B, Gong Z, Li J, Cai H, et al. Change of HA molecular size and boundary lubrication in synovial fluid of patients with temporomandibular disorders. *J Oral Rehabil.* (2010) 37:271–7. doi: 10.1111/j.1365-2842.2009.02048.x
220. Takahashi T, Tominaga K, Takano H, Ariyoshi W, Habu M, Fukuda J, et al. A decrease in the molecular weight of hyaluronic acid in synovial fluid from patients with temporomandibular disorders. *J Oral Pathol Med.* (2004) 33:224–9. doi: 10.1111/j.0904-2512.2004.00024.x
221. Jiang D, Liang J, Fan J, Yu S, Chen S, Luo Y, et al. Regulation of lung injury and repair by Toll-like receptors and hyaluronan. *Nature Med.* (2005) 11:1173–9. doi: 10.1038/nm1315
222. Scanzello CR, Goldring SR. The role of synovitis in osteoarthritis pathogenesis. *Bone.* (2012) 51:249–57. doi: 10.1016/j.bone.2012.02.012
223. Kong J, Yang Y, Sun S, Xie J, Lin X, Ji P. Effect of toll-like receptor 4 on synovial injury of temporomandibular joint in rats caused by occlusal interference. *Medi Inflamm.* (2016) 2016:7694921. doi: 10.1155/2016/7694921
224. Lin X, Xie J, Sun S, Ren X, Kong J, Ji P. Toll-Like Receptor 4 (TLR4) stimulates synovial injury of temporomandibular joint in rats through the activation of p38 mitogen-activated protein kinase (MAPK) signaling pathway. *Med Sci Monit.* (2018) 24:4405–12. doi: 10.12659/MSM.908526
225. Israel HA, Diamond B, Saed-Nejad F, Ratcliffe A. Osteoarthritis and synovitis as major pathoses of the temporomandibular joint: comparison of clinical diagnosis with arthroscopic morphology. *J Oral Maxillofac Surg.* (1998) 56:1023–7. doi: 10.1016/S0278-2391(98)90246-4
226. Israel HA, Langevin CJ, Singer MD, Behrman DA. The relationship between temporomandibular joint synovitis and adhesions: pathogenic mechanisms and clinical implications for surgical management. *J Oral Maxillofac Surg.* (2006) 64:1066–74. doi: 10.1016/j.joms.2006.03.012
227. Hattori T, Ogura N, Akutsu M, Kawashima M, Watanabe S, Ito K, et al. Gene expression profiling of IL-17A-treated synovial fibroblasts from the human temporomandibular joint. *Medi Inflamm.* (2015) 2015:436067. doi: 10.1155/2015/436067
228. Chang SK, Gu Z, Brenner MB. Fibroblast-like synoviocytes in inflammatory arthritis pathology: the emerging role of cadherin-11. *Immunol Rev.* (2010) 233:256–66. doi: 10.1111/j.0105-2896.2009.00854.x
229. Buckley CD, Gilroy DW, Serhan CN. Proresolving lipid mediators and mechanisms in the resolution of acute inflammation. *Immunity.* (2014) 40:315–27. doi: 10.1016/j.immuni.2014.02.009
230. Axmann R, Bohm C, Kronke G, Zwerina J, Smolen J, Schett G. Inhibition of interleukin-6 receptor directly blocks osteoclast formation *in vitro* and *in vivo*. *Arthritis Rheum.* (2009) 60:2747–56. doi: 10.1002/art.24781
231. Kimura A, Kishimoto T. IL-6: regulator of Treg/Th17 balance. *Eur J Immunol.* (2010) 40:1830–5. doi: 10.1002/eji.201040391
232. Takayanagi H, Iizuka H, Juji T, Nakagawa T, Yamamoto A, Miyazaki T, et al. Involvement of receptor activator of nuclear factor kappaB ligand/osteoclast differentiation factor in osteoclastogenesis from synoviocytes in rheumatoid arthritis. *Arthritis Rheum.* (2000) 43:259-69. doi: 10.1002/1529-0131(200002)43:2<259::AID-ANR4>3.0.CO;2-W
233. Kaneyama K, Segami N, Sato J, Yoshimura H, Nishiura R. Expression of receptor activator of nuclear factor-kappaB ligand in synovial tissue: comparison with degradation of articular cartilage in temporomandibular joint disorders. *Oral Surg Oral Med Oral Pathol Oral Radiol Endod.* (2007) 104:e12-7. doi: 10.1016/j.tripleo.2007.02.016
234. Danks L, Komatsu N, Guerrini MM, Sawa S, Armaka M, Kollias G, et al. RANKL expressed on synovial fibroblasts is primarily responsible for bone erosions during joint inflammation. *Ann Rheumat Dis.* (2016) 75:1187–95. doi: 10.1136/annrheumdis-2014-207137
235. Jiao K, Niu LN, Wang MQ, Dai J, Yu SB, Liu XD, et al. Subchondral bone loss following orthodontically induced cartilage degradation in the mandibular condyles of rats. *Bone.* (2011) 48:362–71. doi: 10.1016/j.bone.2010.09.010
236. Taylor KR, Yamasaki K, Radek KA, Di Nardo A, Goodarzi H, Golenbock D, et al. Recognition of hyaluronan released in sterile injury involves a unique receptor complex dependent on Toll-like receptor 4, CD44, and MD-2. *J Biol Chem.* (2007) 282:18265–75. doi: 10.1074/jbc.M606352200
237. Termeer C, Benedix F, Sleeman J, Fieber C, Voith U, Ahrens T, et al. Oligosaccharides of Hyaluronan activate dendritic cells via toll-like receptor 4. *J Exp Med.* (2002) 195:99–111. doi: 10.1084/jem.20001858
238. Termeer CC, Hennies J, Voith U, Ahrens T, Weiss JM, Prehm P, et al. Oligosaccharides of hyaluronan are potent activators of dendritic cells. *J Immunol.* (2000) 165:1863–70. doi: 10.4049/jimmunol.165.4.1863
239. Galandrini R, Galluzzo E, Albi N, Grossi CE, Velardi A. Hyaluronate is costimulatory for human T cell effector functions and binds to CD44 on activated T cells. *J Immunol.* (1994) 153:21–31.
240. Rizzo M, Bayo J, Piccioni F, Malvicini M, Fiore E, Peixoto E, et al. Low molecular weight hyaluronan-pulsed human dendritic cells showed increased migration capacity and induced resistance to tumor chemoattraction. *PLoS ONE.* (2014) 9:e107944. doi: 10.1371/journal.pone.0107944
241. Monasterio G, Guevara J, Ibarra JP, Castillo F, Diaz-Zuniga J, Alvarez C, et al. Immunostimulatory activity of low-molecular-weight hyaluronan on dendritic cells stimulated with Aggregatibacter actinomycetemcomitans or *Porphyromonas gingivalis*. *Clin Invest.* (2019) 23:1887–94. doi: 10.1007/s00784-018-2641-5
242. Tussiwand R, Gautier EL. Transcriptional regulation of mononuclear phagocyte development. *Front Immunol.* (2015) 6:533. doi: 10.3389/fimmu.2015.00533
243. Persson EK, Uronen-Hansson H, Semmrich M, Rivollier A, Hagerbrand K, Marsal J, et al. IRF4 transcription-factor-dependent CD103(+)CD11b(+) dendritic cells drive mucosal T helper 17 cell differentiation. *Immunity.* (2013) 38:958–69. doi: 10.1016/j.immuni.2013.03.009
244. Symons JA, McCulloch JF, Wood NC, Duff GW. Soluble CD4 in patients with rheumatoid arthritis and osteoarthritis. *Clin Immunol Immunopathol.* (1991) 60:72–82. doi: 10.1016/0090-1229(91)90113-O
245. de Jong H, Berlo SE, Hombrink P, Otten HG, van Eden W, Lafeber FP, et al. Cartilage proteoglycan aggrecan epitopes induce proinflammatory autoreactive T-cell responses in rheumatoid arthritis and osteoarthritis. *Ann Rheumat Dis.* (2010) 69:255–62. doi: 10.1136/ard.2008.103978
246. Monasterio G, Castillo F, Rojas L, Cafferata EA, Alvarez C, Carvajal P, et al. Th1/Th17/Th22 immune response and their association with joint pain, imagenological bone loss, RANKL expression and osteoclast activity in temporomandibular joint osteoarthritis: a preliminary report. *J Oral Rehabil.* (2018) 45:589–97. doi: 10.1111/joor.12649
247. Murphy CA, Langrish CL, Chen Y, Blumenschein W, McClanahan T, Kastelein RA, et al. Divergent pro- and antiinflammatory roles for IL-23 and IL-12 in joint autoimmune inflammation. *J Exp Med.* (2003) 198:1951–7. doi: 10.1084/jem.20030896
248. Nakae S, Nambu A, Sudo K, Iwakura Y. Suppression of immune induction of collagen-induced arthritis in IL-17-deficient mice. *J Immunol.* (2003) 171:6173–7. doi: 10.4049/jimmunol.171.11.6173
249. Nakae S, Saijo S, Horai R, Sudo K, Mori S, Iwakura Y. IL-17 production from activated T cells is required for the spontaneous development of destructive arthritis in mice deficient in IL-1 receptor antagonist. *Proc Natl Acad Sci USA.* (2003) 100:5986–90. doi: 10.1073/pnas.1035999100
250. Lurati A, Laria A, Gatti A, Brando B, Scarpellini M. Different T cells' distribution and activation degree of Th17 CD4+ cells in peripheral blood in patients with osteoarthritis, rheumatoid arthritis, and healthy donors: preliminary results of the MAGENTA CLICAO study. *Open Access Rheumatol.* (2015) 7:63–8. doi: 10.2147/OARRR.S81905
251. Yamada H, Nakashima Y, Okazaki K, Mawatari T, Fukushi J, Oyamada A, et al. Preferential accumulation of activated Th1 cells not only in rheumatoid arthritis but also in osteoarthritis joints. *J Rheumatol.* (2011) 38:1569–75. doi: 10.3899/jrheum.101355
252. Nistala K, Adams S, Cambrook H, Ursu S, Olivito B, de Jager W, et al. Th17 plasticity in human autoimmune arthritis is driven by the inflammatory environment. *Proc Natl Acad Sci USA.* (2010) 107:14751-6. doi: 10.1073/pnas.1003852107
253. Penatti A, Facciotti F, De Matteis R, Larghi P, Paroni M, Murgo A, et al. Differences in serum and synovial CD4+ T cells and cytokine profiles to stratify patients with inflammatory osteoarthritis and rheumatoid arthritis. *Arthritis Res Ther.* (2017) 19:103. doi: 10.1186/s13075-017-1305-1
254. Hussein MR, Fathi NA, El-Din AM, Hassan HI, Abdullah F, Al-Hakeem E, et al. Alterations of the CD4(+), CD8 (+) T cell subsets, interleukins-1beta, IL-10, IL-17, tumor necrosis factor-alpha and soluble intercellular adhesion molecule-1 in rheumatoid arthritis and

osteoarthritis: preliminary observations. *Pathol Oncol Res.* (2008) 14:321–8. doi: 10.1007/s12253-008-9016-1
255. Sarkar S, Justa S, Brucks M, Endres J, Fox DA, Zhou X, et al. Interleukin (IL)-17A, F and AF in inflammation: a study in collagen-induced arthritis and rheumatoid arthritis. *Clin Exp Immunol.* (2014) 177:652–61. doi: 10.1111/cei.12376
256. Kaneyama K, Segami N, Sato J, Nishimura M, Yoshimura H. Interleukin-6 family of cytokines as biochemical markers of osseous changes in the temporomandibular joint disorders. *Br J Oral Maxillofac Surg.* (2004) 42:246–50. doi: 10.1016/S0266-4356(03)00258-4
257. Moran EM, Mullan R, McCormick J, Connolly M, Sullivan O, Fitzgerald O, et al. Human rheumatoid arthritis tissue production of IL-17A drives matrix and cartilage degradation: synergy with tumour necrosis factor-alpha, Oncostatin M and response to biologic therapies. *Arthritis Res Ther.* (2009) 11:R113. doi: 10.1186/ar2772
258. Toh ML, Gonzales G, Koenders MI, Tournadre A, Boyle D, Lubberts E, et al. Role of interleukin 17 in arthritis chronicity through survival of synoviocytes via regulation of synoviolin expression. *PLoS ONE.* (2010) 5:e13416. doi: 10.1371/journal.pone.0013416
259. Li GQ, Zhang Y, Liu D, Qian YY, Zhang H, Guo SY, et al. Celastrol inhibits interleukin-17A-stimulated rheumatoid fibroblast-like synoviocyte migration and invasion through suppression of NF-kappaB-mediated matrix metalloproteinase-9 expression. *Int Immunopharmacol.* (2012) 14:422–31. doi: 10.1016/j.intimp.2012.08.016
260. Chen Y, Zhong M, Liang L, Gu F, Peng H. Interleukin-17 induces angiogenesis in human choroidal endothelial cells *in vitro*. *Invest Ophthalmol Vis Sci.* (2014) 55:6968–75. doi: 10.1167/iovs.14-15029
261. Sato K, Suematsu A, Okamoto K, Yamaguchi A, Morishita Y, Kadono Y, et al. Th17 functions as an osteoclastogenic helper T cell subset that links T cell activation and bone destruction. *J Exp Med.* (2006) 203:2673–82. doi: 10.1084/jem.20061775
262. Schaffler MB, Cheung WY, Majeska R, Kennedy O. Osteocytes: master orchestrators of bone. *Calcif Tissue Int.* (2014) 94:5–24. doi: 10.1007/s00223-013-9790-y
263. Xiong J, Piemontese M, Onal M, Campbell J, Goellner JJ, Dusevich V, et al. Osteocytes, not osteoblasts or lining cells, are the main source of the RANKL required for osteoclast formation in remodeling bone. *PLoS ONE.* (2015) 10:e0138189. doi: 10.1371/journal.pone.0138189
264. Kramer I, Halleux C, Keller H, Pegurri M, Gooi JH, Weber PB, et al. Osteocyte Wnt/beta-catenin signaling is required for normal bone homeostasis. *Mol Cell Biol.* (2010) 30:3071–85. doi: 10.1128/MCB.01428-09
265. Shoji-Matsunaga A, Ono T, Hayashi M, Takayanagi H, Moriyama K, Nakashima T. Osteocyte regulation of orthodontic force-mediated tooth movement via RANKL expression. *Sci Rep.* (2017) 7:8753. doi: 10.1038/s41598-017-09326-7
266. Inoue M, Ono T, Kameo Y, Sasaki F, Ono T, Adachi T, et al. Forceful mastication activates osteocytes and builds a stout jawbone. *Sci Rep.* (2019) 9:4404. doi: 10.1038/s41598-019-40463-3
267. Prasadam I, Farnaghi S, Feng JQ, Gu W, Perry S, Crawford R, et al. Impact of extracellular matrix derived from osteoarthritis subchondral bone osteoblasts on osteocytes: role of integrinbeta1 and focal adhesion kinase signaling cues. *Arthritis Res Ther.* (2013) 15:R150. doi: 10.1186/ar4333
268. Wakita T, Mogi M, Kurita K, Kuzushima M, Togari A. Increase in RANKL: OPG ratio in synovia of patients with temporomandibular joint disorder. *J Dental Res.* (2006) 85:627–32. doi: 10.1177/154405910608500709
269. Takayanagi H. Osteoimmunology: shared mechanisms and crosstalk between the immune and bone systems. *Nat Rev Immunol.* (2007) 7:292–304. doi: 10.1038/nri2062
270. Takayanagi H. Osteoimmunology and the effects of the immune system on bone. *Nat Rev Rheumatol.* (2009) 5:667–76. doi: 10.1038/nrrheum.2009.217
271. Kikuta J, Wada Y, Kowada T, Wang Z, Sun-Wada GH, Nishiyama I, et al. Dynamic visualization of RANKL and Th17-mediated osteoclast function. *J Clin Invest.* (2013) 123:866–73. doi: 10.1172/JCI65054
272. Schiffman E, Ohrbach R, Truelove E, Look J, Anderson G, Goulet JP, et al. Diagnostic criteria for temporomandibular disorders (DC/TMD) for clinical and research applications: recommendations of the international RDC/TMD Consortium Network* and orofacial pain special interest groupdagger. *J Oral & Facial Pain Headache.* (2014) 28:6–27. doi: 10.11607/jop.1151
273. Kim YK, Kim SG, Kim BS, Lee JY, Yun PY, Bae JH, et al. Analysis of the cytokine profiles of the synovial fluid in a normal temporomandibular joint: preliminary study. *J Craniomaxillofac Surg.* (2012) 40:e337-41. doi: 10.1016/j.jcms.2012.02.002
274. Takahashi T, Kondoh T, Fukuda M, Yamazaki Y, Toyosaki T, Suzuki R. Proinflammatory cytokines detectable in synovial fluids from patients with temporomandibular disorders. *Oral Surg Oral Med Oral Pathol Oral Radiol Endod.* (1998) 85:135–41. doi: 10.1016/S1079-2104(98)90415-2
275. Kotake S, Udagawa N, Takahashi N, Matsuzaki K, Itoh K, Ishiyama S, et al. IL-17 in synovial fluids from patients with rheumatoid arthritis is a potent stimulator of osteoclastogenesis. The Journal of clinical investigation. (1999) 103:1345-52. doi: 10.1172/JCI5703
276. Tanimoto K, Suzuki A, Ohno S, Honda K, Tanaka N, Doi T, et al. Effects of TGF-beta on hyaluronan anabolism in fibroblasts derived from the synovial membrane of the rabbit temporomandibular joint. *J Dental Res.* (2004) 83:40–4. doi: 10.1177/154405910408300108
277. Kuroda S, Tanimoto K, Izawa T, Fujihara S, Koolstra JH, Tanaka E. Biomechanical and biochemical characteristics of the mandibular condylar cartilage. *Osteoarthr Cartilage.* (2009) 17:1408–15. doi: 10.1016/j.joca.2009.04.025
278. Nakano T, Scott PG. Changes in the chemical composition of the bovine temporomandibular joint disc with age. *Arch Oral Biol.* (1996) 41:845–53. doi: 10.1016/S0003-9969(96)00040-4
279. Jibiki M, Shimoda S, Nakagawa Y, Kawasaki K, Asada K, Ishibashi K. Calcifications of the disc of the temporomandibular joint. *J Oral Pathol Med.* (1999) 28:413–9. doi: 10.1111/j.1600-0714.1999.tb02113.x
280. Takano Y, Moriwake Y, Tohno Y, Minami T, Tohno S, Utsumi M, et al. Age-related changes of elements in the human articular disk of the temporomandibular joint. *Biol Trace Element Res.* (1999) 67:269–76. doi: 10.1007/BF02784426
281. Pufe T, Harde V, Petersen W, Goldring MB, Tillmann B, Mentlein R. Vascular endothelial growth factor (VEGF) induces matrix metalloproteinase expression in immortalized chondrocytes. *J Pathol.* (2004) 202:367–74. doi: 10.1002/path.1527

11

Effects of Sweet Cherry Polyphenols on Enhanced Osteoclastogenesis Associated with Childhood Obesity

Filomena Corbo [1†], Giacomina Brunetti [2†], Pasquale Crupi [3], Sara Bortolotti [4], Giuseppina Storlino [4], Laura Piacente [5], Alessia Carocci [1], Alessia Catalano [1], Gualtiero Milani [1], Graziana Colaianni [4], Silvia Colucci [2], Maria Grano [4], Carlo Franchini [1], Maria Lisa Clodoveo [6], Gabriele D'Amato [7] and Maria Felicia Faienza [5]*

[1] Department of Pharmacy-Drug science, University of Bari Aldo Moro, Bari, Italy, [2] Section of Human Anatomy and Histology, Department of Basic and Medical Sciences, Neurosciences and Sense Organs, University of Bari Aldo Moro, Bari, Italy, [3] CREA-VE, Council for Agricultural Research and Economics–Research Centre for Viticulture and Enology, Turi, Italy, [4] Section of Human Anatomy and Histology, Department of Emergency and Organ Transplantation, University of Bari, Bari, Italy, [5] Paediatric Unit, Department of Biomedical Sciences and Human Oncology, University of Bari Aldo Moro, Bari, Italy, [6] Interdisciplinary Department of Medicine, University of Bari Aldo Moro, Bari, Italy, [7] Neonatal Intensive Care Unit, Di Venere Hospital, Bari, Italy

***Correspondence:**
Giacomina Brunetti
giacomina.brunetti@uniba.it

† These authors have contributed equally to this work

Childhood obesity is associated with the development of severe comorbidities, such as diabetes, cardiovascular diseases, and increased risk of osteopenia/osteoporosis and fractures. The status of low-grade inflammation associated to obesity can be reversed through an enhanced physical activity and by consumption of food enrich of anti-inflammatory compounds, such as omega-3 fatty acids and polyphenols. The aim of this study was to deepen the mechanisms of bone impairment in obese children and adolescents through the evaluation of the osteoclastogenic potential of peripheral blood mononuclear cells (PBMCs), and the assessment of the serum levels of RANKL and osteoprotegerin (OPG). Furthermore, we aimed to evaluate the *in vitro* effects of polyphenol cherry extracts on osteoclastogenesis, as possible dietary treatment to improve bone health in obese subjects. High RANKL levels were measured in obese with respect to controls (115.48 ± 35.20 pg/ml vs. 87.18 ± 17.82 pg/ml; $p < 0.01$), while OPG levels were significantly reduced in obese than controls (378.02 ± 61.15 pg/ml vs. 436.75 ± 95.53 pg/ml, respectively, $p < 0.01$). Lower Ad-SoS- and BTT *Z*-scores were measured in obese compared to controls ($p < 0.05$). A significant elevated number of multinucleated TRAP$^+$ osteoclasts (OCs) were observed in the un-stimulated cultures of obese subjects compared to the controls. Interestingly, obese subjects displayed a higher percentage of CD14$^+$/CD16$^+$ than controls. Furthermore, in the mRNA extracts of obese subjects we detected a 2.5- and 2-fold increase of TNFα and RANKL transcripts compared to controls, respectively. Each extract of sweet cherries determined a dose-dependent reduction in the formation of multinucleated TRAP$^+$ OCs. Consistently, 24 h treatment of obese PBMCs with sweet cherry extracts from the three cultivars resulted in a significant reduction of the expression of TNFα. In conclusion, the bone impairment in obese children and adolescents is sustained by a spontaneous osteoclastogenesis that can be inhibited *in vitro* by the polyphenol content of sweet cherries. Thus, our study opens future perspectives for the use of sweet cherry extracts, appropriately formulated as nutraceutical food, as preventive in healthy children and therapeutic in obese ones.

Keywords: obesity, inflammation, polyphenols, sweet cherry, osteoclastogenesis, CD14+/CD16+ monocytes, osteoporosis, osteopenia

INTRODUCTION

Childhood obesity is one of the major health problems in the western world. It is associated with severe co-morbidities including diabetes, cardiovascular diseases (1, 2), and bone loss, which can occur early in the life (3, 4). It has been reported that the incidence of bone fractures increases in overweight/obese children and adolescents (5). The relationship between childhood obesity and bone impairment has been deepened in animal models. Indeed, Shu et al., found that mice fed with high fat diet (HFD) showed bone loss mainly due to high osteoclastic bone resorption, which is mediated by the increase of pro-osteoclastogenic cytokines and pre-osteoclasts in the bone marrow microenvironment (6).

Osteoclasts (OCs) derive from monocyte precursors which fuse thank to macrophage colony-stimulating factor (MCSF) and receptor activator of nuclear factor kappa-B ligand (RANKL) and become multinucleated cells able to resorb bone. RANKL is mainly produced by cells of the osteoblastic lineage. However, in inflammation also immune cells represent also an important source of the inflammatory cytokines [revised in Dar et al. (7)]. Recently, it has also been reported that bone marrow adipocytes produce RANKL (8), whose action could be inhibited by Osteoprotegerin (OPG), the soluble decoy receptor of RANKL (7). Other cytokines could also support osteoclastogenesis together with RANKL (9), such as TNFα. High levels of this cytokine have been demonstrated in bone diseases as well as in obesity (10–13). This last condition is associated with high levels of pro-inflammatory cytokines, such as interleukins, adipokines, and chemokines, which contribute to the chronic low level of inflammation and oxidative stress which are responsible of the different co-morbidities related to obesity (14, 15). This status of chronic inflammation can be prevented or even reversed by the loss of body weight through a reduction of food intake and enhanced physical activity (16). It has been reported that physical activity directly or indirectly decreased inflammation (17–19). Moreover, eating foods rich in bioactive anti-inflammatory compounds, such as omega-3 fatty acids (FAs) and polyphenols, has been demonstrated to reduce inflammation (20, 21). In particular, the anti-obesity effects of polyphenol-rich diets have been associated to the property of polyphenols to interact with adipose tissues (pre-adipocytes, adipose stem cells, and immune cells).

Sweet cherries are a source of dietary phenolic compounds (~1,500 mg total phenols per kg fresh weight), including phenolic acids (hydroxycinnamic acids) and flavonoids (anthocyanins, flavan-3-ols and flavonols), which are known for their health benefits and important role in preventing several chronic diseases related to oxidative stress (22, 23). Moreover, they show a low glycemic index respect to other fruits and vegetables and represent a source of vitamins, especially vitamin C and minerals, such as potassium, phosphorus, calcium, and magnesium (24, 25).

Studies *in vitro* and *in vivo* have reported that sweet cherries have anti-inflammatory and anti-carcinogenic activity, and characteristics for prevention of cardiovascular disease and diabetes (26).

In the light of these evidences and of the increasing interest on the polyphenol effects on childhood obesity, the aim of this paper were: (a) to deepen the mechanisms of bone impairment in obese children and adolescents, through the evaluation of the serum levels of RANKL and OPG together with the osteoclastogenic potential of peripheral blood mononuclear cells (PBMCs), and (b) to evaluate *in vitro*, the effects of polyphenols from sweet cherry extracts on osteoclastogenesis, as possible dietary treatment to improve bone health in obesity.

MATERIALS AND METHODS

Subjects

Twenty-five obese children with a mean age of 10.8 ± 2.6 years were enrolled at Endocrinology Unit of Pediatric Hospital Giovanni XXIII, University A. Moro of Bari. Inclusion criteria were body mass index (BMI) ≥95th percentile for age and sex. Exclusion criteria were: type 2 diabetes mellitus, secondary or syndromic forms of obesity, hypothyroidism, Cushing disease, viral hepatitis, metabolic or genetic liver diseases, ongoing therapies for chronic systemic diseases. The control group consisted of 21 normal weight healthy children matched for age and gender, recruited on a voluntary basis in the outpatient clinic, who referred to hospital for minor surgery or electrocardiographic record for minor trauma to head, limbs, or chest pain. All the enrolled patients signed an informed consent form. The local ethic committee approved the study. The study was conducted in accordance to the criteria of the declaration of Helsinki. All subjects were in good general health and were not taking drugs in the last 3 months. Serum levels of (25)OH-vitamin D, osteocalcin, calcium, phosphorus, RANKL, OPG, and alkaline phosphatase were measured as previously reported (10). Bone quality was assessed by QUS measurements, performed with a DBM Sonic 1200 bone profiler (Igea S.r.l., Carpi, MO, Italy) employing a sound frequency of 1.25 MHz, as previously described (27).

Cells and Culture Conditions

PBMCs were isolated by centrifugation of peripheral blood samples over Histopaque 1077 density gradient (Sigma Chemical, St. Louis, MO), and cultured in α-MEM (Life Technologies, Paisley, UK) supplemented with 10% fetal bovine serum, 100 IU/ml penicillin, and 100 μg/ml streptomycin (Life Technologies, Inc. Ltd, Uxbridge, UK). To obtain fully differentiated human OCs, the PBMCs were cultured in the presence or absence of 25 ng/ml recombinant human MCSF and 30 ng/ml RANKL (R&D Systems, Minneapolis, MN) for about 20 days. In some experiments, PBMCs were also cultured in the presence of 75 and 100 μg/ml of polyphenol extracts from Giorgia, Bigarreau, and Ferrovia both for mRNA extraction (24 h), MTT assay (24 h) (28), and for osteoclastogenesis (about 20 days) evaluation. The concentrations of the polyphenol extracts were selected according to literature data (29) and calculated according to a previous *in vitro* study on the effect of quercetin-containing cherry extracts on HepG2 cells (30) by considering 440 dalton as the average molecular weight of the compounds in the extracts; then, they were prepared through vacuum drying of the extracts and re-suspension in a suitable medium for the biological assays. Mature OCs were identified as tartrate-resistant acid phosphatase-positive (TRAP) multinucleated cells (Sigma Aldrich, Milan, Italy) containing three or more nuclei. OC resorbing activity was demonstrated by plating the cells on multiwell slides (4×10^5 cells/well) coated with a calcium phosphate film (Millenium Osteologic; Millenium Biologix Inc, Ontario, Canada). This system incorporates a resorbable artificial bone in the form of submicron calcium phosphate films. The photomicrographs were obtained using a Ellipse E400 microscope (Nikon, Tokyo, Japan) equipped with Nikon Plan Fluor 10×/0.30 dicl. The microscope was connected with a Nikon digital camera DxM 1200; the acquisition software was Lucia G version 4.61 (build 0.64) for Nikon Italy.

Flow Cytometry Analysis

Fresh peripheral blood samples from patients and controls were stained with PerCp-CD14 and FITC-CD16 antibodies (all Beckmann Coulter, Milan, Italy). Events were acquired using C6 flow cytometer (Becton Dickinson Immunocytometry System, Mountain View, CA, USA). The area of positivity was determined using an isotype-matched mAb, a total of 10^6 events for each sample were acquired.

RNA Isolation and Real Time-PCR Amplification

Freshly isolated PBMCs of patients and controls, PBMCs treated for 24 h with polyphenol extracts from sweet cherries as well as OCs cultured in the presence of polyphenol extracts from sweet cherries were subjected to mRNA extraction using spin columns (RNeasy, QIAGEN, Hilden, Germany), and reverse-transcription using iScript Reverse Transcription Supermix (Bio-Rad Laboratories, Hercules, CA). The resulting cDNA was amplified using the SsoFast EvaGreen Supermix (Bio-Rad Laboratories) using the Chromo4 Real-Time PCR Detection System (Bio-Rad Laboratories). The following primer pairs were used for the real-time PCR amplification: RANKL S: CGTTGGATCACAGCACAT, RANKL AS: GCTCCTCTT GGCCAGTC; TNFα S: ATCTACTCCCAGGTCCTC, TNFα AS: GATGCGGCTGATGGTGT; calcitonin receptor (CalcR) S: AACAATAGAGCCCAAGCCATTTC, CalcR AS: CCAGCA CAGCCATCCATCC; Cathepsin K (Cath K) S: GGCTCAAGG TTCTGCTAC, Cath K AS: GCTTCCTGTGGGTCTTCTTCC; RANK S: CAGGATGCTCTCATTGGTCAG, RANK AS: AGA AAGGAGGTGTGGATTGC; GAPDH S: TCATCCCTGCCT CTACTG; AS: TGCTTCACCACCTTCTTG.

Reagents and Standards for Chemical Procedures

Formic acid, LC-MS grade water and acetonitrile were purchased from J.T. Baker (Deventer, Holland). Furulic acid, cyanidin-3-O-glucoside chloride, cyanidin-3-O-rutinoside chloride, delphinidin-3-O-glucoside chloride, quercetin-3-O-rutinoside, quercetin-3-O-glucoside, kaempferol-3-O-glucoside, kaempferol-3-O-rutinoside, isorhamnetin-3-O-glucoside, (+)-catechin, (-)-epicatechin, procyanidins B1 and B2, and epicatechin gallate were purchased from Extrasynthese (Genay, France). Cyanidin-3-O-sophoroside chloride, quercetin-4′-O-glucoside, chlorogenic acid, neochlorogenic acid, and cynarin were purchased from Phytolab (Vestenbergsgreuth, Germany).

Fruit Collection

Three sweet cherry cultivars (cv. Ferrovia, Bigarreau, and Giorgia) grown in Apulia region (Southern Italy) was used in this study. Samples were harvested at commercial maturity (1st decade of May—2nd decade of June), on the basis of total soluble solids (TSS), measured as °Brix using a portable refractometer (Atago PR32, Norfolk, Virginia, USA), and titratable acidity (TA) which was determined in the juice by titration with 0.1 N of NaOH (J.T. Baker, Deventer, Holland) to a pH 7 end point (TSS = ~ 17 °Brix; TA = ~ 7 g/L of citric acid equivalents), in 2014 season using 7 years-old sweet cherry trees located in Turi. The trees were trained to a central leader system and planted at a spacing of 4 m × 4 m and were grown under usual conditions of irrigation, fertilization, and pest control (31). Five kg of cherries for each variety were taken on the same day, from four different branches of an individual tree and mixed, then they were frozen in liquid nitrogen and vacuum packed in plastic bags and stored at −80°C for further analysis.

Extraction of Polyphenols From Sweet Cherry and HPLC-MS/MS Analysis

Polyphenols were extracted from cherries and analyzed through a capillary HPLC 1100 coupled with a triple quadrupole QQQ mass detector (Agilent Technologies Palo Alto, CA, U.S.A.), following the procedure proposed in our previous researches (31, 32).

Roughly 100 g of partially defrosted sweet cherry sample were pitted and a homogenate was obtained using an IKA A11—basic homogenizer (IKA—WERKE GMBH & CO.KG—Germany). To avoid compounds degradation, the homogenization was completed in darkness and the sample was placed on ice during the whole procedure (around 5 min). Ten gram of homogenate was put in a glass flask with 10 mL of 1%

hydroxybutyl anisole (BHA) in methanol and 100 μL of ferulic acid internal standard solution (1,000 μg/mL of methanol). Then, the obtained solution was sonicated in an ultrasonic bath of 130 W and 40 kHz (SONICA 2200 EP, SOLTEC, Milano, Italy) for 1 h at 25°C and the liquid phase was separated by filtration under vacuum. The extraction procedure was repeated twice for the solid phase utilizing fresh methanol (10 and 5 mL for 30 min, respectively). Finally, the pooled extracts were concentrated down to 10 mL through a rotavapor Buchi-R-205 under vacuum at 40°C, and stored at −25°C until further analysis.

A Zorbax column SC-C18 (50 × 2.1 mm i.d., particle size 1.8 μm, Agilent Technologies) was used, with the following gradient system: water/formic acid (99:1, v/v) (solvent A) and acetonitrile/formic acid (99:1, v/v) (solvent B), 0.8 min, 95% A−5% B; 2.1 min, 90% A−10% B; 5.6 min, 88% A−12% B; 8 min, 81% A−19% B; 9.2 min 81% A−12% B; 11.2 min 5% A−95% B; 12.8 min 5% A−95%; 13.2 min 95% A−5%; stop time 15 min. The column was kept at 60°C, the flow was maintained at 0.5 mL/min and the sample injection was 1.1 μL. Both positive and negative ESI mode was used for ionization of molecules with capillary voltage at 4,000 V. Nitrogen was used both as drying gas at a flow rate of 8 L/min and as nebulizing gas at a pressure of 30 psi. Temperature of drying gas was 350°C. In the full scan (MS) and product ion (MS/MS) modes, the monitored mass range was from *m/z* 100 to 1,200. Typically, 2 runs were performed during the HPLC-ESI-MS analysis of each sample. First, an MS full-scan acquisition was performed to obtain preliminary information on the predominant *m/z* ratios observed during the elution. An MS/MS full-scan acquisition was then performed: Quadrupole 1 filtered the calculated *m/z* of each compound of interest, while Quadrupole 3 scanned for ions produced by nitrogen collision of these ionized compounds in the chosen range at a scan time of 500 ms/cycle. All data were acquired and processed using Mass Hunter software (version B.01.04; Agilent Technologies). The optimized parameters (fragmentor voltage and collision energy) for each compound together with the mass transitions adopted for multiple reaction monitoring (MRM) are listed in **Table 1S** (Supporting Information). To gauge linearity, calibration curves with five/seven concentration points for each compound were prepared separately. Calibration was performed by linear regression of peak-area ratios of the polyphenols to the relative internal standard vs. the respective standard concentration.

Statistical Analyses

Means and standard deviations of the raw data and regression analysis of calibration samples were carried out using STATISTICA 6.0 software package (StatSoft Inc., Tulsa, OK, U.S.A.).

For statistical analyses of clinical data, the Statistical Package for the Social Sciences (SPSS) for Windows, version 22.0 (SPSS Inc., Chicago, IL, USA) was used. Comparison between groups were performed by *T*-test. Correlations were analyzed with Spearman or Pearson correlation test. The limit of statistical significance was set at 0.05.

TABLE 1 | Characteristics of study population.

	Controls $N = 21$	Obese patients $N = 25$
Gender (male/female)	9/12	9/16
Age (yr)	8.23 ± 3.19	10.8 ± 2.6
Tanner Stage (I, II, III, IV, V)	6,10,4,1,0	8,11,4,2,0
Height SDS	0.36 ± 1.02	0.23 ± 1.48
Weight SDS	0.43 ± 0.87	2.22 ± 0.70**
BMI-SDS	0.25 ± 0.78	2.31 ± 0.41**
Waist circumference (cm)	72.5 ± 7.2	92.04 ± 23.08**
Total cholesterol (mg/dl)	154.8 ± 28.32	164 ± 33.18
HDL (mg/dl)	55.67 ± 9.30	49.08 ± 8.13
LDL (mg/dl)	97.10 ± 21.03	107.54 ± 37.62
Triglycerides (mg/dl)	67.24 ± 19.16	73.00 ± 32.74
Insulin (microU/mL)	9.78 ± 4.50	24.60 ± 12.02**
Glucose (ml/dl)	81.16 ± 7.14	87.22 ± 11.35
HOMA-IR	2.56 ± 0.40	4.93 ± 1.91**
25-OH Vitamin D (ng/ml)	38.64 ± 14.70	29.70 ± 12.89
Osteocalcin (ng/ml)	38.26 ± 19.22	47.44 ± 21.02
PTH (pg/ml)	43.05 ± 15.06	44.07 ± 17.09
Calcium (mg/dl)	9.71 ± 0.40	9.43 ± 0.41
Phosphorus (mg/dl)	4.54 ± 1.4	4.54 ± 0.51
Ad-Sos-Z-score	0.48 ± 0.85	−1.05 ± 1.17*
BTT-Z-score	0.15 ± 0.72	−0.39 ± 1.23*
RANKL (pg/ml)	87.18 ± 17.82	115.48 ± 35.20§
OPG (pg/ml)	436.75 ± 95.53	378.02 ± 61.15§

*SDS, standard deviation score; BMI, body mass index; PTH, parathyroid hormone; Ca, calcium; P, phosphorus; B-ALP, bone alkaline phosphatase; RANKL, receptor activator of nuclear factor kappa-B ligand; OPG, osteoprotegerin. §p < 0.01; *p < 0.05; **p < 0.001.*

RESULTS

Clinical Characteristics

The characteristics of the study population were reported in **Table 1**. Although, in the normal range, lower Ad-SoS- and BTT-*Z*-scores were measured in obese patients compared to controls ($P < 0.05$). The serum levels of 25-OH Vitamin D, calcium, phosphorus, and osteocalcin were comparable to those measured in controls. Interestingly, higher RANKL levels were measured in obese patients with respect to the controls (115.48 ± 35.20 pg/ml vs. 87.18 ± 17.82 pg/ml; $p < 0.01$), while OPG levels were significantly reduced in obese patients than in controls (378.02 ± 61.15 pg/ml vs. 436.75 ± 95.53 pg/ml, respectively, $p < 0.01$). With adjustment for age RANKL levels correlated with waist circumference ($r = 0.144$ $p < 0.022$), and SDS-BMI ($r = 0.129$ $p < 0.038$), whereas OPG levels correlated with waist circumference ($r = -0.348$ $p < 0.0001$), SDS-BMI ($r = -0.381$ $p < 0.0001$), BTT-*Z*-score ($r = 0.208$ $p < 0.002$), HOMA-IR ($r = -0.359$ $p < 0.0001$).

Osteoclastogenesis in Obese Children and Adolescents

OC formation was evaluated in cultures of PBMCs from obese patients and controls. A significant elevated number of multinucleated TRAP^{+} OCs were counted in the un-stimulated cultures of obese patients (**Figure 1B**) compared to the controls (**Figure 1A**), as reported in the histogram (**Figure 1C**). The addition of the pro-osteoclastogenic M-CSF and RANKL in the cultures from patients did not affect the OC number, but they appear larger compared those observed in the un-stimulated cultures (**Figure 1E**). Indeed, the number of large OCs (>10 nuclei) was greater in stimulated compared with un-stimulated cultures from obese patients (35 ± 5 vs. 20 ± 6, $p < 0.01$). Conversely, M-CSF and RANKL are necessary to trigger OC formation in cultures from controls (**Figure 1D**), as reported in the histogram (**Figure 1F**).

To investigate the mechanisms of the enhanced osteoclastogenesis in obese we evaluated both the percentage of $CD14^+/CD16^+$ circulating pre-osteoclasts as well as the levels of the pro-osteoclastogenic cytokines RANKL and TNFα in PBMC extracts. Interestingly, patients displayed a high percentage of $CD14^+/CD16^+$, compared to the controls (**Figure 2**). Furthermore, in mRNA extracts of obese patients we detected a 2.5- and 2-fold increase of TNFα and RANKL transcripts compared to controls, respectively (**Figure 3**).

Effect of Polyphenols From Sweet Cherry on the Spontaneous Osteoclastogenesis of Obese Children and Adolescents

Interestingly, we also evaluated *in vitro* the effect of polyphenol cherry extracts on osteoclastogenesis as possible dietary treatment to improve bone health in obesity.

Polyphenols Content in the Cherries Extracts

Table 1S listed the amount of the main flavonoids (anthocyanins, flavan-3-ols, and flavonols) and chlorogenic acids, which were identified as previously described (31, 32), quantified by HPLC-MS/MS analyses in the tested cherries extracts. The content of the phenolic compounds appeared slightly lesser in the extract of Giorgia (1,391 mg/100 g FW) than Bigarreu and Ferrovia (1,820 and 1,768 mg/100 g FW, respectively), even though both the three varieties were principally characterized by anthocyanins, especially cyanidin-3O-rutinoside, accounting for 19–30% of total polyphenols, and chlorogenic acids (particularly, *trans*-3-O-coumaroylquinic acid and *trans*-3-O-caffeoylquinic acid) ranging between 70 and 80% of the total polyphenols (**Table 1S**).

Polyphenols Effect on Osteoclastogenesis of Obese Children and Adolescents

We investigated the effect of polyphenol extracts from Giorgia, Bigarreau, and Ferrovia on PBMC cultures of patients. We demonstrated that each extract determined a dose-dependent reduction in the formation of multinucleated $TRAP^+$ OCs (**Figures 4A–C**). Furthermore, using the highest dose of polyphenol extracts from Giorgia, Bigarreau, and Ferrovia we demonstrated that the treatment also resulted in a significant reduction of resorption activity (**Figure 4D**), together with a significant reduction of the expression of OC marker genes, such as calcitonin receptor, cathepsin K and RANK (**Figure 4E**). Consistently, 24 h treatment of PBMCs from patients with polyphenol extracts from Giorgia, Bigarreau, and Ferrovia resulted in a significant reduction of the expression of TNFα (**Figure 5A**), whereas RANKL levels were unchanged (**Figure 5B**). Furthermore, by MTT we demonstrated that polyphenol extracts did not significantly affect cell viability of PBMCs from patients (**Figure 6**). These results suggested that polyphenols from sweet cherry inhibit osteoclastogenesis through the reduction of pro-osteoclastogenic cytokines, without affecting cell viability.

DISCUSSION

This study demonstrated that in obese children the reduced bone mineral density (BMD) is associated to the decrease of OPG levels, the increase of RANKL levels, enhanced formation of OCs, of circulating pre-osteoclasts, and pro-osteoclastogenic cytokines. Interestingly, the spontaneous osteoclastogenesis is inhibited *in vitro* by sweet cherry polyphenol extracts.

Previous studies demonstrated that obese subjects showed significantly lower OPG levels respect to the controls (33–35); however no correlation has been reported between OPG and BMI (36, 37). Otherwise, few studies measured higher levels of OPG in obese subjects compared with the controls (38, 39). However, all the previous studies correlated the levels of OPG with the altered HOMA-IR, fasting insulin or glucose. Our study, to our knowledge, is the first demonstrating a direct correlation between OPG levels and BTT-Z score in obese children.

It is known that obesity is associated with bone fragility and the reduced OPG levels could contribute to this status. We also found increased RANKL levels which could explain the bone impairment associated with excess of adipose tissue. Interestingly, we found that RANKL levels positively correlated with waist circumference. The correlation between a central obesity parameter, as the waist circumference, and RANKL levels detected in serum and saliva samples has been previously demonstrated (40). Our data confirmed that visceral fat accumulation represents the main parameter which can predict the entity of bone impairment in obese subjects. These findings also suggest to evaluate bone status in obese subjects with a higher waist circumference than normal values. It is known that RANKL and OPG altered levels have been associated to the altered osteoclastogenesis characterizing bone diseases (41–43). Indeed, it has been demonstrated that anti-RANKL antibody is useful in the treatment of osteoporosis (44). The alterations of OPG and RANKL levels together with the increase of $CD14^+/CD16^+$ circulating pre-osteoclasts and TNFα levels are consistent with the spontaneous osteoclastogenesis of our obese patients as well as of other inflammatory diseases associated with bone loss (45). $CD14^+/CD16^+$ cells have been linked with erosive bone diseases, such as psoriatic arthritis and multiple myeloma (46–48). It is known that $CD14^+/CD16^+$ cells display an enhanced pro-osteoclastogenic activity (47, 48) thus supporting the key role of this cells in the alteration of bone health in obesity. Consistently, rodent models of obesity also demonstrated the increase of OC precursors in the bone marrow (49). Consistently, the ongoing theory sustains that weight gain determines local inflammation

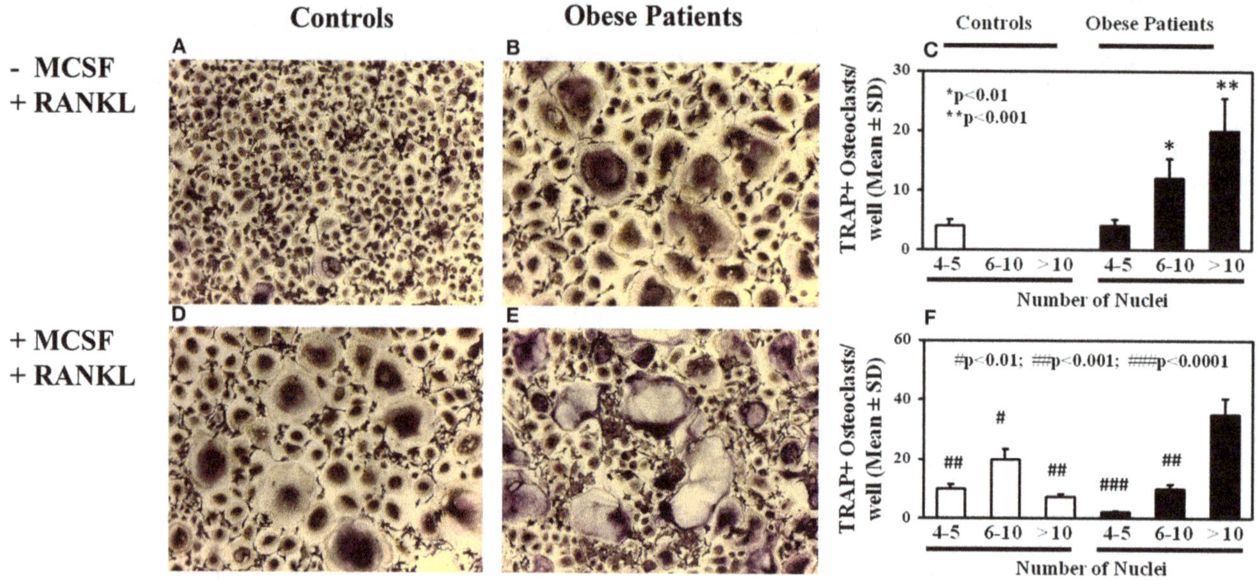

FIGURE 1 | Osteoclastogenesis in obese subjects. Osteoclasts (OCs) identified as tartrate-resistant acid phosphatase-positive (TRAP$^+$) and multinucleated cells with three or more nuclei, differentiated from peripheral blood mononuclear cells (PBMCs) of obese subjects and controls. Few small OCs differentiated in un-stimulated PBMC cultures of a representative control **(A)**, whereas multinucleated TRAP$^+$ OCs differentiated from un-stimulated PBMCs from a representative obese subject **(B)**. The histogram includes OC count deriving from all subjects' cultures, stratified according the number of nuclei per OC **(C)**. In PBMC cultures from the controls, OCs differentiate following MCSF and RANKL addition **(D)**, otherwise in cultures from obese subjects growth factor addition did not further increase osteoclastogenesis **(E)**, compared with the un-stimulated cultures. The histogram reports the results deriving from all the enrolled subjects **(F)**.

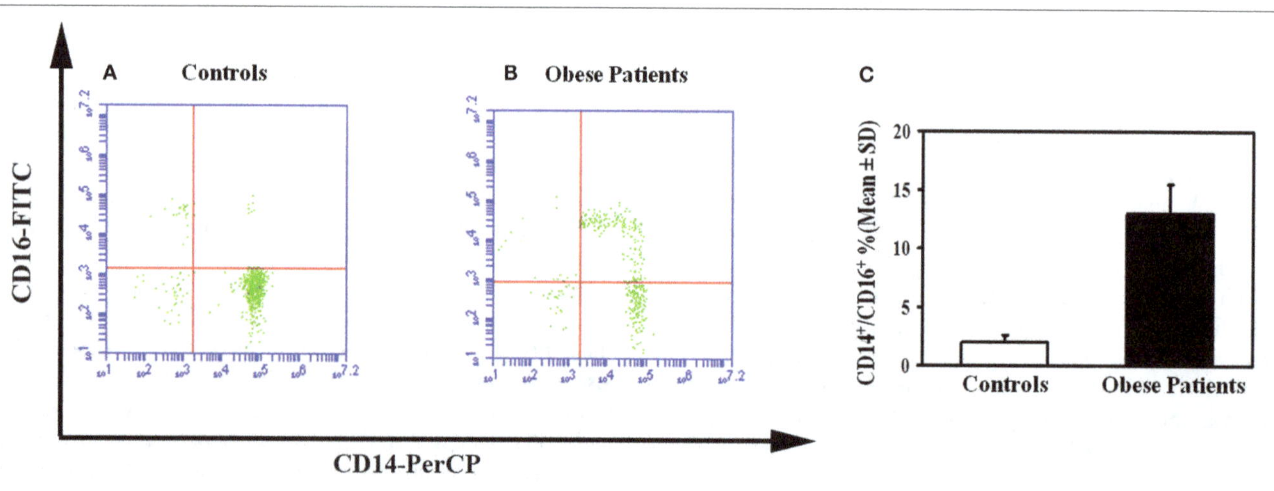

FIGURE 2 | Circulating osteoclast precursors in obese subjects. A representative flow cytometry dot plots displayed the percentage of circulating osteoclast precursors, identified as CD14$^+$/16$^+$ cells in control **(A)** and obese subjects **(B)**. The histograms represent the percentage of CD14$^+$/CD16$^+$ cells measured for all enrolled obese and control subjects by flow cytometry **(C)**.

that stimulate the increased recruitment of circulating pro-inflammatory (Ly6C^{hi}) monocytes, also capable of differentiate in OCs in bone. Recruited monocytes differentiate into an M1 macrophage phenotype which is responsible of the chronic inflammation and thus organ damage associated to obesity (15).

An increased mRNA levels of pro-osteoclastogenic molecules such as RANKL and TNFα has been found in young mice fed with HFD (6). Interestingly, our results also displayed high mRNA levels of TNFα and RANKL in PBMCs from obese subjects. It has been reported that childhood obesity is associated to a state of chronic low-grade inflammation as well as numerous inflammation-related molecules such as TNFα, interleukin 6 (IL-6), and leptin. High levels of these molecules have been linked to co-morbidities associated to obesity (50–53). Furthermore, consisting with our results, transgenic mouse expressing human TNFα determines the augment of OC precursor percentage (54).

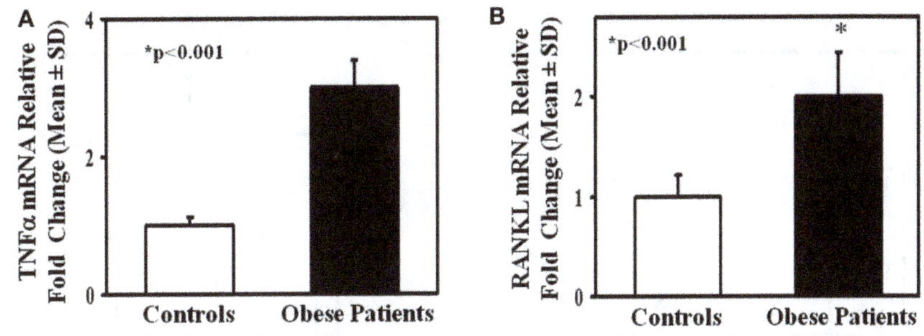

FIGURE 3 | TNFα and RANKL expression in lymphomonocytes from obese subjects. mRNA levels of TNFα **(A)** and RANKL **(B)** in lymphomonocytes from all enrolled controls and obese subjects. Obese subjects expressed higher levels of TNFα and RANKL compared to the controls.

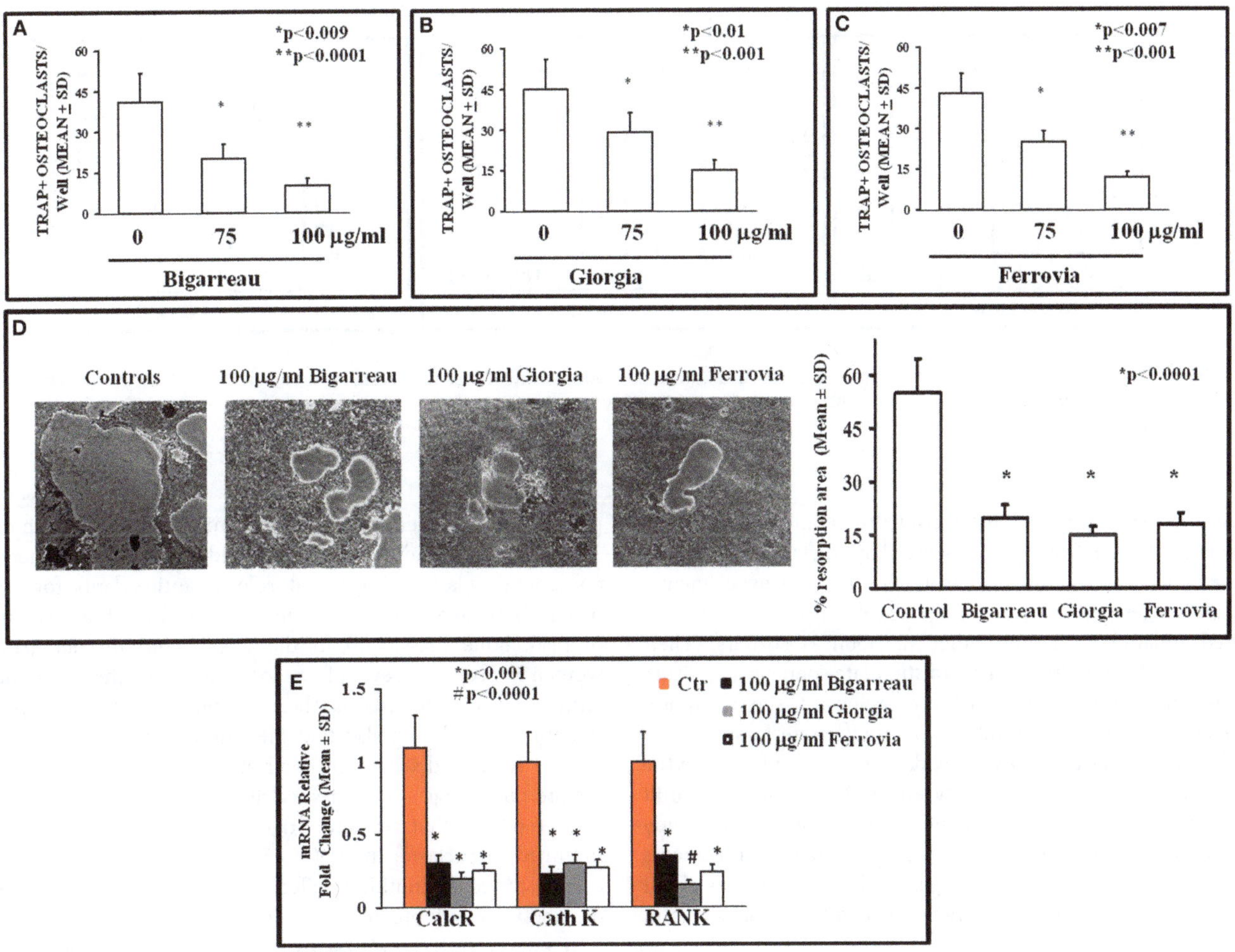

FIGURE 4 | Osteoclastogenesis inhibition by polyphenol extracts from Giorgia, Bigarreau, and Ferrovia. The formation of multinucleated TRAP$^+$ OCs was evaluated in un-stimulated PBMCs from all obese patients cultured in the absence or presence of 75 and 100 µg/ml polyphenol extracts from Bigarreau **(A)**, Giorgia **(B)**, and Ferrovia **(C)**. PBMCs from the patients, cultured on Millenium slides coated with a calcium phosphate film, formed large resorption areas, that were reduced following the treatment with 100 µg/ml polyphenol extracts from Bigarreau, Giorgia, and Ferrovia, as quantified in the histogram **(D)**. The mRNA levels of calcitonin receptor (CalcR), cathepsin K (Cath K), and RANK was evaluated in PBMCs from obese patients cultured in the absence or presence of 100 µg/ml polyphenol extracts from Bigarreau, Giorgia, and Ferrovia **(E)**.

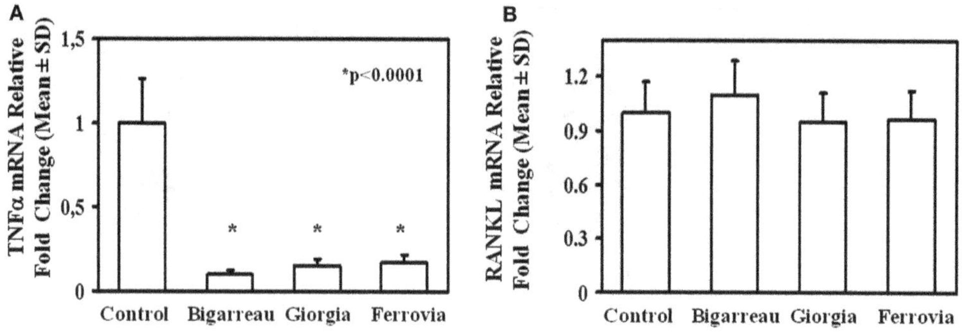

FIGURE 5 | RANKL and TNFα expression in lymphomonocytes from obese subjects. Twenty-four hours treatment of PBMCs from obese subjects with 100 μg/ml polyphenol extracts from Giorgia, Bigarreau, and Ferrovia resulted in a significant reduction of the mRNA levels of TNFα **(A)**, whereas RANKL levels were unchanged **(B)**. The results are referred to all obese subjects.

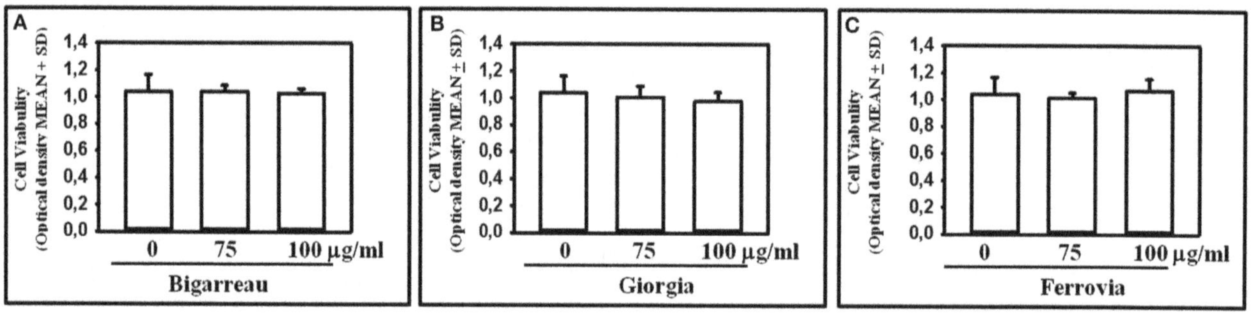

FIGURE 6 | Effect of Polyphenol extracts from Giorgia, Bigarreau, and Ferrovia on PBMC viability. PBMCs were treated for 24 h with 75 and 100 μg/ml polyphenol extracts from Bigarreau **(A)**, Giorgia **(B)**, and Ferrovia **(C)** and analyzed by MTT assay to evaluate cell viability. Results are expressed as mean values of optical density at 570 nm ± standard deviation (SD).

As countermeasure against chronic low-grade inflammation associated to obesity is represented by dietary advice and nutraceuticals (55). Evidences from *in vitro* and experimental models suggest the effects of polyphenols on obesity, obesity-related inflammation, and other metabolic disorders. Their effects include: to induce satiety, to stimulate energy expenditure by inducing thermogenesis in brown adipose tissue, to inhibit adipocyte differentiation and promote adipocyte apoptosis, to modulate lipolysis and activate oxidation (56). Evidence for the effects of polyphenols on obesity and weight control in adult subjects is inconsistent due to the heterogeneity among study populations, intervention period, and polyphenol supplements (57). At the best of our knowledge, there are no studies about the effects of polyphenols extracts on childhood obesity and its comorbidities.

The innovative aspect of this study is related to the inhibition of the spontaneous osteoclastogenesis and reduction of TNFα mRNA levels in PBMC cultures from obese children with the use of polyphenol-rich cherry extracts. This inhibitory effect has been observed with all the three cultivars of sweet cherries, although the content of the phenolic compounds appeared slightly lesser in the extract of Giorgia than Bigarreu and Ferrovia, even though both the three varieties were principally characterized by anthocyanins, especially cyanidin-3O-rutinoside, and chlorogenic acids. These polyphenols' compounds play an important role as antioxidants for bone health, both in young people, in order to favor the formation of peak bone mass, and in the elderly and in menopausal women in order to prevent bone loss. Moreover, the use of these antioxidant compounds has been proposed in anti-resorption therapies considering also that they are able to reduce the OC activity without determining their apoptosis, which is useful to restore physiological bone remodeling (58). Consistently, it has been reported that tea and dried plum polyphenols *in vitro* inhibited osteoclastogenesis (29, 59). Of note, it has also been demonstrated the inhibitory effects of sweet cherry anthocyanins on obesity development in HFD fed mice, by slowing down TNFα and IL-6 levels (60). However, this study did not evaluate the effect on bone, which is known to be negatively affected by obesity as well as by HFD. Conversely, Shen et al., reported that in rats green tea polyphenols improved bone health in HFD-induced obesity by the suppression of bone cell activity (61, 62). Although the positive effect of green tea administration in obese patients has been evaluated in different studies [revised in Suzuki et al. (63)], there were not published data on bone effects. These literature reports together with our findings let us to speculate that also sweet cherry polyphenols can have a protective effect on bone both in HFD fed mice and obese patients.

CONCLUSIONS

Our study, to our knowledge, is the first demonstrating in obese children a spontaneous osteoclastogenesis inhibited by polyphenols from sweet cherry extracts, through the reduction of TNFα, without affecting cell viability. We also demonstrated that the spontaneous osteoclastogenesis observed in PBMCs from obese children is supported by the high percentage of circulating $CD14^{+}/CD16^{+}$ cells and the elevated levels of RANKL and TNFα. Our study opens future perspectives for the use of cherry extracts, appropriately formulated as nutraceuticals as preventive in healthy children and therapeutic in obese ones.

AUTHOR CONTRIBUTIONS

GB, MF, and FC developed the concept and designed the experiments. GC performed most experiments and analyzed data. LP performed cell cultures and ELISA. SB and GS performed flow cytometry. MF and GD provided patients' samples and clinical data. FC, ACi, ACo, GM, MC, PC, and CF developed the chemical part of the paper. GB, MF, FC, and MC wrote the manuscript and all other authors commented on the manuscript.

FUNDING

This work was supported by EU through the Regione Puglia: Avviso aiuti a sostegno dei Cluster Tecnologici Regionali per l'Innovazione—Progetto: PERFORM TECH (PUGLIA EMERGING FOOD TECHNOLOGY)—La sicurezza alimentare mediante l'impiego di tecnologie emergenti per l'elaborazione di prodotti funzionali, recupero di sostanze nutraceutiche dai sottoprodotti e valorizzazione energetica degli scarti (grant number LPIJ9P2).

REFERENCES

1. Faienza MF, Acquafredda A, Tesse R, Luce V, Ventura A, Maggialetti N, et al. Risk factors for subclinical atherosclerosis in diabetic and obese children. *Int J Med Sci.* (2013) 10:338–43. doi: 10.7150/ijms.5181
2. Styne DM, Arslanian SA, Connor EL, Farooqi IS, Murad MH, Silverstein JH, et al. Pediatric obesity-assessment, treatment, and prevention: an endocrine society clinical practice guideline. *J Clin Endocrinol Metab.* (2017) 102:709–57. doi: 10.1210/jc.2017-00561
3. Cao JJ. Effects of obesity on bone metabolism. *J Orthop Surg Res.* (2011) 6:30. doi: 10.1186/1749-799X-6-30
4. Dimitri P. Fat and bone in children - where are we now? *Ann Pediatr Endocrinol Metab.* (2018) 23:62–9. doi: 10.6065/apem.2018.23.2.62
5. Rana AR, Michalsky MP, Teich S, Groner JI, Caniano DA, Schuster DP. Childhood obesity: a risk factor for injuries observed at a level-1 trauma center. *J Pediatr Surg.* (2009) 44:1601–5. doi: 10.1016/j.jpedsurg.2008.11.060
6. Shu L, Beier E, Sheu T, Zhang H, Zuscik MJ, Puzas EJ. High-fat diet causes bone loss in young mice by promoting osteoclastogenesis through alteration of the bone marrow environment. *Calcif Tissue Int.* (2015) 96:313–23. doi: 10.1007/s00223-015-9954-z
7. Dar HY, Azam Z, Anupam R, Mondal RK, Srivastava RK. Osteoimmunology: the Nexus between bone and immune system. *Front Biosci.* (2018) 23:464–92. doi: 10.2741/4600
8. Fan Y, Hanai JI, Le PT, Bi R, Maridas D, DeMambro V, et al. Parathyroid hormone directs bone marrow mesenchymal cell fate. *Cell Metab.* (2017) 25:661–72. doi: 10.1016/j.cmet.2017.01.001
9. Lam J, Takeshita S, Barker JE, Kanagawa O, Ross FP, Teitelbaum SL. TNF-alpha induces osteoclastogenesis by direct stimulation of macrophages exposed to permissive levels of RANK ligand. *J Clin Invest.* (2000) 106:1481–8. doi: 10.1172/JCI11176
10. Brunetti G, Papadia F, Tummolo A, Fischetto R, Nicastro F, Piacente L, et al. Impaired bone remodeling in children with osteogenesis imperfecta treated and untreated with bisphosphonates: the role of DKK1, RANKL, and TNF-α. *Osteoporos Int.* (2016) 27:2355–65. doi: 10.1007/s00198-016-3501-2
11. D'Amelio P, Grimaldi A, Pescarmona GP, Tamone C, Roato I, Isaia G. Spontaneous osteoclast formation from peripheral blood mononuclear cells in postmenopausal osteoporosis. *FASEB J.* (2005) 19:410–2. doi: 10.1096/fj.04-2214fje
12. Ritchlin CT, Haas-Smith SA, Li P, Hicks DG, Schwarz EM. Mechanisms of TNF-alpha- and RANKL-mediated osteoclastogenesis and bone resorption in psoriatic arthritis. *J Clin Invest.* (2003) 111:821–31. doi: 10.1172/JCI16069
13. Arslan N, Erdur B, Aydin A. Hormones and cytokines in childhood obesity. *Indian Pediatr.* (2010) 47:829–39. doi: 10.1007/s13312-010-0142-y
14. Faienza MF, Francavilla R, Goffredo R, Ventura A, Marzano F, Panzarino G, et al. Oxidative stress in obesity and metabolic syndrome in children and adolescents. *Horm Res Paediatr.* (2012) 78:158–64. doi: 10.1159/000342642
15. Kraakman MJ, Murphy AJ, Jandeleit-Dahm K, Kammoun HL. Macrophage polarization in obesity and type 2 diabetes: weighing down our understanding of macrophage function? *Front Immunol.* (2014) 5:470. doi: 10.3389/fimmu.2014.00470
16. Goran MI, Alderete TL. Targeting adipose tissue inflammation to treat the underlying basis of the metabolic complications of obesity. *Nestle Nutr Inst Work Ser.* (2012) 73:49–60. doi: 10.1159/000341287
17. Abramson JL, Vaccarino V. Relationship between physical activity and inflammation among apparently healthy middle-aged and older US adults. *Arch Intern Med.* (2002) 162:1286–92. doi: 10.1001/archinte.162.1 1.1286
18. Geffken DF, Cushman M, Burke GL, Polak JF, Sakkinen PA, Tracy RP. Tracy association between physical activity and markers of inflammation in a healthy elderly population. *Am J Epidemiol.* (2001) 153:242–50. doi: 10.1093/aje/153.3.242
19. Pischon T, Hankinson SE, Hotamisligil GS, Rifai N, Rimm EB. Leisure-time physical activity and reduced plasma levels of obesity-related inflammatory markers. *Obes Res.* (2003) 11:1055–64. doi: 10.1038/oby.2003.145
20. Siriwardhana N, Kalupahana NS, Cekanova M, LeMieux M, Greer B, Moustaid-Moussa N. Modulation of adipose tissue inflammation by bioactive food compounds. *J Nutr Biochem.* (2013) 24:613–23. doi: 10.1016/j.jnutbio.2012.12.013
21. Kalupahana NS, Claycombe KJ, Moustaid-Moussa N. (n-3) Fatty acids alleviate adipose tissue inflammation and insulin resistance: mechanistic insights. *Adv Nutr.* (2011) 2:304–16. doi: 10.3945/an.111.000505
22. Picariello G, De Vito V, Ferranti P, Paolucci M, Volpe M. Species- and cultivar-dependent traits of Prunus avium and Prunus cerasus polyphenols. *J Food Comp Anal.* (2016) 40:50–7. doi: 10.1016/j.jfca.2015.10.002

23. Girelli CR, De Pascali SA, Del Coco L, Fanizzi FP. Metabolic profile comparison of fruit juice from certified sweet cherry trees (Prunus avium L.) of Ferrovia and Giorgia cultivars: a preliminary study. *Food Res Int.* (2016) 90:281–7. doi: 10.1016/j.foodres.2016.11.014
24. Yigit D, Baydas E, Güleryüz M. Elemental analysis of various cherry fruits by wavelength dispersive X-ray fluorescence spectrometry. *Asian J Chem.* (2009) 21:2935–42.
25. Schmitz-Eiberger MA, Blanke MM. Bioactive components in forced sweet cherry fruit (Prunus avium L.), antioxidative capacity and allergenic potential as dependent on cultivation under cover. *LWT Food Sci Technol.* (2012) 46:388–92. doi: 10.1016/j.lwt.2011.12.015
26. Kelley DS, Adkins Y, Laugero KD. A review of the health benefits of cherries. *Nutrients.* (2018) 10:E368. doi: 10.3390/nu10030368
27. Faienza MF, Ventura A, Delvecchio M, Fusillo A, Piacente L, Aceto G, et al. High sclerostin and Dickkopf-1 (DKK-1) serum levels in children and adolescents with type 1 diabetes mellitus. *J Clin Endocrinol Metab.* (2017) 102:1174–81. doi: 10.1210/jc.2016-2371
28. Mori G, Brunetti G, Colucci S, Ciccolella F, Coricciati M, Pignataro P, et al. Alteration of activity and survival of osteoblasts obtained from human periodontitis patients: role of TRAIL. *J Biol Regul Homeost Agents.* (2007) 21:105–14.
29. Oka Y, Iwai S, Amano H, Irie Y, Yatomi K, Ryu K, et al. Tea polyphenols inhibit rat osteoclast formation and differentiation. *J Pharmacol Sci.* (2012) 118:55–64. doi: 10.1254/jphs.11082FP
30. Snyder SM, Zhao B, Luo T, Kaiser C, Cavender G, Hamilton-Reeves J, et al. Consumption of quercetin and quercetin-containing apple and cherry extracts affects blood glucose concentration, hepatic metabolism, and gene expression patterns in obese C57BL/6J high fat-fed mice. *J Nutr.* (2016) 146:1001–7. doi: 10.3945/jn.115.228817
31. Crupi P, Genghi R, Antonacci D. In-time and in-space tandem mass spectrometry to determine the metabolic profiling of flavonoids in a typical sweet cherry (Prunus avium L.) cultivar from Southern Italy. *J Mass Spectrom.* (2014) 49:1025–34. doi: 10.1002/jms.3423
32. Crupi P, Bleve G, Tufariello M, Corbo F, Clodoveo ML, Tarricone L. Comprehensive identification and quantification of chlorogenic acids in sweet cherry by tandem mass spectrometry techniques. *J Food Comp Anal.* (2018) 73:103–11. doi: 10.1016/j.jfca.2018.06.013
33. Ugur-Altun B, Altun A, Gerenli M, Tugrul A. The relationship between insulin resistance assessed by HOMA-IR and serum osteoprotegerin levels in obesity. *Diabetes Res Clin Pract.* (2005) 68:217–22. doi: 10.1016/j.diabres.2004.10.011
34. Holecki M, Zahorska-Markiewicz B, Janowska J, Nieszporek T, Wojaczynska-Stanek K, Zak-Golab A, et al. The influence of weight loss on serum osteoprotegerin concentration in obese perimenopausal women. *Obesity.* (2007) 15:1925–9. doi: 10.1038/oby.2007.229
35. Erol M, Bostan Gayret O, Tekin Nacaroglu H, Yigit O, Zengi O, Salih Akkurt M, et al. Association of osteoprotegerin with obesity, insulin resistance and non-alcoholic fatty liver disease in children. *Iran Red Crescent Med J.* (2016) 18:e41873. doi: 10.5812/ircmj.41873
36. Gannage-Yared MH, Fares F, Semaan M, Khalife S, Jambart S. Circulating osteoprotegerin is correlated with lipid profile, insulin sensitivity, adiponectin and sex steroids in an ageing male population. *Clin Endocrinol.* (2006) 64:652–8. doi: 10.1111/j.1365-2265.2006.02522.x
37. Gannagé-Yared MH, Yaghi C, Habre B, Khalife S, Noun R, Germanos-Haddad M, et al. Osteoprotegerin in relation to body weight, lipid parameters insulin sensitivity, adipocytokines, and C-reactive protein in obese and non-obese young individuals: results from both cross-sectional and interventional study. *Eur J Endocrinol.* (2008) 158:353–9. doi: 10.1530/EJE-07-0797
38. Kotanidou EP, Kotanidis CP, Giza S, Serbis A, Tsinopoulou VR, Karalazou P, et al. Osteoprotegerin increases parallel to insulin resistance in obese adolescents. *Endocr Res.* (2018) 44:1–7. doi: 10.1080/07435800.2018.1480630
39. Suliburska J, Bogdanski P, Gajewska E, Kalmus G, Sobieska M, Samborski W. The association of insulin resistance with serum osteoprotegerin in obese adolescents. *J Physiol Biochem.* (2013) 69:847–53. doi: 10.1007/s13105-013-0261-8
40. Serrano-Piña R, Trujillo-Güiza ML, Scougall Vilchis RJ, Layton-Tovar CF, Mendieta-Zerón H. sRANKL and its correlation with metabolic syndrome parameters in children. *Int J Paediatr Dent.* (2018) 28:633–40. doi: 10.1111/ipd.12422
41. Ventura A, Brunetti G, Colucci S, Oranger A, Ladisa F, Cavallo L, et al. Glucocorticoid-induced osteoporosis in children with 21-hydroxylase deficiency. *Biomed Res Int.* (2013) 2013:250462. doi: 10.1155/2013/250462
42. Brunetti G, Marzano F, Colucci S, Ventura A, Cavallo L, Grano M, et al. Genotype-phenotype correlation in juvenile Paget disease: role of molecular alterations of the TNFRSF11B gene. *Endocrine.* (2012) 42:266–71. doi: 10.1007/s12020-012-9705-0
43. Terpos E, Ntanasis-Stathopoulos I, Gavriatopoulou M, Dimopoulos MA. Pathogenesis of bone disease in multiple myeloma: from bench to bedside. *Blood Cancer J.* (2018) 8:7. doi: 10.1038/s41408-017-0037-4
44. Faienza MF, Chiarito M, D'Amato G, Colaianni G, Colucci S, Grano M, et al. Monoclonal antibodies for treating osteoporosis. *Expert Opin Biol Ther.* (2018) 18:149–57. doi: 10.1080/14712598.2018.1401607
45. de Vries TJ, El Bakkali I, Kamradt T, Schett G, Jansen IDC, D'Amelio P. What are the peripheral blood determinants for increased osteoclast formation in the various inflammatory diseases associated with bone loss? *Front Immunol.* (2019) 10:505. doi: 10.3389/fimmu.2019.00505
46. Wong KL, Yeap WH, Tai JJ, Ong SM, Dang TM, Wong SC. The three human monocyte subsets: implications for health and disease. *Immunol Res.* (2012) 53:41–57. doi: 10.1007/s12026-012-8297-3
47. Chiu YG, Shao T, Feng C, Mensah KA, Thullen M, Schwarz EM, et al. CD16 (FcRgammaIII) as a potential marker of osteoclast precursors in psoriatic arthritis. *Arthritis Res Ther.* (2010) 12:R14. doi: 10.1186/ar2915
48. Bolzoni M, Ronchetti D, Storti P, Donofrio G, Marchica V, Costa F, et al. IL21R expressing CD14+CD16+ monocytes expand in multiple myeloma patients leading to increased osteoclasts. *Haematologica.* (2017) 102:773–84. doi: 10.3324/haematol.2016.153841
49. Ootsuka T, Nakanishi A, Tsukamoto I. Increase in osteoclastogenesis in an obese Otsuka Long-Evans Tokushima fatty rat model. *Mol Med Rep.* (2015) 12:3874–80. doi: 10.3892/mmr.2015.3811
50. Singer K, Lumeng CN. The initiation of metabolic inflammation in childhood obesity. *J Clin Invest.* (2017) 127:65–73. doi: 10.1172/JCI88882
51. Martí A, Marcos A, Martínez JA. Obesity and immune function relationships. *Obes Rev.* (2001) 2:131–40. doi: 10.1046/j.1467-789x.2001.00025.x
52. Dedoussis GV, Kapiri A, Samara A, Dimitriadis D, Lambert D, Pfister M, et al. Expression of inflammatory molecules and associations with BMI in children. *Eur J Clin Invest.* (2010) 40:388–92. doi: 10.1111/j.1365-2362.2010.02277.x
53. Reinehr T, Stoffel-Wagner B, Roth CL, Andler W. High-sensitive C-reactive protein, tumor necrosis factor alpha, and cardiovascular risk factors before and after weight loss in obese children. *Metabolism.* (2005) 54:1155–61. doi: 10.1016/j.metabol.2005.03.022
54. Yao Z, Li P, Zhang Q, Schwarz EM, Keng P, Arbini A, et al. Tumor necrosis factor-alpha increases circulating osteoclast precursor numbers by promoting their proliferation and differentiation in the bone marrow through up-regulation of c-Fms expression. *J Biol Chem.* (2006) 281:11846–55. doi: 10.1074/jbc.M512624200
55. Yarla NS, Polito A, Peluso I. Effects of olive oil on TNF-α and IL-6 in humans: implication in obesity and frailty. *Endocr Metab Immune Disord Drug Targets.* (2018) 18:63–74. doi: 10.2174/1871530317666171120150329
56. Rupasinghe HPV, Sekhon-Loodu S, Mantso T, Panayiotidis MI. Phytochemicals in regulating fatty acids -oxidation: potential underlying mechanisms and their involvement in obesity and weight loss. *Pharmacol Ther.* (2016) 165:153–63. doi: 10.1016/j.pharmthera.2016.06.005
57. Castro-Barquero S, Lamuela-Raventós RM, Doménech M, Estruch R. Relationship between mediterranean dietary polyphenol intake and obesity. *Nutrients.* (2018) 10:1523. doi: 10.3390/nu10101523
58. Domazetovic V, Marcucci G, Iantomasi T, Brandi ML, Vincenzini MT. Oxidative stress in bone remodeling: role of antioxidants. *Clin Cases Miner Bone Metab.* (2017) 14:209–16. doi: 10.11138/ccmbm/2017.14.1.209
59. Bu SY, Lerner M, Stoecker BJ, Boldrin E, Brackett DJ, Lucas EA, et al. Dried plum polyphenols inhibit osteoclastogenesis by downregulating NFATc1 and inflammatory mediators. *Calcif Tissue Int.* (2008) 82:475–88. doi: 10.1007/s00223-008-9139-0
60. Wu T, Tang Q, Yu Z, Gao Z, Hu H, Chen W, et al. Inhibitory effects of sweet cherry anthocyanins on the obesity development in C57BL/6 mice. *Int J Food Sci Nutr.* (2014) 65:351–9. doi: 10.3109/09637486.2013.854749

61. Shen CL, Chyu MC, Cao JJ, Yeh JK. Green tea polyphenols improve bone microarchitecture in high-fat-diet-induced obese female rats through suppressing bone formation and erosion. *J Med Food.* (2013) 16:421–7. doi: 10.1089/jmf.2012.0199
62. Shen CL, Han J, Wang S, Chung E, Chyu MC, Cao JJ. Green tea supplementation benefits body composition and improves bone properties in obese female rats fed with high-fat diet and caloric restricted diet. *Nutr Res.* (2015) 35:1095–105. doi: 10.1016/j.nutres.2015.09.014
63. Suzuki T, Pervin M, Goto S, Isemura M, Nakamura Y. Beneficial effects of tea and the green tea catechin epigallocatechin-3-gallate on obesity. *Molecules.* (2016) 21:E1305. doi: 10.3390/molecules21101305

12

Modulatory Effects of Plant Polyphenols on Bone Remodeling: A Prospective View from the Bench to Bedside

Vanessa Nicolin [1], Nunziatina De Tommasi [2], Stefania Lucia Nori [2], Fulvia Costantinides [3], Federico Berton [3] and Roberto Di Lenarda [1]*

[1] Clinical Department of Medical, Surgical and Health Sciences, University of Trieste, Trieste, Italy, [2] Pharmacy-DIFARMA Department, University of Salerno, Fisciano, Italy, [3] School of Dental Sciences, University of Trieste, Trieste, Italy

Correspondence:
Vanessa Nicolin
nicolin@units.it

During the past, a more comprehensive knowledge of mechanisms implicated in bone resorption processes has driven researchers to develop a compound library of many small molecules that specifically interfere with the genesis of osteoclast precursors cells. Natural compounds that suppress osteoclast commitment may have therapeutic value in treating pathologies associated with bone resorption like osteoporosis, rheumatoid arthritis, bone metastasis, and periodontal disease. The present review is focused on the current knowledge on the polyphenols derived from plants that could be efficacious in suppressing osteoclast differentiation and bone resorption.

Keywords: biomolecules, polyflavonoids, bone remodeling, titanium implant, coating surfaces

INTRODUCTION

Bone Cells and Cell Guest Outsider

The strength and integrity of the human skeleton depends on a delicate balance between bone resorption and formation. Bone resorption represents a final step due to the interaction between cells that involve resorption of bone (osteoclasts, OC), and that synthetize bone matrix (osteoblasts, OB). Bone remodeling allows to adapt bone tissue to mechanical forces and to maintain phosphocalcic homeostasis through coordinated steps of formation and resorption (1, 2).

This equilibrium is close controlled by physical parameters (i.e., mechanical stimulations) and several polypeptides (hormones, cytokines) (3, 4). In addition, bone remodeling cycle maintains the integrity of the skeleton through the balanced action of its cell types.

Cells responsible for bone resorption include (1) bone-forming osteoblast, a cell that produces the organic bone extracellular matrix; (2) the bone resorbing osteoclast that dissolves bone mineral and enzymatically degrades extracellular matrix and inorganic components (5); (3) osteocyte, the maturative phase of osteoblast that acts as a mechanosensor and like an endocrine cell (6); (4) the bone lining cell, that probably may have a role in coupling bone resorption to bone formation (7).

Basically, osteoblasts and osteoclasts (and their precursors) are the central players of bone remodeling and each factor that affects these cells, in the end, affects all the process.

Numerous signaling pathways carry on the activities of osteoblast and osteoclast cells and these include nuclear factor kappa-light-chain-enhancer of activated B cells (RANkL) and Bone Morphogenetic Protein (BMP) (8). RANkL/RANK signaling axes regulates osteoclast recruitment and sustenance in normal bone modeling and remodeling and is adversely regulated by osteoprotegerin (OPG) (9).

An asymmetry between bone resorption and formation can result in bone diseases for instance in osteoporosis and in other bone resorbing pathologies.

Osteoporosis appears to be related with an impairment of bone mass through the reduction of osteogenesis and an enhancement of osteoclastic bone resorption, which results in bone fractures (10). At the present treatment options are limited, having issues with their efficacy, and long-term use. For example, the antiresorptive drugs are efficacious in reducing fracture risk (11, 12). Anti-resorptive agents, such as bisphosphonates and denosumab decrease bone loss through the inhibition of the differentiation and catabolic activity of osteoclasts in part by promoting osteoclast apoptosis. Since bone formation is coupled to bone resorption, inhibition of bone resorption is followed by a decrease in osteoblast activity that affects to adequately restore bone mass and bone quality due to increased microdamage collagen formation (13).

By considering papers on adverse effects of pharmacotherapy (estrogens, bisphosphonates) in the treatment of osteoporosis, there is an increasing request for complementary and alternative medicine.

Plant based therapies (i.e., Polyphenols) are safe options at the common treatment of osteoporosis thanks to diminished side effects and costs; in this context various plant components have been assessed for their potential role in the management of osteoporosis. Polyphenols are phytochemicals normally found in the plant kingdom, whose several biological effects have been reported to be protective against chronic diseases, including neurodegenerative and cardiovascular pathologies, cancer, and bone resorption pathologies (14). Depending on the number of phenol rings they comprehend and on the radicals bound to them, polyphenols can be split into different groups: phenolic acids, flavonoids, stilbenes, tannins, coumarins, and lignans. Recent papers based on molecular characteristics of dietary polyphenols have outlined the advantage in their prevention and management of bone resorption diseases (15). Polyphenols can safeguard bone integrity through the decreasing of oxidative stress, the reduction of inflammation by proinflammatory signaling and the modulation of osteoblastogenesis/osteoclastogenesis, by an osteoimmunological action.

The aim of this review paper was achieved on the development of osteoclast-targeting plant polyphenols that could be a great value for the prevention or treatment of bone resorption.

METHODS

Studies for this narrative review were screened using the online database PubMed. Keywords used to search for articles included bone, polyphenols, iicarin, green tea polyphenols, anthocyanins, phloridzin, oleuropein, resveratrol, quercitrin, plorydzin, dried plum, citrus flavonoid, osteoblasts, osteoclasts, bone remodeling, bone resorption, periodontal disease, osteoporosis, oral health. Articles were selected based on the two aspects of the review (cellular and molecular behavior—clinical relevant scenarios). To discuss the cellular characteristics of the bone, milieu articles were selected based on how well they delineate the subject matter. Experimental studies dealing with the impact of polyphenols activity on bone cellular signaling were included. For the remaining section, were included studies based on the broadest spectrum of clinical applications presented and on the strength of evidence provided. Since the topic is relative newborn in its clinical utilization, most of the selected studies were *in vitro*.

POLYPHENOL COMPOUNDS AND BONE METABOLISM

Polyphenols are natural molecules derived from plants isolated and characterized in the fruits, and vegetables. Bioactive phenolic compounds were known as health benefit components due to their antioxidant and anti-inflammatory features. Up to now, there are almost 8,000 recognized polyphenols of which ~500 are biologically active. They can be obtained from plentiful natural sources and even from food/ beverage industrial products with low costs, thus using resources in a feasible way (16). They can preserve bone health by the action of five possible mechanisms: (i) by decreasing of bone loss through the activity of antioxidants, (ii) by diminishing bone loss through anti-inflammatory action, (iii) by improving osteoblastogenesis, (iv) by reducing osteoclastogenesis, and (v) through osteoimmunological activity. Many flavonoids substances have displayed positive impact on bone metabolism. For example, dietary soy isoflavones suppress bone depletion in rodents and post-menopausic women (17). One of the most studied bioactive compounds during recent years is iicarin, a heavy flavonoid component of Chinese tea, which has been reported to have intriguing osteogenic properties both *in vitro* and *in vivo* (18–21).

Recent researches have identified molecular targets in cell signaling pathways that influence bone structure. Some bioactive compounds seem to have bone anabolic action, which has important implications beyond the inhibition of bone resorption through suppressing osteoclast activation. Probably, the positive actions of these compounds are mainly due to their antioxidant characteristics, since they can act as scavengers of reactive oxygen species (ROS). Considering these properties polyphenols could affect bone metabolism through impairment of inflammatory mediators (22), such as cytokines, primarily involved in supporting osteoclast differentiation and resorption (23), consequently enabling to a decrease in bone resorption (**Figure 1**). Curcumin, for example, can enhance several aspects of bone health in subjects with osteoporosis by acting on different steps in the recruitment and activation of osteoclast cells, increasing mineral density and mechanical strength. Mechanisms that have been suggested involve the downregulation of NF-κB, RANKL, NO production of reactive oxygen species and inflammatory cytokine synthesis (24, 25).

Moreover, a lot of research has recently focused on the use of plum extract due to its high polyphenol content. Graef et al. (26) demonstrated that the polyphenolic extract from dried plums is responsible for reducing osteoclast differentiation and activity through a process of downregulation of osteoclast differentiation acting on the primary bone marrow-cells. In according with

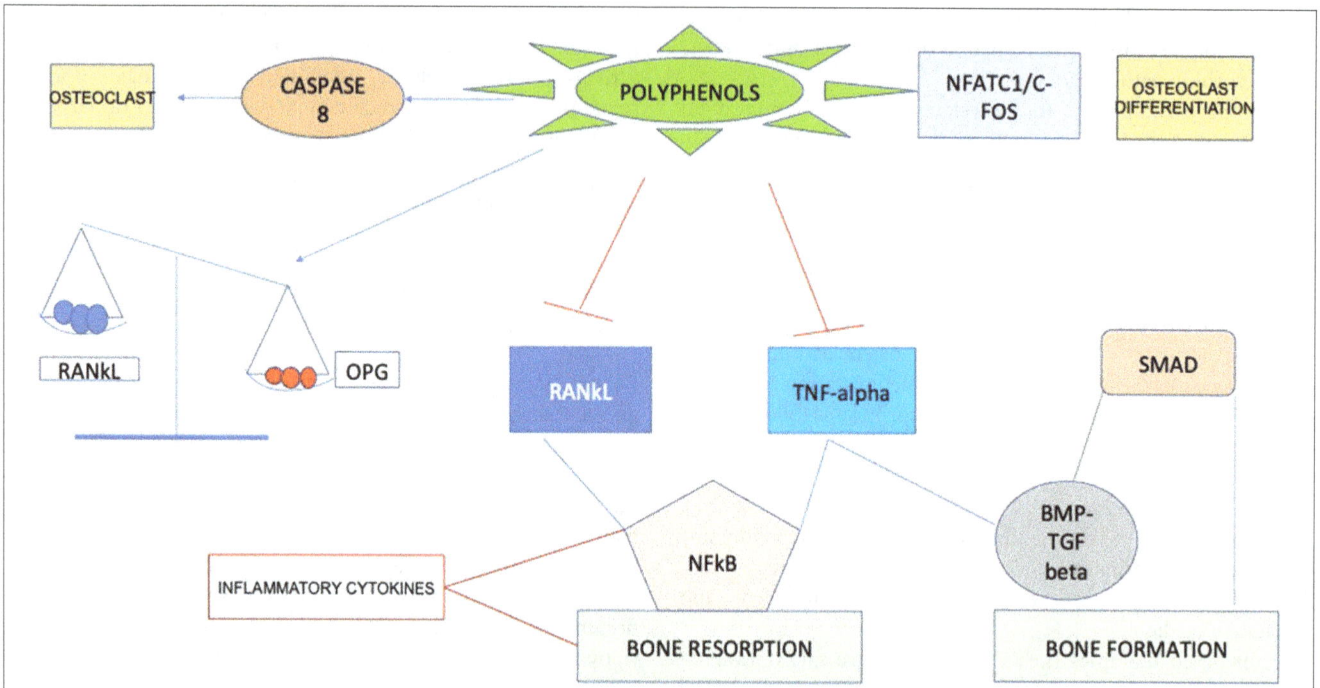

FIGURE 1 | Schematic pathway illustrating the action of polyphenols on bone remodeling.

other studies, this which was mediated through the suppression of Nfatc1, that is the regulator of osteoclast differentiation process (27).

CLINICAL ASPECTS

Osteoporosis

Strategies to avoid osteoporosis include decreasing bone loss induced by acute post-menopause estrogen deficiency. As for other chronic diseases, there is increasing indication that inflammation could be part of the etiology of osteoporosis (28). In particular, oxidative stress regulates the promotion of an enhancement in bone resorption, differentiation, and activity of osteoclast cells, so it has a substantial influence on the incidence of osteoporosis. In general, oxidative stress is described as the state of asymmetry between pro-oxidants and antioxidants. It is assumed that there is a correlation between reactive oxygen species (ROS) and its pathogenesis (29). Polyphenols are able of scavenging ROS and downregulating inflammatory cytokine, including osteoclast differentiation factors, including OPG, TNF-α, RANKL (30). For these reasons, antioxidant-rich foods may represent a possible approach for slowing down age-related bone mass reduction and enhancing bone remodeling. Dietary polyphenols have been related with bone health, which may be in part imputable to their antioxidant capability. For this reason, complementary and alternative medicine has generated interest as a natural chance linked to disease prevention. Natural antioxidant supplementation has been investigated to support the reduction of bone loss caused by oxidative stress (31).

Green tea, for instance, is well-known for its content in phenolic compounds including (−)-epigallocatechin 3-gallate (EGCG), (−)-epicatechin gallate (ECG), (−)-epicatechin (EC), and (−)-epigallocatechin (**Figure 2A**). Shen et al. (32, 33) reported that green tea polyphenols inlet reduces degeneration of bone microarchitecture in rats with chronic inflammation by the downregulation of TNF-α modulating cancellous and endocortical bone compartments. Between Green tea active components, epigallocatechin gallate has attracted attention for its potential health benefits and this molecule was largely investigated for its effect on osteoporosis. The bone formation was affected by EGCG through the enhancement of the alkaline phosphatase activity in osteoblastic cells and bone mineralization, related to the suppression of the osteoclast cells differentiation and of the formation of oxidative stress-induced calcium stone formation in rats (34).

Vester et al. (35) demonstrated that stimulation of primary human osteoblasts with low doses of green tea extracts during oxidative stress over 21 days improved mineralization and had beneficial effect on extra-cellular matrix production with higher gene expression of osteocalcin and collagen1α1 during osteoblasts differentiation.

Anthocyanins are water-soluble glycosides including a variety of compounds comprising pelargonidin, cyanidin, delphinidin, peonidin, petunidin, malvidin (**Figure 3**) (36). The health effects of anthocyanins are mainly due to their ability to impair oxidative stress (37). Anthocyanin chalcones and quinoidal bases with a double bond linked to the keto group are antioxidants in scavenging free radicals (38). Therefore, berry food and drinks could diminish the effects of age-related bone loss and decrease the risk of osteoporosis in humans (39).

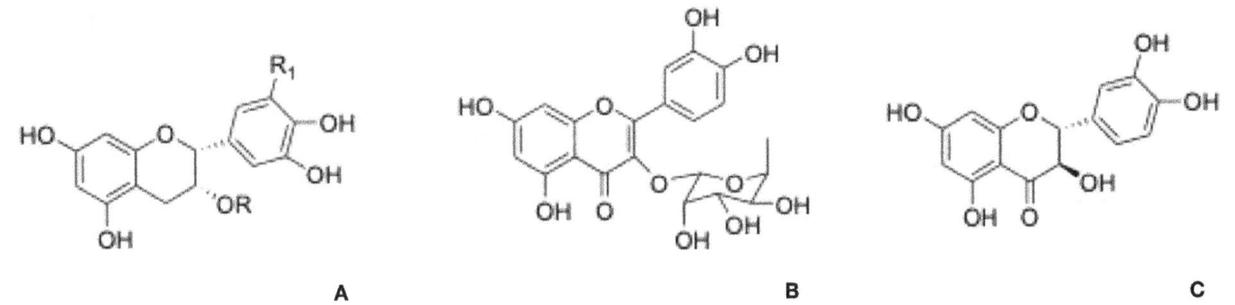

COMPOUND	R	R1
ECGC	Gallic acid	OH
ECG	Gallic acid	H
EC	H	H
EGC	H	OH

FIGURE 2 | (A) Structures of main green tea polyphenols. **(B)** Quercitrin. **(C)** Taxifolin.

In other studies, Devareddy et al. reported that 5% blueberry treatment (w/w) for 100 days inhibited the loss of whole-body bone mineral density due to the ovariectomy in rats, and suppressed femoral mRNA levels of bone turnover biomarkers that were enhanced by estrogen deficiency (40).

Phloridzin, a dihydrochalcone contained in apples, apples juice, and purees, has been demonstrated to contribute to the antioxidant activity (**Figure 4A**). The activity of phloridzin on glucose uptake and diabetes has been explored and reported in many research works (41). The phlorizdin intake displayed a protection against ovariectomy-induced osteopenia under inflammatory patterns by the downregulation of inflammation markers and bone resorption (42).

In a murine model, Kim et al. found that phloretin (not glucoside form of phloridzin) inhibited receptor activator of NF-κB ligand (RANKL)-induced formation of multinucleated osteoclasts and diminished bone resorption area produced during the osteoclast differentiation process (43).

Oleuropein (**Figure 4B**), a secoiridoids esterified with hydroxytyrosol found in the olive tree and derivates, is well-known for its pharmacological activities including antioxidant, anti-inflammatory, anti-cancer, antimicrobial, and antiviral, cardioprotective against acute adriamycin cardiotoxicity, anti-ischemic, and hypolipidemic (44, 45). Puel et al. displayed the dose-dependent bone-sparing effect of oleuropein showing a reduction of bone loss and at the same time a downregulation of inflammatory biomarkers in ovariectomized rats (46).

Resveratrol (**Figure 4C**) is a stilbene phytoalexin found in many plant species and it is crucial polyphenol found in red wine. It has been considered that dietary resveratrol could affect as an antioxidant, promoting nitric oxide production, platelet aggregation and enhancing high-density lipoprotein cholesterol. In addition, resveratrol was shown to be a chemo preventive agent and exhibits anti-inflammatory, neuroprotective, and antiviral properties (28, 47).

The PGF2α-effect on OPG synthesis was suppresses by resveratrol through the inhibition of the MAP kinase pathways in osteoblasts (48).

Also, resveratrol downregulates bone morphogenic protein-4 (BMP-4) and stimulates VEGF synthesis through the inhibition of p70 S6 kinase in osteoblasts (49) via sirtuin-1 (SIRT1) activation (50).

The effect of above described compounds on osteoblast and osteoclast activity, are summarized in **Table 1** (16, 19, 20, 26, 29, 35, 37, 39, 43–45, 50–52).

Periodontal Disease

Periodontitis is a devastating inflammatory disease of tooth-supporting tissues, which are composed by cementum, periodontal ligament, and alveolar bone, due to imbalance between oxidative stress and antioxidant activity.

Of note, inflammatory stimulation by periodontal bacteria increases the production of crevicular fluid and modulate the production of leukocytes, which, in order to deactivate periodontal pathogens, liberate single oxygen, and hypochlorous acid into the crevicular fluid (53).

The subsequent oxidative stress is counteracted by the antioxidant activity of ascorbate, albumin, and urate

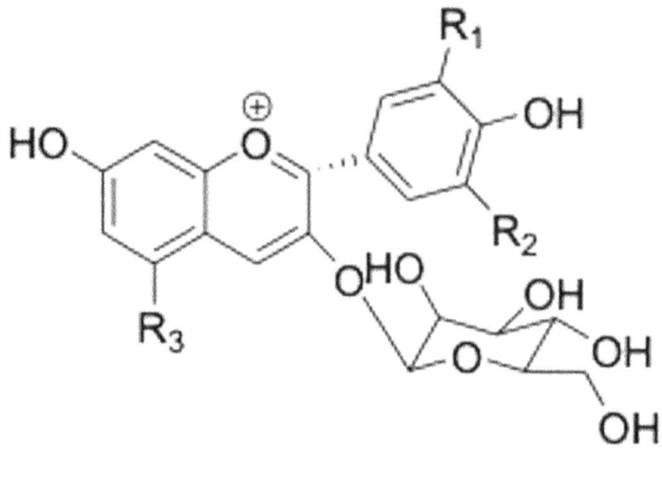

ANTHOCYANIN	R_1	R_2	R_3
Delphinidin 3-glucoside	OH	OH	H
Delphinidin 3,5-diglucoside	OH	OH	glucoside
Cyanin 3-glucoside	OH	H	H
Cyanin 3,5-glucoside	OH	H	glucoside
Pelargonin 3-glucoside	H	H	H
Pelargonin 3,5-glucoside	H	H	glucoside

FIGURE 3 | Structures of main anthocyanins.

characteristic of the crevicular fluid and derived from plasma. When there is instability between oxidative stress and antioxidant activity, periodontal tissue demolition may appear. These remarks suggest that antioxidant rich diets might protect periodontal tissue from development and progression of pathologies, particularly in subjects exposed to environmental and dietary sources of oxidative stress (54, 55).

Based on clinical studies about the biochemical properties delivery of polyphenols formulations there is emerging line of natural therapies for periodontitis that may maximize and improved oral health among more populations. Actually, administration of tea polyphenols, by holding green or black tea, in the mouth for 2–5 min enhance the antioxidant capacity of saliva, and daily use of two fresh grapefruits for 2 weeks increases the phagocytic capability of the polymorphonuclear leucocytes inside the gingival crevicular fluid (56).

Following these suggestions polyphenoids may be employed in dentistry as a prophylaxis against bacterial infection and plaque formation, and as adjuvant therapies to aid post-operative healing of dental sockets and other traumatized tissues. Remarkable, in a recent study researchers find out that quercitrin, a glicoside of quercetin, and ramnose (**Figure 2B**) present in tartary buckwheat and in the bark of several oak, was found bioactive *in vitro* on human gingival fibroblasts, downregulating the gene expression of markers linked to inflammation and overexpressing genes that modulate different categories of collagen (57).

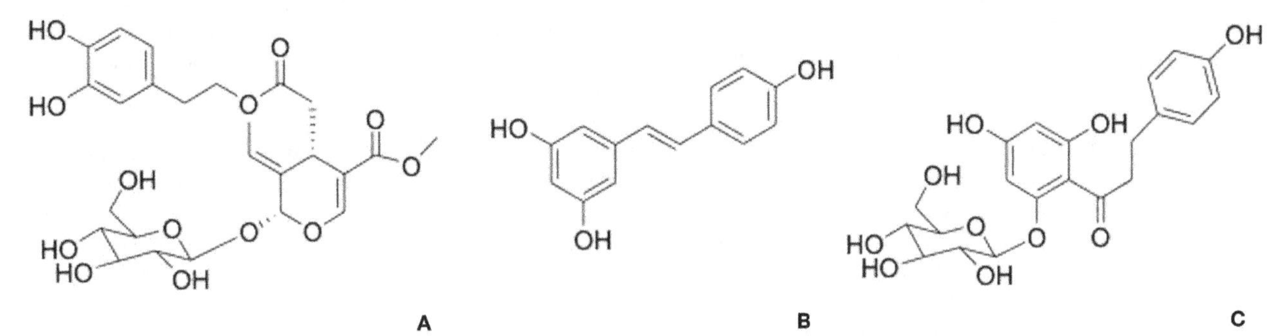

FIGURE 4 | Structures of phloridzin (A), oleuropien (B), and resveratrol (C).

TABLE 1 | Effect of different polyphenols on osteoclasts and osteoblasts activity *in vitro*.

Compound	Effect on osteoclasts	Effect on osteoblasts
Icarin	− (20)	+ (19)
Green tea polyphenols	− (16)	+ (35)
Anthocyanins	− (29)	+ (37)
Phloridzin	− (43)	+ (39)
Oleuropein	− (45)	+ (44)
Resveratrol	− (51)	+ (50)
Dried plum	− (26)	+ (52)

−, Reduced cellular activity.
+, Enhanced cellular activity.

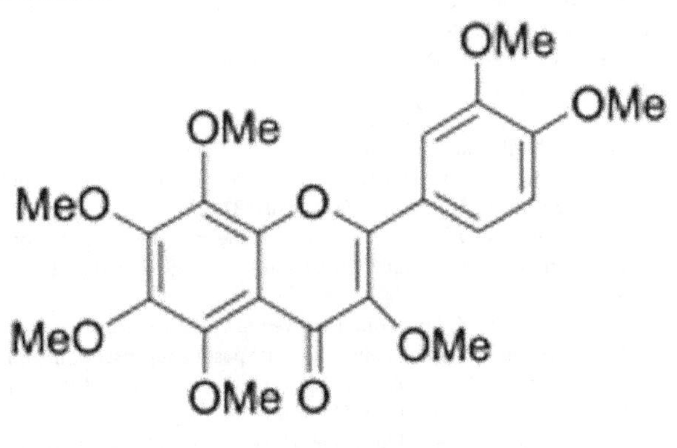

FIGURE 5 | Structure of 3,5,6,7,8,3,4-Heptamethoxyflavone.

Matsumoto et al. have reported that a citrus flavonoid 3,5,6,7,8,3′,4′-Heptamethoxyflavone (HMF) (**Figure 5**) found in Valencia oranges clearly suppressed the osteoclast formation and PGE2 production induced by IL-1. In mouse calvarial organ cultures, HMF attenuated the bone resorption elicited by LPS. HMF inhibits bone resorption induced by inflammation preserving bone mass and contributing to keep away from tooth loss (58).

POTENTIAL APPLICATIONS IN ORAL MEDICAL DEVICES

Due to recent progression in molecular biology and in the bone remodeling pathways many polyphenols are believed promising molecules able to act on osteoblast differentiation and on mineralization without the high financial impact of other osteoinductive factors.

These results are correlated with an exciting application of flavonoids like bioactive surfaces that could be an option to the use of growth factors i.e., in oral medical devices (59). Noteworthy, the use of growth factors, such as BMPs, in biomedical devices has lately gained several negative points regarding its stability, administration, bioactivity, and bioavailability. They are frequently very expensive and very limited in respect on the regulatory approval (60). By another side, flavonoid compounds are cheap, bioavailable, easy to find in daily food and, for this reason, probably easily be translated into clinical applications. For this rationale plant-derived products represent an innovative and interesting candidates for biomaterial applications, including dental research fields. Biomolecules can be believed as promising field relating to the improving of the bioactivity of biomaterial, and a safe substitute to pharmaceuticals, animal-derived compounds or growth factors. With the aim to attempt to obtain a faster osteointegration to speed up the overall treatment process, the use of biomimetic agents represents an interesting research area related with implant dentistry. For example, the functionalization with flavonoids conferred an osteopromotive characteristic to the Titanium surface as discussed by Cordoba et al. (61). In their study, researchers created a bioactive interface based on the covalent immobilization of flavonoids taxifolin (**Figure 2C**) and quercitrin on titanium surfaces.

POLYPHENOLS SAFETY AND TOXICITY

The consumption of food polyphenols such as flavonoids has been associated with a wide range of health benefits both disease preventive and therapeutic agents, including optimizing cardiometabolic health, cancer prevention, and to a lesser extent positively impacting brain functioning in humans.

Diet-derived polyphenols are considered safe based on their long history of use as food or as traditional medicines, recently it is becoming the idea that these specialized metabolites could have toxic effects at pharmacological concentrations, and in several diseases or polypharmaceutical contexts (62).

The risk of toxic effects is increased using pharmacological doses in prevention/treatment and supplement situations and genetic polymorphisms or molecule-drug interactions that decrease/increase the bioavailability. Few reports on toxicity of these compounds are reported, therefore investigations of the side effects of polyphenols is necessary.

CONCLUSIONS

Bone pathologies majorly including osteoporosis osteoarthritis and oral diseases are becoming frequent with the growth in the aging population, a fact which is frightening if we consider the estimations that by 2030 20% of Europeans and 30% of the US population will be over the age of 65. There are only few standard therapies available for the treatment and prevention of these pathologies so a possible protective effect by natural molecules in multifactorial dysmetabolic disease could be a substitute to rise above side effects of conventional therapies.

Majority of the clinical researches underlined in this review, would attempt to demonstrate the relationship between polyphenols intake and bone turnover regulation. However, in spite of abundant *in vitro* and *in vivo* animal models, up to the present time, there is an absence of consistent human studies relating with polyphenol consumption. Although it was largely described the main role of antioxidative mechanism of polyphenols in prevention and treatment of bone remodeling diseases, it would be required more studies focused on the application of these compounds as therapeutic alternative in bone resorption diseases.

AUTHOR CONTRIBUTIONS

VN selected studies and wrote the manuscript and takes responsibility for the manuscript. ND, SN, FC, FB, and RD analyzed and compared literature data, and edited the manuscript. All authors approved the manuscript.

REFERENCES

1. Raggatt LJ, Partridge NC. Cellular and molecular mechanisms of bone modeling. *J Biol Chem.* (2010) 285:25103–8. doi: 10.1074/jbc.R109.041087
2. Chambers TJ, Fuller K. How are osteoclasts induced to resorb bone? *Ann NY Acad Sci USA.* (2011) 1240:1–6. doi: 10.1111/j.1749-6632.2011.06249.x
3. Boyle WJ, Simonet WS, Lacey DL. Osteoclast differentiation and activation. *Nature.* (2003) 423:337–42. doi: 10.1038/nature01658
4. Husheem M, Nyman JK, Vaaraniemi J, Vaananen HK, Hentunen TA. Characterization of circulating human osteoclast progenitors: development of *in vitro* resorption assay. *Calcif Tissue Int.* (2005) 76:222–30. doi: 10.1007/s00223-004-0123-z
5. Teitelbaum SL. Osteoclasts: what do they do and how do they do it? *Am J Pathol.* (2007) 170:427–35. doi: 10.2353/ajpath.2007.060834
6. Bonewald LF, Johnson ML. Osteocytes, mechanosensing and Wnt signaling. *Bone.* (2008) 42:606–15. doi: 10.1016/j.bone.2007.12.224
7. Everts V, Delaissé JM, Korper W, Jansen DC, Tigchelaar-Gutter W, Saftig P, et al. The bone lining cell: its role in cleaning Howship's lacunae and initiating bone formation. *J Bone Miner Res.* (2002) 17:77–90. doi: 10.1359/jbmr.2002.17.1.77
8. Nishimura R, Hata K, Matsubara T, Wakabayashi M, Yoneda T. Regulation of bone and cartilage development by network between BMP signalling and transcription factors. *J Biochem.* (2012) 151:247–54. doi: 10.1093/jb/mvs004
9. Boyce BF, Xing L. Functions of RANKL/RANK/OPG in bone modeling and remodeling. *Arch Biochem Biophys.* (2008) 473:139–46. doi: 10.1016/j.abb.2008.03.018
10. Weitzmann MN, Pacifici R. Estrogen deficiency and bone loss: an inflammatory tale. *J Clin Invest.* (2006) 116:1186–94. doi: 10.1172/JCI28550
11. Adler RA, El-Hajj Fuleihan G, Bauer DC, Camacho PM, Clarke BL, Clines GA, et al. Managing osteoporosis in patients on long-term bisphosphonate treatment: report of a task force of the American Society for Bone and Mineral Research. *J Bone Miner Res.* (2016) 31:16–35. doi: 10.1002/jbmr.2708
12. Faienza MF, Chiarito M, D'Amato G, Colaianni G, Colucci S, Grano M, et al. Monoclonal antibodies for treating osteoporosis. *Opin Biol Ther.* (2018) 18:149–57. doi: 10.1080/14712598.2018.1401607
13. Sims NA, Ng KW. Implications of osteoblast-osteoclast interactions in the management of osteoporosis by antiresorptive agents denosumab and odanacatib. *Curr Osteoporos Rep.* (2014) 12:98–106. doi: 10.1007/s11914-014-0196-1
14. Scalbert A, Manach C, Morand C, Rémésy C, Jiménez L. Dietary polyphenols and the prevention of diseases. *Crit Rev Food Sci Nutr.* (2005) 45:287–306. doi: 10.1080/1040869059096
15. Weaver CM, Alekel DL, Ward WE, Ronis MJ. Flavonoid intake and bone health. *J Nutr Gerontol Geriatr.* (2012) 31:239–53. doi: 10.1080/21551197.2012.698220
16. Austermann K, Baecker N, Stehle P, Heer M. Putative effects of nutritive polyphenols on bone metabolism *in vivo*-evidence from human studies. *Nutrients.* (2019) 11:871. doi: 10.3390/nu11040871
17. Messina M. A brief historical overview of the past two decades of soy and isoflavone research. *J Nutr.* (2010) 140:1350S–4S. doi: 10.3945/jn.109.118315
18. Zhang G, Qin L, Shi Y. Epimedium-derived phytoestrogen flavonoids exert beneficial effect on preventing bone loss in late postmenopausal women: a 24-month randomized, double-blind and placebo-controlled trial. *J Bone Miner Res.* (2007) 22:1072–9. doi: 10.1359/jbmr.070405
19. Huang Z, Cheng C, Wang J, Liu X, Wei H, Han Y, et al. Icariin regulates the osteoblast differentiation and cell proliferation of MC3T3-E1 cells through microRNA-153 by targeting Runt-related transcription factor 2. *Exp Ther Med.* (2018) 15:5159–66. doi: 10.3892/etm.2018.6127
20. Kim B, Lee KY, Park B. Icariin abrogates osteoclast formation through the regulation of the RANKL-mediated TRAF6/NF-κB/ERK signaling pathway in Raw264.7 cells. *Phytomedicine.* (2018) 51:181–90. doi: 10.1016/j.phymed.2018.06.020
21. Huang J, Yuan L, Wang X, Zhang TL, Wang K. Icaritin and its glycosides enhance osteoblastic, but suppress osteoclastic, differentiation and activity *in vitro*. *Life Sci.* (2007) 81:832–40. doi: 10.1016/j.lfs.2007.07.015
22. Bodet C, Chandad F, Grenier D. Cranberry components inhibit interleukin-6, interleukin-8, and prostaglandin E production by lipopolysaccharide-activated gingival fibroblasts. *Eur J Oral Sci.* (2007) 115:64–70. doi: 10.1111/j.1600-0722.2007.00415.x

23. Yao Z, Xing L, Qin C. Osteoclast precursor interaction with bone matrix induces osteoclast formation directly by an interleukin-1-mediated autocrine mechanism. *J Biol Chem.* (2008) 283:9917–24. doi: 10.1074/jbc.M706415200
24. Ozaki K, Kawata Y, Amano S, Hanazawa S. Stimulatory effect of curcumin on osteoclast apoptosis. *Biochem Pharmacol.* (2000) 59:1577–81. doi: 10.1016/S0006-2952(00)00277-X
25. Bharti AC, Takada Y, Aggarwal BB. Curcumin (diferuloylmethane) inhibits receptor activator of NF-kappa B ligand-induced NF-kappa B activation in osteoclast precursors and suppresses osteoclastogenesis. *J Immunol.* (2004) 172:5940–47. doi: 10.4049/jimmunol.172.10.5940
26. Graef JL, Rendina-Ruedy E, Crockett EK, Ouyang P, Wu L, King JB, et al. Osteoclast differentiation is downregulated by select polyphenolic fractions from dried plum via suppression of MAPKs and Nfatc1 in mouse C57BL/6 primary bone marrow cells. *Curr Dev Nutr.* (2017) 1:e000406. doi: 10.3945/cdn.117.000406
27. Smith BJ, Bu SY, Wang Y, Rendina E, Lim YF, Marlow D, et al. A comparative study of the bone metabolic response to dried plum supplementation and PTH treatment in adult, osteopenic ovariectomized rat. *Bone.* (2014) 58:151–9. doi: 10.1016/j.bone.2013.10.005
28. de Vries TJ, El Bakkali I, Kamradt T, Schett G, Jansen IDC, D'Amelio P. What are the peripheral blood determinants for increased osteoclast formation in the various inflammatory diseases associated with bone loss? *Front Immunol.* (2019) 19:505. doi: 10.3389/fimmu.2019.00505
29. Domazetovic V, Marcucci G, Iantomasi T, Brandi ML, Vincenzini MT. Oxidative stress in bone remodeling: role of antioxidants. *Clin Cases Miner Bone Metab.* (2017) 14:209–16. doi: 10.11138/ccmbm/2017.14.1.209
30. Léotoing L, Wauquier F, Guicheux J, Miot-Noirault E, Wittrant Y, Coxam V. The polyphenol fisetin protects bone by repressing NF-κB and MKP-1-dependent signaling pathways in osteoclasts. *PLoS ONE.* (2013) 8:e68388. doi: 10.1371/journal.pone.0068388
31. Horcajada MN, Offord E. Naturally plant-derived compounds: role in bone anabolism. *Curr Mol Pharmacol.* (2012) 5:205–18. doi: 10.2174/1874467211205020205
32. Shen CL, Yeh JK, Stoecker BJ, Chyu MC, Wang JS. Green tea polyphenols mitigate deterioration of bone microarchitecture in middle-aged female rats. *Bone.* (2009) 44:684–90. doi: 10.1016/j.bone.2008.11.018
33. Shen CL, Yeh JK, Cao JJ, Wang JS. Green tea and bone metabolism. *Nutr Res.* (2009) 29:437–56. doi: 10.1016/j.nutres.2009.06.008
34. Oka Y, Iwai S, Amano H, Irie Y, Yatomi K, Ryu K, et al. Tea polyphenols inhibit rat osteoclast formation and differentiation. *J Pharmacol Sci.* (2012) 118:55–64. doi: 10.1254/jphs.11082FP
35. Vester H, Holzer N, Neumaier M, Lilianna S, Nüssler AK, Seeliger C. Green Tea Extract (GTE) improves differentiation in human osteoblasts during oxidative stress. *J Inflamm.* (2014) 11:15. doi: 10.1186/1476-9255-11-15
36. Slatnar A, Jakopic J, Stampar F, Veberic R, Jamnik P. The effect of bioactive compounds on *in vitro* and *in vivo* antioxidant activity of different berry juices. *PLoS ONE.* (2012) 7:e47880. doi: 10.1371/journal.pone.0047880
37. Aqil F, Gupta A, Munagala R, Jeyabalan J, Kausar H, Sharma RJ, et al. Antioxidant and antiproliferative activities of anthocyanin/ellagitannin-enriched extracts from *Syzygium cumini* L. (Jamun, the Indian Blackberry). *Nutr Cancer.* (2012) 64:428–38. doi: 10.1080/01635581.2012.657766
38. Wang H, Cao G, Prior RL. Oxygen radical absorbing capacity of anthocyanins. *J Agric Food Chem.* (1997) 45:304–9. doi: 10.1021/jf960421t
39. Hubert PA, Lee SG, Lee SK, Chun OK. Dietary polyphenols, berries, and age-related bone loss: a review based on human, animal, and cell studies. *Antioxidants.* (2014) 3:144–58. doi: 10.3390/antiox3010144
40. Devareddy L, Hooshmand S, Collins JK, Lucas EA, Chai SC, Arjmandi BH. Blueberry prevents bone loss in ovariectomized rat model of postmenopausal osteoporosis. *J Nutr Biochem.* (2008) 19:694–9. doi: 10.1016/j.jnutbio.2007.09.004
41. Ehrenkranz JRL, Lewis NG, Kahn CR, Roth J. Phlorizin: a review. *Diabetes Metab Res Rev.* (2005) 21:31–8. doi: 10.1002/dmrr.532
42. Puel C, Quintin A, Mathey J, Obled C, Davicco M, Lebecque P, et al. Prevention of bone loss by phloridzin, an apple polyphenol, in ovariectomized ratsunder inflammation conditions. *Calcif Tissue Int.* (2005) 77:311–8. doi: 10.1007/s00223-005-0060-5
43. Kim JL, Kang MK, Gong JH, Park SH, Han SY, Kang YH. Novel antiosteoclastogenic activity of phloretin antagonizing RANKL-induced osteoclast differentiation of murine macrophages. *Mol Nutr Food Res.* (2012) 56:1223–33. doi: 10.1002/mnfr.201100831
44. Santiago-Mora R, Casado-Díaz A, De Castro MD, Quesada-Gómez JM. Oleuropein enhances osteoblastogenesis and inhibits adipogenesis: the effect on differentiation in stem cells derived from bone marrow. *Osteoporos Int.* (2011) 22:675–84. doi: 10.1007/s00198-010-1270-x
45. Chin KY, Ima-Nirwana S. Olives and bone: a green osteoporosis prevention option. *Int J Environ Res Public Health.* (2016) 13:E755. doi: 10.3390/ijerph13080755
46. Puel C, Mathey J, Agalias A, Kati-Coulibaly S, Mardon J, Obled C, et al. Dose-response study of effect of oleuropein, an olive oil polyphenol, in an ovariectomy/inflammation experimental model of bone loss in the rat. *Clin Nutr.* (2006) 25:859–68. doi: 10.1016/j.clnu.2006.03.009
47. Sharma S, Anjaneyulu M, Kulkarni SK, Chopra K. Resveratrol, a polyphenolic phytoalexin, attenuates diabetic nephropathy in rats. *Pharmacology.* (2006) 76:69–75. doi: 10.1159/000089720
48. Kuroyanagi G, Otsuka T, Yamamoto N, Matsushima-Nishiwaki R, Nakakami A, Mizutani J, et al. Down-regulation by resveratrol of basic fibroblast growth factor-stimulated osteoprotegerin synthesis through suppression of Akt in osteoblasts. *Int J Mol Sci.* (2014) 15:17886–900. doi: 10.3390/ijms151017886
49. Kondo A, Otsuka T, Kuroyanagi G, Yamamoto N, Matsushima-Nishiwaki R, Mizutani J, et al. Resveratrol inhibits BMP-4-stimulated VEGF synthesis in osteoblasts: suppression of S6 kinase. *Int J Mol Med.* (2014) 33:1013–18. doi: 10.3892/ijmm.2014.1626
50. Zhao M, Ko SY, Garrett IR, Mundy GR, Gutierrez GE, Edwards JR. The polyphenol resveratrol promotes skeletal growth in mice through a sirtuin 1-bone morphogenic protein 2 longevity axis. *Br J Pharmacol.* (2018) 175:4183–92. doi: 10.1111/bph.14477
51. Murgia D, Mauceri R, Campisi G, De Caro V. Advance on resveratrol application in bone regeneration: progress and perspectives for use in oral and maxillofacial surgery. *Biomolecules.* (2019) 9:E94. doi: 10.3390/biom9030094
52. Graef JL, Rendina-Ruedy E, Crockett EK, Ouyang P, King JB, Cichewicz RH, et al. Select polyphenolic fractions from dried plum enhance osteoblast activity through BMP-2 signaling. *J Nutr Biochem.* (2018) 55:59–67. doi: 10.1016/j.jnutbio.2017.09.014
53. Battino M, Bullon P, Wilson M, Newman H. Oxidative injury and inflammatory periodontal diseases: the challenge of anti-oxidants to free radicals and reactive oxygen species. *Crit Rev Oral Biol Med.* (1999) 10:458–76. doi: 10.1177/10454411990100040301
54. Brunetti G, Colucci S, Pignataro P, Coricciati M, Mori G, Cirulli N, et al. T cells support osteoclastogenesis in an *in vitro* model derived from human periodontitis patients. *J Periodontol.* (2005) 76:1675–80. doi: 10.1902/jop.2005.76.10.1675
55. Ritchie CS, Kinane DF. Nutrition, inflammation, and periodontal disease. *Nutrition.* (2003) 19:475–6. doi: 10.1016/S0899-9007(02)01043-2
56. Staudte H, Sigusch BW, Glockmann E. Grapefruit consumption improves vitamin C status in periodontitis patients. *Br Dent J.* (2005) 4:213–7. doi: 10.1038/sj.bdj.4812613
57. Gomez-Florit M, Monjo M, Ramis JM. Identification of quercitrin as potential therapeutic agent for periodontal applications. *J Periodontol.* (2014) 85:966–74. doi: 10.1902/jop.2014.130438
58. Matsumoto C, Inoue H, Tominari T, Watanabe K, Hirata, M, Miyaura C et al. Heptamethoxyflavone, a citrus flavonoid, suppresses inflammatory osteoclastogenesis and alveolar bone resorption. *Biosci Biotechnol Biochem.* (2015) 79:155–8. doi: 10.1080/09168451.2014.952616
59. Wang Z, Wang D, Yang D, Zhen W, Zhang J, Peng S. The effect of icariin on bone metabolism and its potential clinical application. *Osteoporos Int.* (2018) 29:535–44. doi: 10.1007/s00198-017-4255-1

60. Junker R, Dimakis A, Thoneick M, Jansen JA. Effects of implant surface coatings and composition on bone integration: a systematic review. *Clin Oral Impl Res.* (2009) 4:185–206. doi: 10.1111/j.1600-0501.2009.01777.x
61. Cordoba A, Satue M, Gomez-Florit M, Hierro-Oliva M, Petzold C; Lyngstadaas SP, et al. Flavonoid-modified surfaces: multifunctional bioactive biomaterials with osteopromotive, anti-inflammatory, and anti-fibrotic potential. *Adv Health Mater.* (2014) 4:540–9. doi: 10.1002/adhm.2014 00587
62. Soto-Vaca A, Gutierrez A, Losso JN, Xu Z, Finley JW. Evolution of phenolic compounds from color and flavor problems to health benefits. *J Agric Food Chem.* (2012) 60:6658–77. doi: 10.1021/jf300861c

13

How Autoantibodies Regulate Osteoclast Induced Bone Loss in Rheumatoid Arthritis

Ulrike Steffen[†]*, Georg Schett*[*‡] *and Aline Bozec*[*‡]

Department of Internal Medicine 3, University of Erlangen-Nuremberg, Erlangen, Germany

***Correspondence:**
Georg Schett
georg.schett@uk-erlangen.de
Aline Bozec
aline.bozec@uk-erlangen.de

[†] *Former name: Ulrike Harre*

[‡] *These authors have contributed equally to this work*

Rheumatoid arthritis (RA) is a chronic inflammatory disease, characterized by autoimmunity that triggers joint inflammation and tissue destruction. Traditional concepts of RA pathogenesis have strongly been focused on inflammation. However, more recent evidence suggests that autoimmunity *per se* modulates the disease and in particular bone destruction during the course of RA. RA-associated bone loss is caused by increased osteoclast differentiation and activity leading to rapid bone resorption. Autoimmunity in RA is based on autoantibodies such as rheumatoid factor (RF) and autoantibodies against citrullinated proteins (ACPA). These autoantibodies exert effector functions on immune cells and on bone resorbing osteoclasts, thereby facilitating bone loss. This review summarizes potential pathways involved in increased destruction of bone tissue in RA, particularly focusing on the direct and indirect actions of autoantibodies on osteoclast generation and function.

Keywords: rheumatoid factor (RF), autoantibodies against citrullinated proteins (ACPA), osteoclasts, rheumatoid arthritis, cytokines

INTRODUCTION

Skeletal homeostasis is maintained by continuous removal and replacement of bone throughout life. This process is controlled by the coordinated activity of specific bone cells. Osteoclasts are highly specialized multinucleated cells derived from hematopoietic precursors of the myeloid lineage with the capacity to resorb bone [reviewed in Tanaka et al. (1)]. Osteoclast formation is controlled by the action of soluble mediators, such as receptor activator of nuclear factor-κB ligand (RANKL; also known as TNFSF11), macrophage colony-stimulating factor 1 (M-CSF), and negative regulators, such as the decoy receptor for RANKL, osteoprotegerin (OPG). These cytokines are provided by cells of the osteoblast lineage and immune cells located within the bone microenvironment [reviewed in Schett (2)]. Bone resorption also liberates growth factors deposited in bone, which can act locally on osteoblasts and immune cells.

In parallel to osteoclast-mediated bone resorption, bone formation results from the proliferation of skeletal stem cells and their differentiation into osteoblast. Their fate is to either stay as bone lining cells or to be embedded into the bone matrix as osteocytes [reviewed in Bonewald (3)]. The osteoblast cell lineage includes osteoblast precursors, bone lining cells and osteocytes. Each of them express specific signals that regulate resident cells within the bone marrow. In addition to the crosstalk between different types of bone cells, there is a tight interaction between bone and immune cells, which is still not fully characterized. The importance of this interaction is reflected by diseases, such as rheumatoid arthritis (RA), in which immune activation is linked to bone loss.

RA is a chronic systemic autoimmune disease affecting about 1% of the population worldwide [reviewed in McInnes and Schett (4)]. It is associated with pain, joint swelling, progressive disability and systemic comorbidity. One of the major consequences of RA is the degradation of cartilage and bone tissue. This process results in joint destruction, which leads to significant loss of life quality for the patients. RA-associated bone loss is characterized by three different manifestations: (i) local erosions in the inflamed joints, where bone and cartilage are in direct contact with the inflamed synovium, (ii) periarticular bone loss of trabecular and cortical bone close to sites of inflammation, and (iii) systemic osteopenia and osteoporosis [reviewed in Zerbini et al. (5)]. All three forms of bone loss are caused by altered bone homeostasis with increased osteoclast generation and activity resulting in accelerated bone resorption, while osteoblast-mediated bone formation is suppressed. The reasons for enhanced osteoclast activity have been in the focus of extensive research. Aside from direct inter-cellular interactions and systemic effects of inflammatory cytokines, autoantibodies have been found to play a major role both via directly influencing osteoclasts, as well as, through the induction of inflammatory cytokines released by macrophages.

In this review, we will summarize the current knowledge on autoantibody-mediated bone loss in RA. We will focus on the direct effects of autoantibodies on osteoclasts and pre-osteoclasts as well as indirect effects via cytokines released by activated macrophages. In addition, we will discuss the implications of antibody glycosylation.

THE REGULATION OF OSTEOCLAST ACTIVITY AND DIFFERENTIATION BY AUTOANTIBODIES

Autoantibodies in RA

Although the causes of RA are diverse and not completely understood, it is clear that disease specific autoantibodies constitute an important trigger. The main autoantibodies associated with RA are the rheumatoid factor (RF) and autoantibodies against citrullinated proteins (ACPA). RF is directed against the Fc part of IgG and mainly occurs as IgM. However, to a smaller extent, RF can also be detected as IgG or IgA. Up to 70% of RA patients are RF positive. Of note, RF is also found in a subset of healthy people, especially in the elderly, in patients with other rheumatic diseases (e.g., Sjögren's syndrome or systemic lupus erythematosus) or in patients with viral infections like hepatitis C (6, 7). Although RF is positively associated with increased bone erosion, especially in ACPA positive patients (8, 9), there are no data available about its direct effects on cytokine production or osteoclastogenesis. As RF is directed against IgG, it might lead to a constant basal inflammation by the formation of random IgG complexes or enhance the size of existing immune complexes formed by other autoantibodies. Indeed, the addition of monoclonal IgM-RF increased the production of the pro-inflammatory cytokine TNF-α by macrophages after treatment with ACPA-containing IgG from RA patients (10), suggesting a synergistic interaction of ACPA and RF.

In contrast to RF, ACPA are highly specific for RA with a very low prevalence in healthy people (11, 12). ACPA provide diagnostic value in predicting disease severity and the likelihood to develop bone erosions in RA patients (13). ACPA are detectable up to 10 years before clinical onset of RA (14). Some months before the occurrence of clinical symptoms, ACPA broaden their epitope recognition and isotype usage profile and change their glycosylation toward a more inflammatory phenotype (14–16). In 2010, ACPA have been included into the diagnostic criteria for RA by the American College of Rheumatology (ACR) and European League Against Rheumatism (EULAR) (17). ACPA recognize a variety of citrullinated proteins with citrullinated vimentin, α-enolase, fibrinogen and collagen being the most prominent antigens. Citrullination is a post-translational modification of a positively charged arginine residue into a partially negatively charged citrulline residue. As this process changes the net charge of a protein, neo epitopes appear, that can be recognized by the immune system resulting in autoantibody formation. Citrullination is performed by enzymes of the peptidylarginine deiminase (PAD) family and occuring physiologically during the formation of neutrophil extracellular traps (NETs), apoptosis and skin keratinization [reviewed in Baka et al. (18)]. In addition, the bacterium *Porphyromonas gingivalis* (which is involved in periodontitis) releases PAD (19). Bacterial PAD is suspected to contribute to protein citrullination and ACPA formation, but more research is needed to truly confirm a relationship between periodontitis and RA [reviewed in Araujo et al. (20) and Potempa et al. (21)]. Another trigger of citrullination, especially in the lung, is smoking [reviewed in Klareskog et al. (22)].

Apart from ACPA, a couple of other autoantibodies against posttranslational modifications (AMPA) have been found in the last years, such as autoantibodies against carbamylated proteins (anti-CarP) (23) or autoantibodies against acetylated proteins (24). All groups of autoantibodies can be detected independently of each other in patients with RA. According to a meta-analysis evaluating 25 studies, ACPA are present in 47–88% of RA patients (13). Anti-CarP could be detected in 39–58% of RA patients and in 8–16% of RA patients that are ACPA negative (23, 25, 26), but also in about 7% of osteoarthritis patients and 3,6% of healthy controls (11).

Epidemiological Evidence for Autoantibody-Mediated Bone Loss in RA

Bone loss is strongly associated with ACPA positivity in RA patients (27–29). Higher ACPA titers correlate with increased systemic osteopenia, indicating that ACPA might contribute to bone loss, either directly or via increased systemic inflammation. In the last years, several studies tried to disentangle direct ACPA-mediated effects from inflammation with inconclusive results. Llorente et al. described that the presence of ACPA was associated with baseline bone mass independently of disease activity in a cohort of early RA patients (30), suggesting direct effects of ACPA on the bone. This was further confirmed by studies describing that ACPA positive individuals without clinical signs of RA display signs of bone loss in metacarpal joints (31, 32). However, subclinical inflammation can't be fully excluded in these studies. Ten Brinck et al. reported that ACPA positive RA patients only exhibited bone resorption in the presence of local inflammation (33). However, general inflammation alone seems insufficient to induce bone loss, since patients with ACPA positive RA displayed the most severe form of bone loss when compared to patients suffering from other inflammatory diseases like seronegative RA, psoriatic arthritis or inflammatory bowel disease (34). These studies indicate that an interplay of direct and indirect effects of ACPA on bone homeostasis leads to local and systemic bone loss. We will discuss the mechanisms by which ACPA affect bone later in this review.

Like ACPA, anti-CarP are associated with higher disease severity and increased bone erosion (23, 26, 35), but more research is needed to elucidate its underlying mechanisms. The fact that ACPA fine specificity does not seem to correlate with disease progression and bone erosion (36, 37) strongly suggests common mechanisms for all AMPA to mediate bone loss, most likely via the conserved Fc part of IgG.

FcγR Signaling in Immune Cells and in Osteoclasts

Humans possess five classical FcγR: FcγRI, FcγRIIA, FcγRIIB FcγRIIIA, and FcγRIIIB that differ in their IgG binding capacity and downstream signaling pathways [reviewed in Nimmerjahn and Ravetch (38), Ghazizadeh (39), Nimmerjahn and Ravetch (40), and Ono (41)]. FcγRI is the only known high-affinity FcγR that is able to bind uncomplexed IgG while all other FcγR need the crosslinking effects of immune complexes to become activated. Activation of FcγRI, FcγRIIA and FcγRIIIA results in the phosphorylation of either an intrinsic immunoreceptor tyrosine-based activation motif (ITAM) domain (as for FcγRIIA) or an ITAM domain supplied by accessory proteins, typically the Fc-receptor common γ-chain (FcRγ-chain) (**Figure 1A**). This phosphorylation leads to the recruitment and activation of spleen tyrosine kinase (Syk) and its downstream targets. The most important events after FcγR activation are calcium influx and the engagement of the rat sarcoma (RAS)- rapidly accelerated fibrosarcoma (RAF)- mitogen-activated protein kinase (MAPK) pathway, resulting in antigen uptake, phagocytosis, cellular activation, and the release of pro-inflammatory cytokines by immune cells. Activating FcγRs have one potent inhibitory opponent: FcγRIIB, which contains an intrinsic immunoreceptor tyrosine-based inhibition motif (ITIM) domain. The ITIM domain interferes with ITAM signaling through engagement of src homology 2-containing inositol phosphatase (SHIP) or src homology 2 domain-containing protein tyrosine phosphatases (SHPs) that inhibit calcium influx by hydrolyzing phosphoinositide intermediates. FcγRIIIB, expressed on neutrophils, has a glycosylphosphatidylinositol (GPI) anchor without a signaling domain (44). The mechanisms by which FcγRIIIB transduces signals are still unknown.

Osteoclasts belong to the myeloid cell lineage and share many features with macrophages. Like macrophages, osteoclasts and their precursors express FcγR (45–47) with FcγRI, FcγRIIB and FcγRIIIA being significantly upregulated during human *ex vivo* osteoclastogenesis (46). It is not clear whether FcγR possess a role in bone homeostasis. However, activation of FcγR with crosslinked antibodies enhanced osteoclastogenesis from murine bone marrow cells (47). This suggests that FcγR regulate osteoclast activity and bone resorption. Of

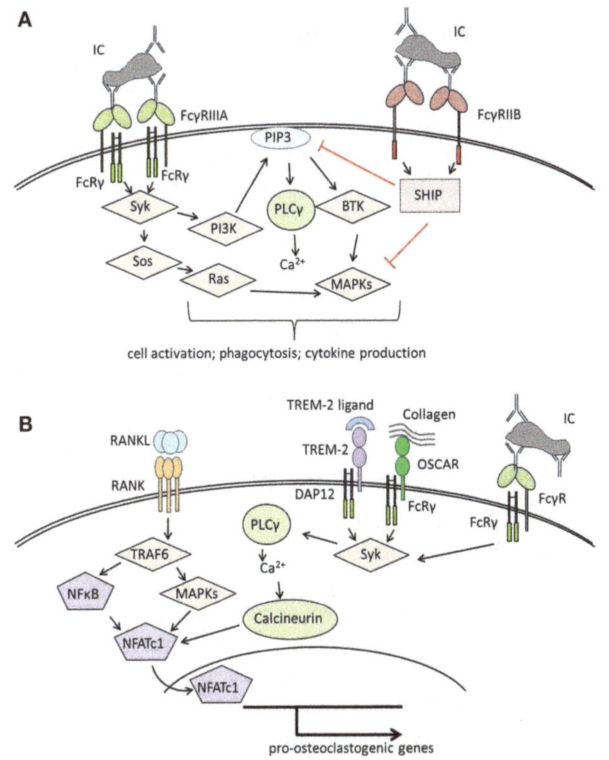

FIGURE 1 | Overview of signaling pathways of **(A)** Fcγ receptors (FcγRs) on immune cells and **(B)** co-stimulatory molecules involved in osteoclastogenesis. **(A)** Crosslinking of activating FcγR (here FcγRIIIA) results in Syk activation starting various signaling pathways that lead to immune cell activation and effector functions like phagocytosis or cytokine production. The distinct signaling pathways have been reviewed in detail in Nimmerjahn and Ravetch (40), Rosales (42). **(B)** Binding of RANKL to RANK leads to the activation of TRAF6, NFκB, and several MAP kinases resulting in the activation of NFATc1, the master transcription factor for pro-osteoclastogenic genes. For a stable NFATc1 activation, costimulatory signals provided by several receptors associated to the accessory molecules DAP12 or FcRγ, like TREM-2 or OSCAR are needed [reviewed in detail in Humphrey and Nakamura (43)]. These receptors lead to Syk activation with subsequent calcium influx enhancing NFATc1 activation. In a similar way, binding of immune complexes to FcγR initiates co-stimulatory signals, thereby enhancing osteoclastogenesis. BTK, Bruton's tyrosin kinase; DAP12, DNAX activation protein of 12kDa; FcRγ, Fc receptor gamma chain; IC, immune complex; MAPKs, mitogen-activated protein kinases; NFATc1, nuclear factor of activated T cells cytoplasmic 1; NFκB, nuclear factor kappa-light-chain-enhancer of activated B cells; OSCAR, Osteoclast-associated immunoglobulin-like receptor; PI3K, phosphatidylinositol-3 kinase; PIP3, phosphatidylinositol 3,4,5-trisphosphate; PLCγ, phospholipase Cγ; SHIP, SH2 domain-containing inositol 5'-phosphatase; Syk, spleen tyrosine kinase; Sos, son of Sevenless; TRAF6, TNF receptor associated factor 6; TREM-2, triggering receptor expressed on myeloid cells 2.

note, osteoclast development is strongly dependent on co-stimulatory signals provided by the accessory protein FcRγ-chain (that is also used by FcγR) and its functional analog DNAX activation protein of 12 kDa (DAP12) (**Figure 1B**). Mice lacking both proteins display a severe osteopetrotic phenotype with impaired osteoclast function (48, 49). FcRγ-chain is likely involved in osteoblast-osteoclast and osteoclast-matrix interactions as it is associated with paired immunoglobulin-like receptor A (PIR-A) and osteoclast-associated receptor (OSCAR) (48, 50). DAP12 associates with TREM-2 and signal-regulatory protein b1 (SIRPb1), which seems to be necessary for the communication between osteoclast precursors (48, 51). Both accessory proteins might enhance the effects of RANKL-signaling by amplifying calcium influx required for the activation of the pro-osteoclastogenic transcription factor, NFATc1 (48).

Direct Actions of ACPA on Osteoclastogenesis

The described positive effects of FcγR signaling on osteoclastogenesis suggest that autoantibodies or autoimmune complexes could directly enhance osteoclast development and hence osteoclast-mediated bone loss in patients with RA. Indeed, we found that affinity-purified autoantibodies against citrullinated vimentin from RA patients, but not ACPA-depleted serum IgG were able to enhance osteoclastogenesis and bone resorption in *ex vivo* osteoclastogenesis assays as well as in recombination activation gene 1 (RAG1)-deficient mice (52). This effect was based on direct binding of autoantibodies to osteoclasts and their precursors resulting in the release of the pro-inflammatory cytokine TNF-α. In later studies, Krishnamurthy and colleagues suggested similar pro-osteoclastogenic effects of ACPA using polyclonal ACPA, purified with a cyclic citrullinated peptide (CCP)-column as well as monoclonal ACPA (53). While the results with polyclonal anti-CCP antibodies confirmed the original findings with polyclonal antibodies against citrullinated vimentin, the monoclonal antibody preparations were later demonstrated to not recognize citrullinated proteins and therefore have to be viewed with caution.

In a murine model of antigen-induced arthritis, immunization against and subsequent challenge with citrullinated vimentin induced stronger periarticular bone loss than immunization against and challenge with methylated bovine serum albumin (mBSA) (54). This effect was independent from inflammation, as mBSA induced more severe synovitis. Similarly, mice immunized with autologous citrullinated type II mouse collagen developed arthritis and bone loss correlating with serum ACPA levels (55).

Together, these studies indicate a direct effect of ACPA on osteoclastogenesis and bone loss. Whether this pro-osteoclastic effect is indeed based on antigen-antibody binding or is preferentially mediated by FcγR remains to be determined.

Impact of Immune Complexes on Osteoclastogenesis

Recently, we found that under certain circumstances not only ACPA, but basically any kind of IgG containing immune complex can increase osteoclast number and bone resorption *in vitro* as well as *in vivo* via binding to FcγR (46, 56). In a murine model of inflammatory arthritis, the osteoclast specific deletion of FcγRIV resulted in a protection from aberrant osteoclast generation and bone erosion in inflamed joints, while inflammation itself was not affected, indicating that inflammatory cytokines alone are not sufficient to induce bone loss in inflammatory arthritis (47). Mice with a global deletion of the inhibitory FcγRIIB exhibit an osteoporotic phenotype even under steady state conditions due to an increase in osteoclast number (57). FcγRIIB is an important regulator of B cells and its deletion leads to a massive induction of autoantibodies (58) that could enhance osteoclastogenesis. Indeed, despite no difference in osteoclast numbers generated *ex vivo* from wildtype and FcγRIIB deficient bone marrow, the addition of sera from FcγRIIB-deficient mice resulted in an increased osteoclastogenesis. This effect could be blocked by IgG depletion or deletion of FcγRIII.

Indirect Effects of Autoantibodies on Osteoclastogenesis by Induction of Proinflammatory Cytokines

In addition to the direct action of autoantibodies on osteoclastogenesis, the release of inflammatory cytokines by macrophages upon autoantibody stimulation has been identified to enhance osteoclast differentiation and function (**Figure 2**). The disequilibrium between pro- and anti-inflammatory cytokine activities facilitates the induction of chronic inflammation and joint damage. It is less known though, how cytokines are organized within a hierarchical regulatory network. Macrophages are considered to play a seminal part in cytokine production in the joints of patients with RA and represent a major source for most of the prominent mediators of disease, such as tumor necrosis factor (TNF)-α and interleukin (IL)-6, but also other cytokines and chemokines involved in the disease process, such as IL-1β, IL-8, and chemokine (C-C motif) ligand 2 (CCL2) (59).

Autoantibodies and their immune complexes may play a central role in shaping a pro-inflammatory environment. Indeed, complexes of ACPA and RF induce robust cytokine production from human macrophages (60–62). This effect is mediated by FcγR signaling on macrophages inducing a strong activation signal for cytokine release (63). In particular, macrophages pre-exposed to M-CSF are sensitive to immune complex-mediated cytokine production. In the synovial membrane of RA patients, M-CSF is present in large amounts (64). We recently showed that treatment of human monocytes with ACPA antibodies or RF leads to the production of the cytokines TNF-α, IL-1β, IL-6, and IL-8 (65). This induction of pro-inflammatory cytokines can enhance osteoclast differentiation (**Figure 2**).

TNF-α is among the most potent cytokines to stimulate osteoclastogenesis. On one hand, TNF-α can induce TRAP positive cells in the absence of RANKL through the induction of the NF-κB pathway (66). On the other hand, TNF-α induces RANK expression by osteoclast precursors (67). In addition, TNF-α and RANKL cooperate to induce osteoclast formation in a TRAF-6 independent pathway through TRAF-3 signaling (68). In addition, TNF-α can indirectly regulate osteoclasts through various stimuli of the stromal cells, for examples by production of RANKL or other cytokines (69).

Like TNF-α, IL-6 is a powerful molecule to induce osteoclast differentiation (70). IL-6 binds the IL-6 receptor, comprising

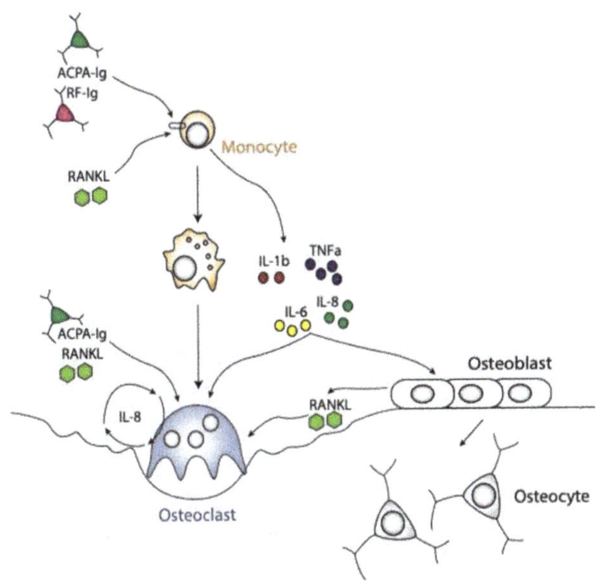

FIGURE 2 | Schematic representations of osteoclast differentiation regulated by ACPA or RF antibodies induced cytokines produced by the monocytic lineages. The cytokines, like TNFa, IL1b, IL6, and IL8 are produced by monocyte lineage challenge with ACPA or RF autoantibodies. All these cytokines are directly able to enhance osteoclast formation. Moreover, they can also regulate stromal cells to secrete RANKL, which in turn will induce osteoclast differentiation. It is also well-known that ACPA can influence IL8 secretion by osteoclasts them-selves which will enhance osteoclastogenesis in an autocrine manner.

the subunit gp130 that is also required for other cytokines. IL-6R induction leads to STAT3 phosphorylation, followed by JAK, which finally induces osteoclast markers (70). Its role is quite contradictory, because one report described that IL-6 inhibits RANKL-induced osteoclastogenesis. It is likely that IL-6 independently regulates different pathways such as NF-κB, ERK or JNK, leading to alternative regulation of osteoclastogenesis (71, 72). In the treatment of human RA, TNF-α, and IL-6 antagonists ameliorate RA equally, indicating that both cytokines are key drivers of synovitis. Of note, the T cell costimulation inhibitor abatacept (cytotoxic T-lymphocyte associated antigen 4 (CTLA4) is most effective in patients with high ACPA and RF autoantibodies (73, 74). Tanaka et al. showed that immune complexes increased CD80/86 expression on monocyte lineages, rendering them sensitive to abatacept (75) which might explain the strong efficacy of abatacept in ACPA positive RA patients. Interestingly, abatacept treatment not only regulates monocytes but also osteoclast differentiation (76).

Implications of Antibody Glycosylation

IgG has one conserved Fc-glycosylation site located at asparagine-297 in the CH2 domain of the heavy chain (**Figure 3**). This glycosylation is critical for the correct conformation of the Fc part and regulates the binding affinity of IgG to FcγR [reviewed in Arnold et al. (77)]. Elimination of the glycan either by enzymatic deglycosylation or by mutation of asparagine-297 to alanine results in a loss of FcγR binding and hence effector functions (78–80). The glycan core structure is strongly conserved and consists of a heptamer of mannose and N-acetyl glucosamine residues. This core structure can be extended by galactose, terminal sialic acid, bisecting N-acetylglucosamine, and core fucose, resulting in a huge variety of theoretically possible glycoforms [reviewed in Zauner et al. (81)]. The exact composition of the Fc glycan determines whether IgG exerts rather pro- or anti-inflammatory effects on immune cells. Especially galactose and terminal sialic acid have been shown to render IgG more anti-inflammatory. 35–45% of random serum IgG from healthy donors is monogalactosylated and 16–27% is bigalactosylated (82). Galactosylation decreases with age (83). During pregnancy, galactosylation is increased and correlates with pregnancy-induced remission of RA (84–86). Only about 10–20% of human serum IgG is sialylated (87, 88), but this low percentage seems to be enough to sustain an anti-inflammatory environment under healthy conditions. It is believed that sialylated IgG actively suppresses immune cells via receptors of the C-type lectin superfamily, such as dendritic cell specific ICAM-grabbing non-integrin (DC-SIGN) (with the murine ortholog SIGNR-1) and the dendritic cell immunoreceptor (DCIR) (89, 90). In addition to Fc glycosylation, about 15–25% of IgG contain Fab glycosylation sites [reviewed in Zauner et al. (81)]. These sites emerge during somatic hypermutation. So far it is unclear if Fab glycosylation has a functional role.

Of note, ACPA display less terminal sialic acid compared to total IgG. ACPA from synovial fluid are even less sialylated (91). The low sialic acid content of ACPA and probably also of other autoantibodies seems to play a key role for the development of clinical disease and bone erosion. In a murine model of collagen induced arthritis, we found that mice fed with sialic acid precursor N-acetylmannosamine did not only display higher sialylation of IgG1, but also have a lower incidence, lower arthritis scores and less bone destruction (46). In addition, it was shown that mice lacking IL-23 do not develop collagen-induced arthritis despite the induction of collagen autoantibodies (92). Autoantibody titers and affinity were not changed compared to wildtype mice, but autoantibodies from IL-23 deficient mice contained more sialic acid. Enzymatic removal of terminal sialic acid resulted in higher arthritis scores, demonstrating the importance of antibody glycosylation for IgG activity. The importance of glycosylation for autoantibody-mediated bone loss is further demonstrated by the fact that even pooled serum IgG from healthy donors is able to enhance osteoclastogenesis and bone resorption after complexation and enzymatic removal of sialic acid (46).

So far it is not completely understood how antibody glycosylation is regulated. The IL-23-T_H17 axis seems to play a crucial role in autoantibody sialylation by the regulation of the enzyme ST6 beta-galactoside α-2,6-sialyltransferase 1 (St6Gal1) that attaches sialic acid to terminal galactose residues (92). Also estrogen positively regulates St6Gal1 expression and postmenopausal women with RA receiving hormone replacement therapy displayed significantly increased Fc sialylation of IgG (93).

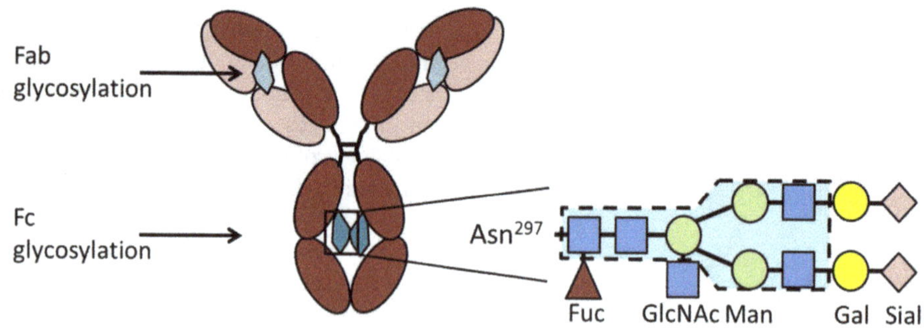

FIGURE 3 | IgG glycosylation. IgG contains a conserved glycosylation site at the asparagine (Asn)^{297} in the CH2 domain of the heavy chain. The Fc glycan (depicted in petrol) consists of a conserved heptamer (shaded in blue) that can be extended by various additional sugar residues. Here we show a fully processed glycan containing all sugar residues possible. In addition to the Fc glycan, some IgG molecules contain a glycosylation site in the Fab region (depicted in light petrol) that occurs stochastically due to the introduction of a new glycosylation site during somatic hypermutation. Asn, asparagine; Gal, galactose; GlcNAc, N-acetylglucosamine; Fuc, fucose; Man, mannose; Sial, sialic acid.

Conclusions and Future Research Agenda

Within the last years, evidence emerged that disease-associated autoantibodies play an important role in the development of bone loss in RA. Especially ACPA have been shown to contribute to aberrant osteoclast formation and activation either by direct stimulation of osteoclast precursors or the induction of a cytokine storm mainly by macrophages. Furthermore, low Fc sialylation of ACPA contributes to their inflammatory and pro-osteoclastogenic phenotype.

The majority of studies addressing autoantibody-mediated bone loss has been performed in mice or *in vitro* models and might incompletely reflect the human situation. There are interesting human studies suggesting that ACPA induce bone loss in the absence of inflammation. However, additional human studies are needed to clarify to what extent ACPA contribute to bone loss in RA patients.

Furthermore, beside the hyperactivation of osteoclasts, an impairment of osteoblast development and function is found in RA patients that aggravates bone loss. To date there is no report showing a direct action of ACPA or RF autoantibodies on osteoblast differentiation or activity, although the FcγRs have been shown to be expressed by stromal cells (47). It would be essential to further develop *in vivo* and *in vitro* experiments delineating the molecular actions of autoantibodies on bone formation.

Beside ACPA, a variety of antibodies directed against modified proteins (AMPA) have been discovered in the last years. Most prominent are anti-CarP, but also antibodies against proteins that have undergone acetylation, oxidation, or malondialdehyde-acetaldehyde addition have been described in RA patients [reviewed in Chang and Nigrovic (94)]. It is likely that other autoantibodies against posttranslational modifications, such as anti-CarP affect osteoclastogenesis and bone loss as well. However, there are no mechanistic data available so far. In addition, there are other autoantibodies known that act via completely different mechanisms than the ones described in this article. For example autoantibodies against OPG function as enhancers of osteoclastogenesis by neutralizing OPG [reviewed in Hauser and Harre (95)]. These autoantibodies are found in autoimmune diseases, such as RA and celiac disease and seem to be a feature that is independent of the original disease drivers. Nevertheless, it might be important to check for the presence of these autoantibodies, especially in patients that are not responding to the current therapies.

Based on the fact that ACPA are associated with increased bone loss in RA, one would wish to control autoimmunity in RA and to induce seroconversion or at least lowering of ACPA levels by treatment. Such approaches are for instance B cell depletion by rituximab or inhibition of T cell co-stimulation with abatacept, which are approved therapies in RA and which significantly lower ACPA levels (96). However, whether modifying autoantibody levels has clinical value in controlling disease, remains to be determined. Aside from antibody reduction, the triggers promoting the induction of effector function of autoantibodies are also targets for future interventions. Given the fact that Fc glycosylation (and especially sialylation) controls the pathogenicity of autoantibodies, it will be interesting to know whether one can control IgG sialylation in RA patients. This might be an important step toward tolerance induction and disease cure.

In addition, in the last years, more attention has been laid on the role of the mucosal immune system during RA initiation and propagation [reviewed in Caminer et al. (97) and Wells et al. (98)]. Dysregulations of microbiota and the gut barrier function might trigger the series of events that deregulate T and B cell responses resulting in autoimmunity in RA patients.

AUTHOR CONTRIBUTIONS

All authors listed have made a substantial, direct and intellectual contribution to the work, and approved it for publication.

ACKNOWLEDGMENTS

This study was supported by the Deutsche Forschungsgemeinschaft: DFG BO-3811/5-1; BO-3811/6-1; CRC1181 project A01; HA 8163/1-1; FOR2886 (TP2, TP3, and TP4); the SPP2084 μBone; the Interdisciplinary Center for Clinical Research (IZKF) grant D23.

REFERENCES

1. Tanaka Y, Nakayamada S, Okada Y. Osteoblasts and osteoclasts in bone remodeling and inflammation. *Curr Drug Targets Inflamm Allergy.* (2005) 4:325–8. doi: 10.2174/1568010054022015
2. Schett G. Osteoimmunology in rheumatic diseases. *Arthritis Res Ther.* (2009) 11:210. doi: 10.1186/ar2571
3. Bonewald LF. The role of the osteocyte in bone and nonbone disease. *Endocrinol Metab Clin North Am.* (2017) 46:1–18. doi: 10.1016/j.ecl.2016.09.003
4. McInnes IB, Schett G. The pathogenesis of rheumatoid arthritis. *N Engl J Med.* (2011) 365:2205–19. doi: 10.1056/NEJMra1004965
5. Zerbini CAF, Clark P, Mendez-Sanchez L, Pereira RMR, Messina OD, Una CR, et al. Biologic therapies and bone loss in rheumatoid arthritis. *Osteopor Int.* (2017) 28:429–446. doi: 10.1007/s00198-016-3769-2
6. Nakken B, Papp G, Bosnes V, Zeher M, Nagy G, Szodoray P. Biomarkers for rheumatoid arthritis: from molecular processes to diagnostic applications-current concepts and future perspectives. *Immunol Lett.* (2017) 189:13–18. doi: 10.1016/j.imlet.2017.05.010
7. Palazzi C, Buskila D, D'Angelo S, D'Amico E, Olivieri I. Autoantibodies in patients with chronic hepatitis C virus infection: pitfalls for the diagnosis of rheumatic diseases. *Autoimmun Rev.* (2012) 11:659–63. doi: 10.1016/j.autrev.2011.11.011
8. Aletaha D, Alasti F, Smolen JS. Rheumatoid factor determines structural progression of rheumatoid arthritis dependent and independent of disease activity. *Ann Rheum Dis.* (2013) 72:875–80. doi: 10.1136/annrheumdis-2012-201517
9. Hecht C, Englbrecht M, Rech J, Schmidt S, Araujo E, Engelke K, et al. Additive effect of anti-citrullinated protein antibodies and rheumatoid factor on bone erosions in patients with RA. *Ann Rheum Dis.* (2015) 74:2151–6. doi: 10.1136/annrheumdis-2014-205428
10. Sokolove J, Johnson DS, Lahey LJ, Wagner CA, Cheng D, Thiele GM, et al. Rheumatoid factor as a potentiator of anti-citrullinated protein antibody-mediated inflammation in rheumatoid arthritis. *Arthritis Rheumatol.* (2014) 66:813–21. doi: 10.1002/art.38307
11. van Delft MAM, van Beest S, Kloppenburg M, Trouw LA, Ioan-Facsinay A. Presence of autoantibodies in erosive hand osteoarthritis and association with clinical presentation. *J Rheumatol.* (2018) 46:101–5. doi: 10.3899/jrheum.180256
12. Wegner N, Lundberg K, Kinloch A, Fisher B, Malmstrom V, Feldmann M, et al. Autoimmunity to specific citrullinated proteins gives the first clues to the etiology of rheumatoid arthritis. *Immunol Rev.* (2010) 233:34–54. doi: 10.1111/j.0105-2896.2009.00850.x
13. Jilani AA, Mackworth-Young CG. The role of citrullinated protein antibodies in predicting erosive disease in rheumatoid arthritis: a systematic literature review and meta-analysis. *Int J Rheumatol.* (2015) 2015:728610. doi: 10.1155/2015/728610
14. Kokkonen H, Mullazehi M, Berglin E, Hallmans G, Wadell G, Ronnelid J, et al. Antibodies of IgG, IgA and IgM isotypes against cyclic citrullinated peptide precede the development of rheumatoid arthritis. *Arthritis Res Ther.* (2011) 13:R13. doi: 10.1186/ar3237
15. Suwannalai P, van de Stadt LA, Radner H, Steiner G, El-Gabalawy HS, Zijde CM, et al. Avidity maturation of anti-citrullinated protein antibodies in rheumatoid arthritis. *Arthritis Rheum.* (2012) 64:1323–8. doi: 10.1002/art.33489
16. van der Woude D, Rantapaa-Dahlqvist S, Ioan-Facsinay A, Onnekink C, Schwarte CM, Verpoort KN, et al. Epitope spreading of the anti-citrullinated protein antibody response occurs before disease onset and is associated with the disease course of early arthritis. *Ann Rheum Dis.* (2010) 69:1554–61. doi: 10.1136/ard.2009.124537
17. Aletaha D, Neogi T, Silman AJ, Funovits J, Felson DT, Bingham CO III, et al. 2010 rheumatoid arthritis classification criteria: an American College of Rheumatology/European League Against Rheumatism collaborative initiative. *Ann Rheum Dis.* (2010) 69:1580–8. doi: 10.1002/art.27584
18. Baka Z, Gyorgy B, Geher P, Buzas EI, Falus A, Nagy G. Citrullination under physiological and pathological conditions. *Joint Bone Spine.* (2012) 79:431–6. doi: 10.1016/j.jbspin.2012.01.008
19. McGraw WT, Potempa J, Farley D, Travis J. Purification, characterization, and sequence analysis of a potential virulence factor from Porphyromonas gingivalis, peptidylarginine deiminase. *Infect Immun.* (1999) 67:3248–56.
20. Araujo VM, Melo IM, Lima V. Relationship between periodontitis and rheumatoid arthritis: review of the literature. *Mediators Inflamm.* (2015) 2015:259074. doi: 10.1155/2015/259074
21. Potempa J, Mydel P, Koziel J. The case for periodontitis in the pathogenesis of rheumatoid arthritis. *Nat Rev Rheumatol.* (2017) 13:606–20. doi: 10.1038/nrrheum.2017.132
22. Klareskog L, Malmstrom V, Lundberg K, Padyukov L, Alfredsson L. Smoking, citrullination and genetic variability in the immunopathogenesis of rheumatoid arthritis. *Semin Immunol.* (2011) 23:92–8. doi: 10.1016/j.smim.2011.01.014
23. Shi J, Knevel R, Suwannalai P, van der Linden MP, Janssen GM, van Veelen PA, et al. Autoantibodies recognizing carbamylated proteins are present in sera of patients with rheumatoid arthritis and predict joint damage. *Proc Natl Acad Sci USA.* (2011) 108:17372–7. doi: 10.1073/pnas.1114465108
24. Juarez M, Bang H, Hammar F, Reimer U, Dyke B, Sahbudin I, et al. Identification of novel antiacetylated vimentin antibodies in patients with early inflammatory arthritis. *Ann Rheum Dis.* (2016) 75:1099–107. doi: 10.1136/annrheumdis-2014-206785
25. Ospelt C, Bang H, Feist E, Camici G, Keller S, Detert J, et al. Carbamylation of vimentin is inducible by smoking and represents an independent autoantigen in rheumatoid arthritis. *Ann Rheum Dis.* (2017) 76:1176–83. doi: 10.1136/annrheumdis-2016-210059
26. Montes A, Regueiro C, Perez-Pampin E, Boveda MD, Gomez-Reino JJ, Gonzalez A. Anti-carbamylated protein antibodies as a reproducible independent type of rheumatoid arthritis autoantibodies. *PLoS ONE.* (2016) 11:e0161141. doi: 10.1371/journal.pone.0161141
27. Hafstrom I, Ajeganova S, Forslind K, Svensson B. Anti-citrullinated protein antibodies are associated with osteopenia but not with pain at diagnosis of rheumatoid arthritis: data from the BARFOT cohort. *Arthritis Res Ther.* (2019) 21:45. doi: 10.1186/s13075-019-1833-y
28. Orsolini G, Caimmi C, Viapiana O, Idolazzi L, Fracassi E, Gatti D, et al. Titer-dependent effect of anti-citrullinated protein antibodies on systemic bone mass in rheumatoid arthritis patients. *Calcif Tissue Int.* (2017) 101:17–23. doi: 10.1007/s00223-017-0253-8
29. Sargin G, Kose R, Senturk T. Relationship between bone mineral density and anti-citrullinated protein antibody and rheumatoid factor in patients with rheumatoid arthritis. *Eur J Rheumatol.* (2019) 6:29–33. doi: 10.5152/eurjrheum.2018.18099
30. Llorente I, Merino L, Ortiz AM, Escolano E, Gonzalez-Ortega S, Garcia-Vicuna R, et al. Anti-citrullinated protein antibodies are associated with decreased bone mineral density: baseline data from a register of early arthritis patients. *Rheumatol Int.* (2017) 37:799–806. doi: 10.1007/s00296-017-3674-9
31. Keller KK, Thomsen JS, Stengaard-Pedersen K, Nielsen AW, Schiottz-Christensen B, Svendsen L, et al. Local bone loss in patients with anti-citrullinated peptide antibody and arthralgia, evaluated with high-resolution peripheral quantitative computed tomography. *Scand J Rheumatol.* (2018) 47:110–116. doi: 10.1080/03009742.2017.1333629
32. Kleyer A, Finzel S, Rech J, Manger B, Krieter M, Faustini F, et al. Bone loss before the clinical onset of rheumatoid arthritis in subjects with anticitrullinated protein antibodies. *Ann Rheum Dis.* (2014) 73:854–60. doi: 10.1136/annrheumdis-2012-202958
33. Ten Brinck RM, Toes REM, van der Helm-van Mil AHM. Inflammation functions as a key mediator in the link between ACPA and erosion development: an association study in Clinically Suspect Arthralgia. *Arthritis Res Ther.* (2018) 20:89. doi: 10.1186/s13075-018-1574-3
34. Simon D, Kleyer A, Englbrecht M, Stemmler F, Simon C, Berlin A, et al. A comparative analysis of articular bone in large cohort of patients with chronic inflammatory diseases of the joints, the gut and the skin. *Bone.* (2018) 116:87–93. doi: 10.1016/j.bone.2018.07.017
35. Ceccarelli F, Perricone C, Colasanti T, Massaro L, Cipriano E, Pendolino M, et al. Anti-carbamylated protein antibodies as a new biomarker of erosive joint damage in systemic lupus erythematosus. *Arthritis Res Ther.* (2018) 20:126. doi: 10.1186/s13075-018-1622-z
36. Scherer HU, van der Woude D, Willemze A, Trouw LA, Knevel R, Syversen SW, et al. Distinct ACPA fine specificities, formed under the

influence of HLA shared epitope alleles, have no effect on radiographic joint damage in rheumatoid arthritis. *Ann Rheum Dis.* (2011) 70:1461–4. doi: 10.1136/ard.2010.146506

37. van Beers JJ, Willemze A, Jansen JJ, Engbers GH, Salden M, Raats J, et al. ACPA fine-specificity profiles in early rheumatoid arthritis patients do not correlate with clinical features at baseline or with disease progression. *Arthritis Res Ther.* (2013) 15:R140. doi: 10.1186/ar4322
38. Nimmerjahn F, Ravetch JV. Antibody-mediated modulation of immune responses. *Immunol Rev.* (2010) 236:265–75. doi: 10.1111/j.1600-065X.2010.00910.x
39. Ghazizadeh S, Bolen JB, Fleit HB. Tyrosine phosphorylation and association of Syk with Fc gamma RII in monocytic THP-1 cells. *Biochem J.* (1995) 305(Pt 2):669–74. doi: 10.1042/bj3050669
40. Nimmerjahn F, Ravetch JV. Fcgamma receptors as regulators of immune responses. *Nat Rev Immunol.* (2008) 8:34–47. doi: 10.1038/nri2206
41. Ono M, Bolland S, Tempst P, Ravetch JV. Role of the inositol phosphatase SHIP in negative regulation of the immune system by the receptor Fc(gamma)RIIB. *Nature.* (1996) 383:263–6. doi: 10.1038/383263a0
42. Rosales C. Fcgamma receptor heterogeneity in leukocyte functional responses. *Front Immunol.* (2017) 8:280. doi: 10.3389/fimmu.2017.00280
43. Humphrey MB, Nakamura MC. A comprehensive review of immunoreceptor regulation of osteoclasts. *Clin Rev Allergy Immunol.* (2016) 51:48–58. doi: 10.1007/s12016-015-8521-8
44. Selvaraj P, Rosse WF, Silber R, Springer TA. The major Fc receptor in blood has a phosphatidylinositol anchor and is deficient in paroxysmal nocturnal haemoglobinuria. *Nature.* (1988) 333:565–7. doi: 10.1038/333565a0
45. Harre U, Keppeler H, Ipseiz N, Derer A, Poller K, Aigner M, et al. Moonlighting osteoclasts as undertakers of apoptotic cells. *Autoimmunity.* (2012) 45:612–9. doi: 10.3109/08916934.2012.719950
46. Harre U, Lang SC, Pfeifle R, Rombouts Y, Fruhbeisser S, Amara K, et al. Glycosylation of immunoglobulin G determines osteoclast differentiation and bone loss. *Nat Commun.* (2015) 6:6651. doi: 10.1038/ncomms7651
47. Seeling M, Hillenhoff U, David JP, Schett G, Tuckermann J, Lux A, et al. Inflammatory monocytes and Fcgamma receptor IV on osteoclasts are critical for bone destruction during inflammatory arthritis in mice. *Proc Natl Acad Sci USA.* (2013) 110:10729–34. doi: 10.1073/pnas.1301001110
48. Koga T, Inui M, Inoue K, Kim S, Suematsu A, Kobayashi E, et al. Costimulatory signals mediated by the ITAM motif cooperate with RANKL for bone homeostasis. *Nature.* (2004) 428:758–63. doi: 10.1038/nature02444
49. Kaifu T, Nakahara J, Inui M, Mishima K, Momiyama T, Kaji M, et al. Osteopetrosis and thalamic hypomyelinosis with synaptic degeneration in DAP12-deficient mice. *J Clin Invest.* (2003) 111:323–32. doi: 10.1172/JCI200316923
50. Kim N, Takami M, Rho J, Josien R, Choi Y. A novel member of the leukocyte receptor complex regulates osteoclast differentiation. *J Exp Med.* (2002) 195:201–9. doi: 10.1084/jem.20011681
51. Paradowska-Gorycka A, Jurkowska M. Structure, expression pattern and biological activity of molecular complex TREM-2/DAP12. *Hum Immunol.* (2013) 74:730–7. doi: 10.1016/j.humimm.2013.02.003
52. Harre U, Georgess D, Bang H, Bozec A, Axmann R, Ossipova E, et al. Induction of osteoclastogenesis and bone loss by human autoantibodies against citrullinated vimentin. *J Clin Invest.* (2012) 122:1791–802. doi: 10.1172/JCI60975
53. Krishnamurthy A, Joshua V, Haj Hensvold A, Jin T, Sun M, Vivar N, et al. Identification of a novel chemokine-dependent molecular mechanism underlying rheumatoid arthritis-associated autoantibody-mediated bone loss. *Ann Rheum Dis.* (2016) 75:721–9. doi: 10.1136/annrheumdis-2015-208093
54. Engdahl C, Bang H, Dietel K, Lang SC, Harre U, Schett G. Periarticular bone loss in arthritis is induced by autoantibodies against citrullinated vimentin. *J Bone Mineral Res.* (2017) 32:1681–91. doi: 10.1002/jbmr.3158
55. Dusad A, Duryee MJ, Shaw AT, Klassen LW, Anderson DR, Wang D, et al. Induction of bone loss in DBA/1J mice immunized with citrullinated autologous mouse type II collagen in the absence of adjuvant. *Immunol Res.* (2014) 58:51–60. doi: 10.1007/s12026-013-8479-7
56. Grotsch B, Lux A, Rombouts Y, Hoffmann AC, Andreev D, Nimmerjahn F, et al. Fra1 controls rheumatoid factor autoantibody production by bone marrow plasma cells and the development of autoimmune bone loss. *J Bone Miner Res.* (2019) 2019:e3705. doi: 10.1002/jbmr.3705
57. Negishi-Koga T, Gober HJ, Sumiya E, Komatsu N, Okamoto K, Sawa S, et al. Immune complexes regulate bone metabolism through FcRgamma signalling. *Nat Commun.* (2015) 6:6637. doi: 10.1038/ncomms7637
58. Bolland S, Ravetch JV. Spontaneous autoimmune disease in Fc(gamma)RIIB-deficient mice results from strain-specific epistasis. *Immunity.* (2000) 13:277–85. doi: 10.1016/S1074-7613(00)00027-3
59. Haringman JJ, Gerlag DM, Zwinderman AH, Smeets TJ, Kraan MC, Baeten D, et al. Synovial tissue macrophages: a sensitive biomarker for response to treatment in patients with rheumatoid arthritis. *Ann Rheum Dis.* (2005) 64:834–8. doi: 10.1136/ard.2004.029751
60. Anquetil F, Clavel C, Offer G, Serre G, Sebbag M. IgM and IgA rheumatoid factors purified from rheumatoid arthritis sera boost the Fc receptor- and complement-dependent effector functions of the disease-specific anti-citrullinated protein autoantibodies. *J Immunol.* (2015) 194:3664–74. doi: 10.4049/jimmunol.1402334
61. Clavel C, Ceccato L, Anquetil F, Serre G, Sebbag M. Among human macrophages polarised to different phenotypes, the M-CSF-oriented cells present the highest pro-inflammatory response to the rheumatoid arthritis-specific immune complexes containing ACPA. *Ann Rheum Dis.* (2016) 75:2184–91. doi: 10.1136/annrheumdis-2015-208887
62. Laurent L, Clavel C, Lemaire O, Anquetil F, Cornillet M, Zabraniecki L, et al. Fcgamma receptor profile of monocytes and macrophages from rheumatoid arthritis patients and their response to immune complexes formed with autoantibodies to citrullinated proteins. *Ann Rheum Dis.* (2011) 70:1052–9. doi: 10.1136/ard.2010.142091
63. Clavel C, Nogueira L, Laurent L, Iobagiu C, Vincent C, Sebbag M, et al. Induction of macrophage secretion of tumor necrosis factor alpha through Fcgamma receptor IIa engagement by rheumatoid arthritis-specific autoantibodies to citrullinated proteins complexed with fibrinogen. *Arthritis Rheum.* (2008) 58:678–88. doi: 10.1002/art.23284
64. Firestein GS, Xu WD, Townsend K, Broide D, Alvaro-Gracia J, Glasebrook A, et al. Cytokines in chronic inflammatory arthritis. I. Failure to detect T cell lymphokines (interleukin 2 and interleukin 3) and presence of macrophage colony-stimulating factor (CSF-1) and a novel mast cell growth factor in rheumatoid synovitis. *J Exp Med.* (1988) 168:1573–86. doi: 10.1084/jem.168.5.1573
65. Bozec A, Luo Y, Engdahl C, Figueiredo C, Bang H, Schett G. Abatacept blocks anti-citrullinated protein antibody and rheumatoid factor mediated cytokine production in human macrophages in IDO-dependent manner. *Arthritis Res Ther.* (2018) 20:24. doi: 10.1186/s13075-018-1527-x
66. Azuma Y, Kaji K, Katogi R, Takeshita S, Kudo A. Tumor necrosis factor-alpha induces differentiation of and bone resorption by osteoclasts. *J Biol Chem.* (2000) 275:4858–64. doi: 10.1074/jbc.275.7.4858
67. Komine M, Kukita A, Kukita T, Ogata Y, Hotokebuchi T, Kohashi O. Tumor necrosis factor-alpha cooperates with receptor activator of nuclear factor kappaB ligand in generation of osteoclasts in stromal cell-depleted rat bone marrow cell culture. *Bone.* (2001) 28:474–83. doi: 10.1016/S8756-3282(01)00420-3
68. Yao Z, Lei W, Duan R, Li Y, Luo L, Boyce BF. RANKL cytokine enhances TNF-induced osteoclastogenesis independently of TNF receptor associated factor (TRAF) 6 by degrading TRAF3 in osteoclast precursors. *J Biol Chem.* (2017) 292:10169–79. doi: 10.1074/jbc.M116.771816
69. Kitaura H, Zhou P, Kim HJ, Novack DV, Ross FP, Teitelbaum SL. M-CSF mediates TNF-induced inflammatory osteolysis. *J Clin Invest.* (2005) 115:3418–27. doi: 10.1172/JCI26132
70. Kudo O, Sabokbar A, Pocock A, Itonaga I, Fujikawa Y, Athanasou NA. Interleukin-6 and interleukin-11 support human osteoclast formation by a RANKL-independent mechanism. *Bone.* (2003) 32:1–7. doi: 10.1016/S8756-3282(02)00915-8
71. Feng W, Liu H, Luo T, Liu D, Du J, Sun J, et al. Combination of IL-6 and sIL-6R differentially regulate varying levels of RANKL-induced osteoclastogenesis through NF-kappaB, ERK and JNK signaling pathways. *Sci Rep.* (2017) 7:41411. doi: 10.1038/srep41411
72. Yoshitake F, Itoh S, Narita H, Ishihara K, Ebisu S. Interleukin-6 directly inhibits osteoclast differentiation by suppressing receptor activator of NF-kappaB signaling pathways. *J Biol Chem.* (2008) 283:11535–40. doi: 10.1074/jbc.M607999200

73. Pers YM, Fortunet C, Constant E, Lambert J, Godfrin-Valnet M, De Jong A, et al. Predictors of response and remission in a large cohort of rheumatoid arthritis patients treated with tocilizumab in clinical practice. *Rheumatology.* (2014) 53:76–84. doi: 10.1093/rheumatology/ket301
74. Alten R, Nusslein HG, Mariette X, Galeazzi M, Lorenz HM, Cantagrel A, et al. Baseline autoantibodies preferentially impact abatacept efficacy in patients with rheumatoid arthritis who are biologic naive: 6-month results from a real-world, international, prospective study. *RMD Open.* (2017) 3:e000345. doi: 10.1136/rmdopen-2016-000345
75. Tanaka M, Krutzik SR, Sieling PA, Lee DJ, Rea TH, Modlin RL. Activation of Fc gamma RI on monocytes triggers differentiation into immature dendritic cells that induce autoreactive T cell responses. *J Immunol.* (2009) 183:2349–55. doi: 10.4049/jimmunol.0801683
76. Bozec A, Zaiss MM, Kagwiria R, Voll R, Rauh M, Chen Z, et al. T cell costimulation molecules CD80/86 inhibit osteoclast differentiation by inducing the IDO/tryptophan pathway. *Sci Transl Med.* (2014) 6:235ra60. doi: 10.1126/scitranslmed.3007764
77. Arnold JN, Wormald MR, Sim RB, Rudd PM, Dwek RA. The impact of glycosylation on the biological function and structure of human immunoglobulins. *Annu Rev Immunol.* (2007) 25, 21–50. doi: 10.1146/annurev.immunol.25.022106.141702
78. Collin M, Shannon O, Bjorck L. IgG glycan hydrolysis by a bacterial enzyme as a therapy against autoimmune conditions. *Proc Natl Acad Sci USA.* (2008) 105:4265–70. doi: 10.1073/pnas.0711271105
79. Kao D, Danzer H, Collin M, Gross A, Eichler J, Stambuk J, et al. A Monosaccharide residue is sufficient to maintain mouse and human IgG subclass activity and directs IgG effector functions to cellular Fc receptors. *Cell Rep.* (2015) 13:2376–85. doi: 10.1016/j.celrep.2015.11.027
80. Lux A, Yu X, Scanlan CN, Nimmerjahn F. Impact of immune complex size and glycosylation on IgG binding to human FcgammaRs. *J Immunol.* (2013) 190:4315–23. doi: 10.4049/jimmunol.1200501
81. Zauner G, Selman MH, Bondt A, Rombouts Y, Blank D, Deelder AM, et al. Glycoproteomic analysis of antibodies. *Mol Cell Proteomics.* (2013) 12:856–65. doi: 10.1074/mcp.R112.026005
82. Kaneko Y, Nimmerjahn F, Ravetch JV. Anti-inflammatory activity of immunoglobulin G resulting from Fc sialylation. *Science.* (2006) 313:670–3. doi: 10.1126/science.1129594
83. Parekh R, Roitt I, Isenberg D, Dwek R, Rademacher T. Age-related galactosylation of the N-linked oligosaccharides of human serum IgG. *J Exp Med.* (1988) 167:1731–6. doi: 10.1084/jem.167.5.1731
84. Bondt A, Selman MH, Deelder AM, Hazes JM, Willemsen SP, Wuhrer M, et al. Association between galactosylation of immunoglobulin G and improvement of rheumatoid arthritis during pregnancy is independent of sialylation. *J Proteome Res.* (2013) 12:4522–31. doi: 10.1021/pr400589m
85. Rook GA, Steele J, Brealey R, Whyte A, Isenberg D, Sumar N, et al. Changes in IgG glycoform levels are associated with remission of arthritis during pregnancy. *J Autoimmun.* (1991) 4:779–94. doi: 10.1016/0896-8411(91)90173-A
86. van de Geijn FE, Wuhrer M, Selman MH, Willemsen SP, de Man YA, Deelder AM, et al. Immunoglobulin G galactosylation and sialylation are associated with pregnancy-induced improvement of rheumatoid arthritis and the postpartum flare: results from a large prospective cohort study. *Arthritis Res Ther.* (2009) 11:R193. doi: 10.1186/ar2892
87. Selman MH, Derks RJ, Bondt A, Palmblad M, Schoenmaker B, Koeleman CA, et al. Fc specific IgG glycosylation profiling by robust nano-reverse phase HPLC-MS using a sheath-flow ESI sprayer interface. *J Proteomics.* (2012) 75:1318–29. doi: 10.1016/j.jprot.2011.11.003
88. Anumula KR. Quantitative glycan profiling of normal human plasma derived immunoglobulin and its fragments Fab and Fc. *J Immunol Methods.* (2012) 382:167–76. doi: 10.1016/j.jim.2012.05.022
89. Anthony RM, Wermeling F, Karlsson MC, Ravetch JV. Identification of a receptor required for the anti-inflammatory activity of IVIG. *Proc Natl Acad Sci USA.* (2008) 105:19571–8. doi: 10.1073/pnas.0810163105
90. Massoud AH, Yona M, Xue D, Chouiali F, Alturaihi H, Ablona A, et al. Dendritic cell immunoreceptor: a novel receptor for intravenous immunoglobulin mediates induction of regulatory T cells. *J Allergy Clin Immunol.* (2014) 133:853–63e5. doi: 10.1016/j.jaci.2013.09.029
91. Scherer HU, van der Woude D, Ioan-Facsinay A, el Bannoudi H, Trouw LA, Wang J, et al. Glycan profiling of anti-citrullinated protein antibodies isolated from human serum and synovial fluid. *Arthritis Rheum.* (2010) 62:1620–9. doi: 10.1002/art.27414
92. Pfeifle R, Rothe T, Ipseiz N, Scherer HU, Culemann S, Harre U, et al. Regulation of autoantibody activity by the IL-23-TH17 axis determines the onset of autoimmune disease. *Nat Immunol.* (2017) 18:104–13. doi: 10.1038/ni.3579
93. Engdahl C, Bondt A, Harre U, Raufer J, Pfeifle R, Camponeschi A, et al. Estrogen induces St6gal1 expression and increases IgG sialylation in mice and patients with rheumatoid arthritis: a potential explanation for the increased risk of rheumatoid arthritis in postmenopausal women. *Arthritis Res Ther.* (2018) 20:84. doi: 10.1186/s13075-018-1586-z
94. Chang MH, Nigrovic PA. Antibody-dependent and -independent mechanisms of inflammatory arthritis. *JCI Insight.* (2019) 4:278. doi: 10.1172/jci.insight.125278
95. Hauser B, Harre U. The role of autoantibodies in bone metabolism and bone loss. *Calcif Tissue Int.* (2018) 102:522–32. doi: 10.1007/s00223-017-0370-4
96. Wunderlich C, Oliviera I, Figueiredo CP, Rech J, Schett G. Effects of DMARDs on citrullinated peptide autoantibody levels in RA patients-A longitudinal analysis. *Semin Arthritis Rheum.* (2017) 46:709–14. doi: 10.1016/j.semarthrit.2016.09.011
97. Caminer AC, Haberman R, Scher JU. Human microbiome, infections, and rheumatic disease. *Clin Rheumatol.* (2017) 36:2645–53. doi: 10.1007/s10067-017-3875-3
98. Wells PM, Williams FMK, Matey-Hernandez ML, Menni C, Steves CJ. 'RA and the microbiome: do host genetic factors provide the link? *J Autoimmun.* (2019) 99:104–15. doi: 10.1016/j.jaut.2019.02.004

14

HGMB1 and RAGE as Essential Components of Ti Osseointegration Process in Mice

*Claudia Cristina Biguetti[1], Franco Cavalla[1,2], Elcia Varize Silveira[3], André Petenuci Tabanez[1], Carolina Favaro Francisconi[1], Rumio Taga[1], Ana Paula Campanelli[1], Ana Paula Favaro Trombone[3], Danieli C. Rodrigues[4] and Gustavo Pompermaier Garlet[1]**

[1] Department of Biological Sciences, Bauru School of Dentistry, University of São Paulo, São Paulo, Brazil, [2] Department of Conservative Dentistry, School of Dentistry, University of Chile, Santiago, Chile, [3] Department of Biological and Allied Health Sciences, Universidade Sagrado Coração, Bauru, Brazil, [4] Department of Bioengineering, University of Texas at Dallas, Dallas, TX, United States

***Correspondence:**
Gustavo Pompermaier Garlet
garletgp@usp.br

The release of the prototypic DAMP High Mobility Group Box 1 (HMGB1) into extracellular environment and its binding to the Receptor for Advanced Glycation End Products (RAGE) has been described to trigger sterile inflammation and regulate healing outcome. However, their role on host response to Ti-based biomaterials and in the subsequent osseointegration remains unexplored. In this study, HMGB1 and RAGE inhibition in the Ti-mediated osseointegration were investigated in C57Bl/6 mice. C57Bl/6 mice received a Ti-device implantation (Ti-screw in the edentulous alveolar crest and a Ti-disc in the subcutaneous tissue) and were evaluated by microscopic (microCT [bone] and histology [bone and subcutaneous]) and molecular methods (ELISA, PCR array) during 3, 7, 14, and 21 days. Mice were divided into 4 groups: Control (no treatment); GZA (IP injection of Glycyrrhizic Acid for HMGB1 inhibition, 4 mg/Kg/day); RAP (IP injection of RAGE Antagonistic Peptide, 4 mg/Kg/day), and vehicle controls (1.5% DMSO solution for GZA and 0.9% saline solution for RAP); treatments were given at all experimental time points, starting 1 day before surgeries. HMGB1 was detected in the Ti-implantation sites, adsorbed to the screws/discs. In Control and vehicle groups, osseointegration was characterized by a slight inflammatory response at early time points, followed by a gradual bone apposition and matrix maturation at late time points. The inhibition of HMGB1 or RAGE impaired the osseointegration, affecting the dynamics of mineralized and organic bone matrix, and resulting in a foreign body reaction, with persistence of macrophages, necrotic bone, and foreign body giant cells until later time points. While Control samples were characterized by a balance between M1 and M2-type response in bone and subcutaneous sites of implantation, and also MSC markers, the inhibition of HMGB1 or RAGE caused a higher expression M1 markers and pro-inflammatory cytokines, as well chemokines and receptors for macrophage migration until later time points. In conclusion, HMGB1 and RAGE have a marked role in the osseointegration, evidenced by their influence on host inflammatory immune response, which includes macrophages migration and M1/M2 response, MSC markers expression, which collectively modulate bone matrix deposition and osseointegration outcome.

Keywords: DAMPs, pre-clinical studies, inflammation, HMGB1, bioengineering, osseointegration, implants, osteoimmunology

INTRODUCTION

Ti-based devices, such as dental implants, are classically used in dentistry, due to their osseointegration capacity that is translated into remarkable clinical success (1–3). However, understanding of the molecular interactions at Ti/host interface, which drive a beneficial equilibrium between immune/inflammatory response and the subsequent bone apposition toward Ti surface remains unclear (3).

A recent study performed an extensive molecular and histological characterization of Ti mediated osseointegration in C57Bl/6 mice, demonstrating a highly orchestrated and transient inflammatory response coordinated with the early stages of osseointegration (4). In view of the dominance of innate immunity elements in the host response that paves the way for osseointegration, in a process where numerous inflammation- and bone healing-related molecules are up-regulated (5, 6), macrophages have been regarded as central determinants of osseointegration outcome (7, 8). Indeed, macrophages can exert key regulatory functions by secreting a range of different mediators (chemokines, cytokines, enzymes, and growth factors) in the inflammatory microenvironment, which consequently influence the intensity and duration of immune response, affecting healing (9, 10). Recent studies suggest macrophages polarization into M1 or M2 phenotypes as a crucial step for determining the success or failure of biomaterial osseointegration, since the dominance of a M1-type response is related to chronic inflammation and fibrous encapsulation of Ti instead of successful osseointegration (7, 9, 11, 12).

Therefore, initial steps of the host inflammatory immune response that will shape macrophages fate in the biomaterial-implantation site seem an essential component for a successful osseointegration outcome. Macrophage polarization around biomaterials begins immediately post-implantation, with biomaterial surface recognition and a transient polarization state, which are influenced by varying microenvironmental cues, some of which are biomaterial-based (9). Thus, it has been supposed that the type and quantity of proteins adsorbed on a biomaterial is influenced by its surface morphological cues and chemistry, which may affect its recognition by macrophages consequently influencing their phenotypic polarization (9, 13).

Considering the candidate proteins for adsorption on Ti surface, damage associated molecular patterns (DAMPs) are a group of endogenous intracellular or extracellular molecules, which are released from their original sites into the microenvironment upon breakage of tissue components caused by trauma or stress, acting as local "danger signals" that trigger host response (14, 15). After their release from damaged tissues, DAMPs are recognized by a number of pattern recognition receptors (PRRs) primarily expressed on macrophages (10, 16, 17). Among several DAMPs/PRRs pathways already described in the literature, the interaction of High Mobility Group Box 1 (HMGB1), the prototypical and most well-characterized DAMP, with the Receptor for Advanced Glycation End Products (RAGE), has been associated with the activation of inflammatory responses and wound healing (18, 19). Indeed, while HMGB1, alone or associated with other molecules, can play pleiotropic functions by activating multiple receptors (TLR4 and TLR2, RAGE, CXCR4) (18, 20, 21). It is also important to mention that HMGB1 is a redox-sensitive molecule and consequently, redox status of its cysteine residues (Cys23, Cys45, and Cys106) is strongly affected by a pro-oxidative and pro-inflammatory environment, since various reactive oxygen species (ROS) are released in inflammatory environments (22, 23). Then, biphasic actions on HMGB1 (pro-inflammatory activity or immune tolerance/healing) may depends on the environment where this molecule is released. In this context, it has been suggested that oxidized or reduced forms of HMGB1 might differently affect the HMGB1 binding into different receptors and induce that biphasic actions (23). For example, oxidized form of HMGB1 accumulates during resolution of inflammation and tissue regeneration in liver, serving as a feedback mechanism to control its proinflammatory activity (22).

RAGE constitute the major receptor for HMGB1 (24–26). Importantly, the axis HMGB1/RAGE is related with several cellular effects which are important to inflammatory and healing outcomes, such as induction of inflammatory response and angiogenesis, tissue remodeling, and stimulation of cellular differentiation for regeneration (19, 27–31). In the context of M1/M2, evidence from *in vivo* studies point that HMGB1 can facilitate M1 macrophage phenotype in certain inflammatory disease models (32, 33), mainly based on HMGB1 interactions with TLR receptors (32). However, other *in vitro* (26) and *in vivo* disease models (34, 35) suggested that HMGB1 can enhance the activity of M2 macrophages, especially in a manner RAGE-dependent (26, 35). Importantly, despite the growing focus on macrophages role in healing, HMGB1/RAGE is a potential trigger of the overall host inflammatory immune response at biomaterials implantation sites, which theoretically can involve other cell besides the macrophages. Indeed, is still unclear how HMGB1/RAGE can trigger and regulate host responses in different inflammatory contexts.

Considering the influence of DAMPs regulating biomaterial incorporation, it has been demonstrated by *in vitro* studies that remaining HMGB1 within xenogeneic biologic scaffolds (after manufacturing processes) affects the response of monocytes/macrophages to the biomaterial and consequently can affect the inflammatory response, such as a bioactive molecule (36). On the other hand, in metallic and permanent biomaterial incorporation, the molecules driving the host response are theoretically exclusively released by host, such as hypothesized by recent reviews in biomaterials science literature (15, 37). Therefore, DAMPs are suggested to be released from tissue damage immediately after biomaterial implantation, possibly interacting with the surface and influencing the innate inflammatory response in the site of biomaterial implantation (15, 38). However, no previous studies have demonstrated the presence of endogenous DAMPs in biomaterials implantation sites, as well their putative role remains to be demonstrated in a cause-and-effect manner.

In face of all evidences for the role of HMGB1 and its cognate receptor RAGE in modulating inflammatory and healing responses, the release of HMGB1 after Ti implant placement could be a critical step for triggering inflammation and healing outcomes in osseointegration sites. Thus, in this present study, we investigated the role of HMGB1 during Ti-mediated oral osseointegration in C57Bl/6 mice, by means of a cause-effect study of pharmacological inhibition of HMGB1 or its cognate receptor RAGE.

MATERIALS AND METHODS

Material Preparation

Titanium implant screws (titanium-6 aluminum-4 vanadium alloy, NTI-Kahla GmbH Rotary Dental Instruments, Kahla, Thüringen, Germany) of Ø 0.6 mm were cut at a length of 1.5 mm. Also, machined 6AL-4V Tinanium discs (Ti-discs) of Ø 6 and 2 mm thick from commercially pure grade 2 alloy were used for subcutaneous implantation. All material were sterilized by autoclaving before surgical procedures, as previously described for oral osseointegration model in C57Bl/6 mice (4).

Animals

Experimental groups comprised C57Bl/6 male mice (10-weeks-old, 25 g of weight in average), bred and maintained in the animal facilities of University of São Paulo, cared according to the recommendations in the Guide for the Care and Use of Laboratory Animals of the National Institutes of Health (39) were used in this study. The experimental protocols were performed according to ARRIVE guidelines (40) and National Institutes of Health guide for the care and use of Laboratory animals (NIH Publications No. 8023, revised 1978), with approval by the local Institutional Committee for Animal Care and Use (CEEPA-FOB/USP, #012/2014). Mice were provided sterile water *ad libitum* and were fed with sterile standard solid mice chow (Nuvital, Curitiba, PR, Brazil) during all experimental periods of this study, except throughout the first 72 h post-Ti implantation for oral osseointegration model, in which diet was crumbled. Experimental groups for oral osseointegration were comprised by 10 animals per group/time point (3, 7, 14, and 21 days), with 6 animals per group/time point for microscopic analysis (microCT, histological, and birefringence analysis) and 4 for molecular (Real Time PCR array) assays; an additional 1 day time point group with 6 animals per group was used for protein elution and HMGB1 quantification. Experimental groups for subcutaneous Ti disc implantation were comprised by 5 animals per group/time point (3, 7, and 14 days) and Ti-disc was implanted in left and right side of animal dorsa, comprising 10 biological samples for each group/time point: 5 Ti disc samples (Ti discs containing the surrounding tissues) from the left side for microscopic analysis (histological, birefringence analysis, and immunohistochemistry) and 5 Ti disc samples from the right side for molecular analysis (Real Time PCR array) and protein elution (an additional 1 day time point was evaluated for HMGB1 quantification). All experimental groups (oral osseointegration and subcutaneous implantation) were divided according to each treatment: Control (no treatment); GZA, IP injection of glycyrrhizic acid (Sigma Aldrich) 200 mg/Kg/24 h for HMGB1 inhibition; vehicle control for GZA (intraperitoneal [IP] injection of 1.5% DMSO solution); RAP, IP injection of RAGE antagonistic peptide (RAP, Merck Millipore, USA) 4 mg/Kg/24 h as previously described (41, 42); and vehicle control for RAP, IP injection of saline solution 0.9%. Mice received daily IP injections of drugs/vehicle, starting 1 day before the surgical procedure and continuing toward the end of experimental periods. No antibiotics and anti-inflammatory drugs were administered to the animals after implantation surgery, in order to avoid interferences on investigated inflammatory/immunological pathways (4).

Experimental Protocol for Oral Osseointegration Model

The Ti-implant placement in edentulous alveolar crest of the oral cavity of C57Bl/6 mice was performed as previously described (4, 43). Briefly, mice were anesthetized previous to the surgery by ketamine chloride 80 mg/kg (Dopalen, Agribrands Brasil, Paulínia, SP, Brazil) and xylazine chloride 160 mg/kg (Anasedan, Agribrands Brasil, Paulínia, SP, Brazil). Then, the mouse was placed in dorsal decubitus position under a stereomicroscope (DF Vasconcellos, São Paulo, SP, Brazil), and oral mucosa was cleaned using topical chlorhexidine solution for 1 min. An incision of 2 mm width parallel to the palatal crease and 1 mm in front of the left first maxillary molar was made and the subjacent bone was drilled using a Ø 0.50 mm pilot drill (NTI-Kahla GmbH Rotary Dental Instruments, Kahla, Thüringen, Germany) at 600 rpm using a surgical motor (NSK-Nakanishi International, Kanuma,Tochigi, Japan). The Ti-implant was screwed down in the implant bed using a castro viejo micro needle holder (Fine Science Tools, British Columbia, CA, USA). The right edentulous alveolar crest was used as Control side, without implant placement. Importantly, animals with early failure related to the surgical procedure (loss of primary stability upon placement) were immediately detected and were not included in the sample size; being only Ti implantations with complete absence of device mobility included in the sample for subsequent analysis, as previously characterized (4). At the end of experimental periods, mice were euthanized and maxillae were removed for microscopic (microtomographic, histological, histomorphometric) or molecular analysis. Samples selected for microscopic analysis were fixed in PBS-buffered formalin (10%) solution (pH 7.2) for 48 h at room temperature, washed overnight in running water and maintained in alcohol fixative (70% hydrous ethanol) until the conclusion of the μCT scanning. Then, the specimens were decalcified in 4.13% EDTA (pH 7.2) following histological processing protocols. Samples for molecular analysis were stored in RNA later (Ambion, Austin, TX, USA) solutions following previous protocols (44, 45), samples for HMGB1 quantification were submitted to protein elution protocol and subsequently frozen for posterior protein assay (46, 47).

Experimental Protocol for Ti Implantation on Subcutaneous Tissue

Mice were anesthetized as previous described for oral osseointegration model. Then, a longitudinal incision was performed in the animal dorsa, were one Ti-disc was implanted in each side. Immediately down from Ti implantation, while the control region remained intact. Ti discs containing the surrounding tissues, as well control samples were collected from the left side for microscopic and from the right side for molecular analysis (Real Time PCR array). Samples collected for microscopic analysis were fixed in PBS-buffered formalin (10%) solution (pH 7.2) for 24 h at RT, then washed over-night in running water and processed for routine histology. Samples collected for molecular analysis were stored in RNAlater (Ambion, Austin, TX, USA) solutions for Real Time PCR array. For protein assay (i.e., HMGB1 detection), Ti-screws, and Ti-discs retrieved after implantation were submitted to protein elution protocol for posterior protein assay (46, 47).

ELISA Assay for HMGB1 Detection

Ti-screws (implanted in bone) and Ti-discs (implanted into subcutaneous tissue) were retrieved from implantantion sites at different time points submitted to a protein elution protocol (46, 47). Briefly, Ti devices were subjected to five consecutive washes with 200 μl of double-distilled water and a final wash with 100 mM NaCl in 50 mM Tris-HCl to remove unadsorbed proteins. The absorbed proteins eluate was obtained by three consecutive submersions of the devices in a solution containing 4% SDS, 100 mM DTT, and 0.5 M TEAB, as previously (46, 47). Total protein of the serum was quantified for subsequent normalization (Pierce Protein Assay Kit), and HMGB1 was measured by ELISA according to the protocol recommended by the manufacturer (MyBioSource). The results were expressed as mean values ± standard deviation nanogram (ng) of protein per milligram of tissue, and represent values of duplicates of each sample obtained in two independent experiments.

Micro-Computed Tomography (μCT) Assessment

Mice maxillae containing the Ti-implants were scanned by Skyscan 1176 System (Bruker Microct, Kontich, Belgium) at 80 kV, 300 μA, 180 degrees of rotation, and exposure range of 1 degree. After scanning and previous reconstructions (NRecon software, Bruker Microct, Kontich, Belgium), representative three-dimensional images were obtained by CT-Vox 2.3 software, while quantitative evaluation of bone to implant interface was assessed using CTAn 1.1.4.1 software (Bruker Microct, Kontich, Belgium) based in previous standardization for measuring bone implant contact volume by means of microCT (4). Briefly, for quantification of bone volume proportion (BV/TV, %) at the implant-bone interface area, a cylindrical region of interest (ROI) with a diameter of 700 μm was set and the bone volume quantification was performed only considering bone implant contact region. After binarization and separation between titanium body and bone by the difference of hyperdensities, BV/TV was acquired.

Histomorphometry

The mice maxillae used for microCT scanning were processed for histological analysis following standardized procedures (4, 45, 48). For both, osseointegration model (maxillae) and subcutaneous, semi-serial sections considering the implantation area were cut with 4 μm thickness. A total of six samples (biological replicates) and nine semi-serial sections (technical replicates) from the central region of implantation sites in the maxilla were taken for hematoxylin and eosin [H&E] staining. For subcutaneous sites, a total of five samples (biological replicates) and eight semi-serial sections (technical replicates) were considered for histomorphometry. The histomorphometry was performed by a single calibrated investigator with a binocular microscope (Olympus Optical Co., Tokyo, Honshu, Japan) using a 100x immersion objective. Six histological fields *per* each HE section, comprising the region adjacent to thread spaces (for osseointegration) or Ti disc space (for subcutaneous), were observed under a 100 points grid in a quadrangular area, by using Image J software (Version 1.51, National Institutes of Health, Bethesda, MD, USA). Points were quantified coinciding with the following structures found in the osseointegration sites or in implant failure sites: blood clot, inflammatory cells, blood vessels, fibroblasts and fibers, osteoblasts, osteoclasts, bone matrix, necrotic bone and foreign body giant cells (FBGC), and other elements (empty spaces left by implant space). For subcutaneous, were quantified structures involving inflammatory and healing process surrounding the Ti-disc space (presence of blood clot, inflammatory cells, fibers, fibroblasts, and blood vessels). Results were presented as the mean area density for each structure considered in each examined group.

Birefringence Analysis

A total of six different samples (biological replicates) and four semi-serial sections (technical replicates) for each sample were used for picrosirius red staining and birefringence analysis of the osseointegration model in the maxillae. For each semi-serial section, three histological fields were evaluated comprising the central region of bone to implant contact. In subcutaneous tissue, five samples (biological replicates) and four semi-serial sections (technical replicates) for each sample were analyzed. For each section, six histological fields were analyzed surrounding the Ti disc space. All specimens were analyzed at 40x magnification through polarizing lens coupled to a binocular inverted microscope (Leica DM IRB/E, Leica Microsystems Wetzlar GmbH, Wetzlar, Germany) and images were captured with a Leica Imaging Software (LAX, Leica Microsystems Wetzlar GmbH, Wetzlar, Germany). As previously described (4, 45, 48), green birefringence color indicates thin fibers; yellow and red colors at birefringence analysis indicate thick collagen fibers. Three fields from each section were analyzed through polarizing lens coupled to a binocular inverted microscope (Leica DM IRB/E, Leica Microsystems Wetzlar GmbH, Wetzlar, Germany), by using 40x magnification immersion objective. Images were captured with a Leica Imaging Software (LAX, Leica Microsystems Wetzlar GmbH, Wetzlar, Germany) and the quantification of birefringence brightness was performed using the software AxioVision 4.8 (Carl Zeiss Microscopy GmbH, Jena, Germany) considering green, yellow, and red spectra pixels2. Mean values of four sections from each animal were calculated and submitted to statistical analysis.

Immunohistochemistry and Quantification of Immunolabeled Inflammatory Cells

A total of five samples (biological replicate) from subcutaneous tissue and three semi-serial sections (technical replicate) of each sample surrounding the Ti implant were used for individual immunodetection of Ly6g-GR1 (sc-168490), F4/80 (a pan marker for murine macrophages, sc-26642), CD80 (M1 macrophage, sc-376012), and CD206 (M2 macrophage, sc-34577), all primary antibodies purchased from Santa Cruz Biotechnology (Santa Cruz Biotechnology, Santa Cruz, CA, USA). Immunohistochemistry protocol was performed as previously described (48). Briefly, histological sections were rehydrated and retrieved the antigens by boiling the histological slides in 10 mM sodium citrate buffer pH 6 for 30 min at 100°C. Subsequently, the sections were pre-incubated with 3% Hydrogen Peroxidase Block (Spring Bioscience Corporation, CA, USA) and subsequently incubated with 7% NFDM to block serum proteins. All primary antibodies were diluted at 1:100 in diluent solution for 1 h at room temperature. Universal immuno-enzyme polymer method was used and sections were incubated in immunohistochemical staining reagent for 30 min at room temperature. The identification of antigen–antibody reaction was performed using 3-3'-diaminobenzidine (DAB) and counterstaining with Mayer's hematoxylin. Positive controls were performed by using mouse spleen for F4/80, CD80, and CD206 macrophages while Ly6g-Gr1+ were directly visualized in the inflamed tissues post-surgical trauma. The analysis of immunolabeled cells (Gr, F4/80, CD80, CD206) was performed by a single calibrated investigator using a 100x magnification, considering six histological fields per section, comprising subcutaneous tissue surrounding the Ti-disc. Three samples (biological replicate) for each experimental period and strains were used for quantitative analysis and a total of three sections of each biological replicate were quantified. A grid image was superimposed on the histological photomicrographs, with 10 parallel lines and 100 points in a quadrangular area, by using Image J software (Version 1.51, National Institutes of Health, Bethesda, MD, USA). Only the points coincident with the immunolabeled cells were considered in cell counting and the mean for each section was obtained for statistical analysis.

Real Time PCR Array Reactions

Maxillae and subcutaneous tissue from all experimental groups and time points were dissected and samples containing only the region of the implant bed were storage in RNA stabilization solution (RNAlater, Thermofisher, Waltham, MA, USA) until Real Time PCR array reactions. Samples from the right side (without implant placement) of maxillae and samples from the down right side of subcutaneous tissue (control region remained intact) were used and a Control. Real Time PCR array reactions were performed as previously described (4, 44, 45), using initially a pool of four samples (biological replicates) from all experimental time-points for each group for maxilla and four samples (biological replicates) for subcutaneous tissue. For all experiments, were performed two technical replicates. Pool analysis were performed in order to select targets in which expression variation presented a significant variation compared to the Control side. Subsequently, upregulated targets were analyzed regarding their kinetics of expression for specific time points (3, 7, 14, and 21days) after implant placement. Briefly, the extraction of total RNA from implantation sites and controls was performed with RNeasy kit (Qiagen Inc, Valencia, CA, USA) according to manufacturers' instructions. The integrity of RNA samples was checked by 2100 Bioanalyzer (Agilent Technologies, Santa Clara, CA, USA), and the complementary DNA was synthesized using 3 μg of RNA through a reverse transcription reaction (QuantiTectRTkit, Qiagen Inc, Valencia, CA, USA) (44). The Real Time PCR array was performed in a Viia7 instrument (LifeTechnologies, Carlsbad, CA, USA) using custom panels for "wound healing" (PAMM-121), "inflammatory cytokines and receptors" (PAMM-011), and "Osteogenesis" (PAMM-026) (SABiosciences, Frederick, MD, USA) for gene expression profiling, followed by data analysis with the RT2 Profiler software (SABiosciences, Frederick, MD, USA) for normalizing the initial geometric mean of three constitutive genes (GAPDH, ACTB, Hprt1), following normalizing the Control group; as previously described (4). Data are expressed as heat map fold change relative to the Control group.

Statistical Analysis

Statistical treatment of quantitative data was performed using GraphPad Prism 5.0 software (GraphPad Software Inc., San Diego, CA, USA). Normally distributed data were analyzed using ANOVA followed by Bonferroni's multiple comparison *post-hoc* tests or student's *t*-test where applicable. For non-normal distributions, data were analyzed by means Kruskal-Wallis test (followed by Dunn's test) and Mann-Whitney test. The statistical significance of the experiment involving Real Time PCR array was evaluated by the Mann-Whitney test, and the values tested for correction of Benjamini and Hochberg (49). Values of $p <$ 0.05 were considered statistically significant.

RESULTS

Detection of HMGB1 on Sites of Bone and Subcutaneous Implantation

HMGB1 was found to be present in the protein adsorption layer characteristically formed in biomaterials surface after implantation (**Figure 1**), as demonstrated by the protein elution from both Ti-screws implanted in bone and Ti-discs implanted in subcutaneous tissue. HMGB1 was present in relatively high

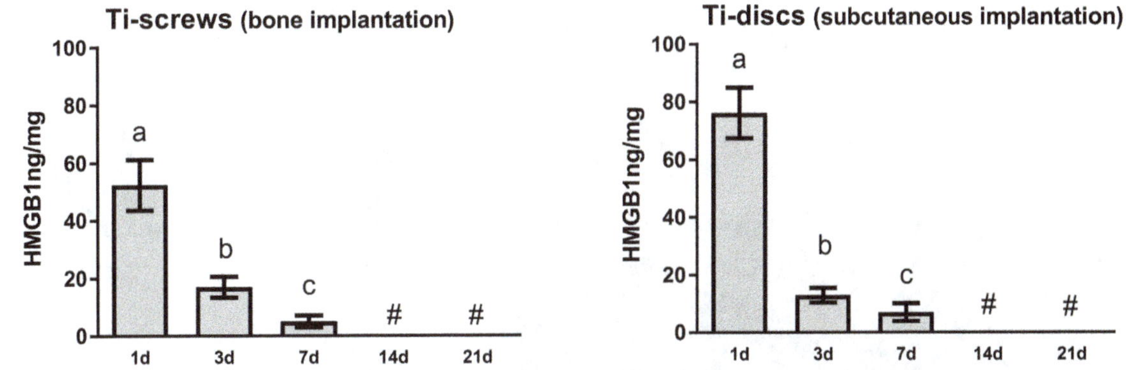

FIGURE 1 | HMGB1 detection in the sites of bone Ti implantation. Ti-screws (implanted in bone) and Ti-discs (implanted into subcutaneous tissue) were retrieved from implantantion sites at 1, 3, 7, 14, and 21 days. Samples were submitted to a protein elution protocol followed by the HMGB1 quantification by ELISA according to the protocol recommended by the manufacturer (MyBioSource). The results were expressed as mean values ± standard deviation nanogram (ng) of protein per milligram of tissue, from a total of five animals/samples (biological replicates) and two technical replicates *per* each group and time point. Different letters indicate significant statistical differences ($p < 0.05$) among time periods in each group, symbol #represent "undectable levels" (Kruskal-Wallis followed by Dunn's test).

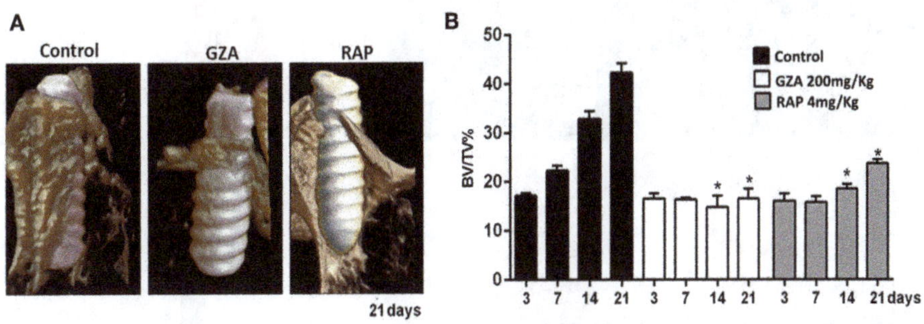

FIGURE 2 | Micro-computed tomography (μCT) analysis of oral osseointegration model in C57Bl/6 mice under HMGB1 or RAGE inhibition. Mice received Ti-screw implantation in the edentulous ridge of maxilla and were divided in according to each treatment: Control (C group, with no treatment); Glycyrrhizic Acid at a dosage of 200 mg/Kg/day (GZA group); or RAGE antagonistic peptide at dosage of 4 mg/Kg/day (RAP group). **(A)** Three-dimensional representative images obtained with the CT-Vox software at 21 days post Ti implantation from Control, GZA, and RAP groups. **(B)** Quantitative analysis of bone volume/tissue volume (BV/TV, %) in the interface bone-Ti along days 3, 7, 14, and 21 post implantation for Control, GZA, and RAP groups. Results are presented as the mean and SD from a total of six biological replicates from each group and time point. Symbol *indicates significant statistical differences ($p < 0.05$) in comparison with control.

concentration in the 1 d time point, followed by a gradual decrease in 3 and 7 days' time points, being non-detectable at the 14 and 21 days' time-points (**Figure 1**), being this pattern similar in bone and subcutaneous implantation sites.

μCT Assessment of Osseointegration

Qualitative and quantitative analyses of mineralized bone matrix revealed a non-significant quantity of bone around Ti threads at 3 days among all groups, whose bone detected around Ti threads characterized the native bone supporting the Ti-implant (**Figures 2A,B**). Detectable, but not statistically significant newly formed bone matrix was observed at 7 days (22.33 ± 1.93) compared to 3 days (17.18 ± 1.11) post Ti-implantation in the Control group, and osseointegration was achieved throughout a gradual and proportion of bone apposition (BV/TV, %) around implant threads at 14 days (32.88 ± 3.16%) and 21 days (42.25 ± 3.86%; **Figure 2B**). On the other hand, the inhibition of HMGB1 and RAGE, in GZA and RAP treated animals, showed a significantly reduced BV/TV around Ti threads at 14 and 21 days compared to the Control group (**Figure 2B**), and DMSO and Saline Solution vehicles treated group as well (data not shown). The mean of BV/TV around implant threads in the GZA treated animals was 14.76 ± 4.06% at 14 days and 16.58 ± 3.40% at 21 days, while in RAP treated animals was 18.53 ± 1.60% at 14 days and 23.69 ± 1.40% at 21 days. The GZA and RAP vehicle control treated groups also achieved osseointegration with no statistical differences compared to the Control (data not shown).

Birefringence of Collagen Fibers on Granulation Tissue and Bone Matrix During Osseointegration

To comprehensively analyze the impact of HGMB1 or RAGE inhibition on organic bone matrix maturation on oral osseointegration in mice, we quantified green, yellow and red spectrum fibers from the bone matrix and initial granulation tissue for all groups (**Figures 3A,B**). All groups showed a negligible quantity of collagen fibers starting at 3 days around the Ti threads, emitting birefringence in the green spectrum (i.e.,

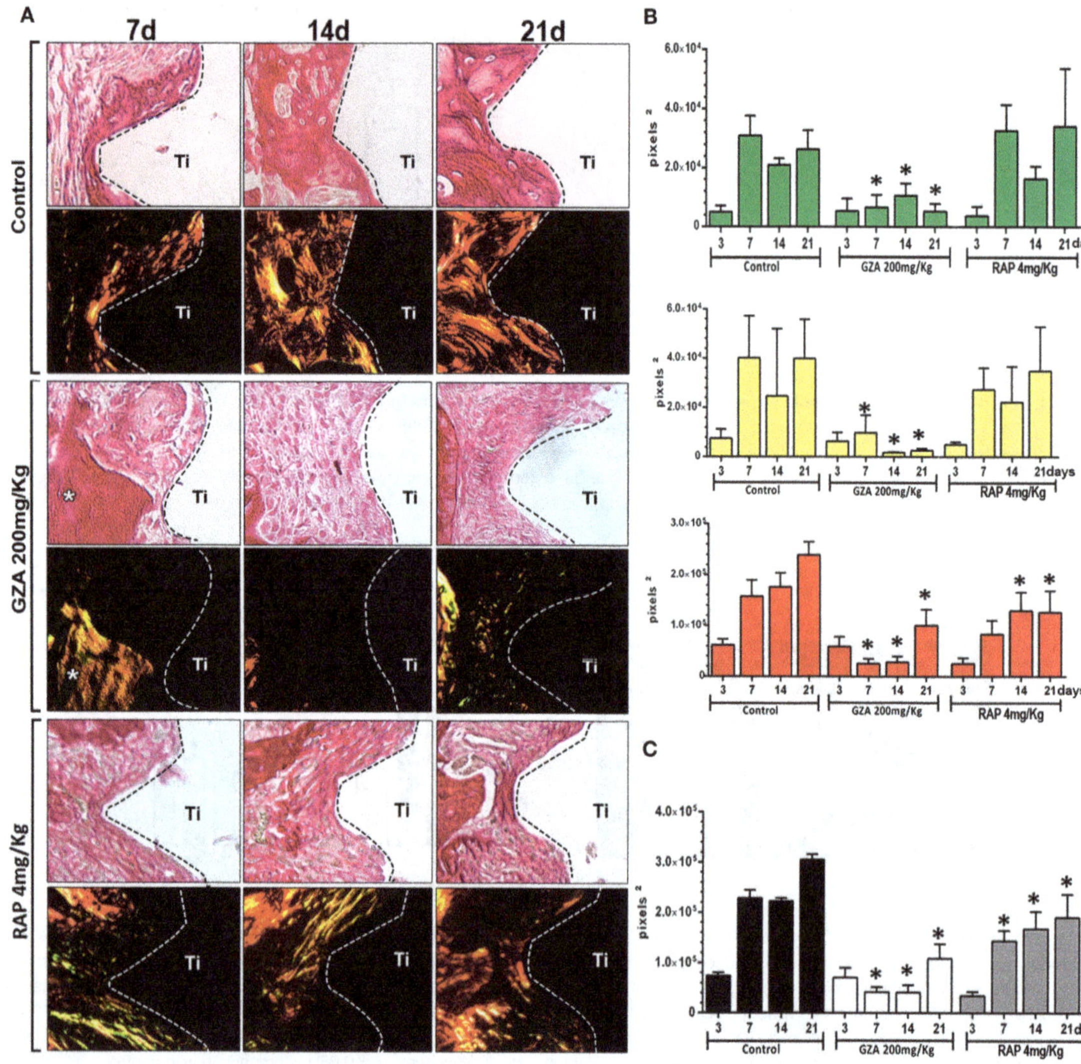

FIGURE 3 | Birefringence analysis of collagen fibers along osseointegration model in C57Bl/6 mice under HMGB1 or RAGE inhibition. Mice received Ti-screw implantation in the edentulous ridge of maxilla and were divided in according to each treatment: Control (C group, with no treatment); Glycyrrhizic Acid at a dosage of 200 mg/Kg/day (GZA group); or RAGE antagonistic peptide at dosage of 4 mg/Kg/day (RAP group). **(A)** Representative sections from oral osseointegration process upon polarized and conventional light, to evaluate collagen fibers maturation along days 3, 7, 14, and 21 post-Ti-screw implantation in the different experimental groups. As visualized upon polarized light, green birefringence color indicates thin fibers; yellow and red colors at birefringence analysis indicate thick collagen fibers. Original magnification 40x. **(B)** Intensity of birefringence measured from Image-analysis software (AxioVision, v. 4.8, CarlZeiss) to identify and quantify area of collagen from each birefringence color (pixels 2) and **(C)** total area of collagen fibers (pixel2) throughout experimental periods. Results are presented as the mean and SD of pixels2 for each color in the birefringence analysis, from a total of six animals/samples (biological replicates) and four technical replicates *per* each group and time point. Symbol *indicates a statistically significant difference vs. control ($p < 0.05$).

immature and thinner fibers). From 7 to 21 days, the Control group showed a significant increase in yellow and red collagen fibers, suggesting organic bone matrix maturation. Conversely, inhibition of HMGB1 in GZA treated mice caused a drastic impairment of bone collagen fibers formation, with significantly reduced amount of all birefringent type of fibers from 7 to 21 days compared to the Control. Under inhibition of RAGE (RAP treated mice), there was also impaired formation and maturation of collagen fibers, with a significantly reduced amount of total fibers at 14 and 21 days compared to the Control. No significant differences were observed in the dynamics of collagen fibers formation and maturation during osseointegration between GZA and RAP Control vehicle treated groups (data not shown).

Histopathological Description and Histomorphometry of Healing Components During Osseointegration

Histopathological analysis revealed osseointegration in the Control group, with intramembranous bone healing following overlapping phases from 3 to 21 days post Ti-implant placement in mice (**Figure 4**). Similar histological dynamics of

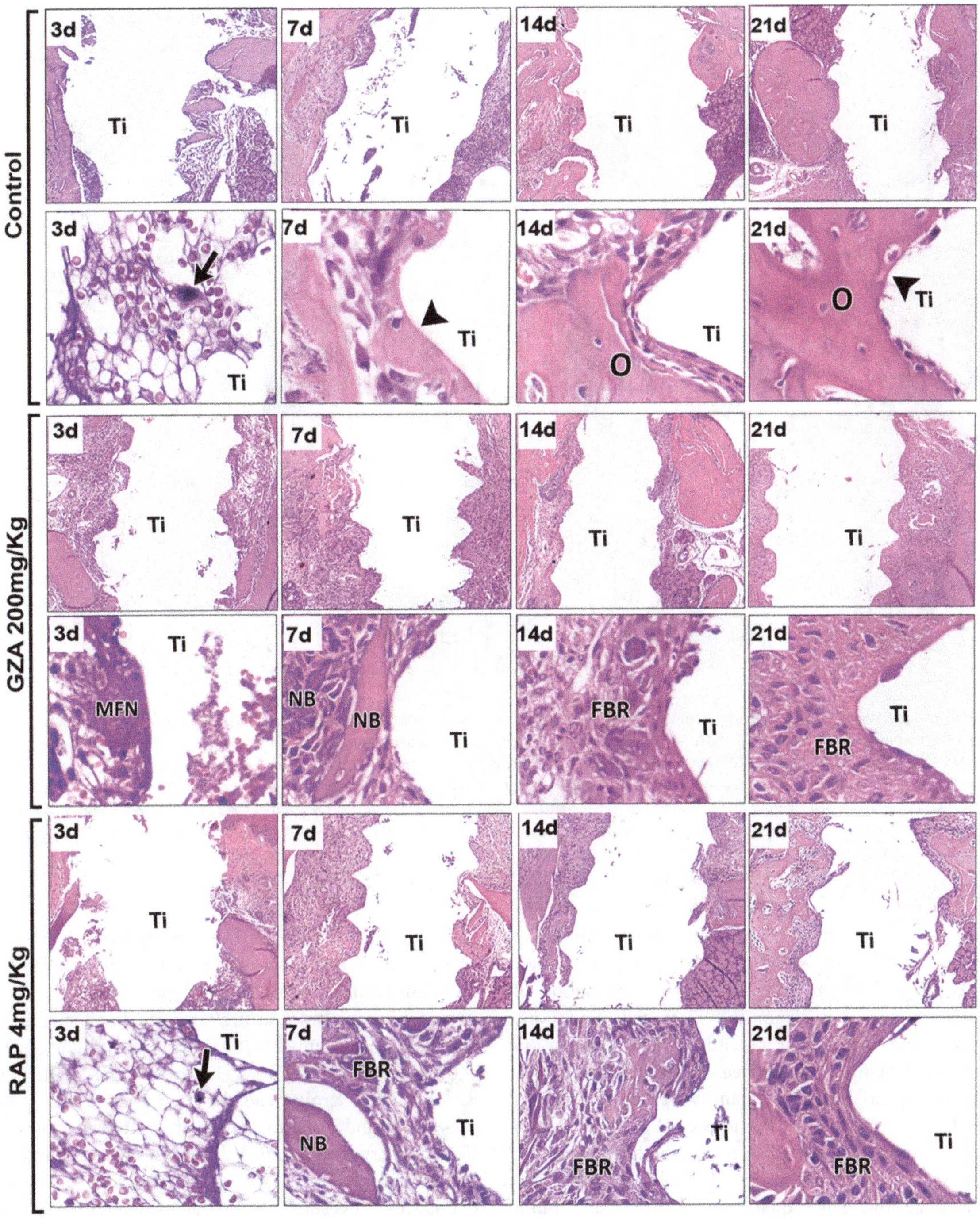

FIGURE 4 | Histopathological analysis along oral osseointegration model in C57Bl/6 mice under HMGB1 or RAGE inhibition. Mice received Ti-screw implantation in the edentulous ridge of maxilla and were divided in according to each treatment: Control (C group, with no treatment); Glycyrrhizic Acid at a dosage of 200 mg/Kg/day (GZA group); or RAGE antagonistic peptide at dosage of 4 mg/Kg/day (RAP group). Chronology of oral osseointegration is observed throughout days 3, 7, 14, and 21 days. Histological slides were stained with H&E and images were captured at 10 and 100x magnification. Ti, Ti screw space; BC, Blood clot; Arrows, fibrin supporting cell migration; Arrowheads, bone/Ti contact region; O, osseointegration; MFN, Malformed fibrin network; NB, Necrotic bone; FBR, Foreign Body Reaction.

osseointegration were observed in the GZA or RAP vehicle treated groups (data not shown). On the other hand, both experimental groups treated with RAP or GZA, exhibited failure of osseointegration, with the typical presence of fibrous connective tissue and foreign body giant cells (FBGC) formation at 14 and 21 days post-Ti implantation. At 3 days, the bone-implant interface in the Control group was filled predominantly by a blood clot (**Figure 5A**) providing support for cell infiltration

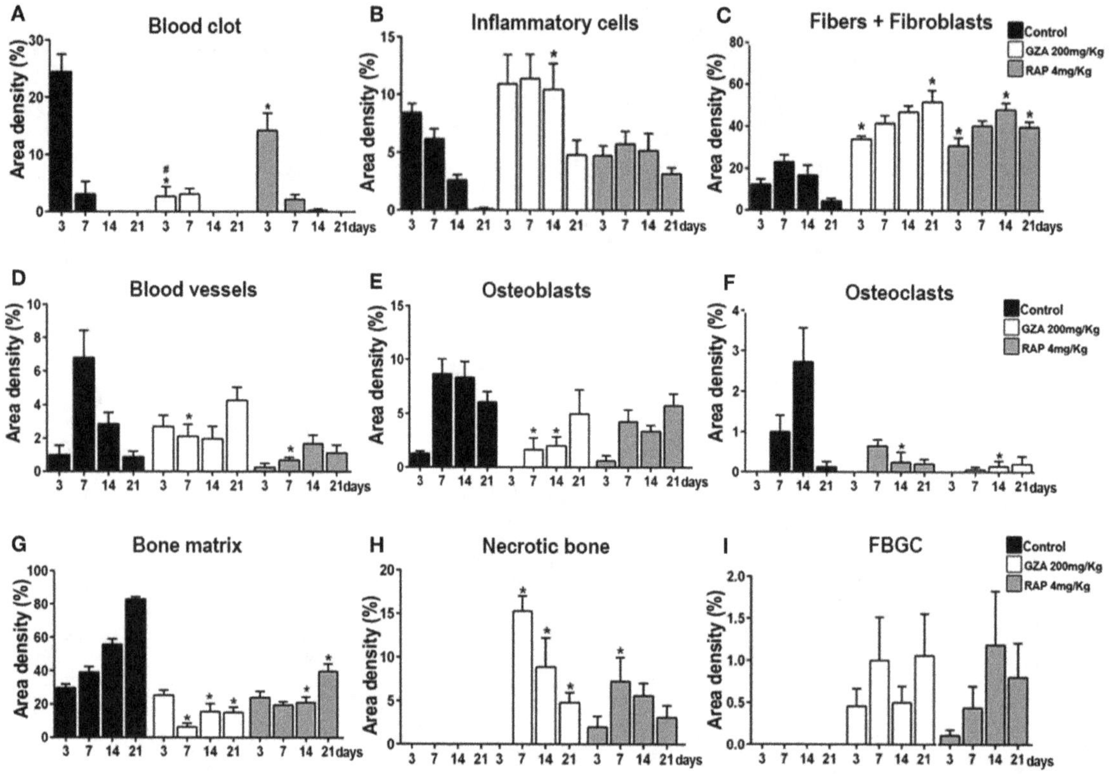

FIGURE 5 | Histomorphometric analysis of healing components along oral osseointegration model in C57Bl/6 mice under HMGB1 or RAGE inhibition. Mice received Ti-screw implantation in the edentulous ridge of maxilla and were divided in according to each treatment: Control (C group, with no treatment); Glycyrrhizic Acid at a dosage of 200 mg/Kg/day (GZA group); or RAGE antagonistic peptide at dosage of 4 mg/Kg/day (RAP group). Results are presented as the means (± SD) of area density for each component related to osseointegration process: **(A)** Blood Clot, **(B)** Inflammatory cells, **(C)** Fibers + Fibroblasts, **(D)** Blood vessels, **(E)** Osteoblasts, **(F)** Osteoclasts, **(G)** Bone matrix, **(H)** Necrotic Bone, and **(I)** FBGC. Results are presented as the mean and SD from a total of six animals/samples (biological replicates) and nine semi-serial sections (technical replicates) *per* each group and time point. Symbol *indicate a statistically significant difference vs. control, #indicate differences between RAP and GZA groups ($p < 0.05$).

(**Figure 4**, arrow). At 7 days, increased quantities of granulation tissue components were observed (blood vessels, fibroblasts, and fibers; **Figures 5C,D**), as well an initial differentiation of osteoblasts and bone matrix from the Ti threads and bone edges (**Figure 4**, arrowheads). At 14 and 21 days, granulation tissue components significantly decreased around Ti threads spaces, followed by an increased quantity of osteoblasts and bone matrix in the same regions (**Figures 4, 5E,G**) resulting in direct contact between implant and bone (**Figure 4**, arrowheads). Furthermore, Control and vehicle groups exhibited osteoclastic resorption lacunae and a few quantities of osteoclasts found around bone debris and pre-existing bone during 3 and 7 days post Ti implantation, followed by osteoclastic remodeling of newly formed bone at 14 and 21 days.

Comparatively to the osseointegration observed in the Control group, RAP treated mice also showed a suitable blood clot formation the bone-implant interface, but in a slighted reduced number, surrounded by an eosinophilic and slight matrix of fibrin network, with identifiable support for cell migration (**Figure 4**, arrows). On the other hand, the inhibition of HMGB1 in GZA treated mice resulted in a disorganized blood clot, with agglomerated platelets (#) and red blood cells separated from the malformed fibrin networks (MFN) (**Figure 4**, GZA group and **Supplementary Figure 1**) and a drastically reduced area density of this component (**Figure 5A**). Both RAP and GZA treated mice showed necrotic/non-viable bone persisting at 7–21 days post Ti-implantation, as well a foreign body reaction (FBR) with the presence of FBGC (**Figures 4, 5H,I**). The inhibition of RAGE in RAP group leaded to a negligible higher quantity of osteoblasts and bone formation in scattered areas surrounding Ti thread spaces compared to HMGB1 inhibition in GZA group (**Figures 4, 5E**). No statistical differences were observed in quantitative results for other elements (empty spaces, artifacts and Ti space; data not shown).

Gene Expression Patterns in Osseointegration Under HGMB1 or RAGE Inhibition

A pool of samples from all periods post-Ti implantation were initially analyzed by means of an exploratory Real Time PCR array (**Figure 6**), considering molecules involved in inflammatory response and bone healing (growth factors; immunological/inflammatory markers; extracellular matrix,

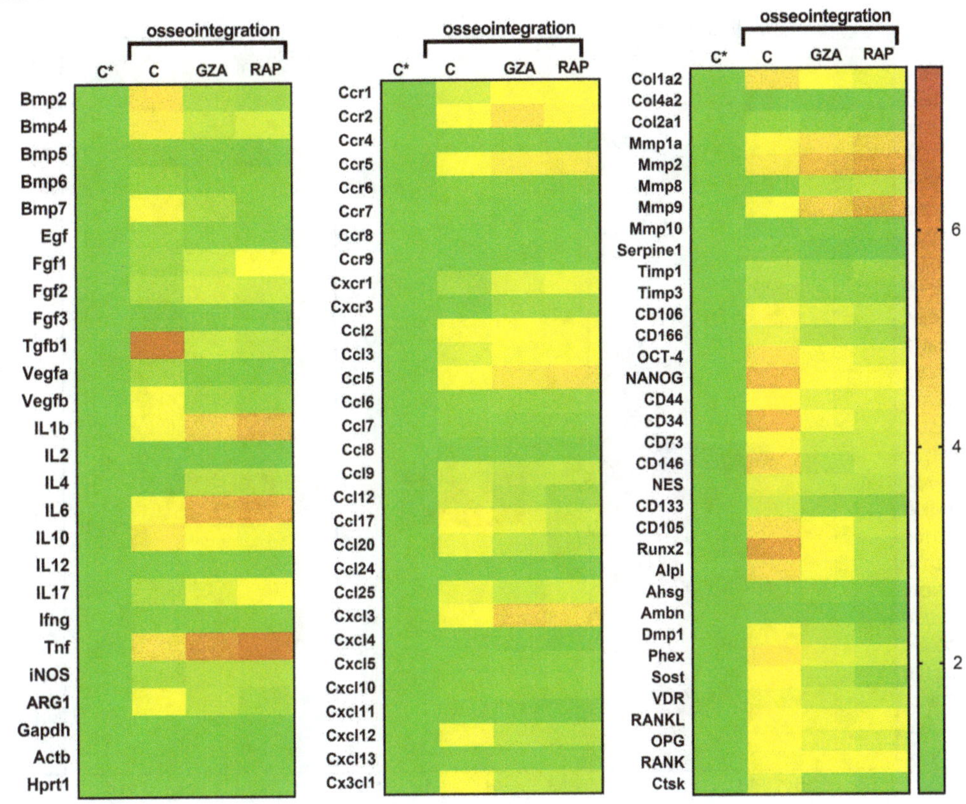

FIGURE 6 | Gene expression patterns in the osseointegration sites under HMGB1 or RAGE inhibition. Mice received Ti-screw implantation in the edentulous ridge of maxilla and were divided in according to each treatment: Control (C group, with no treatment); Glycyrrhizic Acid at a dosage of 200 mg/Kg/day (GZA group); or RAGE antagonistic peptide at dosage of 4 mg/Kg/day (RAP group) Right side without Ti-screw implantation was used as tissue control and represented as **C***. Molecular analysis of the gene expression patterns in the region of Ti screw implantation was comprised of an initial exploratory analysis by Real Time PCR array for each experimental group (Control, RAP and GZA), considering a pool of four samples (biological replicates) and two technical replicates from all the experimental periods (3, 7, 14, 21 days). Real Time PCR array analysis was performed with the VIA7 system (Applied Biosystems Limited, Warrington, Cheshire, UK) using a customized qPCR array comprised of the major targets from the Osteogenesis, Inflammatory Cytokines & Receptors and Wound Healing panels of the PCRarrayRT2 Profiler (SABiosciences/QIAGEN, Gaithersburg, MD, USA). Results are depicted as the fold increase change (and the standard deviation) in mRNA expression from triplicate measurements in relation to the control samples and normalized by internal housekeeping genes (GAPDH, HPRT, β-actin).

MSC, and bone markers). Experimental groups (C, GZA, and RAP) were depicted as the fold increase change in relation to Control samples (C*), which are from the right side of maxilla of C57Bl/6 untreated mice, without surgery. Next, targets with a significant expression significant variation expression in pooled samples were analyzed according to their kinetics of expression during experimental periods (**Figure 7**).

For oral osseointegration model, among growth factors, TGFβ1, and VEGFb were significantly upregulated in C group, such as several MSC putative markers (OCT-4, NANOG, CD44, CD34, CD73, CD146, CD105, CXCL12); while the inhibition of HMGB1 (GZA group) and RAGE (RAP group) resulted in an important reduction in the mRNA levels for all these targets in pooled samples (**Figure 6**). Considering MSC putative markers, mRNA levels peaked at 3 and 7 days at osseointegration Control group and were significantly increased compared to GZA and RAP treated mice, as well TGFb and CXCL12. A slight upregulation for MSC markers were observed in GZA and RAP group compared to Control samples (C*).

Considering bone markers related to osteoblast differentiation (BMP2, BMP4, BMP7, Runx2, ALPL, DMP1, Phex, Sost, VDR) and bone remodeling (RANKL, OPG, CTSK), were positively upregulated in osseointegration Control group, whereas their expressions were drastically reduced in GZA and RAP group, as observed in pooled samples. On the other hand, RAP group presented an upregulation of FGF1 and FGF2 (**Figure 6**). In the osseointegration Control group, the kinetics of BMP2 mRNA levels peaked at 7 days and BMP4 peaked at 14 days. Runx2 and ALPL were upregulated at 7 and 14 days, significantly decreasing at 21 days, while Phex (a osteocyte differentiation marker) was upregulated at 14 days and 21 days (**Figure 7**).

Considering immunological markers for M1/M2 macrophages, a higher expression of ARG1 and IL10, markers for M2 phenotype, was particularly found in the osseointegration process of the Control group compared to the Control tissue (C*), but it was not observed in GZA and RAP treated mice (**Figure 6**). The mRNA levels of these M2 markers peaked at 7 and 14 days, as well TGFb in osseointegration Control group (**Figure 7**). The majority of chemokines and their receptors involved in inflammatory cells migration (CCR1, CCR2, CCR5, CCL2, CCL3, CCL5, CCL9, CCL12, CCL17, CCL20, CCL25, CXCL3, CXC3CL1) were upregulated in osseointegration

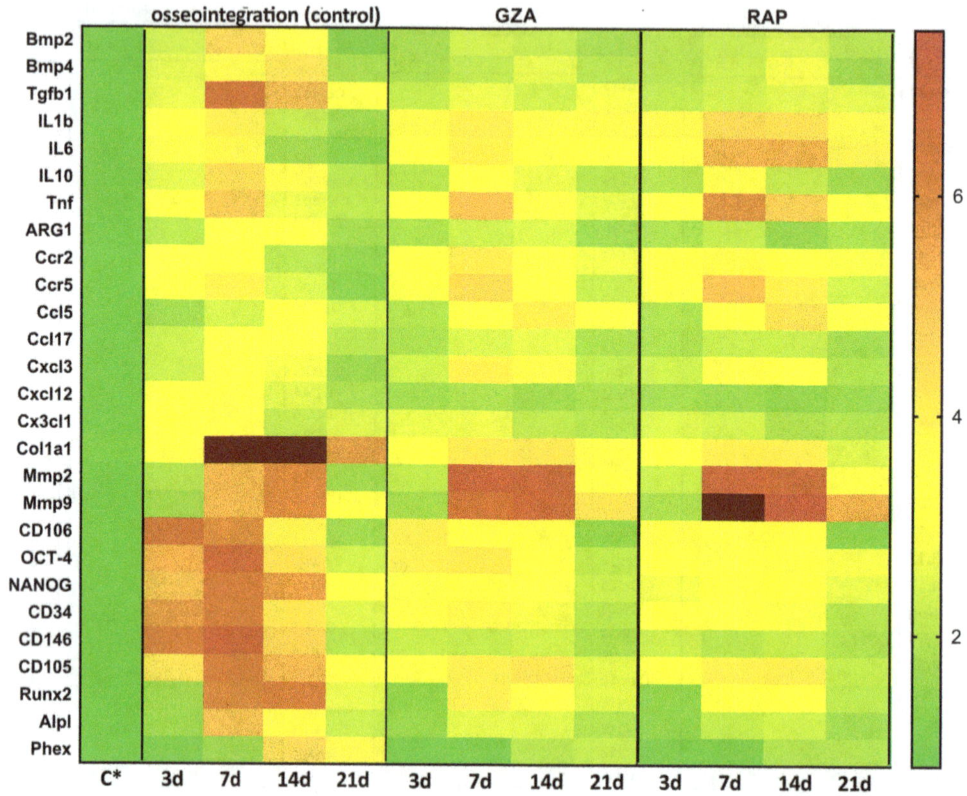

FIGURE 7 | Kinetics of gene expression in the oral osseointegration sites under HMGB1 or RAGE inhibition. Mice received Ti-screw implantation in the edentulous ridge of maxilla and were divided in according to each treatment: Control (C group, with no treatment); Glycyrrhizic Acid at a dosage of 200 mg/Kg/day (GZA group) or RAGE antagonistic peptide at dosage of 4 mg/Kg/day (RAP group). Right side without Ti-screw implantation was used as tissue control and represented as **C***. Molecular analysis of the gene expression in the region of Ti screw implantation was performed following each experimental time point (3, 7, 14, and 21 days), considering four samples (biological replicates) and two technical replicates *per* each group and time point. Targets with a significant expression variation in the previous Real Time PCR array from pooled samples were selected. Real Time PCR array analysis was performed with the VIA7 system (Applied Biosystems Limited, Warrington, Cheshire, UK) using a customized qPCR array comprised of the major targets from the Osteogenesis, Inflammatory Cytokines & Receptors and Wound Healing panels of the PCRarrayRT2 Profiler (SABiosciences/QIAGEN, Gaithersburg, MD, USA). Results are depicted as the fold increase change (and the standard deviation) in mRNA expression from triplicate measurements in relation to the control samples and normalized by internal housekeeping genes (GAPDH, HPRT, β-actin).

sites in the Control group. On the other hand, GZA and RAP treated mice presented a higher expression of CCR2, CCR5, CCL5, and CXCL3 compared to the osseointegration C group in pooled samples (**Figure 6**). Also, pro-inflammatory cytokines were differentially expressed in osseointegration C group compared to the GZA and RAP groups (**Figures 6**, **7**). While pro-inflammatory cytokines (IL1b, IL6, TNF), as well chemokine receptors (CCR2, CCR5) and chemokines (CCL5, CXCL3) were upregulated in early time points (3 and 7 days) in the osseointegration group, their mRNA levels remained upregulated in late time points (14 and 21 days) in GZA and RAP groups.

Finally, among the extracellular matrix markers, Col1a1, MMP2, and MMP9 were upregulated in all experimental groups (**Figure 6**). However, the kinetics of these markers were differently regulated comparing GZA an RAP groups to the osseointegration C group (**Figure 7**). In this way, mRNA levels of Col1a1 were significantly upregulated in the osseointegration Control sites at 7 and 14 days compared to GZA and RAP groups. On the other hand, GZA and RAP treated mice presented higher mRNA levels for MMP2 and MMP9 compared to the Control osseointegration sites (**Figure 7**).

Histomorphometric, Birefringence, Immunohistochemical, and Molecular Analysis of Subcutaneous Healing Under Ti Implantation

Control and both GZA and RAP control vehicle treated mice showed a suitable blood clot formation and a slight inflammatory infiltrate at 3 days, followed by a dense connective tissue formation, containing fibroblasts and negligible quantities of inflammatory cells surrounding region of Ti-disc implantation at 14 days (**Figure 8A**). Also, birefringence analysis revealed a yellow/red spectrum of collagen fibers surrounding the Ti at 14 days (**Figure 8B**). On the other hand, the inhibition of HMGB1 by GZA treatment caused a disruption of blood clot formation at 3 days (arrow, **Figure 8**) and a persistence

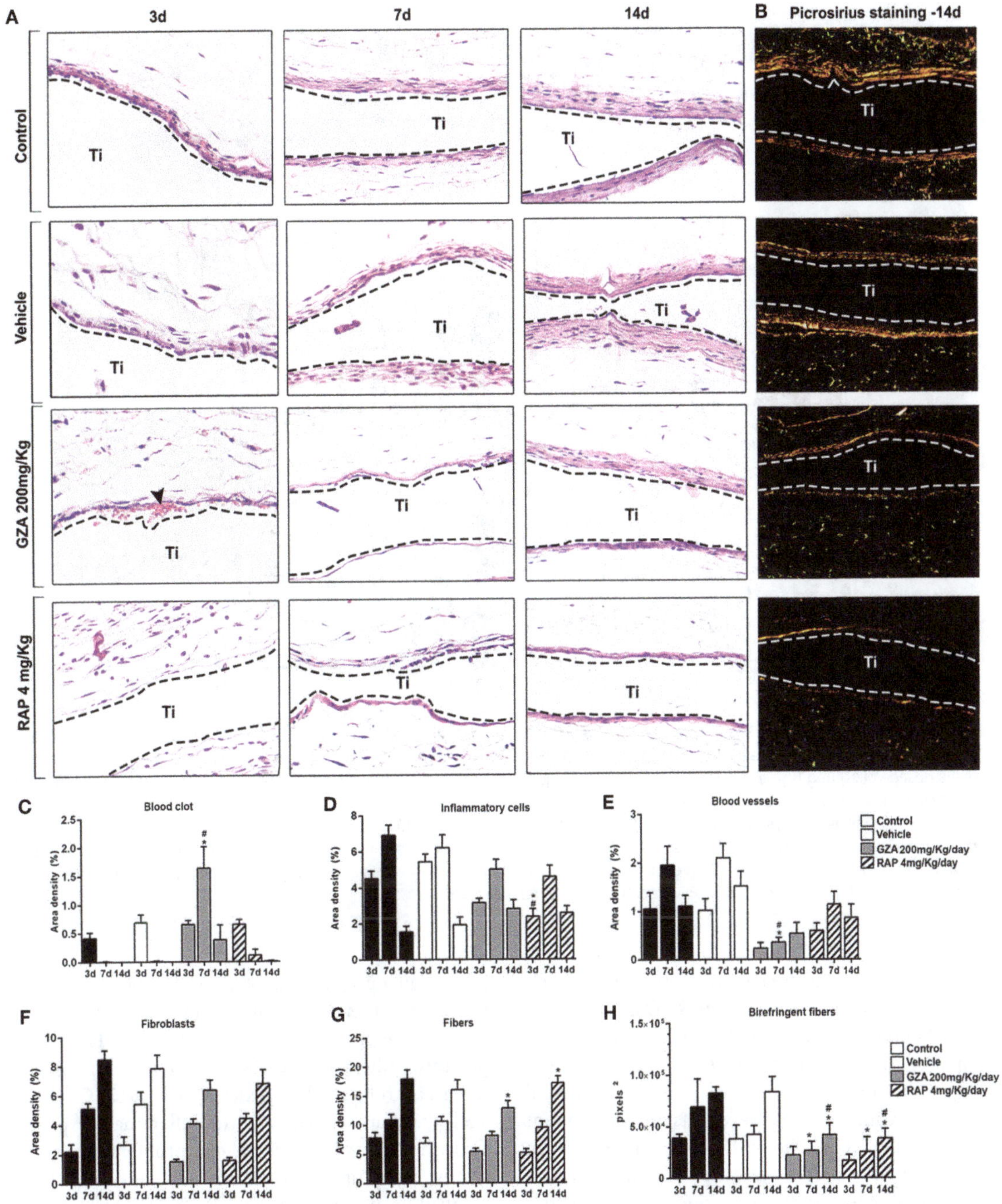

FIGURE 8 | Histophatological, histomorphometric, and birefringence analysis of subcutaneous tissue post implantation of Ti-disc in C57Bl/6 mice under HMGB1 or RAGE inhibition. Mice received Ti-disc implantation in the subcutaneous tissue and were divided in according to each treatment: Control (C group, with no treatment); Vehicle (1.5% DMSO solution); Glycyrrhizic Acid at a dosage of 200 mg/Kg/day (GZA group); or RAGE antagonistic peptide at dosage of 4 mg/Kg/day (RAP group). Vehicle or drugs were administered 1 day before the surgical procedure and were given until the end of experimental periods (3, 7, and 14 days). **(A)** Comparative morphology of the healing phases post Ti disc implantation for each group, stained with H&E (40x magnification) and **(B)** Picrosirius red. **(C–G)** Results from histomorphometry of healing parameters (blood clot, inflammatory cells, fibroblasts, fibers, and blood vessels) are presented as the mean of area density for each structure measured in each examined group. Results are presented as the mean and SD from a total of five animals/samples (biological replicates) and eight semi-serial sections (technical replicates) *per* each group and time point. **(H)** Intensity of birefringence performed using image-analysis software (AxioVision, v. 4.8, CarlZeiss) for total area of birefringent collagen fibers (pixels^2). Results are presented as the mean and SD from a total of five animals/samples (biological replicates) and four semi-serial sections (technical replicates) *per* each group and time point. **(C–H)** Symbols indicate statistically significant difference ($p < 0.05$) between experimental groups (GZA and RAP) vs. Control* and experimental groups vs. Vehicle# at the same time point.

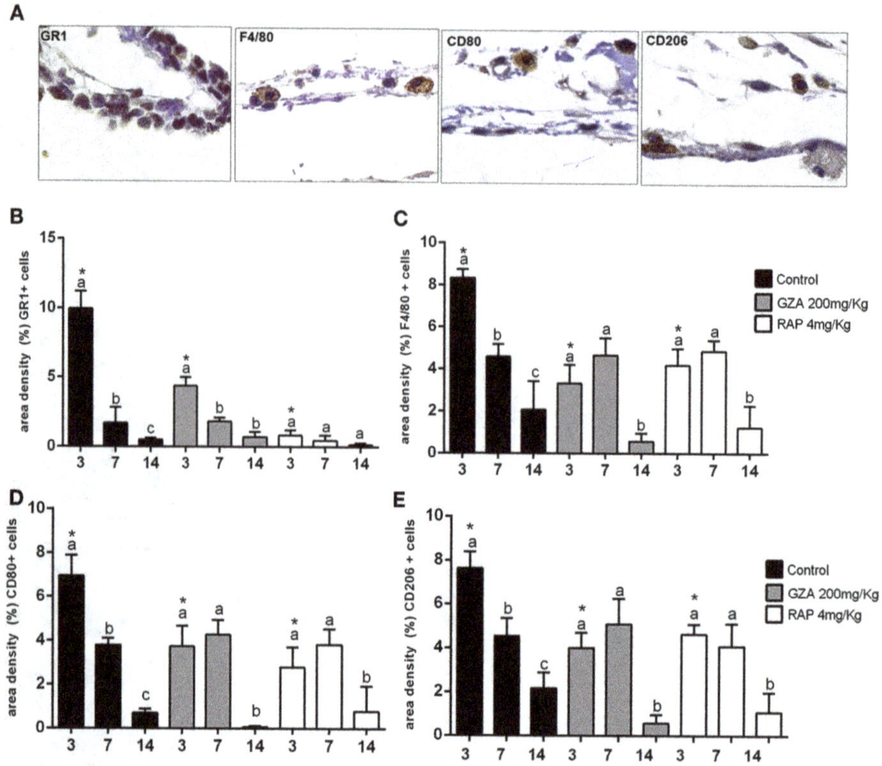

FIGURE 9 | Inflammatory cells recruited to the Ti disc implantation sites in C57Bl/6 mice treated with HMGB1 inhibitor or RAGE antagonist. Mice received Ti-disc implantation in the subcutaneous tissue and were divided in according to each treatment: Control (C group, with no treatment); Vehicle (1.5% DMSO solution); Glycyrrhizic Acid at a dosage of 200 mg/Kg/day (GZA group); or RAGE antagonistic peptide at dosage of 4 mg/Kg/day (RAP group). Vehicles or drugs were administered 1 day before the surgical procedure and were given until the end of experimental periods (3, 7, and 14 days). **(A)** Representative sections of 3 days time point post Ti implantation. Quantitative analysis of **(B)** GR1+, **(C)** F4/80+, **(D)** CD80+cells and **(E)** CD206+ cells was performed for each group at days 3, 7, and 14 days post Ti implantation. Results are presented as the mean and SD from a total of five animals/samples (biological replicates) and three semi-serial sections (technical replicates) *per* each group and time point. Different letters indicate significant differences in each time point ($p < 0.05$); symbol *indicate significant differences between experimental groups (GZA and RAP) vs. control at the same time point.

of blood clot and a decreased area density of blood vessels around Ti disc implantation at 7 days (**Figures 8C,E**). Similarly, both treatments (the inhibition of HMGB1 and the antagonism of RAGE), impaired the host response to the Ti disc by a decreased collagen fiber formation compared to the control and control vehicles, but with no negative effects in the amount of fibroblasts (**Figures 8F,G**). The reduced tissue repair in GZA and RAP could be mainly associated with an ineffective inflammatory response caused by the inhibition of inflammatory signals induced by HMGB1 and RAGE. Immuhistochemistry of GZA and RAP group showed a drastic reduction of GR1+ cells and macrophages (F4/80+ cells, CD80+ cells, CD206+ cells) migration toward the implantation sites at 3 days post Ti implantation compared to the Ti control group (**Figures 9A–E**).

In parallel and in agreement with molecular results for oral osseointegration model, the gene expression patterns in subcutaneous implanted sites on Ti control was also revealed growth factors involved in cell proliferation (FGF1, FGF2, FGF3, TGFb1, EGF) and angiogenesis (VEGFa,b) significantly up-regulated in the Ti Control group compared to the endogenous control (**Supplementary Figure 2**). Consistently, tissue healing and maturation of the ECM was also evidenced in Ti control by a high upregulation of ECM remodeling markers, such as the matrix metalloproteinases (MMP1a, MMP2, MMP9) and their tissue inhibitors TIMPs (TIMP1, TIMP3), as well the protease cathepsin G (CTSG). Among the upregulated cytokines in Ti control samples, CXCL10, CXCL12, CXCL11, IL1β, IL6, TNF were up regulated in the inflammatory phase of healing. Growth factors involved in cell proliferation, mainly for FGF family, were up regulated in GZA and RAP, such as in the Control group, while several ECM formation (Col1a2, Col2a1) and remodeling markers (MMP1a, MMP2, MMP9, TIMP1, TIMP3, CTSG) were down regulated GZA and RAP compared to the control. Importantly, GZA and RAP group presented a downregulation of molecules involved in cell adhesion and migration (CTGF, VTN, ITGA2, ITGA4, ITGA5). All together, these results indicate a role of HMGB1 and RAGE on fibroblasts migration, differentiation, and matrix deposition along tissue repair surrounding a classic biomaterial.

DISCUSSION

Among the several DAMPs and their accompanying PRRs, the interaction of HMGB1 with the receptor RAGE has

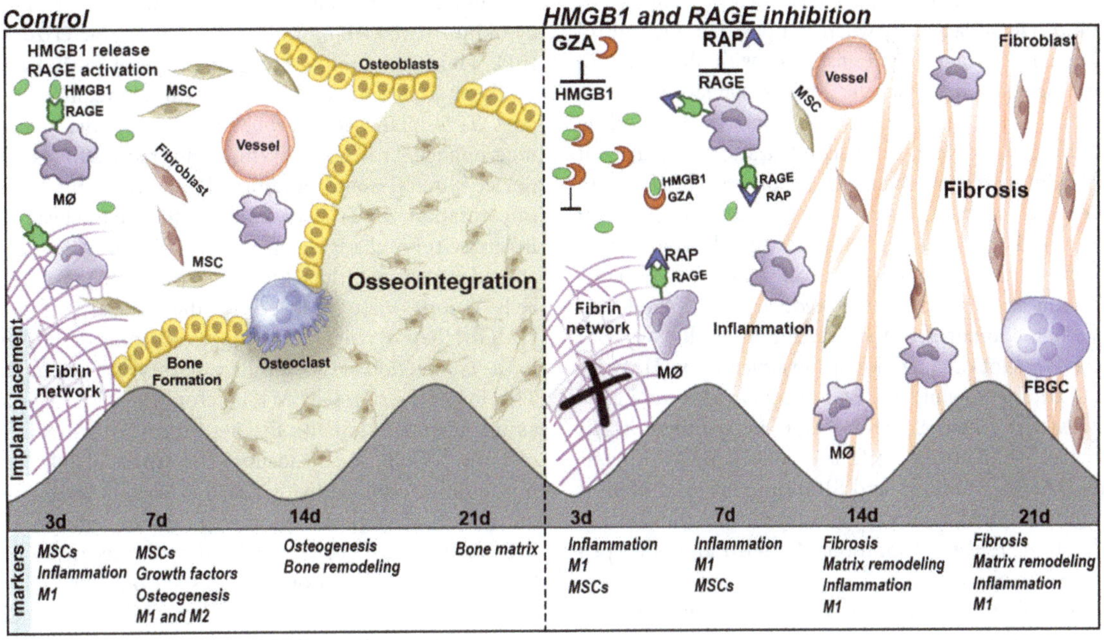

FIGURE 10 | Graphical abstract of proposed roles of HGMB1 and RAGE along oral Ti osseointegration process in mice.

been associated with the activation of inflammatory responses and wound healing, especially in non-infectious environments (18, 19, 22). In this study, the possible involvement of the HMGB1/RAGE pathway in the modulation of host inflammatory immune response at Ti/host interface, and the subsequent influence in the healing and osseointegration processes were investigated. Therefore, to determine the role of HMGB1 and RAGE in the osseointegration process in a cause-and-effect manner, C57Bl/6 mice were subjected to Ti-implant surgical placement in the maxillary edentulous area and were treated with GZA and RAP, respectively, an HMGB1 inhibitor (41) and a RAGE inhibitor (42).

Initially, our results demonstrated that HMGB1 was present in the protein adsorption layer characteristically formed in biomaterials surface after implantation, in both Ti-screws implanted in bone and Ti-discs implanted in subcutaneous tissue (**Figure 1**). Importantly, despite the general assumption that endogenous DAMPs are released upon biomaterials implantation, this is the first actual demonstration that DAMPs (specifically HMGB1) are in fact released and can adsorb to Ti surface. The kinetics of HMGB1 release and adsorption is in agreement with the hypothesis of the injury-triggered release, characterized by high levels in the initial time point followed by a gradual decrease over time (50–52). Also, our results demonstrated that inhibition of both, HMGB1 and RAGE, impaired Ti-mediated osseointegration, as demonstrated by the critical alterations in the dynamics of mineralized and organic bone matrix formation (**Figures 2, 3**). Accordingly, the inhibition of HMGB1 in a model of tooth extraction in mice significantly delayed the bone healing process, but without inhibiting it completely (21). However, it is crucial to consider that in the present study, the presence of a biomaterial is an important variable in the healing site; which may account for the complete impairment of the osseointegration process in comparison with the partial influence of HMGB1 inhibition described in the socket healing (21). Importantly, no previous studies have described possible associations between RAGE blockade and bone healing or osseointegration. It is also important to mention that HMGB1 and RAGE blockade impair the healing of subcutaneous tissue after the grafting of a Ti-disc, reinforcing the role of HMGB1/RAGE axis in the host response to biomaterials and in the subsequent healing response. While the subcutaneous implantation of Ti-devices obviously does not mimic the osseointegration response, it have been considered a valuable model to study biomaterial/host interaction (53), which can be very useful, especially in mice in the view of the very limited dimensions of the Ti implant used for osseointegration analysis, which limits some experimental approaches.

In order to investigate the mechanisms underlying impaired osseointegration due HMGB1 and RAGE inhibition, a series of histomorphometric, and molecular analysis were performed, comparing unsuccessful and successful osseointegration sites. The process of osseointegration starts with the surgical preparation of the bone niche/defect for implant placement, when coagulation proteins from blood are released and then activated to provide the clot formation and consequently a provisional matrix for cell recruitment and migration (15). Accordingly, in the Control group (which achieved osseointegration), an organized blood clot was evidenced at the host/Ti interface at 3 days post-implantation. However, HMGB1 inhibition resulted in disruption of fibrin network formation and impairment of the blood clot structure, followed by a significant decrease in blood clot area density when compared to the Control group. Indeed, HMGB1 acts synergistically with thrombin to promote fibrin deposition and accelerate the coagulation *in vivo*, evidencing its role as an organizer in post-injury wound healing (54). Thus, the initial event of osseointegration impairment due to GZA administration seems to be primarily related to the disruption of the blood clot, since the establishment of a fibrin network in association with Ti threads spaces was drastically compromised upon HMGB1 inhibition. Additionally, RAGE inhibition also resulted in a reduction of blood clot area density when compared to the Control group, but without drastic effects over clot organization as observed upon HMGB1 inhibition. Accordingly, while HMBG1 seems to also act in the clotting process directly (i.e., in a RAGE independent way), RAGE expressed on platelets surface is associated with their activation by DAMPs (HMGB1 and S100 proteins) and platelet aggregation (55, 56), which consequently influence the clotting process, but also the release of additional HMGB1 and other pro inflammatory molecules (56, 57).

In addition to the initial interferences in the clotting process, previous studies demonstrated that HMGB1 promotes the secretion of multiple cytokines in the injured sites, strongly activating and driving the acute inflammatory response (58). Also, it is important to consider that HMGB1 is supposed to play also biphasic actions on injured sites (pro-inflammatory activity or immune tolerance/healing) depending of the environment redox state of its three conserved cysteines (Cys23, Cys45 [Box A], and Cys106 [BoxB]) (23). In this context, it has been proposed that during acute inflammatory response, the release of ROS/RNS induce the active and proinflammatory form of HMGB1 (reduced form of HMGB1); while the oxidation of HMGB1 cause immune tolerance, allowing the healing (22, 23). Considering the receptor RAGE, it is important to mention that two extracellular secreted forms of RAGE can be also present in the environment, besides the conventional receptor, they are endogenous secretory (es) and soluble (s) RAGE, have been identified and play active roles on skeletal biology, mainly related to osteoporosis in aged mice (59). It has been supposed that these RAGE isoforms (mainly sRAGE), could also their ligand-binding ability, acting as decoy receptors preventing ligand binding to RAGE. Importantly, while the analysis of redox modulation of HMGB1 activities, as well of a putative role for sRAGE, are beyond the scope of the present study, since our data point to a role for HMGB1 in osseointegration process, future specific studies focused in such elements may provide additional interesting information to the field.

In this study, HMGB1 or RAGE inhibition disturbed the natural course/fate of inflammatory response after Ti implantation. This resulted in the persistence of inflammatory cells around Ti threads until latter time points, comprising primarily macrophages as suggested by the cellular morphology, while Control mice exhibited the resolution of a transient inflammatory response in early time points (**Figure 4**). Accordingly, the molecular analysis demonstrated that HMGB1 or RAGE inhibition resulted in a persistence of high mRNA levels of CCR2, CCR5, CCL5, which are mainly associated with macrophage migration (48, 60), as well as pro-inflammatory cytokines (IL1b, IL-6, and TNF) that characterize M1 activity (61). Thus, our findings suggest a role of HMGB1 and RAGE on the modulation/resolution of chronic inflammatory response post Ti implantation, probably affecting the overall M1/M2 macrophages response. While the reduced size of the Ti-device limits some additional analysis, the subcutaneous implantation of Ti-discs allowed the characterization of the inflammatory changes upon HMGB1 and RAGE blockade, and demonstrate that the total macrophages, M1 and M2 cells counts were reduced in the absence of a functional HMGB1/RAGE axis. Macrophages are considered key elements in the connection between inflammatory and healing events (11). The initial presence of M1 macrophages has been implicated as an essential step for the activation of acute inflammatory response, while the transitory presence of M2 cells in the proliferative/regenerative phase has been suggested as favorable for the regenerative outcome (11). Conversely, a prolonged M1 activity has been associated with negative outcomes of biomaterial implantation, such as chronically inflamed tissue and severe foreign body reaction (FBR) (37). Considering the osseointegration and subcutaneous results, it is possible to suggest that HMGB1/RAGE axis is required for a proper macrophage chemoattraction after Ti implantation, and that both M1 and M2 responses, and the natural M1/M2 switch along the healing, are compromised by HMGB1 and RAGE inhibition. Accordingly, the molecular analysis of the successful Ti-osseointegration sites in the Control group demonstrated an initial M1-type response followed by a M2-type switch, evidenced by upregulation of M2-type markers (ARG1, TGFb, IL10, and CCL17) (62), which were disrupted by HMGB1/RAGE blockade. These observations are in agreement with previous studies (4, 5, 63). In view of that, the provision of environmental cues that govern the phenotype switch of macrophages and different healing outcomes post biomaterial implantation have been usually based on the biomaterial properties, in a perspective where Ti-based devices might modulate or allow a favorable M1/M2 switch (9). However, we demonstrated that inhibition of a DAMP or its receptor (HMGB1 or RAGE) following biomaterial implantation, can also drastically affect the initial microenvironmental signals for triggering osseointegration, even using a gold standard biomaterial such as a Ti-based device. Significantly, the effects of HMGB1 or RAGE inhibition are not limited to macrophages, as demonstrated by the significant reduction of granulocytes (Gr1+ cells) in the Ti disc implantation. While the main of focus in the cellular aspects of osseointegration (and in the biomaterials in general) have been over macrophages (9, 62), granulocytes are essential elements of early host response (64), and consequently can also theoretically impact the subsequent healing and osseointegration.

The lack of favorable biological microenvironment signals in biomaterial implantation sites can result in persistent chronic inflammation, consequently driving the wound healing around the biomaterial into a foreign body response (FBR) (65). In this manner, HMGB1 and RAGE inhibition drastically reduced the expression of MSC markers and bone markers in the sites of Ti implantation, which was reflected in a fibrotic outcome surrounding Ti threads (**Figures 6, 7**), with features of FBR, such as differentiation of FBGC surrounding the biomaterial and non-viable bone (**Figure 4**), increased expression of MMPs (**Figure 7**), followed by fibrous tissue formation and consequent biomaterial encapsulation (**Figure 4**). As previously proposed by literature, the modulation of host response for desirable biomaterial incorporation outcome is in part surface-based, depending on beneficial biomaterial properties, but signals provided from biomaterial implantation trauma have also been suggested as crucial cues in this process (9). Accordingly to the Control group results, in the presence of a constructive set of external and endogenous factors, including Ti as the external factor and HMGB1 and RAGE as part of endogenous factors, the inflammatory signals triggered post Ti implantation was linked to upregulation of MSC markers (CD206, OCT-4, NANOG, CD44, CD34, CD73, CD146, CD105) at earlier time points (3 and 7 days), and subsequent bone cells differentiation (Runx2, Alp), bone matrix deposition (Col1a1), remodeling (MMP2 and MMP9) (45), and bone maturation (Phex) (66) (**Figure 7**).

The body of this work suggests the participation of HMGB1 in multiple stages of osseointegration process, as a blood clot organizer and inflammatory/healing molecule (**Figure 10**). Several studies have suggested that HMGB1 can act as a regenerative mediator, by triggering inflammation (20), but also as a healing organizer, promoting the recruitment of MSCs, and platelets activation (20, 58). In this cause-effect study, the inhibition of extracellular HMGB1 following biomaterial implantation caused failure of Ti-mediated osseointegration (**Figures 2–5**), which could be associated to its multiple roles acting as a biochemical mediator for clot formation (54, 56, 67), as well as by triggering of signaling inflammatory pathways, which involve the activation of different receptors, such as RAGE. In fact, under the inhibition of RAGE, the immediate extracellular effects of released HMGB1 were maintained, such as confirmed by a suitable blood clot structure in the osseointegration sites at 3 days compared to the HMGB1 inhibition group. However, under the inhibition of RAGE, the HMGB1 cellular effects related to HMGB1/RAGE pathway was blockade, which also resulted in unsuccessful osseointegration.

It is also important to consider the despite the fact that a clear biological effect was observed upon the administration of the RAP and GZA in this study, the dosages used for both inhibitors were based in previous studies carried in C57Bl/6 mice but in different models and kinetics of drug administration (41, 42). Despite the effects observed in our study are compatible with the biological role of HMGB1 and RAGE, confirming the effectiveness of both inhibitions and demonstrating a role for HMGB1 and RAGE in osseointegration process, future studies including a dose-response analysis, may provide additional interesting information to the field. Finally, future studies are required to investigate the inhibition of HMGB1 and/or RAGE only in initial time points during Ti-mediated osseointegration, when these molecules are prevalent and theoretically mainly required, in order to determine their role in each phase of osseointegration.

CONCLUSION

Taken together, our findings suggest that HMGB1 and RAGE actively influence the osseointegration process, by their influence in the balance of host inflammatory immune response, which includes macrophages migration and M1/M2 response, MSC markers expression, and bone deposition (**Figure 10**).

AUTHOR CONTRIBUTIONS

CB and GG contributed to the conception and design, the acquisition, analysis, and interpretation, drafted the manuscript, critically revised the manuscript, gave final approval, and agreed to be accountable for all aspects of work. FC contributed to the acquisition, analysis, and interpretation, drafted the manuscript, critically revised the manuscript, gave final approval, and agreed to be accountable for all aspects of work. ES, APT, and CF contributed to the acquisition, analysis, and interpretation, drafted the manuscript, gave final approval, and agreed to be accountable for all aspects of work. RT, AC, APFT, and DR contributed to the acquisition, analysis, and interpretation, gave final approval, and agreed to be accountable for all aspects of work.

FUNDING

This work was supported by grants #2014/09590-8, #2015/18162-2, #2015/24637-3 from São Paulo Research Foundation (FAPESP), CNPq, and CAPES. DR is supported from the National Institutes of Health (NIH R01 DE026736).

ACKNOWLEDGMENTS

The authors would like to thank Daniele Ceolin, Patricia Germino, and Tania Cestari for their excellent technical assistance.

SUPPLEMENTARY MATERIAL

Supplementary Figure 1 | Histopathological analysis of blood clot in C57Bl/6 mice at 3 days post Ti implantation. Mice received Ti-screw implantation in the edentulous ridge of maxilla and were divided in according to each treatment: Control (C group, with no treatment); Glycyrrhizic Acid at a dosage of 200 mg/Kg/day (GZA group); or RAGE antagonistic peptide at dosage of 4 mg/Kg/day (RAP group). Blood clot is observed throughout days 3, 7, 14, and 21 days. Histological slides were stained with H&E and images were captured at 10 and 100x magnification.

Supplementary Figure 2 | Gene expression patterns post subcutaneous Ti disc implantation in C57Bl/6 mice treated with HMGB1 inhibitor or RAGE antagonist. Mice received Ti-disc implantation in the subcutaneous tissue and were divided in according to each treatment: Control (C group, with no treatment); Glycyrrhizic Acid at a dosage of 200 mg/Kg/day (GZA group); or RAGE antagonistic peptide at dosage of 4 mg/Kg/day (RAP group). Four biological replicates from subcutaneous tissue samples were removed at 3, 7, and 14 days post Ti implantation and a pool of samples from all the experimental time periods in each experimental group was used for a gene expression pattern analysis. Samples of subcutaneous tissue without surgery were used as control. Two technical replicates were considered for each assay. Gene expression was performed by using exploratory analysis by Real Time PCR array, with the VIA7 system (Applied Biosystems, Warrington, UK) and a customized qPCR array comprised of the major targets (Inflammatory Cytokines & Receptors and Wound Healing panels) of the PCRarrayRT2 Profiler (SABiosciences/QIAGEN). Results are depicted as the fold increase change (and the standard deviation) in mRNA expression from triplicate measurements in relation to the control samples and normalized by internal housekeeping genes (GAPDH, HPRT, β-actin).

REFERENCES

1. Adell R, Lekholm U, Rockler B, Branemark PI. A 15-year study of osseointegrated implants in the treatment of the edentulous jaw. *Int J Oral Surg.* (1981) 10:387–416. doi: 10.1016/S0300-9785(81)80077-4
2. Branemark PI, Hansson BO, Adell R, Breine U, Lindstrom J, Hallen O, et al. Osseointegrated implants in the treatment of the edentulous jaw. Experience from a 10-year period. *Scand J Plast Reconstr Surg Suppl.* (1977) 16:1–132.
3. Albrektsson T, Dahlin C, Jemt T, Sennerby L, Turri A, Wennerberg A. Is marginal bone loss around oral implants the result of a provoked foreign body reaction? *Clin Implant Dent Relat Res.* (2014) 16:155–65. doi: 10.1111/cid.12142
4. Biguetti CC, Cavalla F, Silveira EM, Fonseca AC, Vieira AE, Tabanez AP, et al. Oral implant osseointegration model in C57Bl/6 mice: microtomographic, histological, histomorphometric and molecular characterization. *J Appl Oral Sci.* (2018) 26:e20170601.doi: 10.1590/1678-7757-2017-0601
5. Thalji GN, Nares S, Cooper LF. Early molecular assessment of osseointegration in humans. *Clin Oral Implants Res.* (2014) 25:1273–85. doi: 10.1111/clr.12266
6. Agarwal R, Garcia AJ. Biomaterial strategies for engineering implants for enhanced osseointegration and bone repair. *Adv Drug Deliv Rev.* (2015) 94:53–62. doi: 10.1016/j.addr.2015.03.013
7. Hotchkiss KM, Reddy GB, Hyzy SL, Schwartz Z, Boyan BD, Olivares-Navarrete, R. Titanium surface characteristics, including topography and wettability, alter macrophage activation. *Acta Biomater.* (2016) 31:425–34. doi: 10.1016/j.actbio.2015.12.003
8. Gu Q, Yang H, Shi Q. Macrophages and bone inflammation. *J Orthopaedic Transl.* (2017) 10:86–93. doi: 10.1016/j.jot.2017.05.002
9. Sridharan R, Cameron AR, Kelly DJ, Kearney CJ, O'Brien FJ. Biomaterial based modulation of macrophage polarization: a review and suggested design principles. *Mater Today.* (2015) 18:313–25. doi: 10.1016/j.mattod.2015.01.019
10. Mosser DM, Edwards JP. Exploring the full spectrum of macrophage activation. *Nat Rev Immunol.* (2008) 8:958–69. doi: 10.1038/nri2448
11. Brown BN, Ratner BD, Goodman SB, Amar S, Badylak SF. Macrophage polarization: an opportunity for improved outcomes in biomaterials and regenerative medicine. *Biomaterials.* (2012) 33:3792–802. doi: 10.1016/j.biomaterials.2012.02.034
12. Trindade R, Albrektsson T, Wennerberg A. Current concepts for the biological basis of dental implants: foreign body equilibrium and osseointegration dynamics. *Oral Maxillofacial Surg Clin N Am.* (2015) 27:175–83. doi: 10.1016/j.coms.2015.01.004
13. Corradetti B, Taraballi F, Corbo C, Cabrera F, Pandolfi L, Minardi S, et al. Immune tuning scaffold for the local induction of a pro-regenerative environment. *Sci Rep.* (2017) 7:17030. doi: 10.1038/s41598-017-1 6895-0
14. Land WG. The role of damage-associated molecular patterns (DAMPs) in human diseases: part II: DAMPs as diagnostics, prognostics and therapeutics in clinical medicine. *Sultan Qaboos Univ Med J.* (2015) 15:e157-70.
15. Vishwakarma A, Bhise NS, Evangelista MB, Rouwkema J, Dokmeci MR, Ghaemmaghami AM, et al. Engineering immunomodulatory biomaterials to tune the inflammatory response. *Trends Biotechnol.* (2016) 34:470–82. doi: 10.1016/j.tibtech.2016.03.009
16. Fukata M, Vamadevan AS, Abreu MT. Toll-like receptors (TLRs) and Nod-like receptors (NLRs) in inflammatory disorders. *Semin Immunol.* (2009) 21:242–53. doi: 10.1016/j.smim.2009.06.005
17. Sims GP, Rowe DC, Rietdijk ST, Herbst R, Coyle AJ. HMGB1 and RAGE in inflammation and cancer. *Ann Rev Immunol.* (2010) 28:367–88. doi: 10.1146/annurev.immunol.021908.132603
18. Kang R, Chen R, Zhang Q, Hou W, Wu S, Cao L, et al. HMGB1 in health and disease. *Mol Aspects Med.* (2014) 40:1–116. doi: 10.1016/j.mam.2014.05.001
19. Tancharoen S, Gando S, Binita S, Nagasato T, Kikuchi K, Nawa Y, et al. HMGB1 promotes intraoral palatal wound healing through RAGE-dependent mechanisms. *Int J Mol Sci.* (2016) 17:11. doi: 10.3390/ijms17111961
20. Schiraldi M, Raucci A, Munoz LM, Livoti E, Celona B, Venereau E, et al. HMGB1 promotes recruitment of inflammatory cells to damaged tissues by forming a complex with CXCL12 and signaling via CXCR4. *J Exp Med.* (2012) 209:551–63. doi: 10.1084/jem.20111739
21. Aoyagi H, Yamashiro K, Hirata-Yoshihara C, Ideguchi H, Yamasaki M, Kawamura M, et al. HMGB1-induced inflammatory response promotes bone healing in murine tooth extraction socket. *J Cell Biochem.* (2018) 27:26710. doi: 10.1002/jcb.26710
22. Yang H, Lundbäck P, Ottosson L, Erlandsson-Harris H, Venereau E, Bianchi ME, et al. Redox modification of cysteine residues regulates the cytokine activity of high mobility group box-1 (HMGB1). *Mol Med.* (2012) 18:250–9. doi: 10.2119/molmed.2011.00389
23. Janko C, Filipović M, Munoz LE, Schorn C, Schett G, Ivanović-Burmazović I, et al.Redox modulation of HMGB1-related signaling. *Antioxid Redox Signal.* (2014) 20:1075–85. doi: 10.1089/ars.2013.5179
24. Kokkola R, Andersson A, Mullins G, Ostberg T, Treutiger CJ, Arnold B, et al. RAGE is the major receptor for the proinflammatory activity of HMGB1 in rodent macrophages. *Scand J Immunol.* (2005) 61:1–9. doi: 10.1111/j.0300-9475.2005.01534.x
25. Rauvala H, Rouhiainen A. RAGE as a receptor of HMGB1 (Amphoterin): roles in health and disease. *Curr Mol Med.* (2007) 7:725–34. doi: 10.2174/156652407783220750
26. Rojas A, Delgado-Lopez F, Perez-Castro R, Gonzalez I, Romero J, Rojas I, et al. HMGB1 enhances the protumoral activities of M2 macrophages by a RAGE-dependent mechanism. *Tumor Biol.* (2016) 37:3321–9. doi: 10.1007/s13277-015-3940-y
27. Luo Y, Li SJ, Yang J, Qiu YZ, Chen FP. HMGB1 induces an inflammatory response in endothelial cells via the RAGE-dependent endoplasmic reticulum stress pathway. *Biochem Biophys Res Commun.* (2013) 438:732–8. doi: 10.1016/j.bbrc.2013.07.098
28. Lei C, Zhang S, Cao T, Tao W, Liu M, Wu, B. HMGB1 may act via RAGE to promote angiogenesis in the later phase after intracerebral hemorrhage. *Neuroscience.* (2015) 295:39–47. doi: 10.1016/j.neuroscience.2015.03.032
29. Tian X, Sun L, Feng D, Sun Q, Dou Y, Liu C, et al. HMGB1 promotes neurovascular remodeling via Rage in the late phase of subarachnoid hemorrhage. *Brain Res.* (2017) 1670:135–45. doi: 10.1016/j.brainres.2017.06.001
30. Su Z, Wang T, Zhu H, Zhang P, Han R, Liu Y, et al. HMGB1 modulates Lewis cell autophagy and promotes cell survival via RAGE-HMGB1-Erk1/2 positive feedback during nutrient depletion. *Immunobiology.* (2015) 220:539–44. doi: 10.1016/j.imbio.2014.12.009
31. Riuzzi F, Sorci G, Sagheddu R, Donato, R. HMGB1-RAGE regulates muscle satellite cell homeostasis through p38-MAPK- and myogenin-dependent repression of Pax7 transcription. *J Cell Sci.* (2012) 125(Pt 6):1440–54. doi: 10.1242/jcs.092163
32. Su Z, Zhang P, Yu Y, Lu H, Liu Y, Ni P, et al. HMGB1 facilitated macrophage reprogramming towards a proinflammatory M1-like phenotype in experimental autoimmune myocarditis development. *Sci Rep.* (2016) 6:21884. doi: 10.1038/srep21884
33. Tian S, Zhang L, Tang J, Guo X, Dong K, Chen SY. HMGB1 exacerbates renal tubulointerstitial fibrosis through facilitating M1 macrophage phenotype at the early stage of obstructive injury. *Am J Physiol Renal Physiol.* (2015) 308:F69–75. doi: 10.1152/ajprenal.00484.2014
34. Son M, Porat A, He M, Suurmond J, Santiago-Schwarz F, Andersson U, et al. C1q and HMGB1 reciprocally regulate human macrophage polarization. *Blood.* (2016) 128:2218–28. doi: 10.1182/blood-2016-05-7 19757

35. Yang H, Wang H, Levine YA, Gunasekaran MK, Wang Y, Addorisio M, et al. Identification of CD163 as an antiinflammatory receptor for HMGB1-haptoglobin complexes. *JCI Insight.* (2016) 1:7. doi: 10.1172/jci.insight.85375
36. Daly KA, Liu S, Agrawal V, Brown BN, Johnson SA, Medberry CJ, et al. Damage associated molecular patterns within xenogeneic biologic scaffolds and their effects on host remodeling. *Biomaterials.* (2012) 33:91–101. doi: 10.1016/j.biomaterials.2011.09.040
37. Julier Z, Park AJ, Briquez PS, Martino MM. Promoting tissue regeneration by modulating the immune system. *Acta Biomater.* (2017) 53:13–28. doi: 10.1016/j.actbio.2017.01.056
38. Othman Z, Cillero Pastor B, van Rijt S, Habibovic P. Understanding interactions between biomaterials and biological systems using proteomics. *Biomaterials.* (2018) 167:191–204. doi: 10.1016/j.biomaterials.2018.03.020
39. Institute of Laboratory Animal Resources (U.S.). Committee on Care and Use of Laboratory Animals. *Guide for the Care and Use of Laboratory Animals. NIH publication.* Bethesda, MD: U.S. Dept. of Health and Human Services, Public Health Service (2011).
40. Kilkenny C, Browne WJ, Cuthi I, Emerson M, Altman DG. Improving bioscience research reporting: the ARRIVE guidelines for reporting animal research. *Veter Clin Pathol.* (2012) 41:27–31. doi: 10.1371/journal.pbio.1000412
41. Lau A, Wang S, Liu W, Haig A, Zhang ZX, Jevnikar AM. Glycyrrhizic acid ameliorates HMGB1-mediated cell death and inflammation after renal ischemia reperfusion injury. *Am J Nephrol.* (2014) 40:84–95.doi: 10.1159/000364908
42. Arumugam T, Ramachandran V, Gomez SB, Schmidt AM, Logsdon CD. S100P-derived RAGE antagonistic peptide reduces tumor growth and metastasis. *Clin Cancer Res.* (2012) 18:4356–64. doi: 10.1158/1078-0432.CCR-12-0221
43. Mouraret S, Hunter DJ, Bardet C, Brunski JB, Bouchard P, Helms JA. A pre-clinical murine model of oral implant osseointegration. *Bone.* (2014) 58:177–84.doi: 10.1016/j.bone.2013.07.021
44. Araujo-Pires AC, Biguetti CC, Repeke CE, Rodini C Campanelli AP, Trombone AP, et al. Mesenchymal stem cells as active prohealing and immunosuppressive agents in periapical environment: evidence from human and experimental periapical lesions. *J Endodontics.* (2014) 40:1560–5. doi: 10.1016/j.joen.2014.02.012
45. Vieira AE, Repeke CE, Ferreira S Jr., Colavite PM, Biguetti CC, Oliveira RC, et al. Intramembranous bone healing process subsequent to tooth extraction in mice: micro-computed tomography, histomorphometric and molecular characterization. *PLoS ONE.* (2015) 10:e0128021. doi: 10.1371/journal.pone.0128021
46. Romero-Gavilán F, Gomes NC, Ródenas J, Sánchez A, Azkargorta M, Iloro I, et al. Proteome analysis of human serum proteins adsorbed onto different titanium surfaces used in dental implants. *Biofouling.* (2017) 33:98–111. doi: 10.1080/08927014.2016.1259414
47. Kaneko H, Kamiie J, Kawakami H, Anada T, Honda Y, Shiraishi N, et al. Proteome analysis of rat serum proteins adsorbed onto synthetic octacalcium phosphate crystals. *Anal Biochem.* (2011) 418:276–85. doi: 10.1016/j.ab.2011.07.022
48. Biguetti CC, Vieira AE, Cavalla F, Fonseca AC, Colavite PM, Silva RM, et al. CCR2 contributes to F4/80+ cells migration along intramembranous bone healing in Maxilla, but its deficiency does not critically affect the healing outcome. *Front Immunol.* (2018) 9:1804. doi: 10.3389/fimmu.2018.01804
49. Benjamini Y, Hochberg, Y. Controlling the false discovery rate: a practical and powerful approach to multiple testing. *J R Stat Soc Ser B.* (1995) 1:11. doi: 10.1111/j.2517-6161.1995.tb02031.x
50. Liu A, Jin H, Dirsch O, Deng M, Huang H, Bröcker-Preuss M, et al. Release of danger signals during ischemic storage of the liver: a potential marker of organ damage? *Mediators Inflamm.* (2010) 2010:436145. doi: 10.1155/2010/436145
51. Manganelli V, Signore M, Pacini I, Misasi R, Tellan G, Garofalo T, et al. Increased HMGB1 expression and release by mononuclear cells following surgical/anesthesia trauma. *Crit Care.* (2010) 14:R197.doi: 10.1186/cc9316
52. Osoegawa A, Yano T, Yamanaka T, Tagawa T, Shoji F, Yoshino I, et al. Plasma high-mobility group box 1 as an indicator of surgical stress. *Surg Today.* (2011) 41:903–7. doi: 10.1007/s00595-010-4371-4
53. Tilmaciu CM, Mathieu M, Lavigne JP, Toupet K, Guerrero G, Ponche A, et al. *In vitro* and *in vivo* characterization of antibacterial activity and biocompatibility: a study on silver-containing phosphonate monolayers on titanium. *Acta Biomater.* (2015) 15:266–77. doi: 10.1016/j.actbio.2014.12.020
54. Ito T, Kawahara K, Nakamura T, Yamada S, Nakamura T, Abeyama K, et al. High-mobility group box 1 protein promotes development of microvascular thrombosis in rats. *J Thrombosis Haemostasis JTH.* (2007) 5:109–16. doi: 10.1111/j.1538-7836.2006.02255.x
55. Ahrens I, Chen YC, Topcic D, Bode M, Haenel D, Hagemeyer CE, et al. HMGB1 binds to activated platelets via the receptor for advanced glycation end products and is present in platelet rich human coronary artery thrombi. *Thrombosis Haemostasis.* (2015) 114:994–1003. doi: 10.1160/TH14-12-1073
56. Fuentes E, Rojas A, Palomo I. Role of multiligand/RAGE axis in platelet activation. *Thrombosis Res.* (2014) 133:308–14. doi: 10.1016/j.thromres.2013.11.007
57. Fuentes E, Palomo I, Rojas A. Cross-talk between platelet and tumor microenvironment: Role of multiligand/RAGE axis in platelet activation. *Blood Rev.* (2016) 30:213–21. doi: 10.1016/j.blre.2015.11.005
58. Feng L, Xue D, Chen E, Zhang W, Gao X, Yu J, et al. HMGB1 promotes the secretion of multiple cytokines and potentiates the osteogenic differentiation of mesenchymal stem cells through the Ras/MAPK signaling pathway. *Exp Ther Med.* (2016) 12:3941–7.doi: 10.3892/etm.2016.3857
59. Plotkin L, Essex AL, Davis HM. RAGE signaling in skeletal biology. *Curr Osteoporos Rep.* (2019) 17:16–25. doi: 10.1007/s11914-019-00499-w
60. Mack M, Cihak J, Simonis C, Luckow B, Proudfoot AE, Plachy J, et al. Expression and characterization of the chemokine receptors CCR2 and CCR5 in mice. *J Immunol.* (2001) 166:4697–704. doi: 10.4049/jimmunol.166.7.4697
61. Martinez FO, Gordon S. The M1 and M2 paradigm of macrophage activation: time for reassessment. *F1000prime Rep.* (2014) 6:13. doi: 10.12703/P6-13
62. Pajarinen J, Kouri VP, Jamsen E, Li TF, Mandelin J, Konttinen YT. The response of macrophages to titanium particles is determined by macrophage polarization. *Acta Biomater.* (2013) 9:9229–40. doi: 10.1016/j.actbio.2013.06.027
63. Thalji G, Cooper LF. Molecular assessment of osseointegration in vivo: a review of the current literature. *Int J Oral Maxillofac Implants.* (2013) 28:e521–34. doi: 10.11607/jomi.te33
64. Selders GS, Fetz AE, Radic MZ, Bowlin GL. An overview of the role of neutrophils in innate immunity, inflammation and host-biomaterial integration. *Regenerat Biomater.* (2017) 4:55–68. doi: 10.1093/rb/rbw041
65. Anderson JM, Rodriguez A, Chang DT. Foreign body reaction to biomaterials. *Semin Immunol.* (2008) 20:86–100. doi: 10.1016/j.smim.2007.11.004
66. Bonewald LF. The amazing osteocyte. *J Bone Miner Res.* (2011) 26:229–38. doi: 10.1002/jbmr.320
67. Pawlinski R. Platelet HMGB1: the venous clot coordinator. *Blood.* (2016) 128:2376–8. doi: 10.1182/blood-2016-09-738740

15

Interleukin-17A Interweaves the Skeletal and Immune Systems

Mengjia Tang[1†], *Lingyun Lu*[2†] *and Xijie Yu*[1*]

[1] *Department of Endocrinology and Metabolism, Laboratory of Endocrinology and Metabolism, National Clinical Research Center for Geriatrics, West China Hospital, Sichuan University, Chengdu, China,* [2] *Department of Integrated Traditional Chinese and Western Medicine, Laboratory of Endocrinology and Metabolism, West China Hospital, Sichuan University, Chengdu, China*

***Correspondence:**
Xijie Yu
xijieyu@scu.edu.cn;
xijieyu@hotmail.com

[†]*These authors have contributed equally to this work*

The complex crosstalk between the immune and the skeletal systems plays an indispensable role in the maintenance of skeletal homeostasis. Various cytokines are involved, including interleukin (IL)-17A. A variety of immune and inflammatory cells produces IL-17A, especially Th17 cells, a subtype of $CD4^+$ T cells. IL-17A orchestrates diverse inflammatory and immune processes. IL-17A induces direct and indirect effects on osteoclasts. The dual role of IL-17A on osteoclasts partly depends on its concentrations and interactions with other factors. Interestingly, IL-17A exerts a dual role in osteoblasts *in vitro*. IL-17A is a bone-destroying cytokine in numerous immune-mediated bone diseases including postmenopausal osteoporosis (PMOP), rheumatoid arthritis (RA), psoriatic arthritis (PsA) and axial spondylarthritis (axSpA). This review will summarize and discuss the pathophysiological roles of IL-17A on the skeletal system and its potential strategies for application in immune-mediated bone diseases.

Keywords: osteoimmunology, interleukin-17A, osteoclasts, osteoblasts, postmenopausal osteoporosis, rheumatoid arthritis, psoriatic arthritis, axial spondyloarthritis

INTRODUCTION

Over the last 20 years, a growing body of research has focused on the relationship between the skeletal and immune systems. Subsequently, the term "osteoimmunology" was defined for this field of study. Accumulating evidence has shown that multiple components of immune systems including immune organs, multiple immune cells, and immune factors, participate in bone metabolism. In turn, bone cells, including osteoclasts, osteoblasts, bone lining cells, and osteocytes, are indispensable for the regulation of immune systems. The interaction between the skeletal and immune systems constitutes a complex network and is involved in the pathological process of many immune-mediated bone diseases. Recent studies have shown that IL-17A as one of the immune-derived cytokines participates in the regulation of bone metabolism. Understanding the effect of IL-17A on bone metabolism is more conducive to develop new-targeted drugs for immune-related bone diseases. This review will summarize the current knowledge of IL-17A in the skeletal system and will discuss the potential clinical value of IL-17A in immune-mediated bone diseases.

IL-17A SIGNALING PATHWAY AND FUNCTION

The IL-17 family includes six major isoforms: IL-17A, IL-17B, IL-17C, IL-17D, IL-17E, and IL-17F. Six of these isoforms interact with the five receptors (IL-17RA-E), respectively (1). IL-17A was the first member discovered and the most studied of the IL-17 family. Thereafter, following large-scale sequencing of the human and other vertebrate genomes, additional isoforms homologous to IL-17A were found (2). In 1993, Rouvier et al. cloned IL-17 for the first time. IL-17 was initially called the murine cytotoxic T lymphocyte-associated antigen-8 (mCTLA8) and was found to share 57% homology with the open reading frame 13 (ORF13) of Herpesvirus saimiri (HVS) (3). Subsequently, Yao et al. and Fossiez et al. cloned IL-17A in 1995 and 1996, respectively. Humans and mice share 25% amino acid sequence homology in IL-17A (4). IL-17A has been reported to be involved in inflammation and hematopoiesis and its secretion might be restricted to activated memory CD4 $^+$ T cells (4, 5). Current studies indicate that IL-17A is mainly produced by a special CD4$^+$ T cell subtype, Th17 cells (6). In addition, other types of lymphocytes including IL-17$^+$ CD8$^+$ T cells (Tc17 cells) (7), invariant natural killer T (8), Foxp3$^+$ Treg cells (9), γδ T cells (10), lymphoid–tissue inducer (LTi)–like cells (11), innate lymphoid cell (ILC3) (12), and NK cells can produce IL-17A. Besides, lymphocytes, myeloid cells including macrophages/monocytes (13), neutrophils (14), mast cells (15), Paneth cells (16) can secret IL-17A. Moreover, fibroblasts can also produce IL-17A (17). Multiple cytokines affect the expression of IL-17A, IL-1β, tumor necrosis factor (TNF)-β, IL-21, and IL-23 stimulate the expression of IL-17A in T cells (18), while interferon (IFN)-α inhibits the expression of IL-17A in T cells (19). Thus, IL-17A is derived from a variety of immune and inflammatory cells and its expression is regulated by a variety of immune factors.

IL-17A interacts with its receptors to activate downstream regulators and trigger cellular responses. Receptors for IL-17A are ubiquitously expressed on the cellular surface including synoviocytes, chondrocytes, fibroblasts, monocytes/macrophages, mast cells (20, 21). Bone cells including osteoclasts and osteoblasts also express IL-17RA (22). The interaction between IL-17RA and IL-17RC forms a complex to mediate the functions of IL-17A. The binding of IL-17A to the related receptor sites of IL-17RA alters the affinity and specificity of the symmetry receptor site. This response promotes the form of IL-17RA/RC heterodimer and makes an optimal response to mediate the functions of IL-17A homodimers (23, 24). Both IL-17RA and IL-17RC are type I transmembrane proteins. IL-17RA includes two extracellular fibronectin II-like domains and two intracellular "SEFIR" domains (25, 26). The SEFIR is homologous to Toll-IL-1R (TIR) domains found in the TLR/IL-1R family and is crucial for triggering downstream signaling events. IL-17A binds to its heterodimeric receptors complex and then recruits Act1 to activate classic IL-17A signaling cascades through receptor-associated factor 6 (TRAF6) proteins. TRAF6 binding subsequently triggers the mitogen-activated protein kinase (MAPK) pathway, extracellular signal–regulated kinase 1/2 (ERK1/2) pathway, and nuclear factor-κB (NF-κB) pathway. Among the non-classical signaling pathways, IL-17A integrates with epidermal growth factor receptor (EGFR), Notch 1, homolog translocation-associated (NOTCH1), C-type lectin receptor components, and interacts with fibroblast growth factor (FGF) signaling to initiate downstream biological responses (27).

In physiological conditions, IL-17A, as an immune and inflammatory-related factor, plays a protective role in host defenses against many bacterial and fungal pathogens (28). IL-17A activates neutrophils to promote neutrophil recruitment and accumulation (29). Meanwhile, IL-17A also affects the activity of B and T cells to act as a bridge between innate and acquired immune responses. Many studies have suggested that IL-17A is involved in the pathophysiological process of multiple diseases, including inflammatory bowel disease, breast cancer (30), lung cancer (31), cardiovascular system (32), uveitis (33), rheumatoid arthritis (RA), and psoriasis.

EFFECTS OF IL-17A ON THE SKELETAL SYSTEM

Osteoclasts

The skeleton maintains physiological function through a dynamic balance of bone formation and resorption. Osteoclasts derive from the monocyte/macrophage lineage and are key players in bone resorption. IL-17A acts directly on osteoclast precursors. Exposure to IL-17A (0.1–1 ng/ml) induces the expression of colony-stimulating factor-1 receptor (c-Fms) and receptor activator of nuclear factor-κB (RANK) on human peripheral blood mononuclear cells (hPBMCs), thereby promoting more hPBMCs to differentiate into functional osteoclasts. The effect is not dose-dependent, but 1 ng/ml of IL-17A shows the best induction (34). The direct effect of IL-17A on osteoclast precursors seems to be dependent on its concentration. A low concentration of IL-17A (0.5ng/ml) promotes autophagy of osteoclast precursors by activating the RANKL-JNK signaling pathway, thereby enhancing RANKL-induced osteoclast differentiation. However, treatment with a high concentration of IL-17A (5–50 ng/ml) inhibits autophagy and decreases osteoclast formation (35). In addition, a low level of IL-17A can reduce the apoptosis of osteoclasts and thus increases the number of osteoclasts by targeting the RANKL-Beclin1-autophagy-TRAF3 pathway (36). In turn, high levels of IL-17A increase apoptosis of osteoclasts and ultimately reduce pro-osteoclast mediators including cathepsin K, tartrate-resistant acid phosphatase (TRAP), and matrix metalloproteinase (MMP)-9 (36, 37). Interestingly, a higher concentration of IL-17A (100 ng/ml) promotes RANKL-induced polynuclear osteoclast formation and increases the expression of RANK and TRAP (38) (**Figure 1**).

Conversely, IL-17A can regulate osteoclast formation by targeting osteoclast-supporting cells. When activated by IL-17A, human bone marrow-derived mesenchymal stem cells

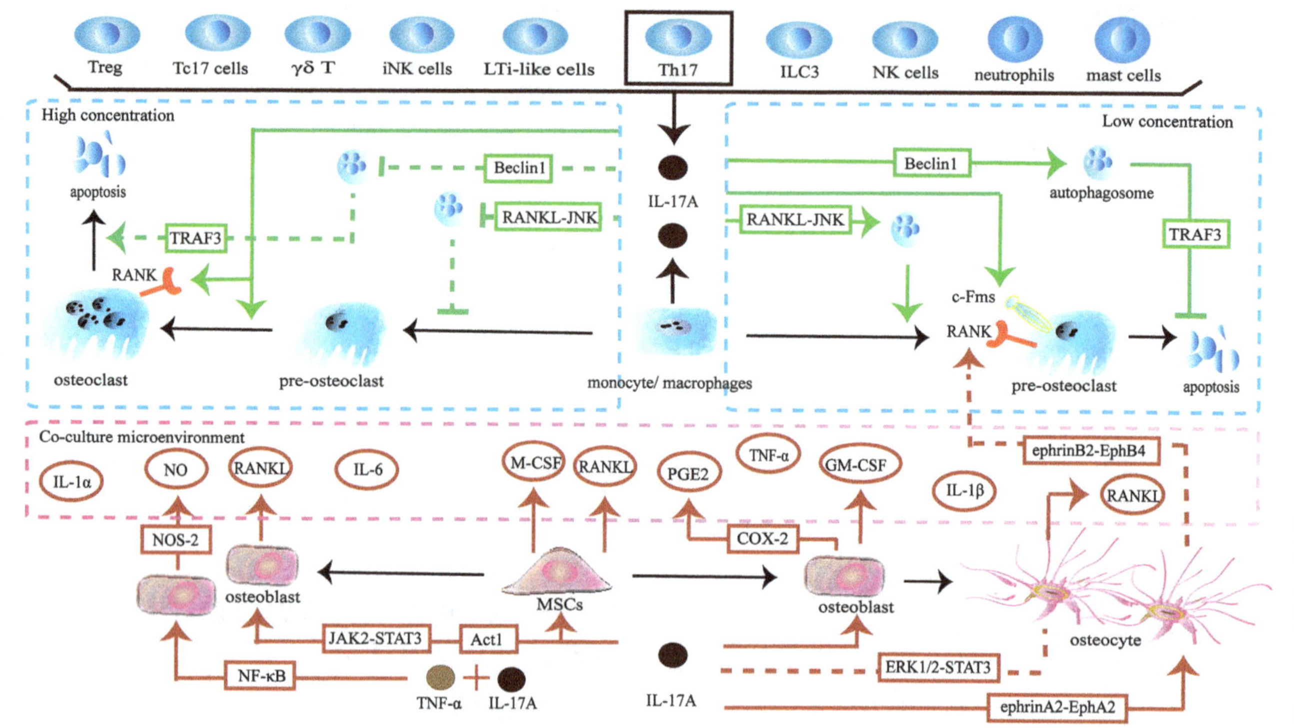

FIGURE 1 | Effects of IL-17A on osteoclasts. ① IL-17A is produced by multiple lymphocytes including Treg cells, IL-17⁺ CD8⁺ T cells (Tc17 cells), γδ T cells, invariant natural killer T (iNK cells), and Th17 cells. Myeloid cells including macrophages/monocytes, neutrophils and mast cells can also secrete IL-17A. Th17 cells are the main source of IL-17A. ② Low concentrations of IL-17A promote osteoclastogenesis through the RANKL-JNK signaling pathway and reduces the apoptosis of osteoclasts through the RANKL-Beclin1-autophagy-TRAF3 pathway. IL-17A increases the expression of c-Fms in osteoclast precursors to promote proliferation and differentiation. IL-17A increases the number of RANK⁺ osteoclast precursors to influence subsequent RANKL-dependent osteoclastogenesis. ③ High concentration of IL-17A (5–50 ng/ml) inhibits osteoclastogenesis through the RANKL-JNK signaling pathway and promotes the apoptosis of osteoclasts through the RANKL-Beclin1-autophagy-TRAF3 pathway. However, a higher concentration of IL-17A (100 ng/ml) increases the number of RANK+ osteoclast precursors and induces polynuclear osteoclast formation. ④ IL-17A acts on osteoclast-supporting cells including mesenchymal stem cells, osteoblasts and osteocytes to produce various cytokines and molecules to regulate osteoclastogenesis indirectly.

(hBM-MSCs) secrete M-CSF and RANKL, thereby supporting osteoclastogenesis (39). When IL-17A binds to its receptors IL-17RA SEFIR/TILL domain on pre-osteoclasts, they trigger Act1 adaptor protein and may activate downstream JAK2-STAT3 signaling to promote the expression of RANKL (40–43). The upregulation of RANKL and the increase the ratio of RANKL/osteoprotegerin (OPG) promotes osteoclastogenesis (44, 45). Moreover, IL-17A stimulates osteoblast precursors to produce cyclooxygenase-2 (COX-2) related-prostaglandin E2 (PGE2), which is a facilitated factor in osteoclasts formation (46). The synergistic effects of IL-17A and TNF-α activate NF-κB-dependent pathways to promote the production of nitric oxide synthase-2 (NOS-2) and nitric oxide (NO). NO triggers the RANKL-RANK pathway to increase osteoclastic bone resorption (47). In addition, IL-17A and TNF-α synergistically induce osteoblast precursors to produce inflammatory factors including IL-1α, IL-1β and IL-6. These cytokines can up-regulate osteoclast activity (48). When activated by IL-17A, osteocytes inhibit the ERK1/2-STAT3 pathway and increase the RANKL/OPG ratio and TNF-α, thereby enhancing osteoclast formation. Furthermore, due to the activation of reversed ephrinA2-EphA2 signaling and suppression of ephrinB2-EphB4 signaling between osteocytes and osteoclast precursors, RANK⁺ bone marrow macrophages (BMMs) are increased, which influences subsequent RANKL-dependent osteoclastogenesis (49). In addition to providing osteoclastic activating factors, IL-17A can promote the expression of inhibitory factors. IL-17A promotes osteoblasts to produce granulocyte-macrophage colony-stimulating factor (GM-CSF), which in turn reduces the expression of RANK in osteoclast precursors and thus may weaken RANKL-RANK signaling to inhibit osteoclastogenesis (50). Moreover, GM-CSF maintains monocytes in an undifferentiated state by downregulating c-Fos, Fra-1, and nuclear factor of activated T cells 1 (Nfatc1) (51) (**Figure 1**).

The *in vitro* effects of IL-17A on osteoclasts are dual. Recent findings indicate that the direct effects of IL-17A on osteoclastogenesis are related to its concentration, but are not dose-dependent. Low concentration of IL-17A promotes osteoclastogenesis, while IL-17A begins to inhibit the formation of osteoclasts as the concentration increases. Strangely, further increases in the concentrations of IL-17A promote osteoclastogenesis. The precise relationship requires further exploration. In addition, IL-17A is involved in osteoclastogenesis *via* other types of cells and factors. The integrated network of cells and the factors they produce makes the specific effects attributable to IL-17A difficult to determine. The dominant effect may vary in different states. Thus, the role of IL-17A needs to be explored in more complex environments *in vivo*.

Osteoblasts

The osteoblast is another important player involved in maintaining bone homeostasis. When IL-17A binds receptors on pre-osteoblasts, it promotes their proliferation in a dose-dependent manner (49, 52, 53). When IL-17A activates TRAF6 and Act1 to initiate Ras-related C3 botulinum toxin substrate 1 guanosine triphosphatase (Rac1 GTPase) and NADPH oxidase 1 (Nox1), the expression of reactive oxygen species (ROS) is upregulated to promote pre-osteoblasts proliferation (39).

Slightly confusingly, the effects of IL-17A on osteoblastic differentiation *in vitro* are fraught with contradictions. A study showed that IL–17A promoted the differentiation of murine pre-osteoblastic MC3T3–E1 through the phosphoinositide 3-kinase-serine/threonine kinases (PI3K-AKT) pathway, whereas another study showed that IL–17A of the same concentration inhibited osteoblastic differentiation of MC3T3-E1 (54, 55). IL-17A can cause an increase in the osteoblastic differentiation of murine calvarial osteoblasts by up-regulating the expression of genes involved in osteoblastic differentiation including Runx2, ALP, osterix, osteocalcin and type I collagen (Colla1), osteoprotegerin (OPG), bone sialoprotein (Ibsp), and osteopontin (Spp1) (43, 44). However, IL-17A inhibits osteogenic differentiation of rat calvarial osteoblast cells by down-regulating expression of genes involved in osteoblastic differentiation including Runx2, ALP, osterix, osteocalcin and type I collagen (56, 57). Different species lead to the expressed differential of IL-17R, which might partly explain this opposite effect (56). When activated by IL-17A, mice bone marrow mesenchymal stem cells (BM-MSCs) secrete IL-6 and IL-1β, thereby activating the AKT, STAT3, and ERK1/2 pathways to promote osteoblastic differentiation (55). However, IL-17A inhibits the Wnt signaling, resulting in reduced levels of osteoblast differentiation markers (osterix and osteocalcin) and early osteocyte markers (Dmp1 and Phex), thereby inhibiting osteoblastic differentiation of BM-MSCs (52). Moreover, IL-17A increases the expression of N-cadherin to inhibit PTHR1-LRP-6 interaction in osteoblasts, which also can inhibit the Wnt-signaling pathway (58) (**Figure 2**).

Studies involving human pre-osteoblasts have indicated that IL-17A could promote bone-derived cells to differentiate into osteoblasts through JAK2/STAT3 signaling (59). In addition, IL-17A promotes the differentiation of hBM-MSCs into osteoblasts and promotes the mineralization of osteoblasts by upregulating bone formation-related gene ALP and Runx2 (39). The synergistic effects of IL-17A and bone morphogenetic protein-2 (BMP-2) promote the osteogenic differentiation of hBM-MSCs (60). Besides, the synergistic effects of IL-17A and TNF-α enhance osteogenic differentiation and mineralization of hBM-MSCs by down-regulating Dickkopf-1 (DKK-1), an inhibitor of the Wnt-signaling pathway (61). Osteoblasts and adipocytes are differentiated from a common pluripotent precursor, the mesenchymal stem cell (MSC). Many studies have suggested the differentiation decision of osteoblasts and adipocytes is delicately balanced and may even have a competitive relationship. IL-17A may steer mesenchymal stem cells into an osteogenic fate. IL-17A activates COX-2-induced prostaglandin E2 to inhibit lipid-related proteins include PPAR-γ, FABP4, and adiponectin. Therefore, the differentiation of hBM-MSCs into adipocytes is reduced (62). However, one study indicated that IL-17A inhibited osteogenic differentiation with up-regulated expression of the Wnt antagonist secreted frizzled-related protein 1 (sFRP1) and down-regulated expression of Wnt3 and Wnt6 in hBM-MSCs (63) (**Figure 2**).

The *in vitro* effects of IL-17A on osteoblasts are difficult to be defined. The effects of IL-17A on osteoblasts may not depend on the concentrations. IL-17A probably exerts distinct roles depending on the *in vitro* model used to assess osteoblast development. In addition, different species may also be partly responsible for the controversial results. It is not excluded that the different experimental methods also influence results. To achieve the precise effects of IL-17A on osteoblasts, the type of *in vitro* model, the correspondence between *in vitro* or *in vivo* effects, and the similarity of the effects between animal models and humans should be considered.

EFFECTS OF IL-17A ON BONE DISEASE

The knockout of IL-17A or its receptors in animal models does not affect bone mass, osteoclast numbers, or osteoblast numbers (34, 40, 64–66). Moreover, neutralizing antibodies directed against IL-17A in wild-type mice also do not influence bone mass (65). These results indicate that IL-17A might not have any effect on bone under normal physiological conditions, and it only plays a role in inflammatory conditions or injury. The involvement of IL-17A in immune-mediated bone disease is worthy of exploration.

Postmenopausal Osteoporosis

Women undergoing natural menopause often experience postmenopausal osteoporosis (PMOP) with a decrease in bone mineral density (BMD) and an increased risk of fractures (67). Estrogen deficiency is the pivotal reason for PMOP. Estrogen deficiency increases osteoclast formation by increasing the number of hematopoietic progenitors and recruiting osteoclast progenitors. Likewise, estrogen deficiency allows prolonged survival of osteoclasts, and the net increase in bone resorption leads to bone loss (68, 69). Recent studies show that osteoimmunology is involved in the pathogenesis of PMOP. Furthermore, T-cell activity is increased while B-cell activity is decreased in postmenopausal women (70, 71). Estrogen deficiency can activate T cells and promotes the production of a variety of immune factors. These factors include IL-6 (72), TNF-α (73), IFN-γ (74), IL-1β, and TNF-β (75), all of which enhance bone loss.

Despite one study showing that the level of serum IL-17A in postmenopausal women with low BMD is not significantly different from that in women with normal BMD (76), other studies have indicated that postmenopausal women with

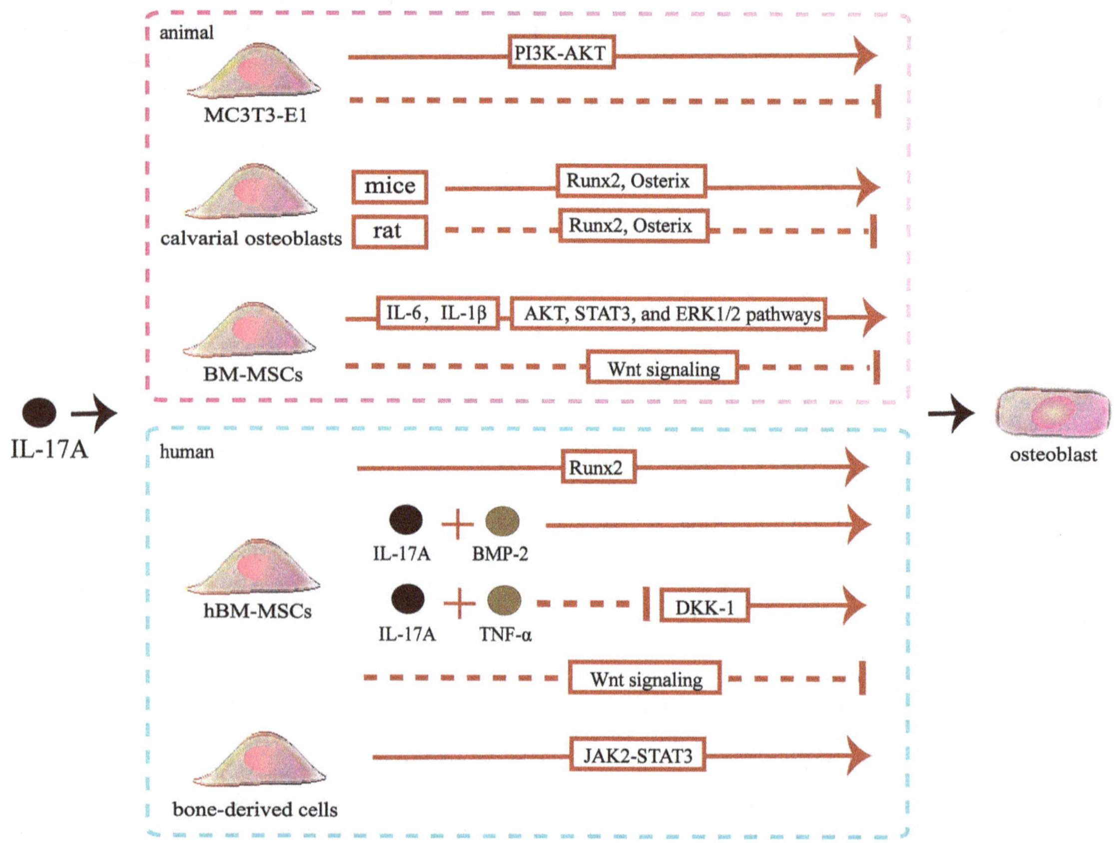

FIGURE 2 | Effects of IL-17A on osteoblasts. ①IL-17A promotes MC3T3-E1 to differentiate into osteoblasts by activating the PI3K-AKT signaling pathways, whereas another study indicated that IL-17A inhibited osteoblastic differentiation of MC3T3-E1. ② IL-17A upregulates Runx2 and osterix expression to promote mice calvarial osteoblast to differentiate into mature osteoblast, whereas downregulates Runx2 and osterix expression to inhibit rat calvarial osteoblast to differentiate into mature osteoblast. ③ IL-17A promotes the secrete of IL-6 and IL-1β to activate the AKT, STAT3, and ERK1/2 pathways and promotes osteoblastic differentiation of bone marrow mesenchymal stem cells (BM-MSCs), whereas IL-17A inhibits osteoblastic differentiation through inhibiting the Wnt signaling pathway.④ IL-17A promotes human BM-MSCs (hBM-MSCs) to differentiate into osteoblasts by upregulating Runx2 expression. IL-17A with bone morphogenetic protein-2 (BMP-2) or with tumor necrosis factor (TNF)-α synergistically enhance osteogenic differentiation. However, IL-17A inhibits osteoblastic differentiation of hBM-MSCs by inhibiting the Wnt signaling pathway. ⑤ IL-17A promotes bone-derived cells to differentiate into osteoblasts by activating the JAK2-STAT3 signaling pathways.

osteoporosis have a higher concentration of serum IL-17A, and have more peripheral blood IL-17-producing CD4$^+$ T-cells (58, 77–80). In postmenopausal women with osteoporosis, the concentration of serum IL-17A is negatively correlated with BMD, but is positively correlated with sRANKL level (78, 79).

In animal studies, ovariectomy (OVX) causes estrogen deficiency and bone loss. The drastic reduction of estrogen increases expression of the differentiation factors of Th17 including STAT3, ROR-α, and ROR-γt, which indicates that more peripheral blood mononuclear cells can differentiate into Th17 and produce IL-17A (80). The level of IL-17A in the bone marrow and blood are increased after OVX (38). IL-17RA knockdown and anti-IL17 antibody injection both protect against bone loss caused by estrogen deficiency (40). Anti-IL-17 antibodies and parathyroid hormone (PTH) can be used in combination to further protect OVX-induced bone loss (58, 81). Anti-IL17 antibodies exert a bone protective effect by inhibiting osteoclast formation, decreasing the apoptosis of osteoblasts and promoting the formation of mineralized nodules. Moreover, the blocking of IL-17A may inhibit osteoblasts to produce osteoclastogenic factors including TNF-α, IL-6, and RANKL in OVX mice (38, 40). Interestingly, anti-IL-17A antibodies have also been reported to reverse the higher frequency of CD4$^+$ T cells and the proliferation of B220$^+$ cells in bone marrow caused by estrogen deficiency. Anti-IL-17A antibodies exert an immuno-protective effect and translate to superior skeletal outcomes (81).

Rheumatoid Arthritis

RA is an autoimmune disease characterized by the upregulation of various immune factors that recruit and activate various immune cells, especially T and B cells to destroy cartilage and bone (82). RA patients have higher levels of IL-17A in synovial tissue and fluid compared with normal subjects (83–85). In a 2-year prospective study, the expression of IL-17A in synovial tissues was associated with increased joint damage progression in RA (86). Except for synovial tissue, RA patients have a higher concentration of serum IL-17A, which is proportional to the severity of RA (87–90). Moreover, the PBMCs of patients with RA produce more IL-17A (91). The increased levels of IL-17A in synovial fluid, serum, PBMCs are associated with the Disease Activity Score of 28 joints (DAS28), and levels of C-reactive protein (CRP), the erythrocyte sedimentation rate (ESR), and rheumatoid factor (RF) expression (92, 93). In addition, evidence suggests that IL-17A is not only related to the progression of the disease but is also associates with the occurrence of the disease. Studies indicate that IL-17A plays an important role in the pre-onset, early, and chronic stages of RA (94, 95).

Collagen-induced arthritis (CIA) is the most common animal model for studies involving RA (96). High levels of IL-17A are detected in $CD4^+$ T cells and γδT cells located in joints of CIA mice (97). Th17 cells are localized adjacent to osteoclasts in the subarticular cartilage and express IL-17A, indicating the involvement of IL-17A in bone destruction of CIA (97). Local injection of IL-17A in the joint increases the morbidity of CIA and joint damage, while local injection of an adenoviral vector expressing murine IL-17A in the joint also accelerates the initiation of CIA and inflammation (98). Treatment with a soluble IL-17R fusion protein or anti-IL-17A antibody prevents bone erosion and the initiation of CIA (99, 100). In the progression of CIA, the local injection of IL-17A in knee-joint promotes arthritis and exacerbates joint damage (101). Anti-IL-17A antibodies ameliorate the severity of arthritis, cartilage damage, and bone loss (97, 102). Combinations that neutralize both TNF-α and IL-17A can also alleviate CIA progression (103). The combination of anti-IL-1β and anti-IL-17A antibodies significantly reduce the severity of arthritis, alleviates bone and cartilage damage, and down-regulates IL-1β, IL-6, IL-17A, IFN-γ, RANKL, and MMP-3 (104, 105). IL-17A plays an important role not only in the pathogenesis but also in the progression of the disease. Moreover, IL-17A is involved in the pathological process of bone erosion and bone loss.

The pathological mechanism of IL-17A may involve the immune activation and an immune cascade reaction in RA. In addition, the activation of osteoclasts promotes bone erosion in RA. Collagen-specific T cells and collagen-specific IgG2a are involved in the development of CIA. IL-17A is responsible for the priming of collagen-specific T cells and collagen-specific IgG2a production (106). Anti-IL-17A significantly reduces splenocytes proliferation and reduces leukocyte recruitment in CIA (105, 107). Anti-IL-17A also down-regulates IL-1β, IL-1, IL-6, IL-17A, and IFN-γ in the joint (104, 105). Increased osteoclast activity in the subchondral, trabecular, and cortical bone erosion areas is observed after local IL-17A overexpression in joint (98, 101, 102).

Several drugs targeting IL-17A are currently being evaluated in clinical trials, but the benefit seems to be not satisfactory for RA. Brodalumab, a human anti-IL-17 receptor A (IL-17RA) monoclonal antibody, did not demonstrate clinical efficacy in active RA patients (108). The humanized anti-IL-17A monoclonal antibody ixekizumab improved the signs and symptoms of RA patients in a phase II study, but the efficacy was not considered robust sufficient to support continued development (109). Bimekizumab is a monoclonal antibody that selectively neutralizes IL-17A and IL-17F. Bimekizumab plus certolizumab pegol further reduced disease activity score 28-joint count C-reactive protein (DAS28(CRP)) for RA patient in a phase II study, but more messages about the efficacy and safety is lack (110). Secukinumab, a fully human monoclonal antibody directed against IL-17A, has advanced in phase III studies. Secukinumab achieved 20% improvement in the American College of Rheumatology criteria (ACR20) at week 24 among patients with active RA, although, studies have suggested that secukinumab may not provide additional benefit beyond the currently approved therapies to such patients and further development was not pursued due to lack well-pleasing efficacy (111–114).

Psoriatic Arthritis

PsA is an immune-mediated chronic inflammatory arthritis associated with psoriasis. PsA presents synovial inflammation, bone destruction, and juxta-articular new bone formation (115, 116). Aberrant cytokine expression of TNF-α, IL-23, IL-22, IL-9, IL-15 is involved in the pathological mechanisms of PsA (117). Serum IL-17A levels are higher in psoriasis patients (118). $IL-17^+$ $CD4^+$ T cells and IL-17A secretion increase in peripheral blood and synovial fluid of PsA (119, 120). Besides $CD4^+$ T cells, IL-17A-producing ILCs are present in the synovial fluid of PsA (121). $IL-17A^+CD8^+$ T cells are enriched in the joints of patients with PsA and have been correlated with disease activity and bone erosion (7).

In the animal model of PsA, increased serum IL-17A is associated with bone loss. The imbalance between osteoblasts and osteoclasts is the main cause for the appearance of PsA in the bone. Skin-resident cells such as keratinocytes, γδT cells, and innate lymphoid cells express IL-17A, which inhibits osteoblasts and osteocytes function through the Wnt signaling (52). In addition, IL-17A may also promote epidermal sheet, keratinocytes and skin resident T cells to produce RANKL (122).

Clinical trials of antagonizing IL-17A in PsA are underway. Secukinumab improves the signs and symptoms of active PsA (123). At the same time, secukinumab inhibits the progression of bone erosions and maintains bone stability (124–127). In 2016, secukinumab became the first targeting IL-17A drug approved by the FDA for the treatment of active PsA. Ixekizumab, an IL-17A specific monoclonal antibody, improved the signs and symptoms of patients with active PsA and inhibited bone damage progression in PsA (128, 129). In 2017, ixekizumab was approved by the FDA for the treatment of PsA. Brodalumab, a fully human monoclonal antibody targeting the IL-17 RA, achieved ACR20 at week 16 among patients with PsA in a phase III study (130). However, the trials were terminated early due to a possible safety concern about suicidal ideation and behavior (131). Bimekizumab, which inhibits both IL-17A and IL-17F, improved ACR50 in patients with active PsA in a phase II trial and phase III trials that are currently underway (132).

Axial Spondyloarthritis

Axial spondyloarthritis (axSpA) is chronic inflammatory bone diseases including non-radiographic axial spondyloarthritis (nr-axSpA) and radiographic axial spondyloarthritis (ankylosing spondylitis [AS]). Bone destruction and new bone formation may occur simultaneously in axSpA. Various types of cytokines including IL-17A, TNF-α and IL-23 are involved in the pathological processes (133, 134). Many studies have indicated that IL-17 is involved in immunopathogenesis of axSpA (135). IL-17$^+$ CD4$^+$ T cells increase in peripheral blood of axSpA and IL-17A synthesis also increases (120, 136–138). Levels of IL-17A in the synovial fluid are elevated in patients with AS (59). Serum IL-17A levels are also higher in AS and elevated IL-17 serum levels may associate with the development of AS (139, 140). A few studies have focused on the role of IL-17 in the processes of axSpA bone damage. IL-17A promotes local mesenchymal stem cell populations to osteoblast differentiation and increases mineralization in AS by JAK2/STAT3 signaling, which may be a mechanism of ankyloses progression (59). Anti-IL-17A treatment prevented bone loss and induced new bone formation in an animal model of pathogenic SpA, mycobacterium tuberculosis-induced disease in B27/hβ2m-transgenic rats (141).

Several IL-17A targeted drugs are currently in clinical trials. Secukinumab and Ixekizumab are both anti-interleukin-17A monoclonal antibodies and have been reported to improve the signs and symptoms of axSpA (142–148). To date, the FDA has approved both antibodies for the treatment of adults with active AS and nr-axSpA with objective signs of inflammation. Netakimab, a humanized monoclonal antibody targeting IL-17A, significantly achieved 20% improvement in Assessment of Spondyloarthritis International Society (ASAS20) response among patients with AS in a phase II study (149). Bimekizumab, a monoclonal antibody that selectively neutralizes IL-17A and IL-17F, achieved ASAS40 response at week 12 in a phase II trial (150). Phase III trials that aim to assess the efficacy and safety of netakimab and bimekizumab in AS patients are currently underway.

CONCLUSION AND PERSPECTIVES

IL-17A is involved in innate immune responses and adaptive immunity. Meanwhile, IL-17A plays an important role in bone homeostasis *via* activation of complex cellular and molecular interactions. IL-17A may exert direct positive or negative effects on osteoclastogenesis depending on its concentration *in vitro*. Osteoblasts are most closely associated with osteoclasts, which both are involved in bone metabolism. IL-17A indirectly regulates osteoclastogenesis by inducing multiple factors derived from the osteoclast-supporting cells. The effects of IL-17A on osteoblasts may depend on the different experimental models of osteoblast development and species tested *in vitro*. These aforementioned cell studies provide evidence supporting the skeletal-regulatory properties of IL-17A and support the concept that IL-17A acts as the link between the skeletal and the immune systems. Future research should focus on the molecular pathways involved and explore the precise reasons for the dual effects of IL-17A in bone cells.

Mechanistic studies have hinted that IL-17A is a bone-destroying cytokine involved in immune-mediated bone diseases, such as PMOP, RA, PsA, and axSpA. IL-17A exerts a negative effect on bone by promoting osteoclastogenesis, excessively activates bone formation, and initiates an immunologic cascade. Indeed anti-IL-17A therapy has produced promising results in clinical trials of RA, PsA, and axSpA, although, few studies have focused on bone damage. A deeper understanding of the molecular mechanisms of IL-17A involved in bone disease may supply novel therapeutic interventions and provide a new thought to prevent bone loss and osteoporosis associated with immune-mediated bone diseases.

AUTHOR CONTRIBUTIONS

XY provided the conception of the manuscript. MT and LL were contributed to perform the literature search and drafted the work. All authors contributed to the article and approved the submitted version.

FUNDING

This work was supported by grants from the National Natural Science Foundation of China [No. 81770875]; the Sichuan University [No. 2018SCUH0093]; the Post-Doctor Research Project, West China Hospital, Sichuan University [No.19HXBH053]; the Health and Family Planning Commission of Sichuan Province [No. 19PJ096]; and the 1.3.5 project for discipline of excellence, West China Hospital, Sichuan University [No. 2020HXFH008, No. ZYJC18003]; the National Clinical Research Center for Geriatrics of West China Hospital (No. Z2018B05).

REFERENCES

1. Liu S. Structural Insights into the Interleukin-17 Family Cytokines and Their Receptors. *Adv Exp Med Biol* (2019) 1172:97–117. doi: 10.1007/978-981-13-9367-9_5
2. Aggarwal S, Gurney AL. IL-17: prototype member of an emerging cytokine family. *J leukocyte Biol* (2002) 71(1):1–8. doi: 10.1189/jlb.71.1.1
3. Rouvier E, Luciani MF, Mattéi MG, Denizot F, Golstein P. CTLA-8, cloned from an activated T cell, bearing AU-rich messenger RNA instability sequences, and homologous to a herpesvirus saimiri gene. *J Immunol* (1993) 150(12):5445–56.
4. Yao Z, Painter SL, Fanslow WC, Ulrich D, Macduff BM, Spriggs MK, et al. Human IL-17: a novel cytokine derived from T cells. *J Immunol* (1995) 155 (12):5483–6.
5. Fossiez F, Djossou O, Chomarat P, Flores-Romo L, Ait-Yahia S, Maat C, et al. T cell interleukin-17 induces stromal cells to produce proinflammatory and hematopoietic cytokines. *J Exp Med* (1996) 183(6):2593–603. doi: 10.1084/jem.183.6.2593
6. Miossec P. IL-17 and Th17 cells in human inflammatory diseases. *Microbes Infect* (2009) 11(5):625–30. doi: 10.1016/j.micinf.2009.04.003
7. Menon B, Gullick NJ, Walter GJ, Rajasekhar M, Garrood T, Evans HG, et al. Interleukin-17+CD8+ T Cells Are Enriched in the Joints of Patients With Psoriatic Arthritis and Correlate With Disease Activity and Joint Damage Progression. *Arthritis Rheumatol* (2014) 66(5):1272–81. doi: 10.1002/art.38376
8. Venken K, Jacques P, Mortier C, Labadia ME, Decruy T, Coudenys J, et al. RORgammat inhibition selectively targets IL-17 producing iNKT and gammadelta-T cells enriched in Spondyloarthritis patients. *Nat Commun* (2019) 10(1):9. doi: 10.1038/s41467-018-07911-6

9. Zhu L, Song H, Zhang L, Meng H. Characterization of IL-17-producing Treg cells in type 2 diabetes patients. *Immunologic Res* (2019) 67(4-5):443–9. doi: 10.1007/s12026-019-09095-7
10. Coffelt SB, Kersten K, Doornebal CW, Weiden J, Vrijland K, Hau C-S, et al. IL-17-producing γδ T cells and neutrophils conspire to promote breast cancer metastasis. *Nature* (2015) 522(7556):345–8. doi: 10.1038/nature14282
11. Crellin NK, Trifari S, Kaplan CD, Cupedo T, Spits H. Human NKp44+IL-22+ cells and LTi-like cells constitute a stable RORC+ lineage distinct from conventional natural killer cells. *J Exp Med* (2010) 207(2):281–90. doi: 10.1084/jem.20091509
12. Triggianese P, Conigliaro P, Chimenti MS, Biancone L, Monteleone G, Perricone R, et al. Evidence of IL-17 producing innate lymphoid cells in peripheral blood from patients with enteropathic spondyloarthritis. *Clin Exp Rheumatol* (2016) 34(6):1085–93.
13. Okamoto N, Homma M, Kawaguchi Y, Kabasawa N, Uto Y, Hattori N, et al. Increased expression of interleukin-17 is associated with macrophages in chronic immune thrombocytopenia. *Int J Clin Exp Pathol* (2018) 11(5):2419–29.
14. Li L, Huang L, Vergis AL, Ye H, Bajwa A, Narayan V, et al. IL-17 produced by neutrophils regulates IFN-gamma-mediated neutrophil migration in mouse kidney ischemia-reperfusion injury. *J Clin Invest* (2010) 120 (1):331–42. doi: 10.1172/JCI38702
15. Hueber AJ, Asquith DL, Miller AM, Reilly J, Kerr S, Leipe J, et al. Mast cells express IL-17A in rheumatoid arthritis synovium. *J Immunol (Baltimore Md 1950)* (2010) 184(7):3336–40. doi: 10.4049/jimmunol.0903566
16. Takahashi N, Vanlaere I, de Rycke R, Cauwels A, Joosten LAB, Lubberts E, et al. IL-17 produced by Paneth cells drives TNF-induced shock. *J Exp Med* (2008) 205(8):1755–61. doi: 10.1084/jem.20080588
17. Sheibanie AF, Khayrullina T, Safadi FF, Ganea D. Prostaglandin E2 exacerbates collagen-induced arthritis in mice through the inflammatory interleukin-23/interleukin-17 axis. *Arthritis Rheum* (2007) 56(8):2608–19. doi: 10.1002/art.22794
18. Golebski K, Ros XR, Nagasawa M, van Tol S, Heesters BA, Aglmous H, et al. IL-1β, IL-23, and TGF-β drive plasticity of human ILC2s towards IL-17-producing ILCs in nasal inflammation. *Nat Commun* (2019) 10(1):2162. doi: 10.1038/s41467-019-09883-7
19. Chalise J, Narendra S, Paudyal B, Magnusson M. Interferon alpha inhibits antigen-specific production of proinflammatory cytokines and enhances antigen-specific transforming growth factor beta production in antigen-induced arthritis. *Arthritis Res Ther* (2013) 15(5):R143. doi: 10.1186/ar4326
20. Nesmond S, Muller C, Le Naour R, Viguier M, Bernard P, Antonicelli F, et al. Characteristic Pattern of IL-17RA, IL-17RB, and IL-17RC in Monocytes/ Macrophages and Mast Cells From Patients With Bullous Pemphigoid. *Front Immunol* (2019) 10:2107:2107. doi: 10.3389/fimmu.2019.02107
21. Zrioual S, Toh ML, Tournadre A, Zhou Y, Cazalis MA, Pachot A, et al. IL-17RA and IL-17RC receptors are essential for IL-17A-induced ELR+ CXC chemokine expression in synoviocytes and are overexpressed in rheumatoid blood. *J Immunol (Baltimore Md 1950)* (2008) 180(1):655–63. doi: 10.4049/ jimmunol.180.1.655
22. Shen F, Gaffen SL. Structure-function relationships in the IL-17 receptor: implications for signal transduction and therapy. *Cytokine* (2008) 41(2):92–104. doi: 10.1016/j.cyto.2007.11.013
23. Krstic J, Obradovic H, Kukolj T, Mojsilovic S, Okic-Dordevic I, Bugarski D, et al. An Overview of Interleukin-17A and Interleukin-17 Receptor A Structure, Interaction and Signaling. *Protein Pept Lett* (2015) 22(7):570–8. doi: 10.2174/0929866522666150520145554
24. Liu S, Song X, Chrunyk BA, Shanker S, Hoth LR, Marr ES, et al. Crystal structures of interleukin 17A and its complex with IL-17 receptor A. *Nat Commun* (2013) 4:1888. doi: 10.1038/ncomms2880
25. Gaffen SL. Structure and signalling in the IL-17 receptor family. *Nat Rev Immunol* (2009) 9(8):556–67. doi: 10.1038/nri2586
26. Gaffen S. IL-17 receptor composition. *Nat Rev Immunol* (2016) 16(1):4. doi: 10.1038/nri.2015.2
27. Li X, Bechara R, Zhao J, McGeachy MJ, Gaffen SL. IL-17 receptor-based signaling and implications for disease. *Nat Immunol* (2019) 20(12):1594–602. doi: 10.1038/s41590-019-0514-y
28. Cypowyj S, Picard C, Maródi L, Casanova JL, Puel A. Immunity to infection in IL-17-deficient mice and humans. *Eur J Immunol* (2012) 42(9):2246–54. doi: 10.1002/eji.201242605
29. Zenobia C, Hajishengallis G. Basic biology and role of interleukin-17 in immunity and inflammation. *Periodontol 2000* (2015) 69(1):142–59. doi: 10.1111/prd.12083
30. Fabre JAS, Giustinniani J, Garbar C, Merrouche Y, Antonicelli F, Bensussan A. The Interleukin-17 Family of Cytokines in Breast Cancer. *Int J Mol Sci* (2018) 19(12):3880. doi: 10.3390/ijms19123880
31. Wu F, Xu J, Huang Q, Han J, Duan L, Fan J, et al. The Role of Interleukin-17 in Lung Cancer. *Mediators Inflammation* (2016) 2016:8494079. doi: 10.1155/2016/8494079
32. Robert M, Miossec P. Effects of Interleukin 17 on the cardiovascular system. *Autoimmun Rev* (2017) 16(9):984–91. doi: 10.1016/j.autrev.2017.07.009
33. Guedes MC, Borrego LM, Proença RD. Roles of interleukin-17 in uveitis. *Indian J Ophthalmol* (2016) 64(9):628–34. doi: 10.4103/0301-4738.194339
34. Adamopoulos IE, Chao CC, Geissler R, Laface D, Blumenschein W, Iwakura Y, et al. Interleukin-17A upregulates receptor activator of NF-kappaB on osteoclast precursors. *Arthritis Res Ther* (2010) 12(1):R29. doi: 10.1186/ar2936
35. Ke D, Fu X, Xue Y, Wu H, Zhang Y, Chen X, et al. IL-17A regulates the autophagic activity of osteoclast precursors through RANKL-JNK1 signaling during osteoclastogenesis in vitro. *Biochem Biophys Res Commun* (2018) 497 (3):890–6. doi: 10.1016/j.bbrc.2018.02.164
36. Xue Y, Liang Z, Fu X, Wang T, Xie Q, Ke D. IL-17A modulates osteoclast precursors' apoptosis through autophagy-TRAF3 signaling during osteoclastogenesis. *Biochem Biophys Res Commun* (2019) 508(4):1088–92. doi: 10.1016/j.bbrc.2018.12.029
37. Kitami S, Tanaka H, Kawato T, Tanabe N, Katono-Tani T, Zhang F, et al. IL-17A suppresses the expression of bone resorption-related proteinases and osteoclast differentiation via IL-17RA or IL-17RC receptors in RAW264.7 cells. *Biochimie* (2010) 92(4):398–404. doi: 10.1016/j.biochi.2009.12.011
38. Tyagi AM, Srivastava K, Mansoori MN, Trivedi R, Chattopadhyay N, Singh D. Estrogen deficiency induces the differentiation of IL-17 secreting Th17 cells: a new candidate in the pathogenesis of osteoporosis. *PloS One* (2012) 7 (9):e44552. doi: 10.1371/journal.pone.0044552
39. Huang H, Kim HJ, Chang EJ, Lee ZH, Hwang SJ, Kim HM, et al. IL-17 stimulates the proliferation and differentiation of human mesenchymal stem cells: implications for bone remodeling. *Cell Death Differ* (2009) 16 (10):1332–43. doi: 10.1038/cdd.2009.74
40. DeSelm CJ, Takahata Y, Warren J, Chappel JC, Khan T, Li X, et al. IL-17 mediates estrogen-deficient osteoporosis in an Act1-dependent manner. *J Cell Biochem* (2012) 113(9):2895–902. doi: 10.1002/jcb.24165
41. Zhang F, Wang CL, Koyama Y, Mitsui N, Shionome C, Sanuki R, et al. Compressive force stimulates the gene expression of IL-17s and their receptors in MC3T3-E1 cells. *Connective Tissue Res* (2010) 51(5):359–69. doi: 10.3109/03008200903456942
42. Funaki Y, Hasegawa Y, Okazaki R, Yamasaki A, Sueda Y, Yamamoto A, et al. Resolvin E1 Inhibits Osteoclastogenesis and Bone Resorption by Suppressing IL-17-induced RANKL Expression in Osteoblasts and RANKL-induced Osteoclast Differentiation. *Yonago Acta Med* (2018) 61 (1):8–18. doi: 10.33160/yam.2018.03.002
43. Wang Z, Tan J, Lei L, Sun W, Wu Y, Ding P, et al. The positive effects of secreting cytokines IL-17 and IFN-γ on the early-stage differentiation and negative effects on the calcification of primary osteoblasts in vitro. *Int Immunopharmacol* (2018) 57:1–10. doi: 10.1016/j.intimp.2018.02.002
44. Kim HJ, Seo SJ, Kim J-Y, Kim Y-G, Lee Y. IL-17 promotes osteoblast differentiation, bone regeneration, and remodeling in mice. *Biochem Biophys Res Commun* (2020) 55(4):1044–50. doi: 10.1016/j.bbrc.2020.02.054
45. Li JY, Yu M, Tyagi AM, Vaccaro C, Hsu E, Adams J, et al. IL-17 Receptor Signaling in Osteoblasts/Osteocytes Mediates PTH-Induced Bone Loss and Enhances Osteocytic RANKL Production. *J Bone mineral Res Off J Am Soc Bone Mineral Res* (2019) 34(2):349–60. doi: 10.1002/jbmr.3600
46. Zhang F, Tanaka H, Kawato T, Kitami S, Nakai K, Motohashi M, et al. Interleukin-17A induces cathepsin K and MMP-9 expression in osteoclasts via celecoxib-blocked prostaglandin E2 in osteoblasts. *Biochimie* (2011) 93 (2):296–305. doi: 10.1016/j.biochi.2010.10.001
47. Van Bezooijen RL, Papapoulos SE, Lowik CW. Effect of interleukin-17 on nitric oxide production and osteoclastic bone resorption: is there dependency on nuclear factor-kappaB and receptor activator of nuclear factor kappaB (RANK)/RANK ligand signaling? *Bone* (2001) 28(4):378–86. doi: 10.1016/s8756-3282(00)00457-9

48. Van bezooijen RL, Farih-Sips HC, Papapoulos SE, Lowik CW. Interleukin-17: A new bone acting cytokine in vitro. *J Bone mineral Res Off J Am Soc Bone Mineral Res* (1999) 14(9):1513–21. doi: 10.1359/jbmr.1999.14.9.1513
49. Liao C, Cheng T, Wang S, Zhang C, Jin L, Yang Y. Shear stress inhibits IL-17A-mediated induction of osteoclastogenesis via osteocyte pathways. *Bone* (2017) 101:10–20. doi: 10.1016/j.bone.2017.04.003
50. Balani D, Aeberli D, Hofstetter W, Seitz M. Interleukin-17A stimulates granulocyte-macrophage colony-stimulating factor release by murine osteoblasts in the presence of 1,25-dihydroxyvitamin D(3) and inhibits murine osteoclast development in vitro. *Arthritis Rheum* (2013) 65 (2):436–46. doi: 10.1002/art.37762
51. Atanga E, Dolder S, Dauwalder T, Wetterwald A, Hofstetter W. TNFalpha inhibits the development of osteoclasts through osteoblast-derived GM-CSF. *Bone* (2011) 49(5):1090–100. doi: 10.1016/j.bone.2011.08.003
52. Uluçkan Ö, Jimenez M, Karbach S, Jeschke A, Graña O, Keller J, et al. Chronic skin inflammation leads to bone loss by IL-17-mediated inhibition of Wnt signaling in osteoblasts. *Sci Transl Med* (2016) 8(330):330ra37. doi: 10.1126/scitranslmed.aad8996
53. Huang W, La Russa V, Alzoubi A, Schwarzenberger P. Interleukin-17A: a T-cell-derived growth factor for murine and human mesenchymal stem cells. *Stem Cells (Dayton Ohio)* (2006) 24(6):1512–8. doi: 10.1634/stemcells.2005-0156
54. Tan J-Y, Lei L-H, Chen X-T, Ding P-H, Wu Y-M, Chen L-L. AKT2 is involved in the IL–17A–mediated promotion of differentiation and calcification of murine preosteoblastic MC3T3–E1 cells. *Mol Med Rep* (2017) 16(5):5833–40. doi: 10.3892/mmr.2017.7315
55. Liao C, Zhang C, Jin L, Yang Y. IL-17 alters the mesenchymal stem cell niche towards osteogenesis in cooperation with osteocytes. *J Cell Physiol* (2020) 235(5):4466–80. doi: 10.1002/jcp.29323
56. Kim YG, Park JW, Lee JM, Suh JY, Lee JK, Chang BS, et al. IL-17 inhibits osteoblast differentiation and bone regeneration in rat. *Arch Oral Biol* (2014) 59(9):897–905. doi: 10.1016/j.archoralbio.2014.05.009
57. Zhang J-R, Pang D-D, Tong Q, Liu X, Su D-F, Dai S-M. Different Modulatory Effects of IL-17, IL-22, and IL-23 on Osteoblast Differentiation. *Mediators Inflammation* (2017) 2017:5950395–. doi: 10.1155/2017/5950395
58. Mansoori MN, Shukla P, Singh D. Combination of PTH (1-34) with anti-IL17 prevents bone loss by inhibiting IL-17/N-cadherin mediated disruption of PTHR1/LRP-6 interaction. *Bone* (2017) 105:226–36. doi: 10.1016/j.bone.2017.09.010
59. Jo S, Wang SE, Lee YL, Kang S, Lee B, Han J, et al. IL-17A induces osteoblast differentiation by activating JAK2/STAT3 in ankylosing spondylitis. *Arthritis Res Ther* (2018) 20(1):115–. doi: 10.1186/s13075-018-1582-3
60. Croes M, Öner FC, van Neerven D, Sabir E, Kruyt MC, Blokhuis TJ, et al. Proinflammatory T cells and IL-17 stimulate osteoblast differentiation. *Bone* (2016) 84:262–70. doi: 10.1016/j.bone.2016.01.010
61. Osta B, Lavocat F, Eljaafari A, Miossec P. Effects of Interleukin-17A on Osteogenic Differentiation of Isolated Human Mesenchymal Stem Cells. *Front Immunol* (2014) 425. doi: 10.3389/fimmu.2014.00425
62. Shin JH, Shin DW, Noh M. Interleukin-17A inhibits adipocyte differentiation in human mesenchymal stem cells and regulates pro-inflammatory responses in adipocytes. *Biochem Pharmacol* (2009) 77 (12):1835–44. doi: 10.1016/j.bcp.2009.03.008
63. Wang Z, Jia Y, Du F, Chen M, Dong X, Chen Y, et al. IL-17A Inhibits Osteogenic Differentiation of Bone Mesenchymal Stem Cells via Wnt Signaling Pathway. *Med Sci Monit Int Med J Exp Clin Res* (2017) 23:4095–101. doi: 10.12659/msm.903027
64. Goswami J, Hernandez-Santos N, Zuniga LA, Gaffen SL. A bone-protective role for IL-17 receptor signaling in ovariectomy-induced bone loss. *Eur J Immunol* (2009) 39(10):2831–9. doi: 10.1002/eji.200939670
65. Li JY, D'Amelio P, Robinson J, Walker LD, Vaccaro C, Luo T, et al. IL-17A Is Increased in Humans with Primary Hyperparathyroidism and Mediates PTH-Induced Bone Loss in Mice. *Cell Metab* (2015) 22(5):799–810. doi: 10.1016/j.cmet.2015.09.012
66. Sato K, Suematsu A, Okamoto K, Yamaguchi A, Morishita Y, Kadono Y, et al. Th17 functions as an osteoclastogenic helper T cell subset that links T cell activation and bone destruction. *J Exp Med* (2006) 203(12):2673–82. doi: 10.1084/jem.20061775
67. Compston JE, McClung MR, Leslie WD. Osteoporosis. *Lancet* (2019) 393 (10169):364–76. doi: 10.1016/S0140-6736(18)32112-3
68. Black DM, Rosen CJ. Clinical Practice. Postmenopausal Osteoporosis. *New Engl J Med* (2016) 374(3):254–62. doi: 10.1056/NEJMcp1513724
69. Zhao R. Immune regulation of osteoclast function in postmenopausal osteoporosis: a critical interdisciplinary perspective. *Int J Med Sci* (2012) 9 (9):825–32. doi: 10.7150/ijms.5180
70. Faienza MF, Ventura A, Marzano F, Cavallo L. Postmenopausal osteoporosis: the role of immune system cells. *Clin Dev Immunol* (2013) 2013:575936. doi: 10.1155/2013/575936
71. D'Amelio P, Grimaldi A, Di Bella S, Brianza SZM, Cristofaro MA, Tamone C, et al. Estrogen deficiency increases osteoclastogenesis up-regulating T cells activity: a key mechanism in osteoporosis. *Bone* (2008) 43(1):92–100. doi: 10.1016/j.bone.2008.02.017
72. Zhong Z, Qian Z, Zhang X, Chen F, Ni S, Kang Z, et al. Tetrandrine Prevents Bone Loss in Ovariectomized Mice by Inhibiting RANKL-Induced Osteoclastogenesis. *Front Pharmacol* (2020) 10:1530. doi: 10.3389/fphar.2019.01530
73. Kim B-J, Bae SJ, Lee S-Y, Lee Y-S, Baek J-E, Park S-Y, et al. TNF-α mediates the stimulation of sclerostin expression in an estrogen-deficient condition. *Biochem Biophys Res Commun* (2012) 424(1):170–5. doi: 10.1016/j.bbrc.2012.06.100
74. Xiong Q, Zhang L, Ge W, Tang P. The roles of interferons in osteoclasts and osteoclastogenesis. *Joint bone Spine Rev du rhumatisme* (2016) 83(3):276–81. doi: 10.1016/j.jbspin.2015.07.010
75. Gao Y, Qian WP, Dark K, Toraldo G, Lin AS, Guldberg RE, et al. Estrogen prevents bone loss through transforming growth factor beta signaling in T cells. *Proc Natl Acad Sci USA* (2004) 101(47):16618–23. doi: 10.1073/pnas.0404888101
76. Mannucci C, Calapai G, Gangemi S. Commentary: Circulatory pattern of cytokines, adipokines and bone markers in postmenopausal women with low BMD. *Front Immunol* (2019) 10:2666. doi: 10.3389/fimmu.2019.02666
77. Zhao R, Wang X, Feng F. Upregulated Cellular Expression of IL-17 by CD4+ T-Cells in Osteoporotic Postmenopausal Women. *Ann Nutr Metab* (2016) 68(2):113–8. doi: 10.1159/000443531
78. Zhang J, Fu Q, Ren Z, Wang Y, Wang C, Shen T, et al. Changes of serum cytokines-related Th1/Th2/Th17 concentration in patients with postmenopausal osteoporosis. *Gynecol Endocrinol Off J Int Soc Gynecol Endocrinol* (2015) 31(3):183–90. doi: 10.3109/09513590.2014.975683
79. Molnár I, Bohaty I, Somogyiné-Vári É. IL-17A-mediated sRANK ligand elevation involved in postmenopausal osteoporosis. *Osteoporosis Int* (2014) 25(2):783–6. doi: 10.1007/s00198-013-2548-6
80. Shukla P, Mansoori MN, Singh D. Efficacy of anti-IL-23 monotherapy versus combination therapy with anti-IL-17 in estrogen deficiency induced bone loss conditions. *Bone* (2018) 110:84–95. doi: 10.1016/j.bone.2018.01.027
81. Tyagi AM, Mansoori MN, Srivastava K, Khan MP, Kureel J, Dixit M, et al. Enhanced immunoprotective effects by anti-IL-17 antibody translates to improved skeletal parameters under estrogen deficiency compared with anti-RANKL and anti-TNF-alpha antibodies. *J Bone mineral Res Off J Am Soc Bone Mineral Res* (2014) 29(9):1981–92. doi: 10.1002/jbmr.2228
82. Smolen JS, Aletaha D, McInnes IB. Rheumatoid arthritis. *Lancet (London England)* (2016) 388(10055):2023–38. doi: 10.1016/s0140-6736(16)30173-8
83. Chabaud M, Durand JM, Buchs N, Fossiez F, Page G, Frappart L, et al. Human interleukin-17: A T cell-derived proinflammatory cytokine produced by the rheumatoid synovium. *Arthritis Rheum* (1999) 42 (5):963–70. doi: 10.1002/1529-0131(199905)42:5<963::aid-anr15>3.0.co;2-e
84. Li N, Wang JC, Liang TH, Zhu MH, Wang JY, Fu XL, et al. Pathologic finding of increased expression of interleukin-17 in the synovial tissue of rheumatoid arthritis patients. *Int J Clin Exp Pathol* (2013) 6(7):1375–9.
85. Ziolkowska M, Koc A, Luszczykiewicz G, Ksiezopolska-Pietrzak K, Klimczak E, Chwalinska-Sadowska H, et al. High levels of IL-17 in rheumatoid arthritis patients: IL-15 triggers in vitro IL-17 production via cyclosporin A-sensitive mechanism. *J Immunol (Baltimore Md 1950)* (2000) 164 (5):2832–8. doi: 10.4049/jimmunol.164.5.2832
86. Kirkham BW, Lassere MN, Edmonds JP, Juhasz KM, Bird PA, Lee CS, et al. Synovial membrane cytokine expression is predictive of joint damage progression in rheumatoid arthritis: a two-year prospective study (the DAMAGE study cohort). *Arthritis Rheum* (2006) 54(4):1122–31. doi: 10.1002/art.21749
87. Siloşi I, Boldeanu MV, Cojocaru M, Biciuşcă V, Pădureanu V, Bogdan M, et al. The Relationship of Cytokines IL-13 and IL-17 with Autoantibodies Profile in Early Rheumatoid Arthritis. *J Immunol Res* (2016) 2016:3109135. doi: 10.1155/2016/3109135

88. Costa CM, Santos M, Pernambuco AP. Elevated levels of inflammatory markers in women with rheumatoid arthritis. *J Immunoassay Immunochem* (2019) 40(5):540–54. doi: 10.1080/15321819.2019.1649695
89. Schofield C, Fischer SK, Townsend MJ, Mosesova S, Peng K, Setiadi AF, et al. Characterization of IL-17AA and IL-17FF in rheumatoid arthritis and multiple sclerosis. *Bioanalysis* (2016) 8(22):2317–27. doi: 10.4155/bio-2016-0207
90. Lee YH, Bae SC. Associations between circulating IL-17 levels and rheumatoid arthritis and between IL-17 gene polymorphisms and disease susceptibility: a meta-analysis. *Postgraduate Med J* (1102) 2017) 93:465–71. doi: 10.1136/postgradmedj-2016-134637
91. Kim KW, Cho ML, Park MK, Yoon CH, Park SH, Lee SH, et al. Increased interleukin-17 production via a phosphoinositide 3-kinase/Akt and nuclear factor kappaB-dependent pathway in patients with rheumatoid arthritis. *Arthritis Res Ther* (2005) 7(1):R139–48. doi: 10.1186/ar1470
92. Roşu A, Mărgăritescu C, Stepan A, Muşetescu A, Ene M. IL-17 patterns in synovium, serum and synovial fluid from treatment-naïve, early rheumatoid arthritis patients. *Romanian J Morphol Embryol = Rev roumaine morphologie embryologie* (2012) 53(1):73–80.
93. El-Maghraby HM, Rabie RA, Makram WK. Correlation between Relative Expression of IL 17 and PERP in Rheumatoid Arthritis Patients and Disease Activity. *Egyptian J Immunol* (2019) 26(2):19–29.
94. Kokkonen H, Söderström I, Rocklöv J, Hallmans G, Lejon K, Rantapää Dahlqvist S. Up-regulation of cytokines and chemokines predates the onset of rheumatoid arthritis. *Arthritis Rheum* (2010) 62(2):383–91. doi: 10.1002/art.27186
95. Raza K, Falciani F, Curnow SJ, Ross EJ, Lee CY, Akbar AN, et al. Early rheumatoid arthritis is characterized by a distinct and transient synovial fluid cytokine profile of T cell and stromal cell origin. *Arthritis Res Ther* (2005) 7(4):R784–95. doi: 10.1186/ar1733
96. Wu S, Meng Z, Zhang Y. Correlation between rheumatoid arthritis and immunological changes in a rheumatoid arthritis rat model. *J Biol Regul Homeostatic Agents* (2018) 32(6):1461–6.
97. Pollinger B, Junt T, Metzler B, Walker UA, Tyndall A, Allard C, et al. Th17 cells, not IL-17+ gammadelta T cells, drive arthritic bone destruction in mice and humans. *J Immunol (Baltimore Md 1950)* (2011) 186(4):2602–12. doi: 10.4049/jimmunol.1003370
98. Lubberts E, Joosten LA, van de Loo FA, Schwarzenberger P, Kolls J, van den Berg WB. Overexpression of IL-17 in the knee joint of collagen type II immunized mice promotes collagen arthritis and aggravates joint destruction. *Inflammation Res Off J Eur Histamine Res Soc [et al]* (2002) 51(2):102–4. doi: 10.1007/bf02684010
99. Bush KA, Farmer KM, Walker JS, Kirkham BW. Reduction of joint inflammation and bone erosion in rat adjuvant arthritis by treatment with interleukin-17 receptor IgG1 Fc fusion protein. *Arthritis Rheum* (2002) 46 (3):802–5. doi: 10.1002/art.10173
100. Lubberts E, Joosten LA, Oppers B, van den Bersselaar L, Coenen-de Roo CJ, Kolls JK, et al. IL-1-independent role of IL-17 in synovial inflammation and joint destruction during collagen-induced arthritis. *J Immunol (Baltimore Md 1950)* (2001) 167(2):1004–13. doi: 10.4049/jimmunol.167.2.1004
101. Lubberts E, van den Bersselaar L, Oppers-Walgreen B, Schwarzenberger P, Coenen-de Roo CJ, Kolls JK, et al. IL-17 promotes bone erosion in murine collagen-induced arthritis through loss of the receptor activator of NF-kappa B ligand/osteoprotegerin balance. *J Immunol (Baltimore Md 1950)* (2003) 170(5):2655–62. doi: 10.4049/jimmunol.170.5.2655
102. Lubberts E, Koenders MI, Oppers-Walgreen B, van den Bersselaar L, Coenen-de Roo CJJ, Joosten LAB, et al. Treatment with a neutralizing anti-murine interleukin-17 antibody after the onset of collagen-induced arthritis reduces joint inflammation, cartilage destruction, and bone erosion. *Arthritis Rheumatic* (2004) 50(2):650–9. doi: 10.1002/art.20001
103. Shen F, Verma AH, Volk A, Jones B, Coleman BM, Loza MJ, et al. Combined Blockade of TNF-α and IL-17A Alleviates Progression of Collagen-Induced Arthritis without Causing Serious Infections in Mice. *J Immunol* (2019) 202 (7):2017–26. doi: 10.4049/jimmunol.1801436
104. Zhang Y, Ren G, Guo M, Ye X, Zhao J, Xu L, et al. Synergistic effects of interleukin-1β and interleukin-17A antibodies on collagen-induced arthritis mouse model. *Int Immunopharmacol* (2013) 15(2):199–205. doi: 10.1016/j.intimp.2012.12.010
105. Li Q, Ren G, Xu L, Wang Q, Qi J, Wang W, et al. Therapeutic efficacy of three bispecific antibodies on collagen-induced arthritis mouse model. *Int Immunopharmacol* (2014) 21(1):119–27. doi: 10.1016/j.intimp.2014.04.018
106. Nakae S, Nambu A, Sudo K, Iwakura Y. Suppression of immune induction of collagen-induced arthritis in IL-17-deficient mice. *J Immunol (Baltimore Md 1950)* (2003) 171(11):6173–7. doi: 10.4049/jimmunol.171.11.6173
107. Chao CC, Chen SJ, Adamopoulos IE, Davis N, Hong K, Vu A, et al. Anti-IL-17A therapy protects against bone erosion in experimental models of rheumatoid arthritis. *Autoimmunity* (2011) 44(3):243–52. doi: 10.3109/08916934.2010.517815
108. Martin DA, Churchill M, Flores-Suarez L, Cardiel MH, Wallace D, Martin R, et al. A phase Ib multiple ascending dose study evaluating safety, pharmacokinetics, and early clinical response of brodalumab, a human anti-IL-17R antibody, in methotrexate-resistant rheumatoid arthritis. *Arthritis Res Ther* (2013) 15(5):R164. doi: 10.1186/ar4347
109. Genovese MC, Greenwald M, Cho CS, Berman A, Jin L, Cameron GS, et al. A phase II randomized study of subcutaneous ixekizumab, an anti-interleukin-17 monoclonal antibody, in rheumatoid arthritis patients who were naive to biologic agents or had an inadequate response to tumor necrosis factor inhibitors. *Arthritis Rheumatol* (2014) 66(7):1693–704. doi: 10.1002/art.38617
110. Glatt S, Taylor PC, McInnes IB, Schett G, Landewé R, Baeten D, et al. Efficacy and safety of bimekizumab as add-on therapy for rheumatoid arthritis in patients with inadequate response to certolizumab pegol: a proof-of-concept study. *Ann Rheumatic Dis* (2019) 78(8):1033–40. doi: 10.1136/annrheumdis-2018-214943
111. Genovese MC, Durez P, Richards HB, Supronik J, Dokoupilova E, Aelion JA, et al. One-year Efficacy and Safety Results of Secukinumab in Patients With Rheumatoid Arthritis: Phase II, Dose-finding, Double-blind, Randomized, Placebo-controlled Study. *J Rheumatol* (2014) 41(3):414–21. doi: 10.3899/jrheum.130637
112. Blanco FJ, Möricke R, Dokoupilova E, Codding C, Neal J, Andersson M, et al. Secukinumab in Active Rheumatoid Arthritis: A Phase III Randomized, Double-Blind, Active Comparator- and Placebo-Controlled Study. *Arthritis Rheumatol* (2017) 69(6):1144–53. doi: 10.1002/art.40070
113. Huang Y, Fan Y, Liu Y, Xie W, Zhang Z. Efficacy and safety of secukinumab in active rheumatoid arthritis with an inadequate response to tumor necrosis factor inhibitors: a meta-analysis of phase III randomized controlled trials. *Clin Rheumatol* (2019) 38(10):2765–76. doi: 10.1007/s10067-019-04595-1
114. Dokoupilová E, Aelion J, Takeuchi T, Malavolta N, Sfikakis PP, Wang Y, et al. Secukinumab after anti-tumour necrosis factor-α therapy: a phase III study in active rheumatoid arthritis. *Scand J Rheumatol* (2018) 47(4):276–81. doi: 10.1080/03009742.2017.1390605
115. de Vlam K, Gottlieb AB, Mease PJ. Current concepts in psoriatic arthritis: pathogenesis and management. *Acta Dermato Venereologica* (2014) 94 (6):627–34. doi: 10.2340/00015555-1833
116. Ritchlin CT, Colbert RA, Gladman DD. Psoriatic Arthritis. *New Engl J Med* (2017) 376(10):957–70. doi: 10.1056/NEJMra1505557
117. Veale DJ, Fearon U. The pathogenesis of psoriatic arthritis. *Lancet (London England)* (2018) 391(10136):2273–84. doi: 10.1016/s0140-6736(18)30830-4
118. Coimbra S, Oliveira H, Reis F, Belo L, Rocha S, Quintanilha A, et al. Interleukin (IL)-22, IL-17, IL-23, IL-8, vascular endothelial growth factor and tumour necrosis factor-α levels in patients with psoriasis before, during and after psoralen-ultraviolet A and narrowband ultraviolet B therapy. *Br J Dermatol* (2010) 163(6):1282–90. doi: 10.1111/j.1365-2133.2010.09992.x
119. Benham H, Norris P, Goodall J, Wechalekar MD, FitzGerald O, Szentpetery A, et al. Th17 and Th22 cells in psoriatic arthritis and psoriasis. *Arthritis Res Ther* (2013) 15(5):R136. doi: 10.1186/ar4317
120. Jandus C, Bioley G, Rivals JP, Dudler J, Speiser D, Romero P. Increased numbers of circulating polyfunctional Th17 memory cells in patients with seronegative spondylarthritides. *Arthritis Rheum* (2008) 58(8):2307–17. doi: 10.1002/art.23655
121. Leijten EF, van Kempen TS, Boes M, Michels-van Amelsfort JM, Hijnen D, Hartgring SA, et al. Brief report: enrichment of activated group 3 innate lymphoid cells in psoriatic arthritis synovial fluid. *Arthritis Rheumatol* (2015) 67(10):2673–8. doi: 10.1002/art.39261
122. Raimondo A, Lembo S, Di Caprio R, Donnarumma G, Monfrecola G, Balato N, et al. Psoriatic cutaneous inflammation promotes human monocyte differentiation into active osteoclasts, facilitating bone damage. *Eur J Immunol* (2017) 47(6):1062–74. doi: 10.1002/eji.201646774

123. McInnes IB, Mease PJ, Kirkham B, Kavanaugh A, Ritchlin CT, Rahman P, et al. Secukinumab, a human anti-interleukin-17A monoclonal antibody, in patients with psoriatic arthritis (FUTURE 2): a randomised, double-blind, placebo-controlled, phase 3 trial. *Lancet (London England)* (2015) 386 (9999):1137–46. doi: 10.1016/s0140-6736(15)61134-5
124. Mease P, van der Heijde D, Landewé R, Mpofu S, Rahman P, Tahir H, et al. Secukinumab improves active psoriatic arthritis symptoms and inhibits radiographic progression: primary results from the randomised, double-blind, phase III FUTURE 5 study. *Ann Rheumatic Dis* (2018) 77(6):890–7. doi: 10.1136/annrheumdis-2017-212687
125. Wu D, Li C, Zhang S, Wong P, Cao Y, Griffith JF, et al. Effect of biologics on radiographic progression of peripheral joint in patients with psoriatic arthritis: meta-analysis. *Rheumatol (Oxford England)* (2020) 59(11):3172–80. doi: 10.1093/rheumatology/keaa313
126. Kampylafka E, d'Oliveira I, Linz C, Lerchen V, Stemmler F, Simon D, et al. Resolution of synovitis and arrest of catabolic and anabolic bone changes in patients with psoriatic arthritis by IL-17A blockade with secukinumab: results from the prospective PSARTROS study. *Arthritis Res Ther* (2018) 20(1):153. doi: 10.1186/s13075-018-1653-5
127. Mease PJ, McInnes IB, Kirkham B, Kavanaugh A, Rahman P, van der Heijde D, et al. Secukinumab Inhibition of Interleukin-17A in Patients with Psoriatic Arthritis. *New Engl J Med* (2015) 373(14):1329–39. doi: 10.1056/NEJMoa1412679
128. Nash P, Kirkham B, Okada M, Rahman P, Combe B, Burmester GR, et al. Ixekizumab for the treatment of patients with active psoriatic arthritis and an inadequate response to tumour necrosis factor inhibitors: results from the 24-week randomised, double-blind, placebo-controlled period of the SPIRIT-P2 phase 3 trial. *Lancet (London England)* (2017) 389(10086): 2317–27. doi: 10.1016/s0140-6736(17)31429-0
129. Mease PJ, van der Heijde D, Ritchlin CT, Okada M, Cuchacovich RS, Shuler CL, et al. Ixekizumab, an interleukin-17A specific monoclonal antibody, for the treatment of biologic-naive patients with active psoriatic arthritis: results from the 24-week randomised, double-blind, placebo-controlled and active (adalimumab)-controlled period of the phase III trial SPIRIT-P1. *Ann Rheumatic Dis* (2017) 76(1):79–87. doi: 10.1136/annrheumdis-2016-209709
130. Mease PJ, Helliwell PS, Hjuler KF, Raymond K, McInnes I. Brodalumab in psoriatic arthritis: results from the randomised phase III AMVISION-1 and AMVISION-2 trials. *Ann Rheumatic Dis* (2020) 80(2):185–93. doi: 10.1136/annrheumdis-2019-216835
131. Foulkes AC, Warren RB. Brodalumab in psoriasis: evidence to date and clinical potential. *Drugs context* (2019) 8:212570. doi: 10.7573/dic.212570
132. Ritchlin CT, Kavanaugh A, Merola JF, Schett G, Scher JU, Warren RB, et al. Bimekizumab in patients with active psoriatic arthritis: results from a 48-week, randomised, double-blind, placebo-controlled, dose-ranging phase 2b trial. *Lancet (London England)* (2020) 395(10222):427–40. doi: 10.1016/s0140-6736(19)33161-7
133. Sieper J, Braun J, Dougados M, Baeten D. Axial spondyloarthritis. *Nat Rev Dis Primers* (2015) 1:15013. doi: 10.1038/nrdp.2015.13
134. Ranganathan V, Gracey E, Brown MA, Inman RD, Haroon N. Pathogenesis of ankylosing spondylitis - recent advances and future directions. *Nat Rev Rheumatol* (2017) 13(6):359–67. doi: 10.1038/nrrheum.2017.56
135. Taams LS, Steel KJA, Srenathan U, Burns LA, Kirkham BW. IL-17 in the immunopathogenesis of spondyloarthritis. *Nat Rev Rheumatol* (2018) 14 (8):453–66. doi: 10.1038/s41584-018-0044-2
136. Jansen DT, Hameetman M, van Bergen J, Huizinga TW, van der Heijde D, Toes RE, et al. IL-17-producing CD4+ T cells are increased in early, active axial spondyloarthritis including patients without imaging abnormalities. *Rheumatol (Oxford England)* (2015) 54(4):728–35. doi: 10.1093/rheumatology/keu382
137. Shen H, Goodall JC, Hill Gaston JS. Frequency and phenotype of peripheral blood Th17 cells in ankylosing spondylitis and rheumatoid arthritis. *Arthritis Rheum* (2009) 60(6):1647–56. doi: 10.1002/art.24568
138. Kenna TJ, Davidson SI, Duan R, Bradbury LA, McFarlane J, Smith M, et al. Enrichment of circulating interleukin-17-secreting interleukin-23 receptor-positive γ/δ T cells in patients with active ankylosing spondylitis. *Arthritis Rheum* (2012) 64(5):1420–9. doi: 10.1002/art.33507
139. Mei Y, Pan F, Gao J, Ge R, Duan Z, Zeng Z, et al. Increased serum IL-17 and IL-23 in the patient with ankylosing spondylitis. *Clin Rheumatol* (2011) 30 (2):269–73. doi: 10.1007/s10067-010-1647-4
140. Liu W, Wu YH, Zhang L, Liu XY, Xue B, Wang Y, et al. Elevated serum levels of IL-6 and IL-17 may associate with the development of ankylosing spondylitis. *Int J Clin Exp Med* (2015) 8(10):17362–76.
141. van Tok MN, van Duivenvoorde LM, Kramer I, Ingold P, Pfister S, Roth L, et al. Interleukin-17A Inhibition Diminishes Inflammation and New Bone Formation in Experimental Spondyloarthritis. *Arthritis Rheumatol* (2019) 71 (4):612–25. doi: 10.1002/art.40770
142. Pavelka K, Kivitz A, Dokoupilova E, Blanco R, Maradiaga M, Tahir H, et al. Efficacy, safety, and tolerability of secukinumab in patients with active ankylosing spondylitis: a randomized, double-blind phase 3 study, MEASURE 3. *Arthritis Res Ther* (2017) 19(1):285. doi: 10.1186/s13075-017-1490-y
143. Baraliakos X, Kivitz AJ, Deodhar AA, Braun J, Wei JC, Delicha EM, et al. Long-term effects of interleukin-17A inhibition with secukinumab in active ankylosing spondylitis: 3-year efficacy and safety results from an extension of the Phase 3 MEASURE 1 trial. *Clin Exp Rheumatol* (2018) 36(1):50–5.
144. Ashany D, Stein EM, Goto R, Goodman SM. The Effect of TNF Inhibition on Bone Density and Fracture Risk and of IL17 Inhibition on Radiographic Progression and Bone Density in Patients with Axial Spondyloarthritis: a Systematic Literature Review. *Curr Rheumatol Rep* (2019) 21(5):20. doi: 10.1007/s11926-019-0818-9
145. Deodhar A, Blanco R, Dokoupilová E, Hall S, Kameda H, Kivitz AJ, et al. Secukinumab improves signs and symptoms of non-radiographic axial spondyloarthritis: primary results of a randomized controlled phase III study. *Arthritis Rheumatol* (2020) 73(1):110–20. doi: 10.1002/art.41477
146. van der Heijde D, Cheng-Chung Wei J, Dougados M, Mease P, Deodhar A, Maksymowych WP, et al. Ixekizumab, an interleukin-17A antagonist in the treatment of ankylosing spondylitis or radiographic axial spondyloarthritis in patients previously untreated with biological disease-modifying anti-rheumatic drugs (COAST-V): 16 week results of a phase 3 randomised, double-blind, active-controlled and placebo-controlled trial. *Lancet (London England)* (2018) 392(10163):2441–51. doi: 10.1016/s0140-6736(18)31946-9
147. Dougados M, Wei JC, Landewé R, Sieper J, Baraliakos X, Van den Bosch F, et al. Efficacy and safety of ixekizumab through 52 weeks in two phase 3, randomised, controlled clinical trials in patients with active radiographic axial spondyloarthritis (COAST-V and COAST-W). *Ann Rheumatic Dis* (2020) 79(2):176–85. doi: 10.1136/annrheumdis-2019-216118
148. Deodhar A, van der Heijde D, Gensler LS, Kim TH, Maksymowych WP, Østergaard M, et al. Ixekizumab for patients with non-radiographic axial spondyloarthritis (COAST-X): a randomised, placebo-controlled trial. *Lancet (London England)* (2020) 395(10217):53–64. doi: 10.1016/s0140-6736(19)32971-x
149. Erdes S, Nasonov E, Kunder E, Pristrom A, Soroka N, Shesternya P, et al. Primary efficacy of netakimab, a novel interleukin-17 inhibitor, in the treatment of active ankylosing spondylitis in adults. *Clin Exp Rheumatol* (2020) 38(1):27–34.
150. van der Heijde D, Gensler LS, Deodhar A, Baraliakos X, Poddubnyy D, Kivitz A, et al. Dual neutralisation of interleukin-17A and interleukin-17F with bimekizumab in patients with active ankylosing spondylitis: results from a 48-week phase IIb, randomised, double-blind, placebo-controlled, dose-ranging study. *Ann Rheumatic Dis* (2020) 79(5):595–604. doi: 10.1136/annrheumdis-2020-216980

16

Osteoimmune Interactions in Inflammatory Bowel Disease: Central Role of Bone Marrow Th17 TNFα Cells in Osteoclastogenesis

Abdelilah Wakkach[1,2], Matthieu Rouleau[1,2] and Claudine Blin-Wakkach[1,2]*

[1] CNRS, UMR 7370, Laboratoire de PhysioMédecine Moléculaire (LP2M), Faculté de Médecine, Nice, France, [2] University Nice Sophia Antipolis, Nice, France

***Correspondence:**
Abdelilah Wakkach
wakkach@unice.fr

Osteoimmunology is an interdisciplinary research field dedicated to the study of the crosstalk between the immune and bone systems. CD4+ T cells are central players in this crosstalk. There is an emerging understanding that CD4+ T cells play an important role in the bone marrow (BM) under physiological and pathological conditions and modulate the differentiation of bone-resorbing osteoclasts. However, identification of the mechanisms that maintain CD4+ T cells in the BM is still a matter of investigation. This article describes the CD4+ T cell populations of the BM and reviews their role as osteoclastogenic population in inflammatory bowel disease.

Keywords: Th17 Cells, osteoclasts, bone marrow, inflammatory bowel diseases, osteoporosis, osteoimmunology

Bone marrow (BM) has long been known to play an important role in the immune system as a central hematopoietic organ. However, its function in T cell-mediated tolerance or immunity remains elusive. In the past, most of immunological studies were focused on T and B cells in the thymus, the lymph nodes, and the spleen considered as the central reservoirs of adaptive immunity. Over time, it became apparent that the immune system has a far more decentralized governing function. Recently, the BM was shown to play several unexpected roles, serving as an important reservoir for memory T cells including pathogenic cells and long-lived plasma cells involved in the maintenance of long-term immunity and pathogenicity.

BONE MARROW RESIDENT CD4+ T CELLS

Memory CD4+ T cells provide rapid and highly effective protective immunity against previously encountered pathogens and can recognize a wide variety of antigens. The concept of systemic memory consists of two major subsets: central memory T (T_{CM}) cells and effector memory T (T_{EM}) cells. Importantly, this identification was done in the blood (1). T_{CM} cells express the chemokine receptor CCR7 and the vascular addressing L selectin (CD62L), which enables them to migrate from the blood to the lymph nodes. T_{EM} cells express low levels of CCR7 and CD62L but have receptors that allow them to access peripheral tissues as, for example, the E-selectin ligand cutaneous lymphocyte antigen (CLA), which grants them access to the skin, and α4β7, an integrin that allows them access to the gut. These memory T cells are called tissue-resident memory T cells (T_{RM}) (2).

In the BM, T cells represent about 3–8% of total nucleated cells. BM T cells reach the BM from the blood and, after homing to the BM, can move back to the blood to migrate to other lymphoid organs (3). The rules governing cell migration to the BM have been investigated mainly in the case of hematopoietic stem cells (HSCs) and revealed the dominant role of the CXCR4–CXCL12 axis in this migration. Analysis of CD4$^+$ T cells from the BM of normal mice or mice affected with inflammatory bowel diseases (IBDs) showed the presence of both T_{CM} and T_{EM} cells that are characterized by a high expression of the chemokine receptors CXCR4 and CCR6 (4, 5). However, the mechanism of recruitment of these T cells in the BM remains elusive. Moreover, the degree to which memory cells are resident (T_{RM}) within the BM versus transiting through it is less clear.

In order for T_{RM} cells to be maintained in the BM, they must adapt to the local environment and ignore signals that may induce their egress outside of the BM. The mechanisms and cells involved in the maintenance of BM T cells represent a matter of active research. BM stroma includes mesenchymal stromal cells (MSCs), endothelial cells, osteoblasts (OBLs), and adipocytes. This stromal cell heterogeneity complicates the understanding of the implication of these cells in the maintenance of immunological memory. It is well recognized that BM stromal cells support hematopoiesis by establishing specialized niches. These niches regulate the fate of HSCs in terms of quiescence, migration, and differentiation (6). The major components of the HSC niches include several MSC populations [CXC12-abundant reticular (CAR) cells and Nestin$^+$ cells] (7), OBLs (8, 9), and endothelial cells (10, 11). In addition, regulatory T cells (12), macrophages (13), and osteoclasts (OCLs) (14, 15) were shown to contribute to the regulation of the HSC niches. MSCs have also been involved in the retention of T cells in the BM. Tokoyoda et al. showed that memory CD4$^+$ T cells are located close to BM stromal cells expressing IL-7 and VCAM1 (16). This was confirmed by Nemoto et al. who reported that in IBD, pathogenic CD4$^+$ T cells are retained in the BM through interactions with IL-7-producing MSCs (17). However, the exact nature of the VCAM1$^+$ and IL-7$^+$ stromal cells and their role in the maintaining of memory CD4$^+$ T cells remain to be elucidated. Adoptive transfer of B and T lymphocytes in mice led to seeding of dendritic cell (DC) clusters with grafted cells in perivascular domains, which were referred to as BM immune niches (18). Overall, these observations suggested the existence of CD4$^+$ T cell niches that remain to be characterized in term of cell composition and regulation. The identification of BM immune niches raises many new questions. Which molecules regulate T cell migration? How are memory CD4$^+$ T cells maintained and for how long? How do they interact with BM stroma under physiological and inflammatory conditions? The identification of BM-specific factors that control T cell functions is likely to have a major impact on translational medicine.

CROSSTALK BETWEEN CD4$^+$ T CELLS AND BONE CELLS

The crosstalk between the immune and bone systems led to the emergence of an interdisciplinary field called osteoimmunology (19). This field emerged from clinical observations reporting that patients presenting an overactivation of the immune system, such as chronic infections and chronic inflammatory diseases, also display bone loss (20–22). The importance of this crosstalk was further confirmed with the identification of the role of activated CD4$^+$ T cells in pathological osteoclastogenesis (23). Its scope has been extended to encompass a wide range of molecular and cellular interactions, including those between immune cells and bone cells, and between bone cells and hematopoietic cells. These interactions are essential for the development of the immune and bone systems (15, 24).

Bone remodeling is a highly regulated process involving complex interactions between the activity of the bone-forming OBLs and the activity of the bone-resorbing OCLs. OCLs are multinucleated cells from the myeloid lineage (monocytes and DCs) (25) that degrade the bone matrix and release growth factors that contribute to the coupling between OCLs and OBLs (26). The mesenchymal-derived OBLs migrate to the eroded sites and initiate new bone formation by the secretion of an extracellular matrix and its calcification. In a physiological state, bone remodeling provides an adequate environment for the development of the immune system and the protection of HSCs (6).

The BM represents a reservoir for memory T cells among which 25% are Foxp3$^+$ regulatory T cells (27). It is also a preferential site for the migration or the selective retention and function of regulatory T cells. This finding provides evidence for an unidentified role of the BM in T-cell homeostasis. Moreover, Tokoyoda et al. have shown that in adult mice, more than 80% of antigen specific memory CD4$^+$ T cells rest in the BM for more than 90 days after immunization and do not proliferate (16). From these observations, we can hypothesize that the immunosuppressive activity of BM regulatory T cells participates in the quiescence of memory T cells as recently shown for CD8$^+$ memory T cells (28). In this study, regulatory T cells suppress proliferation and effector programs during the memory differentiation of CD8$^+$ T cells in the lymph nodes (28). In addition to regulatory T cells, MSCs are also generally considered as immunosuppressive cells. MSCs may suppress T-lymphocyte proliferation and functions both *in vitro* and *in vivo* (29, 30). They produce soluble factors, including TGF-β, able to mediate suppression of T-cell proliferation (31). MSCs can also inhibit T cell proliferation by increasing IL-10 secretion (31). These properties suggest that the immunosuppressive effect of MSCs may participate to the preservation of CD4$^+$ memory T cells in the BM. However, MSCs are a heterogeneous population of cells and their immune suppressive activity has mainly been explored in pathological conditions. It is therefore important to better understand this function to clarify how MSCs may control the quiescence and niche of CD4$^+$ T cells.

To date, the role of CD4$^+$ regulatory T cells and memory T cells on bone cells in physiological conditions remains controversial. It has been reported that Rag1$^{-/-}$ mice lacking T cells have a normal bone phenotype (32), whereas T cell-deficient nude mice display, with age, an increased bone resorption and a decreased bone mineral density (33). T cells are capable of mediating anti-osteoclastogenic signals, as depletion of CD4 and CD8 T lymphocytes in mice *in vivo* enhances vitamin D3-stimulated OCL formation by blocking the production of osteoprotegerin (OPG) by B cells (34). These observations revealed the difficulty to conclude on the role of CD4$^+$ T cells in steady state osteoclastogenesis because they can have direct and indirect effects on

OCL precursors and also because of their heterogeneity. Indeed, Th1, Th2, and Th17 cells have been reported to have opposite effects on OCL differentiation *in vitro*. Th1 and Th2 cells inhibit OCL formation through their production of INF-γ and IL-4, respectively, whereas Th17 cells have an osteoclastogenic helper effect *in vitro* mediated by MSCs (35).

OSTEOIMMUNOLOGY INTERACTIONS IN INFLAMMATORY BOWEL DISEASE

Inflammatory bowel diseases are inflammatory diseases that affect the gastrointestinal tract. There are two main clinical forms of IBD: Crohn's disease which affects any part of gastrointestinal tract and ulcerative colitis in which the pathology mostly affects the colonic mucosa (36). Several factors including genetic factors, gut microbiota, and the host immune system have been described to contribute to IBD (36). Moreover, these diseases are often associated with extra-intestinal manifestations, in particular, bone loss. Indeed, more than 40% of patients with IBD also present bone loss that remains a major extra-intestinal cause of morbidity leading to an impaired quality of life and productivity (37). The prevalence of osteopenia and osteoporosis in patients presenting with IBD ranges from 22–77% to 17–41%, respectively, depending on the population location or the study design. According to the WHO, osteoporosis is defined as a systemic skeletal disease that occurs when bone resorption exceeds bone formation. In low-turnover osteoporosis, bone resorption is normal whereas the synthesis of bone tissue is reduced. In contrast, in high-turnover osteoporosis, the activity of OCL is increased. Osteoporosis associated with chronic inflammation usually follows the high-turnover pattern, whereas corticosteroid-induced osteoporosis is usually of the low-turnover pattern (38).

The association between chronic inflammation and bone destruction has been recognized a long time ago, leading to the hypothesis of the participation of immune cells in the control of bone remodeling (19). A seminal work published in 1999 by Kong et al. established the role of $CD4^+$ T cells in inflammatory osteoclastogenesis. In this study, the authors demonstrated that activated $CD4^+$ T cells produce RANKL and induce the differentiation of OCLs *in vitro* (23). Besides that, ctla4$^{-/-}$ mice, in which T cells are spontaneously activated, displayed a severe osteoporosis. Interestingly, transfer of $CD4^+$ T cells from ctla4$^{-/-}$ mice into lymphocyte-deficient rag1$^{-/-}$ mice caused bone destruction that can be reversed through inhibition of RANKL by OPG (23). One additional study confirmed these observations and identified a common causal link between intestinal inflammation and bone loss showing that activated T cells producing RANKL accumulate in the BM during intestinal inflammation (39). Taken together, these studies suggest that pathogenic $CD4^+$ T cells present in the BM during IBD are potentially osteoclastogenic.

Using a mouse model of colitis, induced in SCID mice by injection of $CD4^+CD45RB$high naive T cells, Nemoto et al. found that a large number of $CD4^+CD44^+CD62L^-$ memory T cells resides in the BM. Transfer of BM memory $CD4^+$ T cells into new recipient SCID mice reproduced colitis. These BM $CD4^+$ cells of colitic mice have therefore been described as "colitogenic memory T cells" (5). Importantly, these resident BM $CD4^+$ memory T cells are closely associated with IL-7-producing stromal cells, and they cannot induce colitis when transferred into IL-7$^{-/-}$ × Rag1$^{-/-}$ mice, suggesting that IL-7 plays an essential role in their maintenance or survival in the BM (5). Recently, the same group has demonstrated that BM MSCs are the major source of IL-7 and play a pathological role in IBD by forming the niche for these colitogenic $CD4^+$ memory T cells (17). However, their osteoclastogenic effect has not been explored.

Although IBD has traditionally been assumed to be a Th1-dependent disease, there is controversy over the role of Th1 on bone homeostasis. IFN-γ has been shown to directly inhibit osteoclastogenesis by interfering with the RANKL–RANK signaling pathway (40). Moreover, *in vitro* differentiated $CD4^+$ Th1 cells have been shown to inhibit OCL formation through their canonical production of IFN-γ (35). In contrast, observations in humans suggested that IFN-γ may promote osteoclastogenesis because it improves bone resorption in osteopetrotic patients treated with IFN-γ (41). IFN-γ is also a physiologic inducer of MHC class II expression by APCs resulting in the activation of T cells that induce bone resorption by their secretion of RANKL and TNF-α (42). Together, these data suggest that IFN-γ inhibits OCL formation through direct targeting of maturing OCLs, while it promotes osteoclastogenesis indirectly by stimulating T cell activation.

Nowadays, it is well known that the inflamed gastrointestinal mucosa of patients with IBD is massively infiltrated with Th17 cells and that Th17-related cytokines are produced in excess (43). Based on this, it is obvious that Th17 cells play an important role in the pathogenesis of IBD, which was previously solely attributed to Th1 cells. However, although a pathogenic role in intestine inflammation has been ascribed to Th17 cells, administration of neutralizing anti-IL-17A antibody to patients with Crohn's disease did not show any therapeutic benefit (44). Moreover, in some patients, it exacerbated the disease suggesting a protective role of IL-17A (44). Thus, despite the role of Th17 cytokines is important in many aspects of intestinal homeostasis and protection from mucosal pathogens, their role in the pathogenesis of IBD remains ambiguous. However, IL-17 represents a potent osteoclastogenic cytokine, and its receptors are expressed by many cell types, including OBLs and OCLs (45). Kotake et al. reported that IL-17 is abundant in rheumatoid synovial fluid and that IL-17 stimulates OCL differentiation by inducing RANKL expression by OBLs (46). It should be noted that the effect of IL-17 is not limited to this direct action on the OBLs. IL-17 facilitates local inflammation by recruiting and activating immune cells, which leads to an abundance of inflammatory cytokines such as TNF-α (46). IL-17-deficient mice are resistant to bone destruction induced by LPS (35). Otherwise, Oostlander et al. suggested a particular role for IL-17 in osteoclastogenesis in Crohn's disease patients (47). More recently, we have shown that BM Th17 T cells expressing high levels of TNFα were able to induce OCL differentiation in IBD mice. This T-cell-induced OCL differentiation could be inhibited by IL-17 blockade (4) suggesting the importance of IL-17A in osteoporosis.

A picture emerged from the literature (48, 49) to define what we believe to be osteoclastogenic T cells: first, osteoclastogenic T cells should not produce a large amount of IFN-γ. Second, they should trigger local inflammation and the production of inflammatory cytokines, including TNF-α, that induce RANK-L expression on MSCs. Third, they should express RANK-L and might directly participate in the increase of osteoclastogenesis.

Recent data indicate that in IBD, Th17 cells-producing TNF-α represent the long-sought-after osteoclastogenic T cell subset that fulfills all the criteria mentioned above (4, 50). In murine models of IBD associated with bone loss, we have shown that Th17-producing TNF-α cells accumulate in the BM, the colon, and spleen and have a potent capacity to induce OCL differentiation without addition of any exogenic osteoclastogenic factors (4). Through their production of RANK-L and TNFα, Th17 cells directly induce the differentiation of precursors into OCLs (4), but they also have a major effect on MSCs through their production of IL-17. Indeed, IL-17 increases RANK-L expression in MSCs leading to increased OCL formation (4, 35, 46). Moreover, in the context of IBD, Th17 cells increase the expression of monocyte chemoattractant protein-1 (MCP-1) and macrophage inflammatory protein 1α (MIP-1α) by MSCs, which may promote the recruitment of inflammatory monocytes (OCL precursors) in the BM and their differentiation into OCLs (4). To translate these finding into human disease, IL-17-producing T cells from the blood of IBD patients are osteoclastogenic cells *in vitro* and increase MIP-1α and MCP-1 expression by human MSCs (4, 47), suggesting their participation to osteoporosis in these patients. Therefore, Th17 cells represent a key target for innovative therapeutic approaches for IBD-associated bone destruction.

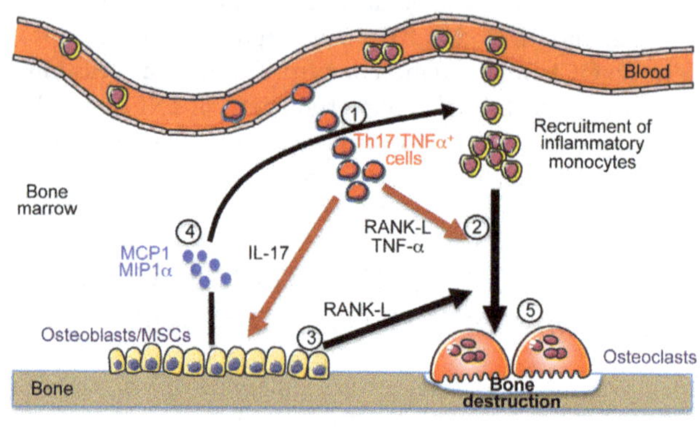

FIGURE 1 | Th17 cells induce bone destruction in IBD. In IBD, Th17 TNFα cells migrate and accumulate in the bone marrow (1). They express RANK-L and TNF-α that participate to osteoclast differentiation (2). They also express IL-17 that stimulates the local inflammation and activates osteoblasts to produce RANK-L inducing osteoclast formation (3) and MCP-1 and MIP-1α chemokines (4) participating to the recruitment of osteoclast precursor cells (monocytes) in the BM that contribute to the increased osteoclastogenesis (5) and to bone destruction.

CONCLUDING REMARKS

Recent advances have contributed to our understanding of the biology of $CD4^+$ T cells in the BM. These T cells fulfill both homeostatic and pathological functions with respect to the bone system. IBD is an immune-mediated disease characterized by systemic Th1 and Th17 responses and bone destruction. Recent studies have revealed that Th17 cells are not only required for the initiation of systemic immune response as they are critical regulators in the chronic inflammation associated with bone destruction, particularly in rheumatoid arthritis. Our recent findings extend these observation to IBD in which the site of inflammation is far from the bone and provide the first characterization of osteoclastogenic Th17 $TNF\text{-}\alpha^+$ cells in the BM linking IBD and bone destruction.

Collectively, we propose that these osteoclastogenic cells, once in the BM, enable the secretion of chemokines and RANKL by stromal cells. This enhances the recruitment of inflammatory monocytes and DCs that differentiate into OCLs and increase the bone resorption leading to osteoporosis as illustrated in **Figure 1**.

AUTHOR CONTRIBUTIONS

AW wrote and reviewed the manuscript. CB-W and MR reviewed the manuscript.

ACKNOWLEDGMENTS

The work of the authors was supported by the "Fondation pour la Recherche Médicale" (Equipe FRM DEQ20130326467), the "Agence Nationale de la Recherche" (ANR), the "Arthritis Fondation," the "Société Française de Rhumatologie" and the "Société Francophone du Diabète" (SFD).

REFERENCES

1. Sallusto F, Lenig D, Förster R, Lipp M, Lanzavecchia A. Two subsets of memory T lymphocytes with distinct homing potentials and effector functions. *Nature* (1999) **401**:708–12. doi:10.1038/44385
2. Mueller SN, Gebhardt T, Carbone FR, Heath WR. Memory T cell subsets, migration patterns, and tissue residence. *Annu Rev Immunol* (2013) **31**:137–61. doi:10.1146/annurev-immunol-032712-095954
3. Di Rosa F, Pabst R. The bone marrow: a nest for migratory memory T cells. *Trends Immunol* (2005) **26**:360–6. doi:10.1016/j.it.2005.04.011
4. Ciucci T, Ibáñez L, Boucoiran A, Birgy-Barelli E, Pène J, Abou-Ezzi G, et al. Bone marrow Th17 TNFα cells induce osteoclast differentiation, and link bone destruction to IBD. *Gut* (2015) **64**:1072–81. doi:10.1136/gutjnl-2014-306947
5. Nemoto Y, Kanai T, Makita S, Okamoto R, Totsuka T, Takeda K, et al. Bone marrow retaining colitogenic CD4+ T cells may be a pathogenic reservoir for chronic colitis. *Gastroenterology* (2007) **132**:176–89. doi:10.1053/j.gastro.2006.10.035
6. Scadden DT. Nice neighborhood: emerging concepts of the stem cell niche. *Cell* (2014) **157**:41–50. doi:10.1016/j.cell.2014.02.013
7. Schajnovitz A, Itkin T, D'Uva G, Kalinkovich A, Golan K, Ludin A, et al. CXCL12 secretion by bone marrow stromal cells is dependent on cell contact and mediated by connexin-43 and connexin-45 gap junctions. *Nat Immunol* (2011) **12**:391–8. doi:10.1038/ni.2017

8. Calvi LM, Adams GB, Weibrecht KW, Weber JM, Olson DP, Knight MC, et al. Osteoblastic cells regulate the haematopoietic stem cell niche. *Nature* (2003) **425**:841–6. doi:10.1038/nature02040
9. Zhang J, Niu C, Ye L, Huang H, He X, Tong W-G, et al. Identification of the haematopoietic stem cell niche and control of the niche size. *Nature* (2003) **425**:836–41. doi:10.1038/nature02041
10. Butler JM, Nolan DJ, Vertes EL, Varnum-Finney B, Kobayashi H, Hooper AT, et al. Endothelial cells are essential for the self-renewal and repopulation of Notch-dependent hematopoietic stem cells. *Cell Stem Cell* (2010) **6**:251–64. doi:10.1016/j.stem.2010.02.001
11. Ding L, Saunders TL, Enikolopov G, Morrison SJ. Endothelial and perivascular cells maintain haematopoietic stem cells. *Nature* (2012) **481**:457–62. doi:10.1038/nature10783
12. Fujisaki J, Wu J, Carlson AL, Silberstein L, Putheti P, Larocca R, et al. In vivo imaging of Treg cells providing immune privilege to the haematopoietic stem-cell niche. *Nature* (2011) **474**:216–9. doi:10.1038/nature10160
13. Chow A, Lucas D, Hidalgo A, Méndez-Ferrer S, Hashimoto D, Scheiermann C, et al. Bone marrow CD169+ macrophages promote the retention of hematopoietic stem and progenitor cells in the mesenchymal stem cell niche. *J Exp Med* (2011) **208**:261–71. doi:10.1084/jem.20101688
14. Kollet O, Dar A, Shivtiel S, Kalinkovich A, Lapid K, Sztainberg Y, et al. Osteoclasts degrade endosteal components and promote mobilization of hematopoietic progenitor cells. *Nat Med* (2006) **12**:657–64. doi:10.1038/nm1417
15. Mansour A, Abou-Ezzi G, Sitnicka E, Jacobsen SEW, Wakkach A, Blin-Wakkach C. Osteoclasts promote the formation of hematopoietic stem cell niches in the bone marrow. *J Exp Med* (2012) **209**:537–49. doi:10.1084/jem.20110994
16. Tokoyoda K, Zehentmeier S, Hegazy AN, Albrecht I, Grün JR, Löhning M, et al. Professional memory CD4+ T lymphocytes preferentially reside and rest in the bone marrow. *Immunity* (2009) **30**:721–30. doi:10.1016/j.immuni.2009.03.015
17. Nemoto Y, Kanai T, Takahara M, Oshima S, Nakamura T, Okamoto R, et al. Bone marrow-mesenchymal stem cells are a major source of interleukin-7 and sustain colitis by forming the niche for colitogenic CD4 memory T cells. *Gut* (2013) **62**:1142–52. doi:10.1136/gutjnl-2012-302029
18. Sapoznikov A, Pewzner-Jung Y, Kalchenko V, Krauthgamer R, Shachar I, Jung S. Perivascular clusters of dendritic cells provide critical survival signals to B cells in bone marrow niches. *Nat Immunol* (2008) **9**:388–95. doi:10.1038/ni1571
19. Arron JR, Choi Y. Osteoimmunology: bone versus immune system. *Nature* (2000) **408**:535–6. doi:10.1038/35046196
20. Stellon AJ, Davies A, Compston J, Williams R. Bone loss in autoimmune chronic active hepatitis on maintenance corticosteroid therapy. *Gastroenterology* (1985) **89**:1078–83.
21. Feldmann M, Brennan FM, Maini RN. Role of cytokines in rheumatoid arthritis. *Annu Rev Immunol* (1996) **14**:397–440. doi:10.1146/annurev.immunol.14.1.397
22. Piepkorn B, Kann P, Forst T, Andreas J, Pfützner A, Beyer J. Bone mineral density and bone metabolism in diabetes mellitus. *Horm Metab Res* (1997) **29**:584–91. doi:10.1055/s-2007-979106
23. Kong Y-Y, Feige U, Sarosi I, Bolon B, Tafuri A, Morony S, et al. Activated T cells regulate bone loss and joint destruction in adjuvant arthritis through osteoprotegerin ligand. *Nature* (1999) **402**:304–9. doi:10.1038/46303
24. Blin-Wakkach C, Wakkach A, Quincey D, Carle GF. Interleukin-7 partially rescues B-lymphopoiesis in osteopetrotic oc/oc mice through the engagement of B220+ CD11b+ progenitors. *Exp Hematol* (2006) **34**:851–9. doi:10.1016/j.exphem.2006.04.003
25. Wakkach A, Mansour A, Dacquin R, Coste E, Jurdic P, Carle GF, et al. Bone marrow microenvironment controls the in vivo differentiation of murine dendritic cells into osteoclasts. *Blood* (2008) **112**:5074–83. doi:10.1182/blood-2008-01-132787
26. Tang Y, Wu X, Lei W, Pang L, Wan C, Shi Z, et al. TGF-beta1-induced migration of bone mesenchymal stem cells couples bone resorption with formation. *Nat Med* (2009) **15**:757–65. doi:10.1038/nm.1979
27. Zou L, Barnett B, Safah H, Larussa VF, Evdemon-Hogan M, Mottram P, et al. Bone marrow is a reservoir for CD4+CD25+ regulatory T cells that traffic through CXCL12/CXCR4 signals. *Cancer Res* (2004) **64**:8451–5. doi:10.1158/0008-5472.CAN-04-1987
28. Kalia V, Penny LA, Yuzefpolskiy Y, Baumann FM, Sarkar S. Quiescence of memory CD8(+) T cells is mediated by regulatory T cells through inhibitory receptor CTLA-4. *Immunity* (2015) **42**:1116–29. doi:10.1016/j.immuni.2015.05.023
29. Nauta AJ, Fibbe WE. Immunomodulatory properties of mesenchymal stromal cells. *Blood* (2007) **110**:3499–506. doi:10.1182/blood-2007-02-069716
30. Anderson P, Souza-Moreira L, Morell M, Caro M, O'Valle F, Gonzalez-Rey E, et al. Adipose-derived mesenchymal stromal cells induce immunomodulatory macrophages which protect from experimental colitis and sepsis. *Gut* (2013) **62**:1131–41. doi:10.1136/gutjnl-2012-302152
31. Sioud M. New insights into mesenchymal stromal cell-mediated T-cell suppression through galectins. *Scand J Immunol* (2011) **73**:79–84. doi:10.1111/j.1365-3083.2010.02491.x
32. Anginot A, Dacquin R, Mazzorana M, Jurdic P. Lymphocytes and the Dap12 adaptor are key regulators of osteoclast activation associated with gonadal failure. *PLoS One* (2007) **2**:e585. doi:10.1371/journal.pone.0000585
33. Li Y, Toraldo G, Li A, Yang X, Zhang H, Qian W-P, et al. B cells and T cells are critical for the preservation of bone homeostasis and attainment of peak bone mass in vivo. *Blood* (2007) **109**:3839–48. doi:10.1182/blood-2006-07-037994
34. Grcević D, Lee SK, Marusić A, Lorenzo JA. Depletion of CD4 and CD8 T lymphocytes in mice in vivo enhances 1,25-dihydroxyvitamin D3-stimulated osteoclast-like cell formation in vitro by a mechanism that is dependent on prostaglandin synthesis. *J Immunol* (2000) **165**:4231–8.
35. Sato K, Suematsu A, Okamoto K, Yamaguchi A, Morishita Y, Kadono Y, et al. Th17 functions as an osteoclastogenic helper T cell subset that links T cell activation and bone destruction. *J Exp Med* (2006) **203**:2673–82. doi:10.1084/jem.20061775
36. Maloy KJ, Powrie F. Intestinal homeostasis and its breakdown in inflammatory bowel disease. *Nature* (2011) **474**:298–306. doi:10.1038/nature10208
37. Tilg H, Moschen AR, Kaser A, Pines A, Dotan I. Gut, inflammation and osteoporosis: basic and clinical concepts. *Gut* (2008) **57**:684–94. doi:10.1136/gut.2006.117382
38. Raisz LG. Pathogenesis of osteoporosis: concepts, conflicts, and prospects. *J Clin Invest* (2005) **115**:3318–25. doi:10.1172/JCI27071
39. Ashcroft AJ, Cruickshank SM, Croucher PI, Perry MJ, Rollinson S, Lippitt JM, et al. Colonic dendritic cells, intestinal inflammation, and T cell-mediated bone destruction are modulated by recombinant osteoprotegerin. *Immunity* (2003) **19**:849–61. doi:10.1016/S1074-7613(03)00326-1
40. Takayanagi H, Ogasawara K, Hida S, Chiba T, Murata S, Sato K, et al. T-cell-mediated regulation of osteoclastogenesis by signalling cross-talk between RANKL and IFN-gamma. *Nature* (2000) **408**:600–5. doi:10.1038/35046102
41. Key LL, Rodriguiz RM, Willi SM, Wright NM, Hatcher HC, Eyre DR, et al. Long-term treatment of osteopetrosis with recombinant human interferon gamma. *N Engl J Med* (1995) **332**:1594–9. doi:10.1056/NEJM199506153322402
42. Gao Y, Grassi F, Ryan M, Pacifici R. IFN-gamma stimulates osteoclast formation and bone loss in vivo via antigen-driven T cell activation. *J Clin Invest* (2007) **117**(1):122–32. doi:10.1172/JCI30074
43. Ray S, De Salvo C, Pizarro TT. Central role of IL-17/Th17 immune responses and the gut microbiota in the pathogenesis of intestinal fibrosis. *Curr Opin Gastroenterol* (2014) **30**:531–8. doi:10.1097/MOG.0000000000000119
44. Hueber W, Sands BE, Lewitzky S, Vandemeulebroecke M, Reinisch W, Higgins PDR, et al. Secukinumab, a human anti-IL-17A monoclonal antibody, for moderate to severe Crohn's disease: unexpected results of a randomised, double-blind placebo-controlled trial. *Gut* (2012) **61**:1693–700. doi:10.1136/gutjnl-2011-301668
45. Van bezooijen RL, Farih-Sips HC, Papapoulos SE, Löwik CW. Interleukin-17: a new bone acting cytokine in vitro. *J Bone Miner Res* (1999) **14**:1513–21. doi:10.1359/jbmr.1999.14.9.1513
46. Kotake S, Udagawa N, Takahashi N, Matsuzaki K, Itoh K, Ishiyama S, et al. IL-17 in synovial fluids from patients with rheumatoid arthritis is a potent stimulator of osteoclastogenesis. *J Clin Invest* (1999) **103**:1345–52. doi:10.1172/JCI5703
47. Oostlander AE, Everts V, Schoenmaker T, Bravenboer N, van Vliet SJ, van Bodegraven AA, et al. T cell-mediated increased osteoclast formation from

peripheral blood as a mechanism for Crohn's disease-associated bone loss. *J Cell Biochem* (2012) **113**:260–8. doi:10.1002/jcb.23352

48. Takayanagi H. Osteoimmunology: shared mechanisms and crosstalk between the immune and bone systems. *Nat Rev Immunol* (2007) **7**:292–304. doi:10.1038/nri2062
49. Jones D, Glimcher LH, Aliprantis AO. Osteoimmunology at the nexus of arthritis, osteoporosis, cancer, and infection. *J Clin Invest* (2011) **121**:2534–42. doi:10.1172/JCI46262
50. Syrbe U, Siegmund B. Bone marrow Th17 TNFα cells induce osteoclast differentiation and link bone destruction to IBD. *Gut* (2015) **64**:1011–2. doi:10.1136/gutjnl-2014-308436

Permissions

All chapters in this book were first published in CPO, by Frontiers; hereby published with permission under the Creative Commons Attribution License or equivalent. Every chapter published in this book has been scrutinized by our experts. Their significance has been extensively debated. The topics covered herein carry significant findings which will fuel the growth of the discipline. They may even be implemented as practical applications or may be referred to as a beginning point for another development.

The contributors of this book come from diverse backgrounds, making this book a truly international effort. This book will bring forth new frontiers with its revolutionizing research information and detailed analysis of the nascent developments around the world.

We would like to thank all the contributing authors for lending their expertise to make the book truly unique. They have played a crucial role in the development of this book. Without their invaluable contributions this book wouldn't have been possible. They have made vital efforts to compile up to date information on the varied aspects of this subject to make this book a valuable addition to the collection of many professionals and students.

This book was conceptualized with the vision of imparting up-to-date information and advanced data in this field. To ensure the same, a matchless editorial board was set up. Every individual on the board went through rigorous rounds of assessment to prove their worth. After which they invested a large part of their time researching and compiling the most relevant data for our readers.

The editorial board has been involved in producing this book since its inception. They have spent rigorous hours researching and exploring the diverse topics which have resulted in the successful publishing of this book. They have passed on their knowledge of decades through this book. To expedite this challenging task, the publisher supported the team at every step. A small team of assistant editors was also appointed to further simplify the editing procedure and attain best results for the readers.

Apart from the editorial board, the designing team has also invested a significant amount of their time inunderstanding the subject and creating the most relevant covers. They scrutinized every image to scout for the most suitable representation of the subject and create an appropriate cover for the book.

The publishing team has been an ardent support to the editorial, designing and production team. Their endless efforts to recruit the best for this project, has resulted in the accomplishment of this book. They are a veteran in the field of academics and their pool of knowledge is as vast as their experience in printing. Their expertise and guidance has proved useful at every step. Their uncompromising quality standards have made this book an exceptional effort. Their encouragement from time to time has been an inspiration for everyone.

The publisher and the editorial board hope that this book will prove to be a valuable piece of knowledge forresearchers, students, practitioners and scholars across the globe.

List of Contributors

Luca Massaccesi
Department of Biomedical Sciences for Health, Università degli Studi di Milano, Milan, Italy

Vincenza Ragone
Research and Develpoment Department, Permedica S.p.A, Merate, Italy

Nadia Papini
Department of Medical Biotechnology and Traslational Medicine, Università degli Studi di Milano Milan, Italy

Giancarlo Goi
Department of Biomedical, Surgical and Dental Sciences, Università degli Studi di Milano, Milan, Italy

Massimiliano Marco Corsi Romanelli
Department of Biomedical Sciences for Health, Università degli Studi di Milano, Milan, Italy
U.O.C SMEL-1 Patologia Clinica San Donato, IRCCS Policlinico San Donato, Milan, Italy

Emanuela Galliera
Department of Biomedical Sciences for Health, Università degli Studi di Milano, Milan, Italy
IRCCS Istituto Ortopedico Galeazzi, Milan, Italy

Lan Xiao and Kenneth Beagley
Institute of Health and Biomedical Innovation, Queensland University of Technology, Brisbane, QLD, Australia
The Australia-China Centre for Tissue Engineering and Regenerative Medicine, Queensland University of Technology, Brisbane, QLD, Australia

Thor Friis
Institute of Health and Biomedical Innovation, Queensland University of Technology, Brisbane, QLD, Australia

Yin Xiao and Yinghong Zhou
Institute of Health and Biomedical Innovation, Queensland University of Technology, Brisbane, QLD, Australia
The Australia-China Centre for Tissue Engineering and Regenerative Medicine, Queensland University of Technology, Brisbane, QLD, Australia
Key Laboratory of Oral Medicine, Guangzhou Institute of Oral Disease, Stomatology Hospital of Guangzhou Medical University, Guangzhou, China

Deniz Ragipoglu, Melanie Haffner-Luntzer, Jochen Kroner, Anita Ignatius and Verena Fischer
Trauma Research Center Ulm, Institute of Orthopedic Research and Biomechanics, Ulm University Medical Center, Ulm, Germany

Anne Dudeck and Martin Voss
Medical Faculty, Institute for Molecular and Clinical Immunology, Otto-von-Guericke University Magdeburg, Magdeburg, Germany

Sebastian Dohnke and Luise Fischer
Osteoimmunology, DFG-Center for Regenerative Therapies Dresden (CRTD), Technische Universität Dresden, Dresden, Germany
Molecular and Cellular Immunology/ ImmuneRegulation, DFG-Center for Regenerative Therapies Dresden (CRTD), Technische Universität Dresden, Dresden, Germany

Karsten Kretschmer and Julia Riewaldt
Molecular and Cellular Immunology/Immune Regulation, DFG-Center for Regenerative Therapies Dresden (CRTD), Technische Universität Dresden, Dresden, Germany

Caroline Herkner, Reni Kitte and Annette I. Garbe
Osteoimmunology, DFG-Center for Regenerative Therapies Dresden (CRTD), Technische Universität Dresden, Dresden, Germany

Paul Humbert, Valérie Trichet, Frédéric Blanchard and Pierre Layrolle
Laboratory Phy-Os, Inserm UMR1238, University of Nantes, Nantes, France

Meadhbh Á. Brennan
Laboratory Phy-Os, Inserm UMR1238, University of Nantes, Nantes, France
Harvard School of Engineering and Applied Sciences, Harvard University, Cambridge, MA, United States

Noel Davison
MERLN Institute for Technology-Inspired Regenerative Medicine, Maastricht University, Maastricht, Netherlands
Instructure Labs, B.V., The Hague, Netherlands

Philippe Rosset
Laboratory Phy-Os, Inserm UMR1238, University of Nantes, Nantes, France
Centre Hospitalier Universitaire de Tours, Tours, France

Mubashir Ahmad, Yasmine Hachemi, Kevin Paxian and Jan Tuckermann
Institute of Comparative Molecular Endocrinology (CME), University of Ulm, Ulm, Germany

Florian Mengele
Institute of Comparative Molecular Endocrinology (CME), University of Ulm, Ulm, Germany
Praxisklinik für Orthopädie,Unfall- und Neurochirurgie Prof. Bischoff/ Dr. Spies/ Dr. Mengele, Neu-Ulm, Germany

Mascha Koenen
Institute of Comparative Molecular Endocrinology (CME), University of Ulm, Ulm, Germany
Department of Immunobiology, Yale School of Medicine, New Haven, CT, United States

Giovanni Lombardi
Laboratory of Experimental Biochemistry & Molecular Biology, IRCCS Istituto Ortopedico Galeazzi, Milan, Italy
Department of Physiology and Pharmacology, Faculty of Rehabilitation and Kinesiology, Gdansk University of Physical Education and Sport, Gdansk, Poland

Ewa Ziemann
Department of Physiology and Pharmacology, Faculty of Rehabilitation and Kinesiology, Gdansk University of Physical Education and Sport, Gdansk, Poland

Giuseppe Banfi
Laboratory of Experimental Biochemistry & Molecular Biology, IRCCS Istituto Ortopedico Galeazzi, Milan, Italy,
Vita-Salute San Raffaele University, Milan, Italy

Maria Papadaki, Vagelis Rinotas, Foteini Violitzi and Eleni Douni
Laboratory of Genetics, Department of Biotechnology, Agricultural University of Athens, Athens, Greece
Division of Immunology, Biomedical Sciences Research Center "Alexander Fleming", Athens, Greece

Trias Thireou
Laboratory of Genetics, Department of Biotechnology, Agricultural University of Athens, Athens, Greece

George Panayotou and Martina Samiotaki
Division of Molecular Oncology, Biomedical Sciences Research Center "Alexander Fleming", Athens, Greece

Julia Löffler, F. Andrea Sass, Agnes Ellinghaus, Georg N. Duda and Anke Dienelt
Julius Wolff Institute and Center for Musculoskeletal Surgery, Charité-Universitätsmedizin Berlin, Corporate Member of Freie Universität Berlin, Berlin Institute of Health, Humboldt-Universität zu Berlin, Berlin, Germany
Berlin Institute of Health Center for Regenerative Therapies, Charité-Universitätsmedizin Berlin, Corporate Member of Freie Universität Berlin, Berlin Institute of Health, Humboldt-Universität zu Berlin, Berlin, Germany

Sebastian Filter and Alexander Rose
Julius Wolff Institute and Center for Musculoskeletal Surgery, Charité-Universitätsmedizin Berlin, Corporate Member of Freie Universität Berlin, Berlin Institute of Health, Humboldt-Universität zu Berlin, Berlin, Germany

Alpdogan Kantarci
Forsyth Institute, Cambridge, MA, United States

Carla Alvarez
Forsyth Institute, Cambridge, MA, United States
Periodontal Biology Laboratory, Faculty of Dentistry, Universidad de Chile, Santiago, Chile

Gustavo Monasterio and Marcela Hernández
Periodontal Biology Laboratory, Faculty of Dentistry, Universidad de Chile, Santiago, Chile

Franco Cavalla
Department of Conservative Dentistry, Faculty of Dentistry, Universidad de Chile, Santiago, Chile

Luis A. Córdova
Department of Oral and Maxillofacial Surgery, Faculty of Dentistry, San Jose's Hospital and Clínica Las Condes, Universidad de Chile, Santiago, Chile

Dominique Heymann
INSERM, UMR 1232, LabCT, CRCINA, Institut de Cancérologie de l'Ouest, Université de Nantes, Université d'Angers, Saint-Herblain, France

Gustavo P. Garlet
Department of Biological Sciences, Bauru School of Dentistry, University of São Paulo, Bauru, Brazil

Pirjo Pärnänen
Department of Oral and Maxillofacial Diseases, University of Helsinki, Helsinki University Hospital, Helsinki, Finland

Timo Sorsa
Department of Oral and Maxillofacial Diseases, University of Helsinki, Helsinki University Hospital, Helsinki, Finland
Department of Oral Diseases, Karolinska Institutet, Stockholm, Sweden

Hsi-Ming Lee and Lorne M. Golub
Department of Oral Biology and Pathology, School of Dental Medicine, Stony Brook University, Stony Brook, NY, United States

Rolando Vernal
Periodontal Biology Laboratory, Faculty of Dentistry, Universidad de Chile, Santiago, Chile
Dentistry Unit, Faculty of Health Sciences, Universidad Autónoma de Chile, Santiago, Chile

Filomena Corbo, Alessia Carocci, Alessia Catalano, Gualtiero Milani and Carlo Franchini
Department of Pharmacy-Drug science, University of Bari Aldo Moro, Bari, Italy

Giacomina Brunetti and Silvia Colucci
Section of Human Anatomy and Histology, Departmemt of Basic and Medical Sciences, Neurosciences and Sense Organs, University of Bari Aldo Moro, Bari, Italy

Pasquale Crupi
CREA-VE, Council for Agricultural Research and Economics-Research Centre for Viticulture and Enology, Turi, Italy

Maria Grano, Graziana Colaianni, Sara Bortolotti and Giuseppina Storlino
Section of Human Anatomy and Histology, Department of Emergency and Organ Transplantation, University of Bari, Bari, Italy

Maria Felicia Faienza and Laura Piacente
Paediatric Unit, Department of Biomedical Sciences and Human Oncology, University of Bari Aldo Moro, Bari, Italy

Maria Lisa Clodoveo
Interdisciplinary Department of Medicine, University of Bari Aldo Moro, Bari, Italy

Gabriele D'Amato
Neonatal Intensive Care Unit, Di Venere Hospital, Bari, Italy

Vanessa Nicolin and Roberto Di Lenarda
Clinical Department of Medical, Surgical and Health Sciences, University of Trieste, Trieste, Italy

Nunziatina De Tommasi and Stefania Lucia Nori
Pharmacy-DIFARMA Department, University of Salerno, Fisciano, Italy

Fulvia Costantinides and Federico Berton
School of Dental Sciences, University of Trieste, Trieste, Italy

Ulrike Steffen, Georg Schett and Aline Bozec
Department of Internal Medicine 3, University of Erlangen-Nuremberg, Erlangen, Germany

Claudia Cristina Biguetti, André Petenuci Tabanez, Carolina Favaro Francisconi, Rumio Taga, Ana Paula Campanelli and Gustavo Pompermaier Garlet
Department of Biological Sciences, Bauru School of Dentistry, University of São Paulo, São Paulo, Brazil

Franco Cavalla
Department of Biological Sciences, Bauru School of Dentistry, University of São Paulo, São Paulo, Brazil
Department of Conservative Dentistry, School of Dentistry, University of Chile, Santiago, Chile

Ana Paula Favaro Trombone and Elcia Varize Silveira
Department of Biological and Allied Health Sciences, Universidade Sagrado Coração, Bauru, Brazil

Danieli C. Rodrigues
Department of Bioengineering, University of Texas at Dallas, Dallas, TX, United States

Mengjia Tang and Xijie Yu
Department of Endocrinology and Metabolism, Laboratory of Endocrinology and Metabolism, National Clinical Research Center for Geriatrics, West China Hospital, Sichuan University, Chengdu, China

Lingyun Lu
Department of Integrated Traditional Chinese and Western Medicine, Laboratory of Endocrinology and Metabolism, West China Hospital, Sichuan University, Chengdu, China

Abdelilah Wakkach, Matthieu Rouleau and Claudine Blin-Wakkach
CNRS, UMR 7370, Laboratoire de PhysioMédecine Moléculaire (LP2M), Faculté de Médecine, Nice, France
University Nice Sophia Antipolis, Nice, France

Index

www.ingramcontent.com/pod-product-compliance
Lightning Source LLC
LaVergne TN
LVHW082159200926
848484LV00008B/2187
* 9 7 9 8 8 8 7 4 0 4 2 6 4 *